Steps Toward a Universal Patient Medical Record:

A Project Plan to Develop One

Steps Toward a Universal Patient Medical Record:

A Project Plan to Develop One

MICHAEL R. MCGUIRE
Care Delivery Consultant

Steps Toward a Universal Patient Medical Record:
A Project Plan to Develop One

Universal Publishers
Boca Raton, Florida • USA
2004

ISBN: 1-58112- 509-7

www.universal-publishers.com

Preface

Why develop a *universal patient medical record* that would be available to all clinicians caring for a patient no matter where the clinician is located in the world? One should be developed because it would benefit patients and benefit mankind, and because it is inevitable.

Healthcare today is oriented toward short-term treatment of medical conditions. I predict this will change in the near future: medical care will become more long-term oriented, preventing as well as treating disease. This will result in a need for a complete medical history for a patient, no matter where the patient was seen for healthcare in a country, or in the world.

A patient's medical history would include *biomarkers* for disease, where biomarkers have been defined by the National Institutes of Health as "cellular, biochemical, molecular, or genetic characteristics or alterations by which a normal, abnormal, or simply biologic process can be recognized, or monitored."(NIH 2004) An individual's genome could provide permanent biomarkers while other biomarkers may change over time. Through biomarkers, diseases could be predicted. A universal patient medical record is a place where such biomarkers for an individual could be stored.

When the paper medical record was first used, medical care was most often performed by a physician who worked individually in the care of a patient. With managed care, national healthcare, and the great mobility of people moving from place to place, care is no longer given by an individual physician but by many. Even when a patient is assigned to a primary care physician in a healthcare organization, care is still often given in teams, and after the primary care physician sends the patient to a specialist, the primary care physician seldom follows up on the patient's care. In all these cases, there is a need for a universal patient medical record that supports communication between these many caregivers, whether they work together or independently in providing a patient's care or work in different healthcare organizations. A universal patient record should thus be centered around an individual, not a healthcare organization nor any single caregiver.

Today, each physician is restricted to providing care in a very specific geographic location of the world. With telecommunications and telemedicine, this need not be so. Healthcare can be accomplished by a physician located anywhere in the world and a patient located anywhere else in the world. Thus, there is a need for remotely located caregivers to be able to concurrently access the same patient medical record.

As evidenced by the AIDS and SARS epidemics and by global warming, the health of each person in the world can be affected by what happens in other parts of the world. There are too few physicians in the world, too few nurses, and too few other healthcare workers. The world must make better use of all its healthcare workers. This can be accomplished through a universal patient medical record.

There would be a complete, immediately available, medical record. When a patient showed up for care with identification, even when unconscious in the emergency department, a universal patient medical record could provide the health history for the patient, informing caregivers of drug allergies, significant health problems, or other information that could improve care or potentially save the patient's life.

The universal patient medical record could save money in many ways, including by automatically capturing charges for medical services as they are identified in the medical record, and by allowing discharge activities to be done concurrently, quicker and thus with less cost. Public health organizations, insurance companies, the patient's personal physician, or other interested parties could be sent information on patient care and charges immediately after care is given or while care is being given, providing information quicker, potentially reducing fraud, providing better care, and quickly identifying public health problems before they get worse. Costs for paper, diagnostic image film, and associated labor, time, and space to transport and store them can be saved.

With a universal patient medical record:

- Better patient care could be provided that avoids medical mistakes due to lack of information due to unavailability of the medical record.
- There would be a single, complete automated patient medical record, rather than many fragmented ones.
- Communications between all types of caregivers would be enhanced, whether they worked on a single treatment for a patient, over many treatments, or over the patient's lifetime.
- There would a single place to permanently store the lifestyles, environmental conditions, and disease biomarkers for an individual. There could then be greater emphasis on individualized preventive care and diseases could be prevented before they occur.
- The lifestyles, environmental conditions, and biomarkers that predict diseases could be better determined as a result of a research database derived from these complete medical records.
- Healthcare workers could work across borders and provide healthcare and provide mentoring even when they were located remotely from each other, or remotely from the patient.
- Public health agencies, caregivers and the public can be more quickly informed about public health problems.
- Money can be saved.

Contents

CHAPTER 1

Introduction

CHAPTER OUTLINE

1.1 THE NEED FOR AN AUTOMATED MEDICAL RECORD

Over a patient's lifetime, a patient may be seen in many different healthcare organizations by many different physicians and nurse practitioners, and thus have many separate paper medical records. There is an urgent need to combine these medical records to produce a single *automated patient medical record.*

Such an automated patient medical record could be designed so it could evolve into a patient medical record that could be used by any healthcare organization in the world and any authorized healthcare provider. This book refers to such a patient medical record as the *universal patient medical record,* or *universal patient record* for short.

Various terms have been used for what this book calls the automated patient medical record, including *electronic medical record, electronic health record, electronic patient record, computer-based patient record (CPR),* and *automated medical record*, with definitions that vary from organization to organization. This book views the term automated patient medical record as an evolving entity, so the term is given a broad definition: "Patient medical records available over a network".

1.2 APPROACH TAKEN BY THIS BOOK

This book shows in detail how the patient medical record could be automated in healthcare organizations to produce such a universal patient record. As an example healthcare organization where automation would first occur, it uses a *Health Maintenance Organization (HMO).*

An HMO is a corporate entity that provides comprehensive health care for each member of the HMO for a fixed periodic payment paid in advance by the member or his employer. This

HMO has its own hospitals and medical offices spread throughout the United States. This is a fictional HMO, but is representative of a very large HMO in the United States. A national healthcare system would have many of the same characteristics as such an HMO, and thus what the reader reads in this book could equally apply to such a national healthcare system.

Because such an automated patient medical record on a large-scale does not yet exist and there may be many forms that it might take, simply describing such a patient medical record in detail would be presumptuous at this time. Instead, this book presents a *project plan* for development of an automated patient medical record in an HMO that could evolve into a universal patient record and presents possible and alternative results of this development effort. This book shows how a universal patient record is likely to evolve and how an automated patient medical record should be designed from the very beginning to be compatible with such a universal patient record.

A project to create a universal patient record, or even an automated patient medical record, is a very large one. This book defines a *project* as a well-defined sequence of steps—with constraints on time, costs, resources and quality—that leads to a clear set of products and goals. The product of our project is an automated patient medical record in an HMO that could evolve into a universal patient record. A *project plan* is a plan to do a particular project.

This project is a very complex one. To do it well, the resulting automated patient medical record must be looked at from **many different points of view** that must be **consistent with each other**. Some of these many mutually consistent points of view are the following: business, patient care and best medical practices, public health, project management and costs, universal patient record, healthcare and computer standards, current and future technology, law and legislation, caregiver workflow, user interfaces, computer software and hardware systems, and research.

1.3 INTENDED READERSHIP

The intended readership of this book are healthcare professionals: physicians, nurses and other caregivers, and healthcare organization managers and public health analysts. The intended readership also includes business and computer professionals: business analysts, system analysts, database analysts, and project managers. More specifically the intended readership of this book is anyone who is interested in the field of *medical informatics*, the use of computers in medical care.

1.4 ORGANIZATION OF THIS BOOK

The next chapter of this book describes in detail how to do any large-scale healthcare project and presents logical steps in such a project. Each chapter thereafter describes a step in a project to develop the automated patient medical record; these chapters each begin with a section labeled "project context" that describes the step in the context of a project.

Throughout the book, important terms will be italicized with these definitions included in the glossary. Because healthcare standards are important to doing any healthcare project, current healthcare standards are presented in the appendix.

Also presented throughout this book are *models,* where a model is a simplified description of a complex process. For example, the models in this book include the following:

- Models of patient care

- Models for doing a complex project

During a project, a model of the project's systems, workflows, or other products as agreed upon so far in a project can be created. This book calls such a model a *conceptual view*. A conceptual view is a vehicle for communication and critique of a project that is updated as more agreements are made on the products of the project.

Key Terms

automated patient medical record
computer-based patient record (CPR)
conceptual view
electronic health record
electronic medical record
electronic patient record
medical informatics
model
project
project plan
universal patient medical record
universal patient record

Study Questions

1. What are other terms for an automated patient medical record?
2. A medical record is centered around what? A healthcare organization? A provider? A patient? A medical department? Discuss.
3. What is the universal patient record?
4. What is a project? What is a project plan?

CHAPTER 2

How to Do a Large-Scale Complex Healthcare Project

CHAPTER OUTLINE

2.1 A LARGE-SCALE HEALTHCARE PROJECT

This book describes how to do a project to create an automated patient medical record in a large health organization that could evolve into a universal patient medical record. This is a very large-scale complex project. This chapter describes in detail how to do any large-scale project in a healthcare organization and provides the structure for the remainder of this book. This chapter is summarized in section 2.11.

2.2 A SUCCESSFUL PROJECT

The purpose of a project is to improve an organization or to fulfill governmental or industry mandates. The characteristics of a successful project within an organization, or within each organization for a multi-organizational project, are the following:

1. **Fulfills organizational needs:** The project fulfills a logical set of important needs of the organization.
2. **Integrated:** The project produces products that work together with pre-existing systems and employee workflows, and other projects, to support the organization.
3. **Adaptable:** The project produces products that can be changed as the organization changes to continue to fulfill the needs of the organization.

2.2.1 Fulfills Organizational Needs

Organizational needs, also called *organizational objectives,* are those things an organization needs to do to run the organization and have a quality organization.

For an organization to be successful, upper management of the organization must continually identify and work toward achieving organizational objectives. For example, for an HMO these *organizational objectives* might be the following: (1) provide excellent patient care, (2) generate sufficient money to run the HMO well and to expand the HMO, and (3) fulfill all the requirements of government and regulatory organizations.

Projects are selected which, together with the existing organization, fulfill these objectives with the greatest benefit to the organization. The objectives for each project, the *project objectives*, must be compatible with, and support, the organizational objectives.

For example, a project to develop a medical billing system, might have the project objective of supporting the collection of money from medical insurers and patients. This supports the organizational objective of generating money for the HMO.

The objectives of doing our project to automate the patient medical record might be the following: (1) to provide better patient care by providing an immediately available patient medical record, (2) to save money for the healthcare organization, (3) to assist healthcare workers in their jobs, and (4) to provide better information to manage the healthcare organization. These four project objectives potentially support all three of the organizational objectives.

To be useful in the evaluation of the success of a project, project objectives must be measurable, so the organization can determine whether these project objectives have been achieved once the project is complete. To measure a project objective, the organization can set targets to be met that can be measured and that lead to the final objectives. Such targets are called *goals* (King 1988). A goal can be set after a particular phase of the project or at the end of the project to measure whether or not an objective is being achieved. For example, a "goal" for a five-year project might be to have an immediately available automated patient record for 40% of the HMO patient visits after three years and 95% of the HMO patient visits at the end of the project. The project's final success can be determined by how closely the project meets the project objectives as measured by the final goals for the project.

Strategies (King 1988) that lead more quickly to the objectives and fulfillment of the goals also need to be established. For example, one strategy might be to create a Clinical Data Repository as a first step in automation of patient medical record. (A Clinical Data Repository is a database that combines clinical data related to a patient from various healthcare organization clinical systems, but is only a portion of the information in the automated patient medical record—see chapter 15.)

2.2.2 Integrated

In addition to producing products that fulfill the needs of the organization, a project must produce products that are integrated. *Integrated* in the context of an organization means that all the employee workflows, automated systems, and other parts of the organization function well together, ideally meeting the totality of the objectives of the organization. Once completed, the products of projects must be integrated into the organization.

For this integration to be done efficiently, there must be communication between these various parts of the organization. Of particular importance to the automated patient medical record system for speed and consistency is that patient and medical information should not have to be entered a second time into an automated system when it is already available—This requires communication between automated systems.

2.2.3 Adaptable

Adaptable means that an organization can change in the future to adapt to new business needs without great difficulty.

The products of a project should be created so they can be easily changed to meet changing organization business requirements. The most efficient way to do this is for business managers to anticipate future changes in the organization at the beginning of the project. This anticipation of the future requires management "vision". In anticipating such future business needs, management assumes a significant probability of being wrong, as anticipating the future is extremely hard to do.

One change this book anticipates is that there will eventually be a single universal patient medical record shared by many different healthcare organizations. This anticipated change should be built into the automated patient medical record project from the very beginning so the automated patient medical record could evolve into a universal patient record.

There are also other ways the project can be made adaptable that do not require anticipating future business requirements, and thus are less risky:

- Use industry-wide standards
- Document why project decisions were made so future decisions can be based upon these decisions
- Think of the products of the project in terms of components where a component can later be replaced without affecting other components—this is called *component adaptability*
- Use a phased approach to doing the project that enables adaptability during the project—this is explained in the next section.

2.3 A PHASED APPROACH

Figure 2.1 presents a phased approach to doing a project. This phased approach to doing a project promotes the three requirements for a successful project: fulfills organizational needs, integration, and adaptability.

Large-scale complex projects such as ours need to be broken into smaller sub-projects, or *phases*. An *overall design* of the entire project is done at the very beginning that includes breaking the project into phases. At the beginning of the second and each later phase there is a determination of whether the overall design has to be re-done because a previous phase or next phase changes the overall design.

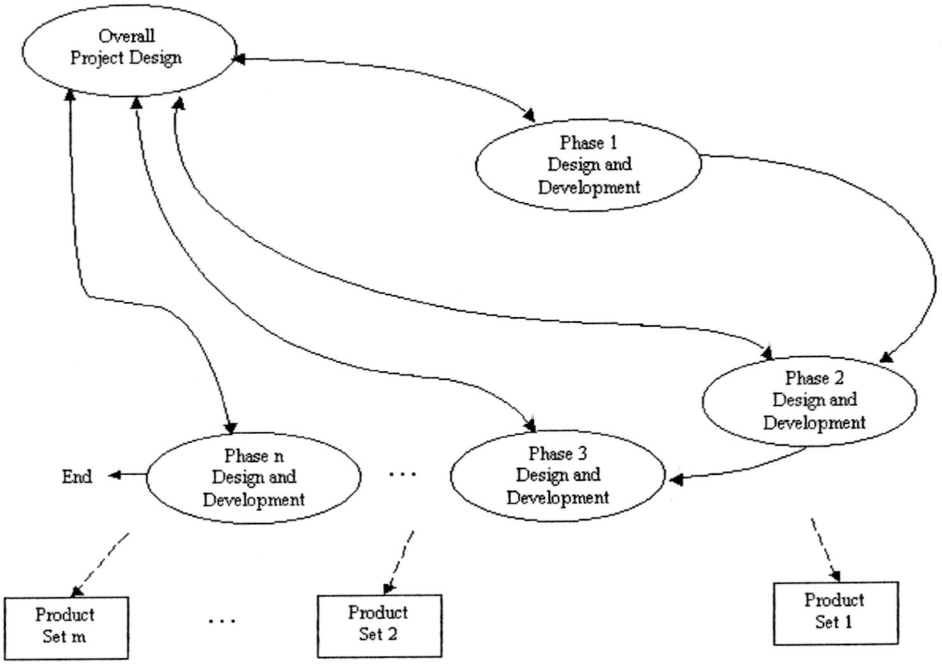

Figure 2.1 A phased approach to doing a project

For example, our project begins with a complete overall design of the automated patient medical record. The project is then broken up into phases to implement the automated patient medical record. One phase might be to interface the automated system to encounter systems that identify encounters such as outpatient visits, inpatient admissions, etc. Another phase might be to integrate a caregiver ordering system. During the design of the caregiver ordering system, it may be discovered that additional encounter information is needed and the overall automated patient medical record system may require some redesign.

The project model pictured in figure 2.1 has a number of advantages over others, foremost of which is always knowing that you are going the right direction to produce the final products. Doing a complete initial overall design allows the final products of the project to be predicted at the beginning, with each phase then developing products or immediate products that can be adapted into producing the next product leading to the final products of the project. Possibly redoing the overall design after an analysis later in the project during the start of a phase allows redirection of the project, with the project personnel again knowing what products to develop. Thus, the people doing and controlling the project always know where they are heading!

Other advantages of this approach are the following: (1) Going from one consistent design to another is much easier than trying to fix an inconsistent design. (2) The final products of a large-scale complex project often cannot be completely defined at the beginning; this project model allows redefinition of the overall products as more is learned about the project over the life of the project. (3) Breaking the project into phases allows the results of the project to be given to the organization at bit at a time, early on, with early payback to the organization—phases can be ordered such that those producing immediate results are done first. (4) The project can be evaluated early on and continuously to determine if it is meeting the project and organizational objectives and goals, with this evaluation possibly resulting in early revision of the project or termination of the project before too much money is spent. (5) This approach minimizes the cost of expensive re-working of the project, as re-working is done as soon as possible, before it becomes too costly. (6) Phases of the project may be done concurrently, effectively using available resources.

Products of a project could include automated systems, changes in the way employees function in doing their work, rewired buildings with installed workstations, etc., or different combinations, or "sets", of these products that function together. Each product set during the lifetime of the project should be adaptable, allowing change of the products to produce the next product set.

The "phased approach" project model in figure 2.1 is similar to project models referred to as the "incremental model" (Whitten 1995), the "iterative model" (Whitten 1995), the "evolutionary delivery method" (Gilb 1988), the "staged model" (Rajlich and Bennett 2000), and the "spiral model" (Boehm 1988).

Doing the overall design up front, and potentially re-doing it again before each phase, insures both that the project meets the needs of the organization and that the final product is integrated and adaptable.

Revisiting the overall design of the project before each phase allows upper management to verify that goals are being met and strategies are being followed to work toward the final objectives of the project. Costs can be reviewed after each phase and kept under control. Return on investment can be evaluated. **It thus allows upper management to have control over the project.**

It will insure adaptability by allowing early redesign of the project if necessary. After each phase, the phase and the overall project can be reviewed, revised, improved or restructured. New or changed requirements can be incorporated.

It will insure that other automated systems using the same information are integrated by allowing redesign of the project as necessary so that all automated systems are properly integrated.

In order to make the model in figure 2.1 somewhat more flexible, we allow the project model to have the following additional characteristics:

- Re-visiting the overall design may involve only reviewing a part, rather than the whole, of the overall design. Prior to simple phases and phases where much was known ahead of time, the review of overall design phase may not be needed at all.
- Phases may be added or changed as a result of revisiting the overall project design.
- Maintenance of a phase, for example a subsystem, occurs immediately after a phase is complete and could result in such significant changes that a new phase is required, with possible revisiting of the overall design.
- Phases may be added or deleted from the project plan for other reasons, for example, because of changes in organizational strategies or cost considerations.
- It may be appropriate to re-visit the overall design to account for multiple upcoming phases, rather than just one.
- Unlike what is shown in figure 2.1, phases can partially or completely overlap one another in time.

This project model is necessary because a large project takes a long time to complete and thus must be broken down into phases to simplify the project and to account for changes in the organization while the project is being done.

Use of this project model is not an excuse to do bad design. In fact, a large complex project is only feasible if the total of the design at each step fits together impeccably. Any significant error in the design may be embedded into the project and require significant re-work to get rid of it. Fixing multiple errors in a large project later on in the project may be cost-prohibitive or impossible. The earlier in a project a problem is detected, the lower the cost to fix it. For example, it has been estimated that fixing a problem early on in a project to create an automated system could be 1% as costly as making the fix after the automated system has been implemented in the organization (Pfleeger 1988).

2.4 THE PLAYERS

Many people, of varying roles, and aptitudes and interests, must be participants in a large project for it to be successful. These many diverse groups must work together as equals with the professionalism of each group respected by the other. The reason this cooperation is required is that a large-scale complex project is a **single organism rather than the sum of its parts**, with any one decision in one part of the project (e.g., a database design decision) potentially affecting any other part of the project (e.g., the user interface, with—in our project—a possible consequential effect on patient care).

Accordingly, this book, unlike many others, does not look at a project from the single point of view of a project manager, but from the points of view of the many participants in a large-scale project.

The most successful projects involve meetings involving a diversity of different categories of people who meet together and learn from each other, creating a group dynamics to exchange information, thus creating a unified product that meets the many diverse needs of the organization (e.g., provide excellent medical care, have good system response time, supply information needed by government and regulatory agencies, record medical supplies used).

There are four important categories of people who should be involved in a large-scale complex project: domain experts, content facilitators, upper management, and process facilitators. *Domain experts* are experts in the project subject area (e.g., patient care and medicine). *Content facilitators* gather information from the domain experts to design and produce the product. *Upper management* pays the bills and determines the organizational objectives for the project. *Process facilitators* work in group meetings to insure that meetings are productive, that group dynamics are established and that participants learn to run their own meetings.

Domain experts include *workers in the organization* (including upper management), who know how the organization functions, *customers* who know how the organization provides services, and experts from *the outside world* who know what happens outside the organization.

In our project developing an automated patient medical record system, the organization will be a particular type of healthcare organization, a Health Maintenance Organization (HMO). An HMO is a corporate entity that provides comprehensive health care for each member of the HMO for a fixed periodic payment paid in advance by the member or his employer; such a payment system is referred to as "capitation". Our HMO has its own hospitals and medical offices spread throughout the United States. This is a fictional HMO, but is representative of a very large HMO that may exist in the United States.

Upper management in our example are management physicians who control the operations of the HMO. Being management physicians, they care very much about quality patient care as well as about the financial health of the HMO.

The workers in the organization include everyone in the HMO, but especially "caregivers", those who provide medical care to patients: physicians, nurses, medical assistants, hospital unit assistants, etc. The customers are the members and patients of the HMO, and a patient's family members. The outside world includes people in the following types of organizations: suppliers, the government, regulatory agencies, software and hardware suppliers, and other healthcare organizations.

Content facilitators for a project include *business analysts*, *system analysts*, *database analysts*, *domain analysts,* members of the *technical staff*, and *project managers*, and *standards analysts*. Business analysts gather information from upper management, workers, customers and outside experts to identify what an improved organization would look like and to identify business requirements that would accomplish these improvements. System analysts take the business requirements and a description of the improved organization to create requirements for automated systems. Part of system analysis is determining new and changed databases—databases are places to save information; database analysts work with system analysts and domain experts or domain analysts to define databases for a project or for an organization, or change existing databases. A domain analyst is an expert in how a particular type of business functions and works with domain experts to facilitate solutions; for example, a domain analyst might be an analyst who is also an expert on provision of medical care and work with domain experts (e.g., the caregivers) in an HMO to reengineer medical care, changing work flows. The technical staff create and implement automated systems. Project managers schedule activities making up the project and guide personnel in their execution. A standards analyst insures that the standards of the organization and of the industry—in our case the healthcare industry—are followed.

For a large-scale complex project, meetings between project members are likely to occur over an extended period of time. For any long-lasting meetings of project group members, there should be a *process facilitator*, or simply "facilitator", to guide the group in making decisions until the participants in the group or sub-group learn how to work together (in which case the whole group assumes the responsibilities of the process facilitator). Along with the participants, the process facilitator develops **processes to be followed during meetings** to enable the group to work efficiently and make decisions (e.g., "It seems that our group has decided upon the following process: Any agreement this week will be written down. During the following week's meeting we will either finalize the agreement or retract the agreement. This allows us to think over our agreements between meetings and discuss the agreements with our various groups."). The process facilitator also teaches the group about *interventions* to be used if the group bogs down; for example, when multiple people are talking at once, the process facilitator might say, "Just a moment, one person at a time. Joe you were first, and then Carol". An excellent book on *facilitation* is (Kaner et al. 1996).

When there are automated systems, members of the technical staff are involved in the procurement, development and implementation of these automated systems. This staff may include the following: *system architects*, people who define how computers and other devices are linked logically and physically, how data is distributed between databases on the computers, and how software is distributed; *capacity planners*, people who get information from business planners on anticipated number of users and customers, and who determine and anticipate the activity within systems and networks, thus identifying hardware and network requirements; *software developers*, who design software; and other data processing personnel such as programmers, programmer/analysts and testers who program and test the software. Additionally, *vendors* may supply off-the-shelf software in place of organizationally developed systems.

The next section describes the different steps (or activities) making up a project and which participants are involved in each step.

2.5 STEPS IN A PROJECT

From my experience, each phase of a project, as well as the overall project design or re-design, can be broken down into the following steps:

- **Business analysis step**: Define the project or phase, and determine business requirements: changes to the organization from the project or a phase from a business point of view. The business analysis step may include the following activities: identify the project or phase; describe the current organization with respect to the project or phase and determine what to change and what to preserve; identify reasons to do the project/phase; identify obstacles; establish a vision for the future; and from all this, identify business requirements.
- **Evaluation step**: For the project as a whole during the overall project design, or for a phase, evaluate the projected value of the project or phase or actual success of the project or phase so far. Determine whether to continue, change course, or terminate the project or phase; included in this process for the overall design is whether to re-do previous phases and re-do plans for future phases.
- **Business reengineering step**: Determine how employees will function differently due to the project or phase. Included in this process is determination of user interfaces for automated systems.
- **System analysis step**: Determine technical requirements for new automated systems and changes to existing automated systems as a result of the project or phase.
- **Project plan step**: For the project, break the project into phases; for a phase, break the phase into tasks in order to develop or implement the phase.
- **Development step**: Based upon information from the system analysis step, develop or make changes to automated systems, or alternatively purchase a vendor system. (This is done only as part of a phase.)
- **Implementation step**: Change the way employees function in the organization together with implementing or changing automated systems in the organization that are part of the project. (This is done only as part of a phase.)

The first five steps are steps occurring both as part of the overall design (or redesign) and of a phase. The last two steps are only part of a phase and produce products of the project. Figure 2.2 in the next section of this book shows these steps within the overall design, and figure 2.3 in the following section shows the steps in a phase.

2.5.1 Overall Design (or Redesign)

The first part of a project is the initial overall design to plan the complete project; the overall design can later be revisited if during a phase it is determined that the phase would cause a change in the overall design of the project. The overall design (redesign) is shown in figure 2.2.

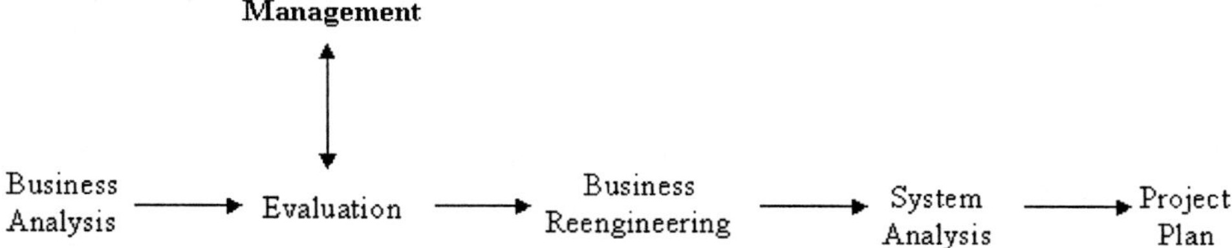

Figure 2.2 Steps Within the Overall Design.

The overall design includes an overall business analysis step to define the project, an evaluation step to inform upper management of the project's feasibility at this point, a business reengineering step to identify changed organizational workflows, a system analysis step to do an initial overall design of automated systems if any, and a project plan step to break the project into phases.

The purposes of the overall design are the following:

- to define the project and its objectives
- to insure that all the component parts of the project, and all its phases, will fit together
- to allow upper management to evaluate whether they will getting what they expect from the project, and allow them to make a decision of whether to terminate, change or go ahead as is with the project.

The initial overall design phase begins with the business analysis step, in which ideas for the project are introduced by upper management or sold to upper management. Upper management must provide strong support and agree to expend the required money. Upper management provides the initial objectives for the project (expected future results from the project), strategies for accomplishing the project, and intermediate goals for the project (e.g., in the third year of the project there will be actual cost savings to the organization as a result of the project). Objectives and strategies for the project are based upon objectives and strategies for the organization: Project objectives must support organizational objectives, and strategies for doing the project must be consistent with organizational strategies. Business requirements are derived from project objectives, where *business requirements* are future required characteristics of the organization that will result from the project.

In continuation of the business analysis step, workers and others describe the current working environment where the changes will occur and the current applicable automated systems. Through a process that includes incorporation of the information from management and workers' ideas for improvements in the organization, a future projected organization as related to the project is described. Additional business requirements are determined by identifying business requirements that produce the future environment from the current one.

Next, a very important evaluation step is completed. The projected future environment is compared against the current environment, and benefits, obstacles and risks, return on investment and other values are determined for the project recorded in a *feasibility study*. Upper management uses the feasibility study to determine whether the project is possible to do and, if so, to compare the project against other projects, evaluating how each project would satisfy organizational objectives relative to its costs, determining which projects should be done and which ones should have priority over other projects.

An additional determinant in the evaluation step is how each project would change the organization. Upper management compares the changes against their *vision* of what they want the organization to look like in the future. If there is a significant difference between the two, upper management may change the project to be more in line with their vision, adding additional business requirements for the project and possibly resulting in a modification of the feasibility study.

If there is a go ahead from upper management to continue with the project, a business reengineering step is done to determine changes to organizational workflows and to determine user interfaces for any new or changed automated systems based upon business requirements. An overall system analysis step is then done to determine automated system requirements from the business requirements and from the identified user interfaces. The business reengineering and system analysis steps closely depend on each other as automated systems could change organizational workflows; thus, the business reengineering and system analysis steps often overlap, with the user interfaces and employee workflows influencing the automated system requirements and the automated system requirements influencing the user interfaces and employee workflows.

Finally, and this is a very difficult step, the project is broken up into phases, or subprojects. (These phases later produce the actual products produced by the project.) The earlier phases should provide the infrastructure, if applicable, for further phases (e.g., the security subsystem and databases for an automated system should be developed early on as these are part of the infrastructure needed to produce the automated system; wiring within buildings and networks should also be created early on to support the automated systems). Ideally, although not necessarily, early phases should provide significant benefits to the organization (e.g., provide revenue for the organization), so that the benefits of the project materialize early on, even if it is later determined that the project should be terminated. Within the overall project plan and at the end of the project, measurable goals should be scheduled to evaluate the progress of the project and to compare the actual versus the expected results of the project.

The initial overall design, even if done without all the necessary information, is very important as it establishes a direction and consistency for the project. Projects where all its parts (i.e., all phases) are done in a consistent manner are much easier to later change, than ones done inconsistently.

Reference (Booker 2000) has shown how important this upfront initial overall design is for enterprise software projects: "Those users who spent more upfront time and effort analyzing their systems, business and process needs fared much better than those who didn't. ... Users who follow these procedures achieved positive outcomes 56 percent of the time vs. only 8 percent for those who failed to conduct such an analysis."

2.5.2 A Phase

The actual creation of the products of the project occurs within the various phases of the project. A project can usually be broken up into phases in many ways.

For example, our project to improve patient care in an HMO through automation of the patient medical record might include the following phases: (1) a phase to standardize clinical systems (pharmacy system, clinical laboratory system, etc.) within the HMO that need to be interfaced with the automated medical record system, (2) a phase to interface these clinical systems, store combined clinical system information, and enable display of it, (3) a phase to automate the patient medical record within the emergency and outpatient clinics creating an outpatient medical record, (4) a phase to automate the patient medical record in the inpatient (i.e., hospital) setting, integrating the inpatient with the outpatient record medical record information.

For each such phase of the project, there is, like in the initial overall design, a set of steps. See figure 2.3 for the steps within a phase. There are the same set of steps plus two additional ones that do not occur in the overall design, a development step and an implementation step: (1) a business analysis step to compare the current working environment to the future one after the phase and to develop resultant business requirements as a result of the phase; (2) a business reengineering step where changed workflows are developed for the phase and, if applicable, user interfaces for new or change automated systems are designed; (3) a system analysis step to identify changes to automated systems or new automated systems for the phase, (4) a project plan step where a detailed project plan for the phase is developed in terms of tasks, including detailed estimated costs for each task and potential problems that must be managed during the phase; (5) a development step, if any, where the automated systems are developed or procured from vendors and customized for the organization, and (6) an implementation step where the new working methods are implemented, workers are retrained, and the automated systems are implemented. As part of the business analysis step of a phase is a determination of whether this phase unexpectedly affects the overall design of the system, requiring that the overall design be re-done.

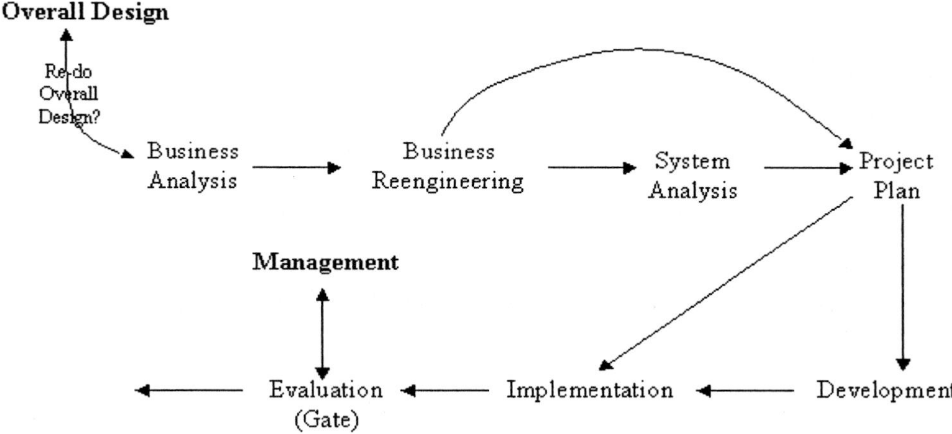

Figure 2.3 Steps Within a Phase.

A phase may not involve automated systems (e.g., a phase to re-wire medical centers) and thus the system analysis step and development step (which design and produce automated systems respectively) may thus be skipped.

Periodically, the whole project must be reviewed, as part of the evaluation step, to determine if goals are being met. Such points in the project are called *gates*. Although figure 2.3 shows the evaluation step (a gate) occurring at the end of a phase, evaluation steps (gates) could occur anywhere in the project. Gates should be pre-planned as part of the overall design project plan step to periodically evaluate the project's progress, allowing management to make decisions on changing, or even terminating the project.

2.5.3 Continuing or Terminating the Project

At an evaluation point during the project, it may be determined that the project should be terminated or revised. If the project is not terminated, the project will eventually reach its scheduled completion point.

People often think of a project being completed once all the products of the project are initially installed, e.g., once the automated patient medical record is installed. But I think that this is the wrong point of view. A project—such as the automated patient medical record system—should be viewed as always being a project until it is decommissioned, as it will likely be continually changing to meet the changing needs of the organization until that time. Changing a system after it is delivered to improve it or to correct errors, referred to as *maintenance*, is always required unless an organization is willing to live with a system that does not quite work correctly.

At the end of a phase, the phase goes into maintenance mode. Once all the products of the project are installed, the entire project goes into maintenance mode.

Maintenance, after an automated system is completed according to the schedule, could consume 70-80% of the costs during the lifetime of the automated system (Martin and Osborne).

2.5.4 The Steps in Detail

2.5.4.1 Business Analysis Step

In the *business analysis step*, business changes to the organization that would result from the project or phase are identified. This is the first step in the initial overall project analysis and in a phase. Figure 2.4 shows this step as it would occur in the initial overall design of the project.

Looking at the needs of the organization and the current environment and systems, upper management identifies potential projects. By analyzing the current environment and systems, management identifies problems in the organization. Based upon these problems and the needs of the organization, upper management identifies potential projects to further the needs and fix the problems.

A project is broken down into phases: sub-projects. Each phase must be identified and described. Each phase in the project also has a business analysis step.

For a project or a phase, upper management identifies *objectives*, *strategies*, and *goals* for the project or phase (King 1988). Objectives are the future positions of the organization expected from the changes resulting from the project or phase. Strategies are ways to accomplish these objectives. Goals are targets to be met and measured at specific points in time that can be used to measure the progress or lack of progress of the project in achieving the project objectives.

For example, for the automated patient medical record project, some project objectives might be to save money for the HMO, to have the patient medical record instantaneously available upon a patient visit, and to have the system calculate all charges to patients and insurance companies automatically. Strategies might include to create a common hardware infrastructure throughout the healthcare organization so the automated medical record system can be easily implemented; to implement the automated patient medical record first in the west coast region of the HMO to implement it the quickest, before rolling it out to other regions; and to immediately work with insurance companies for a data format to transmit healthcare charges to them. One goal related to the objective of saving the company money would be to have a positive return on investment by the third year (where "return on investment" is a comparison of the total costs of the project with the increased revenue accruing from the project.)

These (project or phase) objectives, strategies and goals would later be used to evaluate the progress and success of the project in a later evaluation step. They could also be used to compare this project against other projects, whose project objectives might also be important for the organization, so money can be allocated between the projects according to their value to the organization, or one project can be done instead of the other.

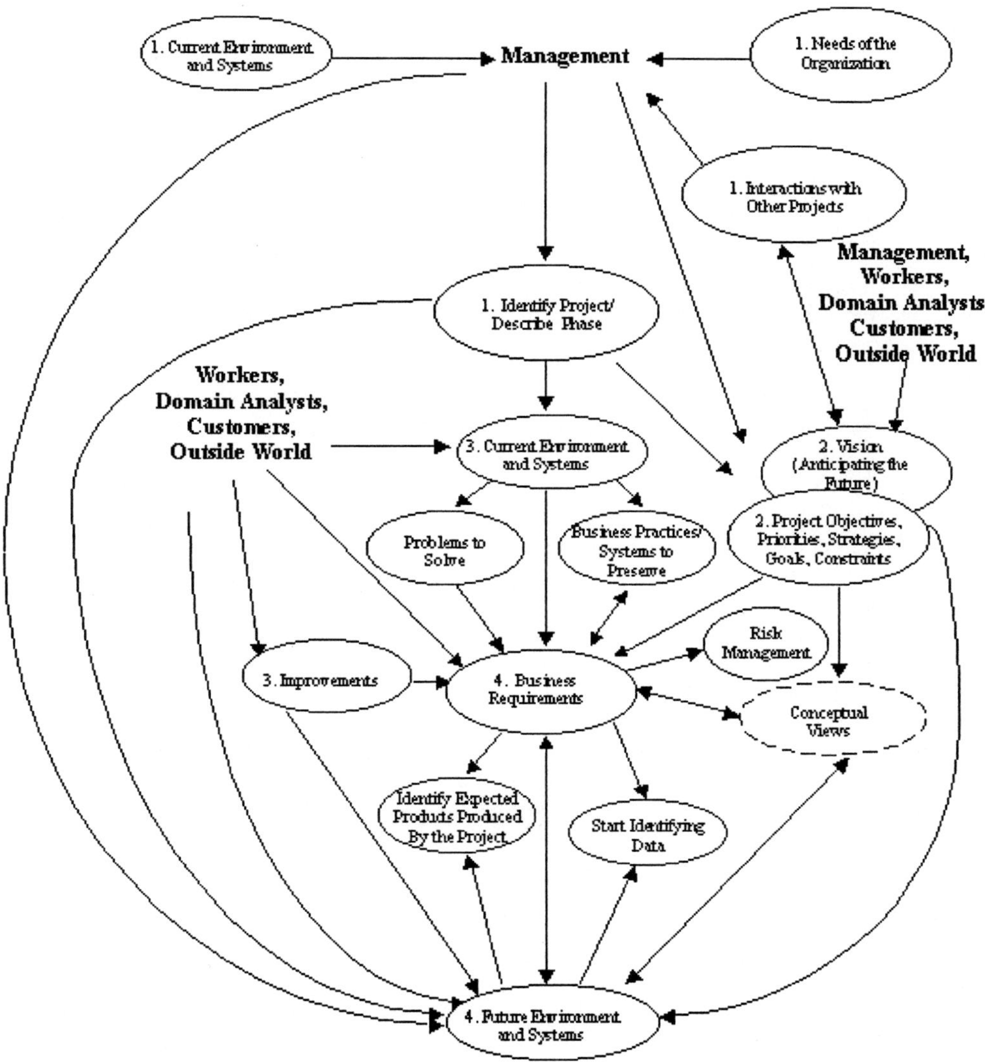

Figure 2.4 Business analysis step in the initial overall design.

Project (or phase) objectives, strategies and goals are derived from objectives, strategies and goals for the organization. This is done by identifying aspects of the project that further these organizational objectives, strategies or goals. These become the project objectives, strategies and goals. For example, if an organizational objective is patient satisfaction and some aspect of doing the project strongly promotes patient satisfaction, then this would become a project objective.

During the business analysis step, upper management identifies *constraints* for the project or phase. The most important constraints are the amount of money and amount of time allocated to the project or phase.

Also, during the business analysis step, a *vision* for the project should be developed. This vision takes ideas from many different sources to predict or define the future of the organization and outside world with respect to the project, in our case with respect to the automated patient medical record. Ideally, by meeting the vision, the product would have an extended life span in that the resulting product would fit into the organization as it changes and, where applicable, the resulting product would later be compatible with, and perhaps could interface with, systems in other organizations. In the case of our automated patient medical record system, this vision might include integration of the automated patient medical record with a possible universal patient health record that would be available to many healthcare organizations both inside and outside the HMO.

Vision, anticipating the future, also applies to determining how this project affects other projects, in the interim and once completed, and how other projects affect this project. This provides upper management with important information to select, evaluate and coordinate projects within the organization.

Vision entails significant risk that the prediction of the future is wrong. Thus *risk management*, planning alternative measures if a prediction turns out to be wrong, is important.

After the development of objectives, strategies and goals, the workers and domain experts would then identify *the current environment and systems* as a baseline for evaluating any changes. From detailed observations and analyses of the current environment and systems, *essential business practices* that must be preserved are identified. The workers could then identify *improvements* they would like to see in the current environment or automated systems. From upper management's ideas for change, objectives, strategies, and goals, from various people's vision of the future, from the worker's list of improvements, and from an analysis done by the workers, upper management, domain experts and business analysts, a proposed *future environment and automated systems* is described.

Finally, the business analysts and domain analysts together with workers and upper management create a list of *business requirements* (changes to the organization together with things to keep the same) to transform the current environment to the future one. Business requirements include both requirements for changing the organization and for creating and changing automated systems.

As a method to clarify ideas, models of systems, workflows, etc. may be created, presenting *conceptual views*, or less abstract, more concrete views, of the systems and working environment. These conceptual views are vehicles for communication and for critique, especially for people who find that working with objectives and business requirements alone is too abstract for them.

When a project or phase involves an automated system, then storage of information on databases is required. Because developing databases is so terribly difficult, a start should be made at the start of the project or phase to identifying items making up the database: business objects (e.g., a physician order), database objects (e.g., order status, order type of a physician order) and relationships between objects (e.g., each caregiver order has an order status such as "in process", "completed", "results returned"), and requirements for new information that is not on any existing database. Existing corporate databases—databases that are currently being used throughout the organization—that could be used by the project should be identified; use of corporate databases is one way of integrating the different parts of the organization.

Finally, expected products of the project, including potential new and changed automated systems, and the need for changed employee workflows, are identified.

The primary product of the business analysis step are business requirements for the project or phase.

Business requirements based upon overcoming *obstacles* should be identified in the business analysis step except for the initial overall design. The reason for this is that the initial overall design should look at the benefits from the project first; if these benefits are not great enough, then it may not be worthwhile to put in the expense of looking at the obstacles also. Thus, for the initial overall design, I made looking at obstacles part of a later evaluation step.

Part of the business analysis step of a phase should involve identifying whether the overall design of the project should be re-done. This is obviously not required in a business analysis step in the overall design.

2.5.4.2 Evaluation Step

Figure 2.5 shows the activities in an *evaluation step* for the initial overall design. The evaluation step occurs as both a part of the overall design and of a phase.

In the evaluation step, the project is evaluated. In the overall design, a projection of the project in the future is made to determine if the project will meet expectations. In a phase, an evaluation is done of the project so far. After this evaluation, it may be decided to go ahead with the project as is, change the project, or terminate the project.

In the overall design, the evaluation is done after the business analysis step (see figure 2.2). In other cases, evaluations can be unscheduled and done any time it is deemed necessary, or, alternatively, they can be pre-scheduled to occur at designated times during the project (for example, in figure 2.3, at the end of the phase).

The business analyst and system analyst present an evaluation of the project or phase to upper management. The business analyst explains the business side of the project and related issues. The system analyst presents the technical and automated system side of the project and related issues.

From this evaluation, upper management determines if they are, or will be, getting what they are paying for. This evaluation compares the changed, or projected future, work environment to the initial work environment and determines if the objectives, goals and vision of the organization are indeed being fulfilled by this change. Evaluation also involves identifying obstacles to the project that must be considered, both for determining if an obstacle makes the project too difficult to do, but also for determining additional business requirements that mitigate the obstacle or a contingency plan that is followed later on in the project if the obstacle does occur. The results of the evaluation step may be termination of the project, changes to the project, or continuing the project as planned.

The evaluation step during the initial overall design is there to ask the question, "Should we continue with the project?" In our project model the evaluation step for the overall design occurs directly after the business analysis step, as enough information has been gathered to make management decisions but an inordinate amount of time, money and effort has not yet been expended.

On the other hand, in our model, the evaluation step in a phase can be scheduled to occur anywhere in any phase or an unscheduled evaluation step could occur when it is decided it is necessary. These evaluation steps are put in less to ask the question "Should we continue with the project?" but more to ask "Where are we? Are we meeting our goals? And if not, what changes to the project do we need to make?"

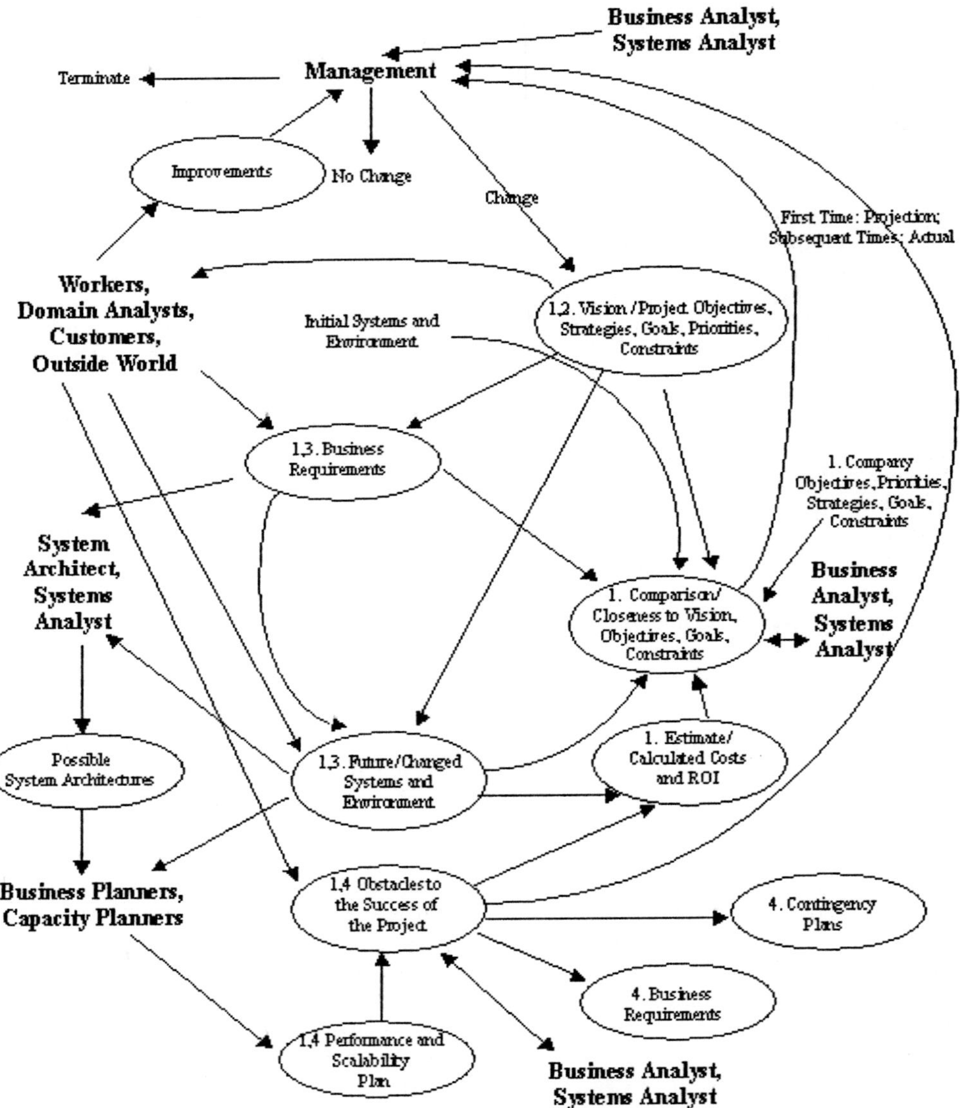

Figure 2.5 Evaluation step for the initial overall design.

The first evaluation point in a project, as part of the initial overall design, is actually done before any changes are implemented; thus, the evaluation is entirely based upon projected changes to the organization due to the project rather than actual changes. Such an evaluation study in the initial overall design before any project changes are implemented falls under the category of a *feasibility study*.

A *feasibility study* (Sommerville 2000) evaluates whether or not the proposed system is feasible and whether or not it could be developed given existing budgetary constraints and obstacles. In other words, based upon business requirements, it determines "Is there at least one solution that is currently feasible?" and if there is, "Is there at least one solution that the organization will be able to afford that benefits the organization?"

The results of an evaluation are reported to higher management. Besides benefits, *obstacles* to the success of the project are also reported to management; these are important to include because project objectives tend to deal with benefits of projects more often than obstacles. Suggested *improvements* in the project from workers are also reported to upper management for possible inclusion in the project.

Higher-level management has to make decisions on whether to continue the project, change the project, or terminate the project. They might make changes in the objectives, strategies, goals, or vision for the project, or on constraints such as the amount of money allocated for the project.

Changes in the objectives, strategies, goals, vision or constraints for the project could result in changes in projections of the future working environment, and new or changed business requirements. These changes are identified by business analysts working in coordination with workers, domain analysts, customers and the outside world.

An obstacle is any actual or potential hindrance to the successful completion of a project. For identified obstacles, additional business requirements might be added to the project. For an unpredictable obstacle, a *contingency plan* may be created, a plan to follow if the obstacle does occur.

Technical obstacles for a large automated system often involve future performance and scalability of the system (e.g., an automated system may be so slow that users would not want to use it). A performance and scalability plan should be started in the evaluation step that anticipates growth of the automated systems, growth in number of customers and changes in technology. This plan should be used during the duration of the project and also afterwards to plan upgrades to hardware and system software systems and record measured bottlenecks in the system so they can be resolved before there are problems. In the evaluation step, the performance and scalability plan would be used to determine whether it is or will be technologically feasible to do the project within the required budget for the project.

The performance and scalability plan is developed by three sets of participants: system architects, business planners and capacity planners. System architects determine possible system architectures, which describe the computer systems running the automated systems, the networks connecting the computers, the distribution of data on databases, and the flow of transactions occurring within the system. Business planners make an estimate of future growth and changes in the organization, including estimates of increases in HMO membership, in number of patients, and in nurses and physicians who work in the HMO. Capacity planners evaluate whether or not the proposed automated systems and system architectures will be able to handle the future growth and changes, taking into account projected future technology and monetary constraints on the project. Possible problems could include slow response time, exceeding the capacity of databases or network connections, or other slow-downs or failures of the automated systems.

2.5.4.3 Business Reengineering Step: Workflows and User Interfaces

Figure 2.6 shows activities in the *business reengineering step*, a step which identifies changes to employee workflows including those for automated systems. For automated systems, user interfaces and elements of future databases are also identified, and interfaces between automated systems may be identified.

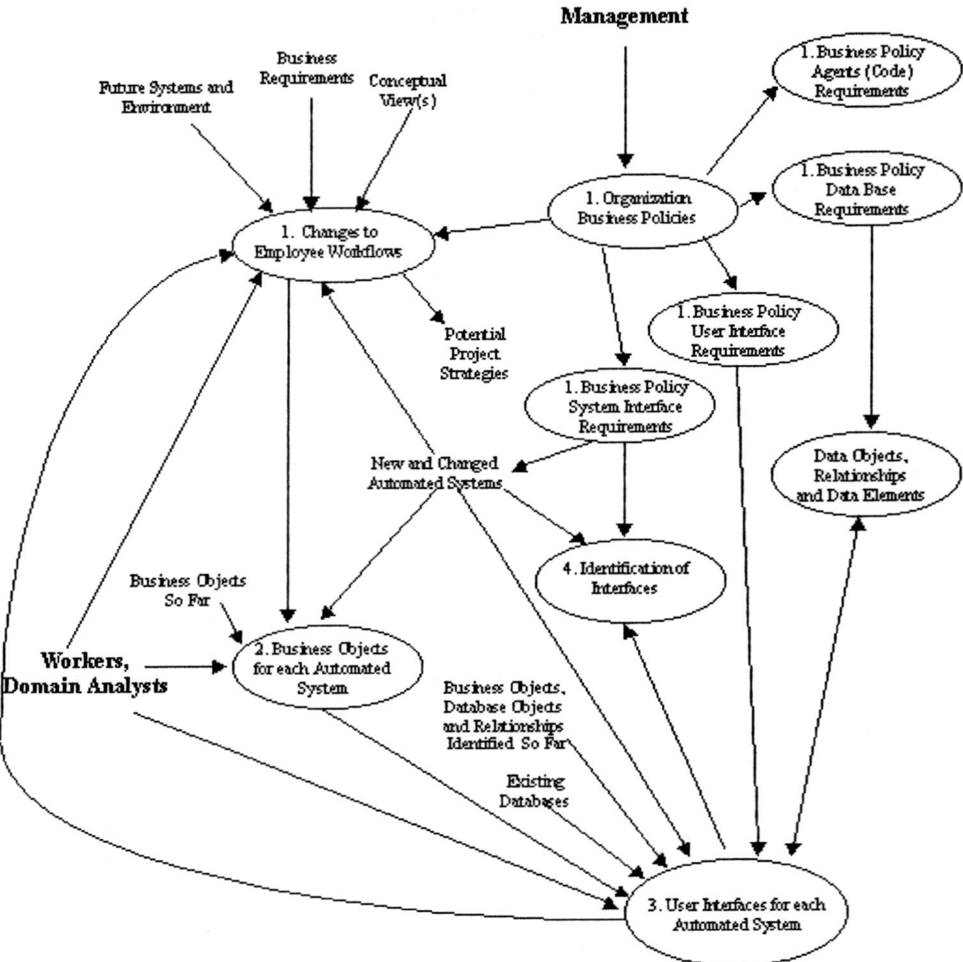

Figure 2.6 Business Reengineering step: workflows and user interfaces.

The business reengineering step applies both for the overall project design and for any phase in the project. For each category of employee in the organization, the future workflow of the employee is identified.

Workflows must take into account management-determined *business policies* for the company, which may have to be revised to account for changes in the organization resulting from the project. For example, one business policy of the HMO might be to have each HMO member pick a *primary care physician*—in medicine, pediatrics, gynecology—to be her or his primary caregiver, also called a *personal physician*. For each business policy, the following should be documented: (1) employee workflows related to the business policy, (2) user interfaces (i.e., information input by users into automated systems) related to the business policy, (3) databases (all the information that needs to be collected and stored) to implement the business policy, (4) *algorithms* to execute the business policy, implemented in code possibly on many different computers, and (5) interfaces between the various computer systems that are required for the business policy. The business policy to associate each healthcare organization member with a primary care physician, for example, might require changes in all five areas to implement in the automated systems: workflows, user interfaces, databases, code and interfaces while other business policies might be implemented purely operationally effecting only employee workflows. **Business policies often cross projects and automated systems**—Documenting business policies looking beyond single projects or automated systems and considering the organization as a whole insures that projects and systems in the organization are integrated.

New and changed automated systems for the project are identified earlier in the business analysis step. Here in the business reengineering step, the user interface for each of these new or changed automated systems, and each category of worker using the system, is determined.

In order to develop user interfaces that best correspond to the business (in this case, patient care), it is best to define "business objects" that a typical user is familiar with in his work. For example, for a person providing patient care, these objects may include "patients", "physician schedules", and "the patient medical record". Chapter 12 identifies many of the business objects for our project and describes in detail the benefits of identifying business objects.

Since, all data in the user interfaces comes from and will be stored on databases or comes from interfaces with other automated systems or from information input in user interfaces, user interfaces must be kept in synchronization with these sources of information. Some of the databases may already exist in the organization while others might have to be created. Interfaces between automated systems (network communication), which pass data between computer systems, also may already exist or have to be created.

The primary purpose of the business reengineering step is to redefine how the organization functions. Thus, this, the business reengineering step, is very important in a project, as the primary purpose of any project is to change the organization to fulfill organizational objectives (e.g., improve patient care, save the HMO money).

2.5.4.4 System Analysis Step

When there are automated systems in the project, the requirements for the automated systems, including software, databases, hardware, interfaces and infrastructure, are determined in the *system analysis step* (see figure 2.7). These requirements for automated systems are determined from the results of previous steps: Business requirements for the systems come from the business analysis step, while business polices—and associated user interfaces for systems, employee workflows, and data requirements (e.g., for databases)—and other user interfaces come from the business reengineering step. System analysts facilitate and record the results of the system analysis step, working with the technical staff, business analysts, domain experts, standards analysts, and vendors.

System requirements are determined in the system analysis step. A *system requirement* is a required characteristic of a new or changed automated system. System requirements include requirements for: *hardware*; *system software* including operating systems, database management systems and network middleware; *application software* for each automated system; *databases*; and *interfaces* between automated systems. System software is generic software that provides support to run computers, while application software is software to support the needs of an organization. An interface is data transferred between automated systems, with the data either being transferred via network connections, or multi-system reading and writing information to and from databases or other data stores.

Interfaces would be designed with the participation of domain experts understanding the meaning of the data transferred and technical experts and automated system users understanding the current automated systems. Software and hardware vendors developing an automated system could be involved. Interfaces could be with systems outside of the initial scope of the project, including systems outside the organization. I propose that all these interfaces be described in an *interface plan* so that information on the interface can be shared by managers on each of the systems that need to be changed.

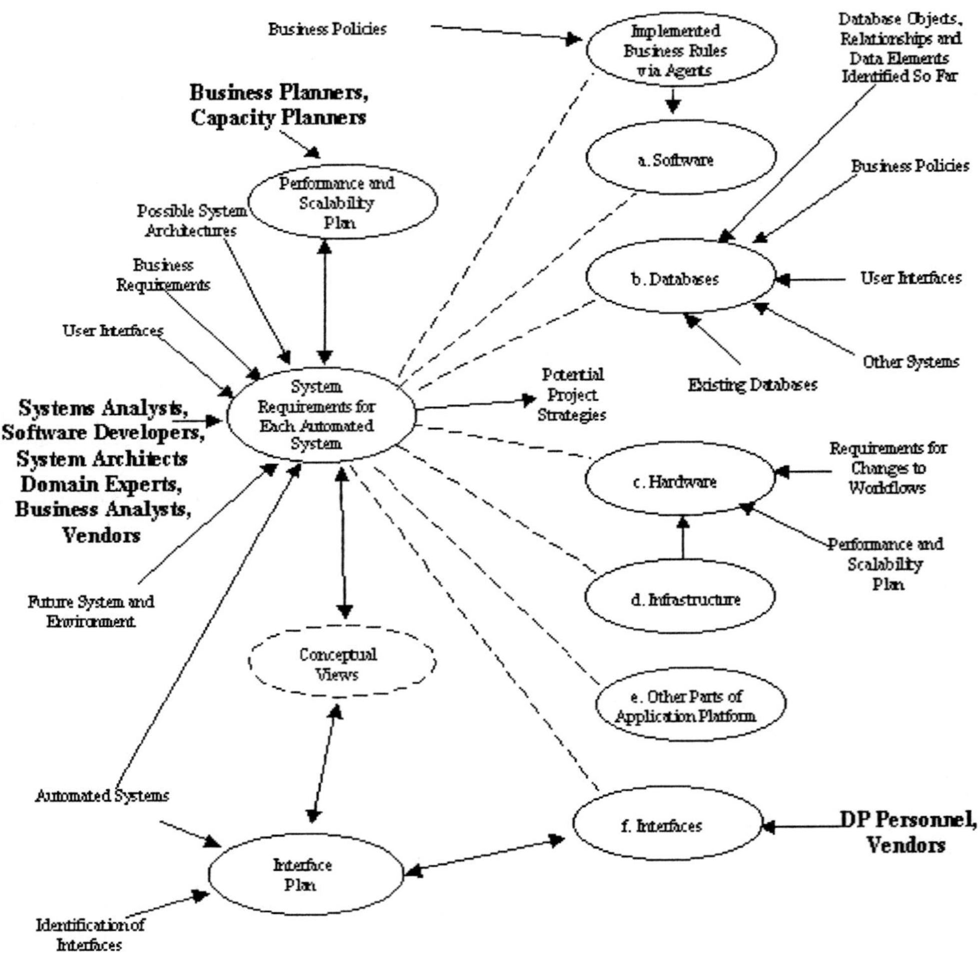

Figure 2.7 System analysis step.

In the business reengineering step, organizational *business policies* associated with the project are identified, with specifications for code and associated tables, interfaces between systems, databases and changes to user interfaces. In this, the system analysis step, the code and tables, interfaces between systems, and databases would be defined in more detail. In this book, an *agent* is a way of categorizing and separating out a set of items implementing an organizational business policy: a combination of code and tables, interfaces between systems, databases, user interfaces (possibly all spread across a number of different software systems), and administrative and operational procedures followed by employees implementing the business policy, so that the business policy could be implemented and changed by the people responsible for the business policy instead of relying totally on technical staff to do so. Part of the system analysis step is defining these agents.

Databases are completely defined in the system analysis step. Databases need to support all automated systems and business policies in the organization, including existing automated systems, and new or changed automated systems that are part of the project. For the system analysis step, database information can most usefully be expressed in terms of *entity-relationship (E-R) diagrams* and *data dictionaries*, as well as by text, describing the required data and relationships between the data—see chapter 13. Data dictionaries exist as documentation tools to describe a database, and also can be used for operational control of the database within a database management system when the database is actually used.

If changes in infrastructure are needed, such as building rewiring or remodeling, these changes are planned during the system analysis step. The planned infrastructure would be implemented during the implementation step. The choice of hardware for the automated systems could be influenced by space considerations within facilities and other infrastructure factors.

Hardware must also be compatible with the way workers actually do their job. Thus, the choice of hardware in this step may be influenced by workflows identified in the previous business reengineering step. For example, respiratory therapists who already carry around lots of equipment from room to room may not be able to carry any additional equipment, such as portable computers, as the total weight of these items may then be too much.

Finally, hardware must be compatible with the performance and scalability requirements identified in the performance and scalability plan. The performance and scalability plan is a document that should be kept up-to-date during and after the project, projecting future hardware capacity needed in the system. This capacity would be expressed in terms of number of users, transaction volumes, and network traffic. When a project has automated systems that will grow in capacity over time, it is extremely important to identify projected long-term capacity and scalability requirements up front during the initial overall design so the systems can be developed and planned accordingly; otherwise, there is the high likelihood that a large-scale automated system could quickly become obsolete due to lack of capacity.

2.5.4.5 Project Plan: Breaking the Project into Phases or Tasks

The *project plan* step occurs in the initial overall design and occurs in each phase. When this step occurs during the initial overall design, the project is broken up into *phases*. When it occurs as part of a phase, the phase is broken up into *tasks*. See figures 2.8.

Doing all aspects of a very large-scale complex project (such as automation of the patient medical record) all at once is risky, and undoubtedly not feasible. During the overall design, the project should be broken up into phases, smaller sub-projects. Likewise, to make a phase simpler, each phase is broken into tasks. For a large project, both the overall project and each phase would have its own project plan and project manager.

In order for such an approach to work, phases (or tasks) that provide the infrastructure needed by later phases (or tasks) should be done first. For example, if creation of an automated patient medical record depends upon information coming from other automated systems, then the interfaces with these systems should be developed early in the project.

Ideally, high payback phases would be done first, so that the benefits from the project can be realized as early as possible. For example, if an automated patient medical record system provides the input for a billing system that would result in an increase in revenues to the HMO, then the phase to integrate the billing system could be done early on so as to create an earlier return on investment for the project.

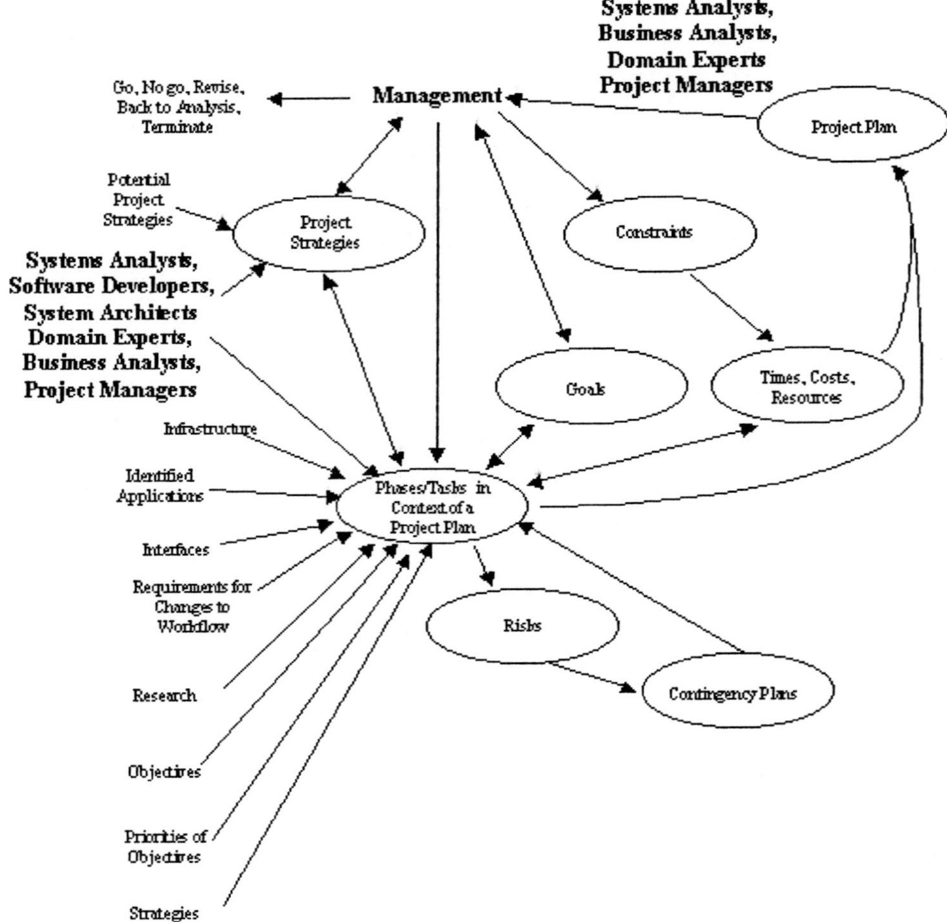

Figure 2.8 Project plan step: breaking the project into phases or a phase into tasks.

What is produced from the project plan step is an *overall project plan* for the project scheduling the phases within the project, and a *project plan* for each phase, each scheduling tasks to accomplish the phase. The primary user of the overall project plan would be the overall project manager, while the primary user of the phase project plan would the phase project manager. *Resources*—people, equipment, rooms, etc.—would be determined and allocated for the initial overall project design, and for each task in each phase.

Once these project plans have been created, intermediate and end-of-project *goals* can be scheduled within the project plans. *Contingency plans* can be scheduled for *risks* (potential obstacles to the project) that can be anticipated ahead of time. Evaluation steps (also called *gates*) can be scheduled anywhere in the project plan of the project or phase to evaluate the status of the project at that particular time during the project.

In order to save money, to fulfill organizational objectives more quickly, or for other reasons, *project strategies* would be developed. Project strategies could change phases, tasks and the project plans. For example, one project strategy might be, early in the project, to minimize any changes to existing interfacing clinical systems, while in the long run to standardize clinical systems throughout the HMO.

2.5.4.6 Development Step: Automated Systems

Figure 2.9 shows the *development step.* In the development step, automated systems are developed or procured from vendors for implementation in the implementation step. The development step only occurs within a phase and not as part of the initial design.

The development step occurs when a phase involves development of an automated system, purchase of an automated system from a vendor, or a change to an existing automated system. It only occurs as a part of a phase of the project, not in the overall design, as the overall design is for planning of the project rather than creation of products of the project.

User interface requirements for the automated systems together with associated changed employee workflows for the organization are defined in the business reengineering step. System requirements for the automated systems (hardware, application code, databases, interfaces with other automated systems, and other parts of the application) are defined in the system analysis step. Specifications for implementation of business policies carried out within the automated systems are produced within the combination of the business reengineering step and the system analysis step; these business policies are implemented through user interfaces, code and data or databases. Business requirements, how the organization is changed business-wise, is determined in a number of different steps, but primarily in the Business Requirements step. Using this information, automated systems are developed or changed to incorporate these requirements.

Sometimes a choice must be made to determine whether to develop a system within the company or to purchase a system or software package from a vendor—in other words, a decision must be made to "build or buy". If the choice is to buy, then there may be many such systems or software packages—*solution alternative analysis* is a method to choose between these purchased systems or packages.

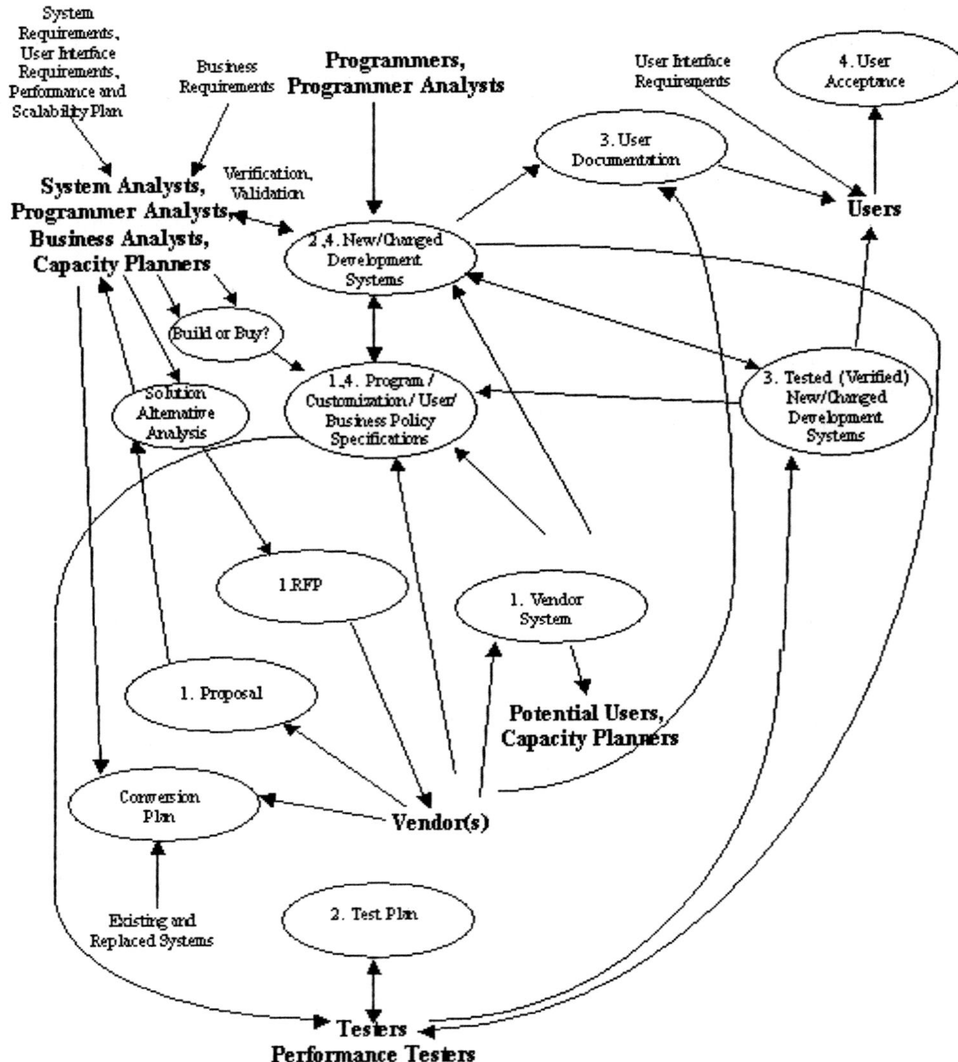

Figure 2.9 Development step: development of automated systems.

If the automated system is developed within the company, then, in the development step, the system, business, and user interface requirements and business policies are used by system analysts and programmer analysts to create *functional and non-functional specifications* for the automated systems, describing programs externally, and *internal design specifications* for the automated system, describing the programs internally. Functional specifications describe individual *functions*—the smallest discrete, complete set of code of an automated system that can be initiated by the user and run to completion to produce a single purpose set of results—while non-functional specifications describe items independent of functions or that apply to multiple functions. These specifications are collectively reviewed by business, management and technical groups and then used to create the code.

If the automated system is to be procured from a vendor, rather than developed within the organization, this process will be somewhat different. The system, business, and user interface requirements and business policies would be used by the systems and business analysts to create a "request for proposal" (RFP) to send to vendors; this would make a request for proposals for systems meeting these requirements. The vendor would write a proposal, including identification of customizations to the system, and send it back to the organization for review.

Based on an evaluation of vendor proposals and the vendor system, analysts, management and other employees may select one of the vendor systems. The evaluation process would probably include management and analysts to evaluate whether the system met business requirements and business policies or could be customized to do so. Potential users would evaluate user interfaces. And capacity planners would evaluate whether or not the vendor system could handle anticipated future network and transaction volumes and could be integrated with other automated systems.

After selection of a vendor system, a contract to use and change the vendor system would be written. The vendor, system analysts and programmer analysts would develop specifications for customization of the vendor product.

In the case of an organizationally developed system, the hardware and system software (including operating systems, databases, and network middleware) is chosen in the system analysis step. In the case of use of a vendor, there are two possibilities: (a) the hardware and system software is determined by what the vendor systems uses; or (b) the hardware and system software is chosen by the organization in the system analysis step and is a requirement put in the RFP.

Organizationally developed application software would be programmed by programmers from the functional, non-functional, and internal design specifications; vendor application software would be customized by the vendor according to agreements with the organization. In either case, the software would then be installed on a *development system*, in other words, an automated system used by the programmers, analysts and testers to develop, modify or test the system rather than one used by the organizational users of the system. The development process usually also requires utility programs to support the programming process and to manage software; examples are compilers and change management programs (where compilers translate programs into a form computers can understand and change management programs keep track of changes in programs).

The development system may be on a single computer or a network of computers, and may, and usually does, include interfaces to development systems for automated systems that would otherwise be outside the scope of the project. These interfaces allow all the development systems to share the same information (rather than creating multiple sets of the same information, which may cause data integrity problems by resulting in systems being out of synchronization with each other).

Additional development systems may be produced to test new ideas or to simulate interfaces with other organizational systems. Such systems may also be on a single computer or a network of computers.

Test plans would be created from the functional, non-functional and internal design specifications, vendor customization specifications, or performance and scalability specifications to test the whole or parts of the development system as it is programmed, installed and integrated. The development system would be tested, resulting in all parts of the system being tested and verified as working correctly. The tested system would be implemented during the implementation step and re-tested during implementation. Testing is also called *validation*.

If errors were found during testing, the program or vendor customization or business policies specifications might have to be updated or the development systems might have to be reprogrammed. In the latter case, the development system would then be re-tested again. This process would continue until the system passed all tests.

During development, the system would also be compared against system, business, user interface, and business policy requirements to determine if these requirements were being fulfilled. This process is called *verification*.

Once the development system passes all tests, it would be available for implementation in the implementation step, where it would be transferred over to a nearly identical hardware and software systems used by the actual organizational users, called *production systems*. Bringing the code to production may involve moving over one or more of the development systems to production, with any remaining production systems remaining the same.

A *conversion plan* may be developed in the development step to be executed in the implementation step. The conversion plan tells how to convert data in existing and replaced production systems to produce the data for the new and changed production system databases.

During the development of an in-house system, capacity planners provide advice on how to create a system that meets performance and scalability requirements. During the procurement of a vendor system, capacity planners provide input to the RFP to identify performance and scalability requirements for the vendor system and to later evaluate vendor systems on how well they meet these requirements. The development system, whether an in-house system or vendor produced system, would be tested to insure that it could handle the required number of system users when it is implemented in production.

2.5.4.7 Implementation Step: Automated Systems and Changed Workflows

Figure 2.10 shows the *implementation step* in which the changes in the organization are implemented. If there are any changed or new automated systems, they are also implemented in this step, moving them from development to production.

Implementation involves installing new or changed automated system(s) developed in the development step, and changing the way workers currently do their jobs according to workflows identified in the business reengineering step. The implementation step could occur without installation of new or changed automated systems, and thus might simply implement new workflows for employees in the organization.

The actual computer systems on which an automated system will eventually be installed must be put in as an early part of implementation, perhaps at the time of the development step. This may involve extensive amounts of money on hardware, rewiring of buildings, or even remodeling or building of buildings. Any hardware selected must be able to handle future capacity and performance requirements.

Based upon the workflow requirements, the organizational working patterns would be changed. These changes could be minor ones, simply automating current manual functions, or could involve "drastic changes" to significantly transform and improve the organization. Drastic changes in the way an organization functions to significantly improve the organization has been termed "business process reengineering" (Champy and Hammer 1993).

Before using a new automated system, workers must be trained in its use and trained in any changes to way their work would be done. The automated system would be physically installed and the workers would use the new automated system in the changed work environment.

As part of installation of an automated system, data in other existing systems and in replaced systems may have to be installed in the automated system's databases, with possible conversion of data from one format to another. This is controlled by the conversion plan created during the development step.

If there is a new automated system replacing an old automated system, then there are several approaches to phasing out the old system and phasing in the new one. Of course, one approach is to just turn off the old one and start the new one. Other approaches would involve running both systems in parallel. See chapter 15 for additional phase out approaches.

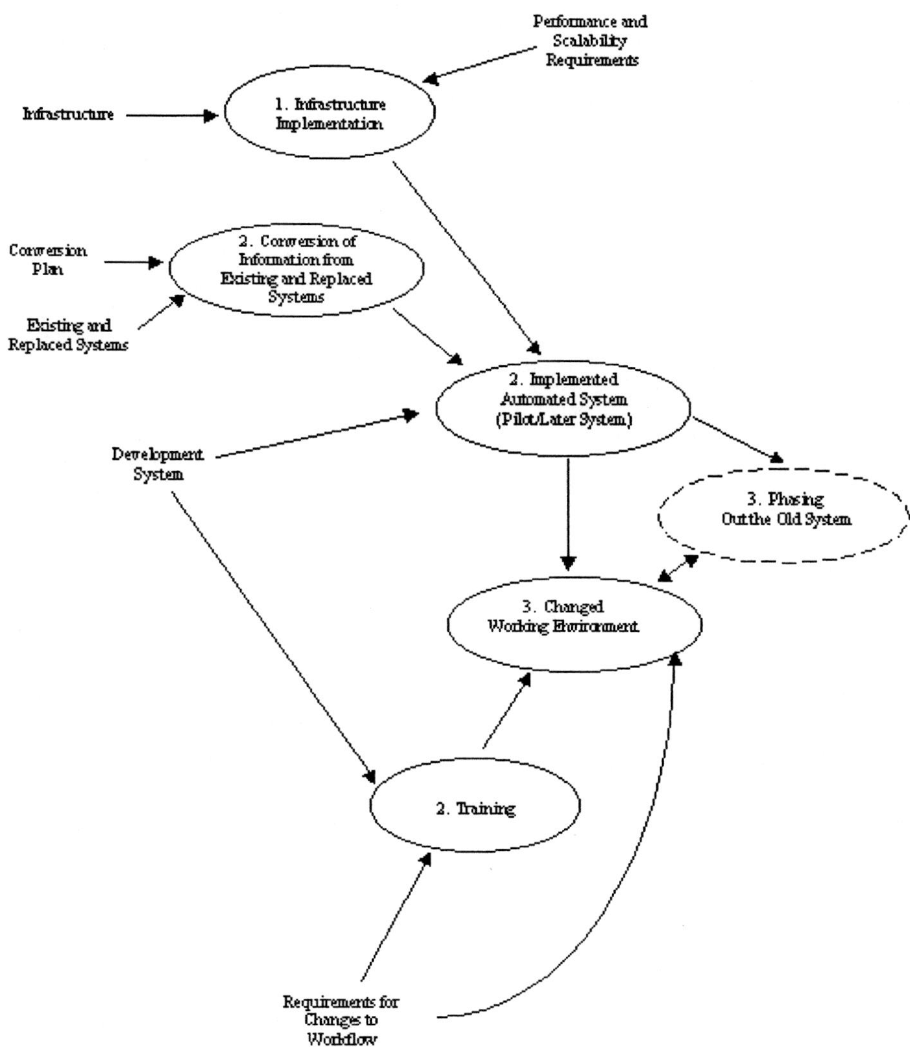

Figure 2.10 Implementation step.

2.6 FLOW OF INFORMATION IN A PROJECT

Figure 2.11 identifies the flow of some of the information during the project.

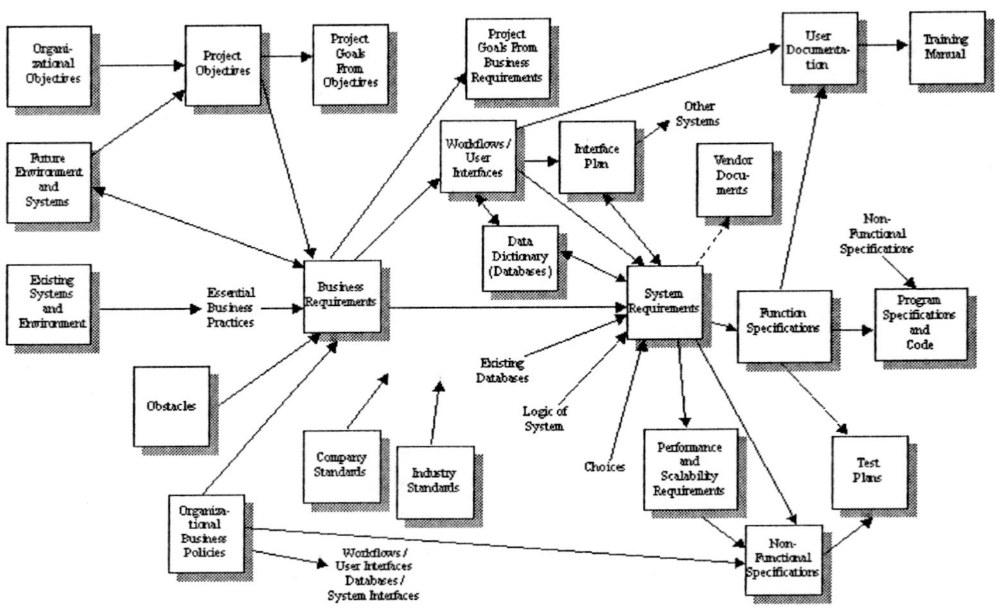

Figure 2.11 Some flows of information during a project.

Project objectives, what the organization hopes to gain from the project, that match *organizational objectives*, are identified; for example, an organizational objective might be to "improve medical care within the HMO" with one corresponding project objective being "to create a complete and always available patient medical record". From these project objectives *business requirements* are derived, where these business requirements are characteristics of the organization after the project that fulfill the project objectives; for example, a corresponding business requirement to the project objective "to create a complete and always available patient medical record" might be "to store each patient's medical record electronically, making the medical record available to caregivers both inside the HMO and within other healthcare organizations".

Goals for the project objectives, ways to measure fulfillment of a project objective or progress toward the project objective, are identified. For example, a goal might be the following: "at the end of the project, HMO members' medical record will be immediately available for at least 99% of the patient visits of HMO members to HMO outpatient clinics as measured by observation of a representative sampling outpatient visits in each HMO facility". Goals can be set up for the end of the project, but also for immediate points in the project.

Additional business requirements are created by identifying *essential business practices* within the current environment and systems that should be preserved, and, at the same time, by identifying *non-essential business practices* that provide little value or that are no longer needed, and thus should be discarded. For example, one essential business practice might be for the HMO to produce required reports to the U.S. Government agency HCFA that identify Medicare patients who have been admitted to the hospital; generation of these reports could be preserved, but with the automated system generating these reports rather than the reports being produced manually. With the inclusion of an automated ordering and results reporting system within the automated patient medical record system, a now unneeded business practice might be the use of couriers to return back clinical test results from the clinical laboratory to the emergency department.

Business requirements are also derived from identified *obstacles* to achieving the changed organization and systems; for example, one obstacle to achieving the changed organization and systems might be "the government mandates certain security requirements for patient information". One business requirement derived from this obstacle might be "to build these government security requirements in the automated patient medical record system".

Organizational *business policies*, sets of rules and procedures for running the organization, are developed by the organization. These business policies may be implemented across many environments and systems. For example, there might be a company business policy to "to have each HMO member pick a primary care physician who would guide patient care for the patient with this primary care physician recorded for the patient in automated systems". Such a policy might be supported by HMO automated systems, including the patient medical record system and many other HMO systems. Such business policies might thus result in additional business requirements for the project, but also changes outside the project, for example, a change to the HMO appointment system to identify members' primary care physicians.

Industry standards—in our case, healthcare standards—and company standards are usually identified in documents for use during the project and use during all other projects. These standards apply to all phases of the project.

When enough business requirements have been developed, a projection of the *future environment and systems* is done. The future environment and systems could be reviewed by upper management to determine if it meets their ideas; as a result of this projection, additional project objectives could be developed, and additional business requirements derived.

Like for a project objective, a business requirement might also have an associated goal to measure progress towards its achievement; for example, for the business requirement to "to reengineer the care process based upon input from physicians" might be the *goal* of "surveying physicians to validate that 95% of them feel they are providing equal or better quality of care than before automation of the patient medical record".

From the business requirements, *workflows* for operations within the organization are established, *user interfaces* for automated systems are determined, and ways the user interfaces mesh with the workflows are identified; a way to associate user interfaces with workflows are called *use cases*. Since user interfaces collect and display data, user interfaces can help determine the data that needs to be stored on *databases*. Additionally, common data within the organization collected within one automated system must be passed to other automated systems via database and network *interfaces* between these systems.

System requirements for the automated systems come from the user interface requirements, the business requirements, the logic of the various automated systems and from discretionary choices. New and changed *automated systems* produced by the project are identified. New *databases* and existing databases to be modified are defined, interfaces with other automated systems are finalized. Requirements for *performance* and *scalability* for the automated systems are identified.

When there are automated systems, it is determined whether to develop each system in-house or to buy it. When an automated system is or may to be bought, then various choices of systems meeting the business and system requirements so far are evaluated doing a solution alternative analysis and generating a *solution alternative analysis* document. The vendors may be asked for information via *Request for Information (RFI)* documents or asked to give presentations of their products. *Requests for Proposals (RFPs)* can be sent to the vendors, with *proposals* being returned by the vendors. The proposals, presentations, and as well as responses to RFIs could be evaluated, again possibly using a solution alternative analysis document. Upon a vendor being chosen and a contract signed, various other vendor documents would ensue.

When an automated system is to be developed in-house, the hardware architecture is determined: hardware, networks and operating systems. *Functional and non-functional specifications* describe the automated system from an external point of view; these specifications are broken up into *functions*, where a function is the smallest discrete, complete set of code of an automated system that can be initiated by the user and run to completion to produce a single purpose set of results. *Internal design specifications* are written to describe the automated system from an internal point of view; program code itself provides additional internal design documentation.

The automated systems—specifically, the software and hardware implementing the systems—are installed in a development system. *Test plans* for each of the programs are created to define how to test each program and how to test the system for performance requirements and scalability; the system is tested using the test plans. Later the automated system is installed in data centers and medical centers. *User documentation* is created to describe how the system and user interface functions. Manuals on how to train the system, *training manuals*, might also be created.

A *requirement* is a required characteristic of the changed organization or of a new or changed automated system resulting from a project. Table 2.1 lists different types of requirements and figure 2.12 shows the relationships between these requirements.

Table 2.1 Project Requirements

Requirement Type	*Description*	*Information Source*	*Characteristics*
Business Requirements	Changes to the business functioning of the organization due to the project.	Upper management, employees, customers, domain experts	Must be consistent and complete; otherwise, missing business requirements will be determined by implication later on by people who should not determine them and/or resulting products will not fit together well.
Business Reengineering Requirements	Employee workflows in the domain of the project, including for any automated systems.	Upper management, employees	Must be consistent with the business requirements.
User Interface Requirements	User interfaces for automated systems, compatible with the workflows.	Employees (in particular automated system users), upper management	Must be useable and consistent with workflows.

Data Base Requirements	Data, data relationships and information needs.	Database analysts (from management, employees and domain experts)	Must both handle all user interfaces and all business requirements.
System Requirements	Hardware and software architecture and overall automated system design, including interfaces to other automated systems.	System architects, domain experts, upper management	Must be reliable, fast, adaptable and integrated, and be appropriate for the user interfaces and system interfaces.
System Functional Requirements	Requirements for each automated system function.	Created by business and system analysts in conjunction with automated system users; used by software developers.	Together with the non-functional requirements, must be consistent with all requirements and produce maintainable code. Must complement the other changes in the organization.
System Non-functional Requirements	Automated system implementation of overall business policies, standards, performance guarantees, and regulations.	Business and system analysts (from upper management, domain experts, system architects, performance analysts); used by software developers.	Together with the functional requirements, must be consistent with all requirements and produce maintainable code. Must complement the functional requirements and all other changes in the organization.
Program Requirements and the Programs	Requirements for each computer program.	Software developers.	Together with the functional and non-functional requirements, must be consistent with all requirements and produce maintainable code. Must complement the other changes in the organization.

As noted in figure 2.12, changing a business requirement after it has been incorporated into automated systems could cost one hundred times as much as making the change in the business analysis step when business requirements are determined.

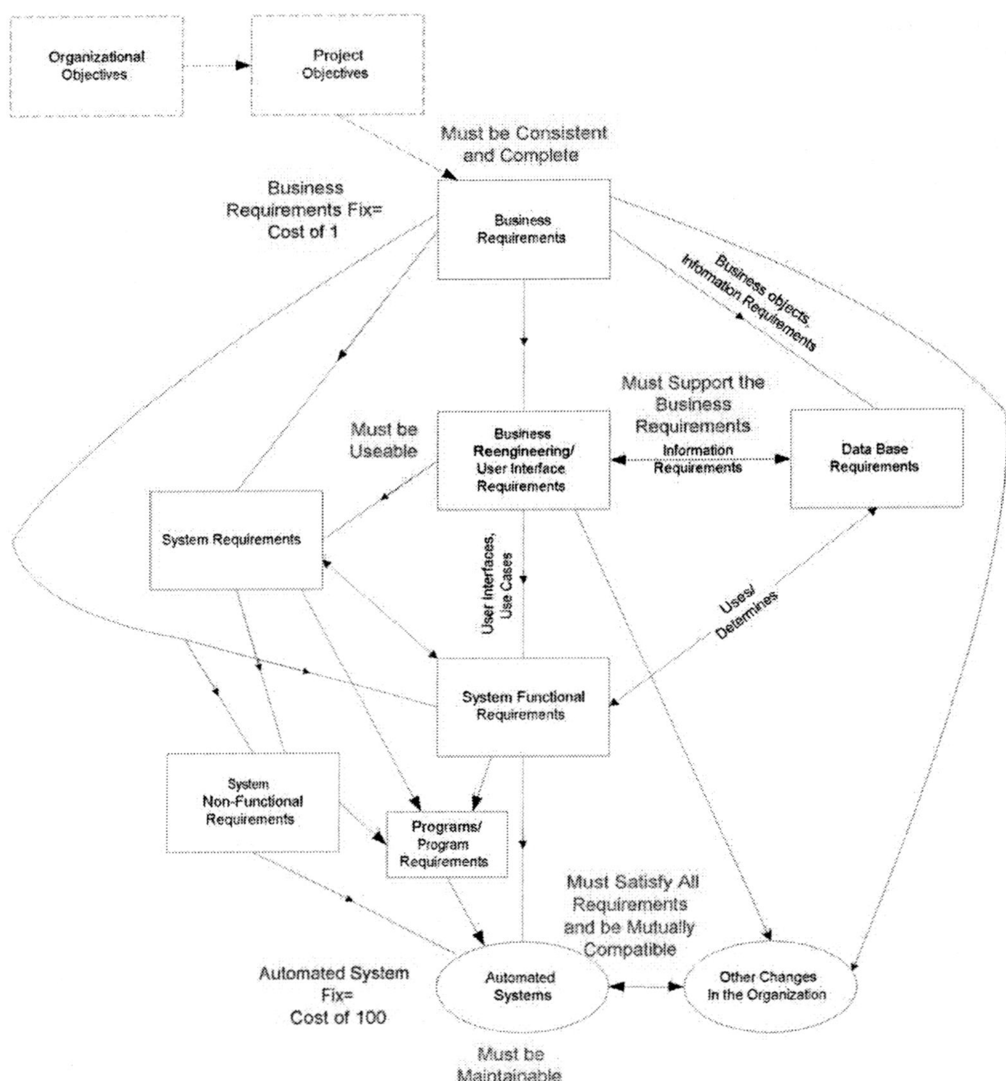

Figure 2.12 Project requirements, their relationships and related products.

Some organizations, especially U.S. government organizations, believe in tracing requirements such as shown in table 2.1 and figure 2.12 from one set of documents to another, including tracing requirements to software code. Requirements tracing is discussed in detail in reference (Jarke 1998). *Requirements traceability* is quite costly and requires significant discipline by those doing the documentation.

Once an automated system is completed, it must be maintained as the system is used. Maintenance involves changing the system for new enhancements and corrections of errors in the system. Keeping and updating all the project documentation after the automated system is implemented is probably not feasible, but it is extremely useful for the maintenance phase to have the following documentation, which is kept up-to-date:

1. **Functional specifications**, describing the external view of the automated system on a function by function basis.
2. **Non-functional specifications**, describing the external view of the automated system for items independent of functions or that apply to multiple functions.
3. **Internal design specifications**, describing the overall internal design of the automated system matching this design with the functional and non-functional specification.
4. **Program code.** Program code should be self-documenting. (Additional documentation on programs is likely to quickly become out-of-date and is usually not useful.)
5. **Data dictionary.** A description of tables, data elements and other items making up the data bases.
6. **Test plans.** Procedures to control testing of the system.
7. **Business policies.** Business policies and the programs, databases, and interfaces implementing the business policies.
8. **User and training manuals.**

2.7 THE ROLES OF PROJECT PARTICIPANTS

During a project to develop a software system, various sets of requirements are developed. Table 2.1 identifies which groups are responsible for developing each of these sets of requirements. It is important that each group stay within its role.

Only employees in the project area and upper management in the organization, are in a position to determine business requirements, business reengineering requirements, and user interface requirements for a project and an organization—such requirements should **not** be determined by software and database designers. However, as bad as it is for software and database designers to determine business, business reengineering, and user requirements, it is equally bad for management and users to determine how a system should be designed or coded, or databases created, as doing so requires specialized capabilities. It is my experience that not following these roles results in non-structured, non-maintainable, or unusable software systems.

On the other hand, software and database designers, as well as system architects, should be facilitators in the identification of business, business reengineering, and user interface requirements, as they need to thoroughly understand these requirements and to insure that inconsistencies in requirements and missing requirements are resolved. They need this deep understanding of the requirements to be able to produce a logical and integrated software and database design that fulfills these requirements.

Viewing employees, upper management, and the organization as "customers" of the "technical community"—of the software and database designers and system architects, who develop software and hardware systems—the IEEE (Institute for Electrical and Electronic Engineers) (IEEE 1998) developed a diagram to explain the interaction between these two groups in the development of requirements for an automated system. See figure 2.13 that was adapted from the IEEE diagram.

What should be developed are *well-formed requirements*, "a statement of system functionality (a capability) that can be validated, that must be met or possessed by a system to solve a customer problem or to achieve a customer objective, and that is qualified by measurable conditions and bounded by constraints (IEEE 1998)." In general, well-formed requirements have the following desirable characteristics: simplicity, clarity, completeness, and consistency. Well-formed requirements are developed by management and employees who will use the system or information from the system, and technical personnel who will define or create the system, working together with content and process facilitators.

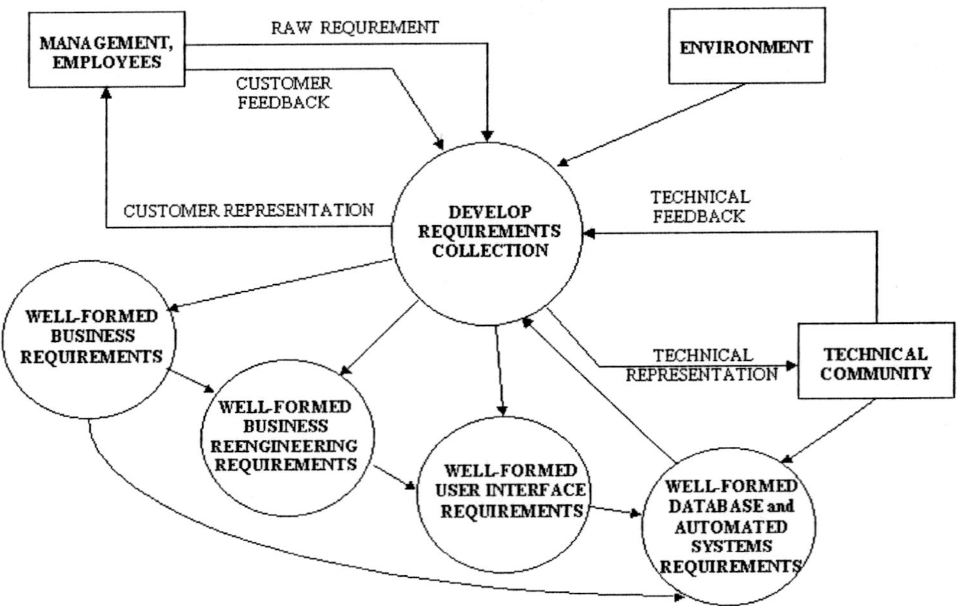

Figure 2.13 Well-formed requirements.

Projects are most effectively done by people of different professional skills working together, sharing and coordinating their differing ideas to produce the products of the project. The group dynamics of an effective project development group is vastly different from the group dynamics of a typical healthcare team: the former has to be democratic to be effective, while healthcare teams are usually controlled from the top. For a project to be done well, the project must encourage this free flow of ideas. "We find comfort among those who agree with us; we find growth among those who don't" (Nemko)—encourage this growth so the best possible agreements can be made.

2.8 CONTROLLING CHANGES

Once major decisions have been made during the project, they should be recorded and put under change control (Whitten 1995). The *change control process* is a formal process where changes are made to *controlled documents* with the agreement of members of a designated *change control board.*

During each step of the project, participants in the step are recording agreements. During this time, the final results of the step remain in flux and may change. But at the end of a project step, these final agreements need to be recorded comprehensively and understandably, with a sign off by all the participants so these results can be used in later steps. For example, if technical requirements for a new automated system are being determined during the system analysis step based upon a set of business and user interface requirements in previous steps, then any later change in these business or user interface requirements would also effect the technical requirements. It is difficult for participants in a step to do their jobs if the results they depend upon change after the participants have already made decisions based upon these results. Thus documentation of the final decisions in a project step should be recorded at the end of a step and placed under change control.

The change control board generally approves or disapproves a change in the project at a high, non-detailed, level. Once the change is approved, it is analyzed by project groups and defined in more detail, with determination of which controlled documents to update.

Within a project group, a walkthrough may be held to review the change for inclusion in the controlled documents. A *walkthrough* is thus a meeting where controlled documents are reviewed in detail.

Controlled documents within a project may include one or more of the following documents:

- organizational objectives, strategies, goals, and priorities of objectives
- project objectives, strategies, goals, constraints, and priorities of objectives
- business requirements and goals
- user workflow requirements
- user interface style guide
- user interface requirements
- system requirements
- organizational business policies
- data dictionary
- interface plan
- programming standards
- functional specifications
- non-functional specifications
- internal design specifications
- program code
- test plans
- performance and scalability requirements
- user documentation, including description of user interfaces
- training manuals.

Suggested changes to systems, both during the project and after project completion, can come from many sources, including from users and upper management. Changes are often prioritized by the change control board or by user groups so the most important ones are done first.

A *help desk* may be set up for the automated systems in a project that consists of designated telephone numbers to which users can call to seek advice and to report errors in the systems.

Errors in systems differ from changes. Errors are identified by differences between the way the system works and the way the program specification, vendor customization specification, project business policies specification, or performance and scalability specification describes the system to work. Changes, on the other hand, are changes to any of these specifications and the corresponding changes to programs. Like for changes, errors are also usually prioritized and are fixed accordingly—but errors are usually given much higher priority than changes. The controlled documents thus have the important purpose of distinguishing errors from changes.

Another form of control of the project is only implementing changes and error corrections to automated systems on a pre-scheduled basis and keeping previous *versions* of the software and other controlled documents. This is referred to as a *release process*, with controlled documents being under release control. If there is a problem in a *release*, the release can be backed out, returning to the previous *version*.

2.9 MEASURING THE SUCCESS OF THE PROJECT

When a project reaches completion, it is deemed successful if all of the following are true (Pinto and Sleven 1988):

The project

- achieves basically all the objectives originally set for it
- is accepted and used by the audience for whom the project was intended
- comes in on-schedule
- comes in on-budget.

The latter two are related to two normal *constraints* on projects that are usually determined by upper management at the beginning of the project: allocated **time** to do the project and the allocated **money** to do the project. To determine whether the project was on-schedule and on-budget these two constraints are compared against the actual time to do the project and the actual cost of the project.

Whether or not *project objectives* have been achieved can be determined by *goals* set up at the start of the project to measure these project objectives at the end of the project. For example, for a project objective to increase member satisfaction with patient care, the goal might be that there be a 15 percent increase in the number of HMO patients who are highly satisfied with patient care after the project is complete as compare with those at the start of the project. Determining whether the project was responsible for the change may be harder to determine.

Surveying and observing users at the end of the project can determine whether or not the project is accepted and used by its intended audience. If the intended users avoid or work around the system, this is an indication of non-acceptance of the system. However, sometimes users are slow to accept major changes, and this determination may have to be deferred until some time after the project is complete.

2.10 THE IMPORTANCE OF INFRASTRUCTURE

It is a human tendency to want quick results. A project should be considered as building for the future, not building for quick results. To build for the future—to build something that lasts—it is important to build the infrastructure first. This takes time, and it takes management realization that something very useful is happening when the infrastructure is being built, despite there appearing to be no useful results out of the project.

Infrastructure is everything in the project that is hidden. There are two types of infrastructure associated with a project: (1) infrastructure for the project itself and (2) infrastructure for the products of the project.

Examples of infrastructure within a project are (1) the hiring or selection of the right people to do the project, (2) the meetings and hard work to design and implement the products of the project, (3) the necessary documentation and the control of this documentation, (4) the computer systems on which systems are developed (4) the training of personnel, (5) change management of software and databases, etc. If money is not spent on project infrastructure, then the quality of resulting products is likely to be much less.

Examples of the infrastructure for the products of a project (e.g., the automated patient medical record system) are (1) the people and facilities to support the product such as help desks and technical personnel, (2) the changes to buildings, including changes to wiring, (3) the training of employees in new workflows or in the use of new automated systems; etc. If money is not spent on the infrastructure for an automated system, then, when the automated system goes down, there are likely to be long periods where no work gets done or where data has a chance of being lost or corrupted. Putting in the infrastructure after the product is implemented almost always costs significantly more money.

Often the infrastructure created for the project can become part of the infrastructure for the products of the project (e.g., controlled documentation and development systems are still needed once the product is implemented; change management of software and databases is still needed).

It is important for management to realize several things about infrastructure:

1. Setting up infrastructure costs lots of money without any apparent results.
2. Without properly setting up the infrastructure for a product of the project, the product will likely eventually function poorly, or even fail.

2.11 SUMMARY

The basic parts of the project approach presented in this chapter are as follows:

- **Identify a potential project:** Identify a potential project and establish a project mission statement.
- **Describe the organization prior to the project:** Describe the current environment and systems with respect to the project.
- **Identify how the organization will benefit from the project:** Determine project objectives based upon organizational objectives.
- **What should the project NOT change?** Identify current business practices to be preserved.
- **How would the organization function after the project?** Describe the changed (i.e., the future) environment and systems.
- **What must be done to make these changes to the organization?** Identify business requirements for the project to achieve the future environment and systems that satisfy the project objectives.

- **What could stop the project from succeeding?** Identify obstacles and how to overcome them (which may add additional business requirements).
- **Is the project worth doing?** Evaluate the project in comparison to other projects in the organization; determine which ones to do (if any) and which ones to change or terminate (if any).
- **How do you measure whether the project is successful?** Identify goals used to measure whether project objectives and business requirements are being achieved or have been achieved.
- **How will employees be working differently after the project?** Determine workflows for the future environment and determine user interfaces or requirements for user interfaces for new and changed automated systems.
- **Describe any new or changed automated systems:** Determine the design of new and changed automated systems.
- **Develop a project plan for the project and any phases (sub-projects) within the project:** Develop a project plan, including estimates of costs. For a large complex project, break the project into phases such that implementation of the phases will accomplish the total project, with consideration that there may have to be, at any point, possible redesign of the project or of previous phases or possible addition of phases to accomplish the overall project. Break phases into tasks. As a result of a phase or phases, intermediate products may be produced, with the final product being the final results of the project. (Infrastructure for the project should be done in the earlier stages of the project.)
- **Develop or procure automated systems, if any:** Develop automated systems in-house or procure them from outside vendors.
- **Make the changes to the organization and implement the products of the project, such as automated systems:** Implement the changed environment and the new and changed automated systems. Do infrastructure first.
- **Monitor and maintain the changes.**

Key Terms

adaptable
business analysis
business analyst
business policies
business reengineering
business requirements
change control
code
content facilitator
contingency plan
controlled documents
database
database analyst
development
development system
domain analyst
domain expert
evaluation
facilitation
feasibility study
goal
implementation
infrastructure
integrated
interface
maintenance
organizational objective
overall design
performance
personal physician
phase
primary care physician
process facilitator
product
production system
project manager
project objective
project plan
requirement
requirements traceability
risk
scalable
solution alternative analysis
standards analyst
strategies
system analysis
system analyst
technical staff
upper management
validation
verification
well-formed requirement
workflow

Study Questions

1. What is the purpose of a project?
2. Why must project objectives support organizational objectives?
3. What does integrated mean? Adaptable mean? If a system is scalable, which of these attributes does it support?
4. If you were upper management, why would you select one project over another?
5. What is the usefulness of doing an initial overall design in a project and later overall redesigns during the project? Why should upper management be included?
6. Why is it important to have a mix of different types of people doing a project? What is (process) facilitation and why is it necessary in a large-scale project?
7. What are the purposes of the Business analysis step? Evaluation step? Business reengineering step? System analysis step? Project plan step? Development step? Implementation step? Maintenance?
8. Why is it important to do infrastructure first for a project?

CHAPTER 3

A Project to Automate the Patient Medical Record in an HMO

CHAPTER OUTLINE

3.1 PROJECT CONTEXT: IDENTIFYING A PROJECT

The management of an organization cares about projects in so far as how they benefit the organization, advancing organizational objectives. For example, for a healthcare organization, these organizational objectives might be to provide quality medical care for its patients at an affordable cost, to follow healthcare industry and government standards and regulations, and to increase healthcare employee and member satisfaction with the healthcare organization.

Potential projects are developed by looking at the way the organization currently functions and determining changes in the way it functions that would promote the organizational objectives (see figure 3.1). For example, within the healthcare organization, it might have been observed that paper medical records are often unavailable or incomplete, adversely impacting patient care.

It seems clear that a project to "automate the patient medical record" would promote the organizational objective of improvement of patient care by providing a complete and always-available patient medical record within the healthcare organization.

A potential project is identified by stating a *project mission*. A *project mission* is a summary of the change to the organization expected to be produced by the project. The mission of the project in this book is to "improve patient care in the HMO through automation of the patient medical record".

In general, when a project mission is stated, it should not include a solution. A *solution* is one of many different alternative ways of accomplishing all or part of a change. As Tom Gilb states in the book *Principles of Software Engineering Management*, "Solutions are never holy; they can and should be changed in the light of new requirements, conflicts with other solutions, or negative practical experience with them" (Gilb 1988). For example, a less solutions-based project mission might be to "improve patient care by creating a complete, always-available patient medical record within the healthcare organization", which might allow for some interim, non-automated solutions

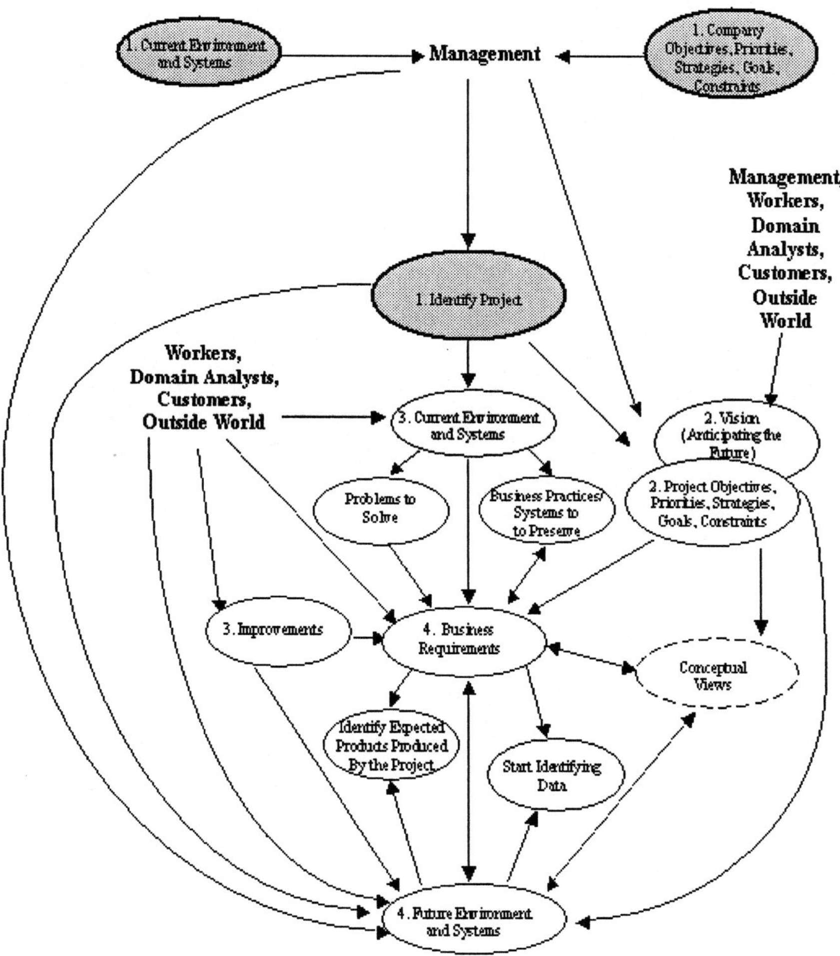

Figure 3.1 Business analysis: project mission.

However, in this case, management considers that the solution "automation the patient medical record" to be an integral part of having a complete, always-available medical record, and they also foresee that automation of the patient medical record could provide other benefits that improve patient care, including electronic ordering and checking for medication errors.

In this book, the healthcare organization in which the patient medical record is to be automated is a large HMO, which has many hospitals and medical office buildings throughout the nation. The HMO is administered both from a single national location and at various regional locations. Upper management are management physicians who administer the HMO.

Key Terms

project mission

solution

Study Questions

1. What is a project mission?

2. Why should the project mission statement normally not identify a solution?

CHAPTER 4

Patient Care Using Paper Medical Records

CHAPTER OUTLINE

4.1 PROJECT CONTEXT: THE CURRENT ENVIRONMENT

The purpose of doing a project is to make beneficial changes to the organization. In order to identify changes that are beneficial, it is first essential to study the current environment with respect to the project.

This purpose of studying the current environment in an organization is to do all of the following:

- To gain an understanding of the organization with respect to the project area
- To clarify problems that the project can resolve
- To identify other alternative, and perhaps more appropriate, projects which can improve the organization and also fix these problems

- To determine essential business practices and automated systems that should be preserved by the project
- To provide a baseline against which the changed organization could later be compared.

4.2 PLAYERS IN PATIENT CARE

The people who receive care in an HMO fall into the following non-exclusive categories:

- *HMO member*: a person who pays a capitation fee—a fixed periodic payment—to the HMO or whose family or employer pays such a fee for the person so the person can receive comprehensive health care from the HMO
- *non-HMO member*: a person who is not a member of the HMO
- *patient*: a person who seeks or comes in for care
- *inpatient*: a patient who receives care in a hospital
- *outpatient*: a patient who receives care outside the hospitals.

The people that provide patient care in an HMO fall into the following categories:

- *outpatient physician*: a physician in the outpatient setting
- *hospitalist/inpatient physician*: a physician in a hospital
- *outpatient nurse*: a nurse in the outpatient setting
- *medical assistant*: a healthcare professional who performs a variety of clinical, clerical and administrative duties within a healthcare setting
- *emergency department (ED) triage nurse*: a nurse who assesses patients' medical problems in the emergency department to determine urgency and priority of care to determine which patient is to be seen next
- *nurse practitioner*: a registered nurse who has completed an advanced training program in primary health care delivery, and may provide primary care for non-emergency patients, usually in an outpatient or community setting
- *physician assistant*: a practitioner trained in aspects of the practice of medicine who works with or under the supervision of a physician to provide diagnostic and therapeutic care
- *inpatient nurse*: a nurse in the hospital
- *unit assistant*: a healthcare professional who performs a variety of clinical, clerical and administrative duties within a unit, or section, of the hospital
- *ED physician*: a physician in the emergency department
- *ED nurse*: a nurse in the emergency department
- *advice nurse*: a nurse who takes patient phone calls and advises the patient on medical conditions according to protocol; the advice nurse informs the patient when self-care is appropriate and when a patient needs to come in and when the patient does not
- *appointment clerk*: a person who takes member phone calls and who may schedule an appointment
- *case manager*: a person specifically assigned to oversee the case management of a member of the healthcare organization, where case management is an organized system

for delivering health care, which includes assessment and development of a plan of care, coordination of services, referrals and follow-ups

- *clinical social worker*: a social worker in the clinical care setting who meets with a patient to provide assistance and advice on care, follow-up care, resources, and caregivers
- *allied health professional*: A person who has received special training in care of a patient or in a supporting activity other than a physician (e.g., training in emergency medical services, respiratory therapy, occupational therapy, home healthcare, clinical laboratory science).
- *health care services representative/ombudsman*: an ombudsman who an HMO member could call to resolve problems, to learn more about how the HMO functions and to learn more about the benefits provided to the member
- *quality manager*: a healthcare professional who evaluates the quality of healthcare in the healthcare organization, who is responsible for the generation of reports for accreditation and government agencies
- *medical researcher*: a healthcare professional who does clinical research such as research into new medications, procedures or best practices for the treatment of various medical conditions
- *ancillary services personnel*: personnel providing support services other than room, board, medical or nursing services to patients, including the following: clinical laboratory, x-ray, physical therapy, injection clinic, pharmacy, optical sales and hearing center
- *medical transcriptionist*: Medical language specialist who transcribes dictation by physicians and other healthcare professionals in order to document patient care.

The people who provide patient care have various types of degrees, licenses and certifications, including the following:

- *doctor of medicine (MD):* A healthcare practitioner who has completed a doctorate degree in medicine and who has a license within a state to practice medicine as a physician
- *board certified specialist*: A physician, nurse, or other healthcare professional who has advanced education and training in a specialty area such as internal medicine, surgery, ophthalmology, etc., each specialty with a qualifying organization which offers qualifying examinations to become "board certified"
- *registered nurse (RN)*: In the U.S., a person who completed a prescribed course of study from an approved nursing education program and who has passed the National Council Licensure Examination for Registered Nurses (NCLEX-RN) exam
- *nurse practitioner (NP):* A registered nurse who has completed an advanced training program in primary health care delivery, and may provide primary care for non-emergency patients, usually in an outpatient or community setting
- *licensed practical nurse (LPN)*: A nurse who is licensed by a state board of nursing after completing an education program and passing the licensure exam who practices under the supervision of a registered nurse.

4.3 PATIENT CARE WORKFLOWS

The following describes the activities of people who provide care within an HMO.

In general, there are no orientation sessions for new members in most HMOs. Usually, a member's first encounter with the HMO is when the patient has a medical problem where the member needs to see an outpatient physician; thus, we begin with a description of outpatient care in an HMO.

4.3.1 Outpatient Care in an HMO

When a member is sick, the patient or a relative telephones to make an appointment or to talk to an advice nurse. The advice nurse gives advice to the patient on self-care and on whether and when the patient should come in, and also makes appointments.

An appointment is made either with a physician, nurse practitioner or physician assistant, with a first appointment for a problem usually being in a primary care department. *Primary care* is a department which would be the first point of contact in the HMO for a given episode of illness. Primary care departments are medicine or family practice for adults, pediatrics or family practice for children, and in some HMOs, gynecology/obstetrics for women. The member is appointed to the HMO facility most conveniently located for the patient.

Based upon HMO and facility protocols, members can choose a primary care physician in medicine, pediatrics or family practice to guide the member's care, also called a "personal physician". Women can also choose a gynecology physician. A member may choose to have a nurse practitioner or physician assistant instead, or decide that he does not want an assigned healthcare provider.

Upon seeing the patient, the primary care physician may refer the patient to a specialist (e.g., dermatologist, urologist, gynecologist, ophthalmologist, etc.) When a primary care physician determines whether the patient sees a specialist, the primary care physician is said to have the role of a "gatekeeper". (Advice nurses, by protocol, can sometimes book the patient directly with a specialty area physician or nurse practitioner, bypassing the gatekeeping process.)

Urgent care clinics may exist in the HMO for seeing the patient after normal business hours for non-emergency situations.

In general, member visits require appointments, with the visits pre-scheduled through a scheduling system that produces daily schedules for the physicians, nurse practitioners, and physician assistants. Although most urgent care clinics also require appointments, they also have a lot of "drop-in" patients, patients who come in without an appointment. For minor problems in the outpatient setting, the patient may see a registered nurse rather than a physician, nurse practitioner or physician assistant.

For same day and next day appointments, the patient's outpatient medical record is ordered at the time of the appointment. For future appointments, the medical record is only ordered by the appointment system the day before; this allows the patient to make an appointment for an earlier date and have the chart available for that appointment. The advice nurse doesn't have a patient medical record (i.e., chart) available to her in the current environment.

During the patient visit, the physician, nurse practitioner, physician assistant and clinic nurses may add information to the patient chart or produce documentation that is later added to the chart. The clinician orders diagnostic tests (e.g., clinical lab tests, x-rays, etc.), but generally does not get the results until the next day; the patient often goes to another location to have a specimen collected (e.g., a blood test, a urine specimen). The clinician also orders medication that the patient later picks up from the pharmacy. An order is on paper with a copy being put in the patient's chart.

An outpatient physician may also provide care for the patient when the patient is not in the medical facility. For example,

- informing the patient of diagnostic test results over the telephone
- approving or disapproving phone-in medication refill requests
- providing consultation advice for a patient after the patient seeks advice from an advice nurse or talks to the physician's nurse.

In these three cases, the physician most often orders the patient's chart. This may require the physician to have to wait up to half a day, or longer if the patient has an appointment with another physician at that time the chart is ordered.

Patients who "drop in", without an appointment, may or may not be seen on the same day. Patients who "drop in" may go through a triage process (for example, run by a registered nurse) to determine if a patient should be seen immediately, should wait to be seen, should go directly to the emergency department, should schedule an appointment for later, or could administer self-care. For drop-in patients, the chart may be ordered; a visit may sometimes occur without the chart.

4.3.2 Care in the Emergency Department in the HMO

When a patient is faced with an emergency medical problem, he may come into the emergency department on his own or with the assistance of his friends or family. This may happen after receiving advice from an advice nurse or from a physician in urgent care who advises the patient to go the emergency department. Patients may also come in via ambulance to the emergency department.

All "walk-in patients" go through a triage process, controlled by a triage nurse. The patient is assessed. The triage nurse creates a list of patients by what time they came in and by urgency of the medical problem and assigns them to available rooms accordingly.

Patient charts within the facility are ordered from the chart room. If the charts are in an outpatient physician's office, they may be retrieved from there.

Generally, before a patient is given care, an extensive interview is conducted and an examination is given, recording all relevant health information for the patient on paper, on a history and physical (H&P) form. The H & P may be started by the triage nurse and continued after the patient is assigned to a room.

Care is then given to the patient. Orders for clinical laboratory tests, diagnostic imaging, or other diagnostic tests are made by a physician or nurse under the supervision of a physician; the patient is usually not discharged until the results come back. Orders for medications are made. The patient is stabilized or procedures are initiated.

The patient is eventually discharged to home, to a hospital, or to an outside medical facility. The patient is given a written set of instructions and follow-up appointments are usually made.

Orders, again, are all on paper. They are included in the patient's chart, either immediately or later.

The *emergency department census* identifies the rooms and names of all patients currently in examination rooms in the emergency department. The emergency department census is generally kept on a board and is updated when a new patient is put in a room, when a patient is discharged and the bed is dirty, or when a bed has been cleaned.

4.3.3 Inpatient Care in the HMO

Most often patients either enter the hospital as a walk-in with a pre-scheduled admission (called a pre-admission) or through the emergency department.

The patient goes through an admission process. This use to be done in the admissions office prior to the patient going into the hospital, but is occurring more and more often in the hospital room. A pre-admission would normally be accomplished ahead of the hospital stay during an outpatient visit. Admission and pre-admission is automated with pre-admission information carried over to the admission.

After the patient is moved to a bed in a room in a unit of the hospital (e.g., a medical-surgery unit), the patient is added to the unit census. On admission or pre-admission, the patient is assigned with an admitting physician and attending physician. The patient's chosen primary care physician may also be involved or, alternatively, a hospitalist may be assigned, a physician who is a specialist in in-patient medicine, who takes over responsibility for the patient's care from the patient's personal care provider during the patient's hospital stay.

Nurses are assigned with patients with consideration of acuity (severity) of the patients' medical conditions. Upon a nursing shift change, other nurses are assigned.

Copies of the complete patient chart are ordered from various places, including outpatient charts. An inpatient chart for the inpatient stay is created. A summary document is created for the inpatient stay from existing chart documents, that includes physician diagnoses, nursing diagnoses, physician orders, etc., that, because it is a summary of information in the chart, is not saved in the chart; often this a trade-name document called the "Kardex".

Nurses create extensive documentation during the inpatient stay that is saved in the inpatient chart. The next section describes many of these documents. Physician documentation and orders are also put in the inpatient chart.

Usually, all patient outpatient medications are taken away and medication administration is highly controlled during the hospital stay. Medications the physician orders are recorded on a medication administration record (MAR), which the nurse uses to identify and record the administration of these medications; often the outpatient medications are reordered and also recorded on the MAR. Medications from the pharmacy for the unit are put on a cart, with the cart being sent to the unit at specified times.

Significant documentation also occurs on discharge, with ordering of medications for the patient when he is discharged and becomes an outpatient; these discharge medications become outpatient medications. The patient is discharged to home or to another medical facility. Outpatient appointments may be scheduled on discharge.

An important document to control inpatient workflow that is not a part of the patient medical record is the inpatient *unit census*, identifying the names and rooms of all patients in the unit, where a unit is a section of the hospital reserved for a particular purpose (e.g., the intensive care unit or ICU). The unit census is generally kept on a board and is updated when a new patient is put in a room, when a patient has been identified to be discharged, or when a patient is actually discharged.

In the emergency department and then the hospital, information of particular importance are *allergies and adverse reactions to medications*, and *advance directives*. Advance directives are written instructions a patient has prepared for medical personnel to inform them of the patient's wishes for treatments and care when the patient is incapacitated, especially regarding life-sustaining treatment if the patient's condition becomes irreversible. If the patient is unconscious or otherwise incapacitated, this information may not be available unless recorded in local charts.

4.4 PAPER MEDICAL RECORD DOCUMENTS

4.4.1 Types of documents

The paper patient chart includes the following parts:

- patient identifier and patient demographics information
- patient clinical data
- patient financial data.

The non-financial portions of the chart will be described.

4.4.1.1 Patient Identifier

A patient identifier is required to select a patient of interest to a caregiver. Currently this patient identifier is most often differs in format and content for each healthcare organization.

Through HIPAA (The Health Insurance Portability and Accountability Act of 1996 for Medicare and Medicaid programs) the U.S. Government enacted into law the requirement for established standards for health-related commerce that was to be implemented by the year 2000. This legislation mandates a standard healthcare identifier for each individual, employer, health plan, and health care provider in the U.S. Although this identifier is for financial transactions, there is the potential of a future patient identifier that could be used in patient medical records across healthcare organizations. The mandate for a standard patient identifier has been indefinitely deferred.

4.4.1.2 Patient Demographics

Patient demographics is information that identifies, locates, or describes a patient. Typical *patient demographics* information is the following:

- name
- addresses
- phone numbers
- sex
- date of birth
- emergency contact information
- race(s) (which is important in some medical decisions)
- religion
- source of payment.

The following additional information may be important in providing care to the patient and might be included along with patient demographics:

- contact information for spouse, parent, person with Durable Power of Attorney for Healthcare or guardian

- for a minor, (1) who is legally able to consent to a child's care, and (2) any special legal constraints, such as a parent who is not allowed to consent to care, who is not allowed to pick up a child from the clinic, or who is not allowed to have access to the child's medical information (Richards and Rathbun 1999)
- advance directives.

Advance directives are written instructions a patient has prepared for medical personnel to inform them of the patient's wishes for treatments and care when the patient is incapacitated, especially regarding life-sustaining treatment if the patient's condition becomes irreversible. An advance directive is a legal document prepared when the individual is competent and able to make decisions.

Of particular importance in California, Texas, and other states bordering Mexico is the following information:

- language preference
- indication of whether or not an interpreter is required.

Some additional demographics information of lesser medical and financial importance is the following:

- marital status
- occupation
- ethnicity
- education
- employment.

4.4.1.3 Patient Clinical Information

Clinical information in the current paper chart consists of documents of varying types. These documents are likely to vary from organization to organization or even from facility to facility in an organization.

What is presented here are documents found in the current paper charts of a large number of healthcare organizations and is assumed for our HMO. Also presented are basic descriptions of the care processes during which this clinical information is created.

Outpatient Clinical Information The typical outpatient chart includes some or all of the documents listed in table 4.1 (Loeb 1992).

Table 4.1 Outpatient Clinical Documents

Document	*Description*
History and Physical	The patient's initial medical examination and evaluation data. This document includes the following: chief complaint (CC), history of present illness (HPI), past medical history (PMH), family history (FH), social history (SH) and marital history, review of systems (ROS), physical exam (PE), assessment, diagnosis (Dx), impression, rule out (R/O), plan, prognosis (Px).

Progress Notes	Documentation for a follow-up visit. The physician's objective findings concerning improvement or aggravation of the condition, any change in treatment or medication, and the patient's own report about the condition.
Physician's Orders	A record of a physician's medical orders.
X-rays, other diagnostic images, EKGs, etc.	
Diagnostic findings	Diagnostic and laboratory data—for example, hematology, pathology, radiology, and X-ray test results and transcriptions.
Correspondence / E-mail	Letters and E-mail conveying clinical information on the patient.
Phone messages	Phone messages conveying clinical information on the patient.
Consent forms	A patient's or patient's guardian's consent for treatment, special procedures or to release information.
Consultation reports	An opinion about the patient's condition by a practitioner other than the primary care physician.

A patient calls in for an appointment or an appointment was made after a previous visit. The patient comes in at the time of the appointment; alternatively, a patient "walks in" and may be seen.

Either after the patient is escorted to a room or just prior, a nurse takes the patient's vital signs and puts this information either on the physical examination part of the *history and physical* form or on a separate *vital sign record*. If not already in the examination room, the patient is escorted to the room.

Figure 4.1 identifies a classical data collection and interpretation strategy known as the *hypothetico-deductive approach* (Shortliffe and Barnett 2001), followed by many physicians and nurse practitioners within the examination room (and which is applicable both for the outpatient and inpatient setting).

This physician or nurse practitioner records examination information on *history and physical (H&P), progress notes* and associated documents referred to as SOAP notes, standing for Subjective, Objective, Assessment and Plan. As a first step in this process, the patient's identity (ID) is verified and the *chief complaint (CC)* is recorded (Becklin and Sunnarborg 1994). Information given by the patient is recorded under the heading *subjective*. A *history of present illness (HPI)* is recorded that would include the following: (1) the symptoms that are troubling the patient, (2) when the symptoms first occurred, (3) the patient's opinions as to the cause of the illness, (4) remedies the patient may have tried, including any medication treatment. From this information the caregiver forms some initial hypotheses on the diagnosis; the set of active hypotheses are referred to as the *differential diagnosis*, a set of possible diagnoses.

The caregiver asks further questions of the patient, including information about *past medical history (PMH)*, past illnesses and treatments administered, past operations, accidents, injuries, congenital problems and allergies; *family history (FH)*, health information about other family members, especially genetic disorders; and *social history (SH)* if applicable, information related to the patient's eating, drinking, smoking habits and occupation. The caregiver then reviews each body system with the patient (e.g., respiratory system) and records it as a *review of systems (ROS)*.

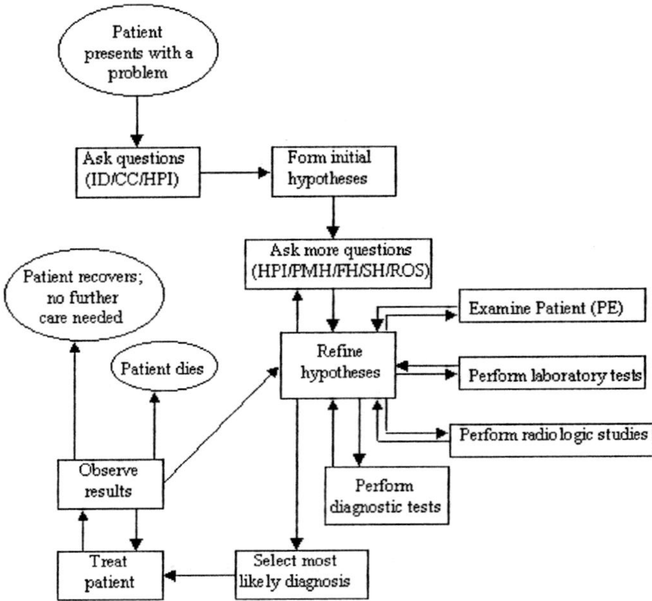

Figure 4.1 A model for patient care (Shortliffe and Barnett 2001).

In order to refine the hypotheses on the diagnosis, the caregiver exams the patient and may order diagnostic tests. The caregiver's examination of the patient is recorded under the heading *objective*. Previously recorded vital signs might be included in this section. Results of the examination are recorded under the heading *physical exam (PE)*, with findings usually separated out by each body area; the physical exam may later include laboratory, X-ray and other diagnostic results that come back on *medical reports* for various *diagnostic findings*, laboratory reports, X-ray reports, etc.

From the subjective and objective findings, including diagnostic test results, the caregiver makes a best determination of *diagnosis (Dx)*, the name of the condition from which the patient is suffering, which is recorded under the heading *assessment*.

The *plan* or treatment section lists a treatment for the patient, which may include the following:

- medications and dosages
- instructions given to patients
- any recommendations for hospitalization or surgery
- any special tests that need to be performed.

The caregiver's *prognosis (Px)*, the caregiver's opinion of what the outcome of the illness will be (e.g., "fair", "good", "poor" or "guarded").

In reality, this data collection and interpretation process for outpatients usually extends beyond the single outpatient visit. The physician or nurse practitioner orders but does not wait for diagnostic test results before forming a preliminary diagnosis. Treatment is determined on this preliminary diagnosis, usually involving a medication program. When the caregiver receives back the diagnostic test results, the caregiver determines whether or not to modify the diagnosis. If the diagnosis needs to be modified, the patient may be called by the physician, the nurse practitioner or his nurse with modified treatment instructions, or the patient may be called to arrange a return visit.

During this process, the caregiver may request an evaluation of the patient from clinical specialists for additional diagnoses and treatment recommendations. This may result in a *referral letter* to the clinical specialist with a *consultation report* being returned from the clinical specialist.

The patient may remain in treatment for a long time over many visits (e.g., chemotherapy for cancer, or treatment for diabetes or other chronic condition). The patient may return many times with a cycle of observation, with possible changing of the diagnosis or treatment.

In the outpatient setting, some HMOs have *advice nurses* who answer patient phone calls and follow protocols based upon patient symptoms. Through a triage process, the advice nurse might have the patient (1) seek an emergency evaluation by coming in within a short period to the Emergency department or the physician's office, (2) come in to see a physician within 24 hours, (3) make a future appointment with a physician, (4) attend a health education class or (5) follow self management. The advice nurse might describe care steps the patient should follow.

In some situations, the advice nurse may request advice of a physician regarding a patient. She might make a phone call to the physician or leave a *phone message* or send an *e-mail message.* The phone message or e-mail message could optionally be put in the chart. At the same time as the phone message or e-mail, any paper chart could be ordered, sending it to the physician. Upon receiving the physician's advice, the advice nurse would later call back the patient or alternatively, the physician or a nurse could call back the patient.

An *appointment clerk* in an HMO makes appointments following protocols. An appointment could be made for a patient upon the patient calling in or made for the patient after the patient's visit to schedule a follow-up appointment. Upon protocol, a patient calling in could be transferred to an advice nurse.

An important document to control outpatient workflow that is not a part of the patient medical record is the *outpatient schedule*. Schedules are for a particular physician, nurse, room or piece of equipment identifying by time all patients scheduled to see that person, room or piece of equipment (i.e., and thus identifying all patients who have an appointment with the person or object). There is generally one schedule for each date the person works or the room or piece of equipment is used. Schedules might also identify who shows up for an appointment and who does not, who cancels, and who does not have an appointment but will be seen. The outpatient schedule is thus a very important workflow document for outpatient clinics.

Inpatient Clinical Information The typical inpatient chart includes some or all of the documents listed in table 4.2 (Loeb 1992) and is assumed in our HMO. The inpatient care process involves admitting and caring for the patient, and may include the admissions department personnel, physicians, nurses, and unit assistants.

Table 4.2 Inpatient Clinical Documents

Document	*Description*
Face sheet	Information identifying the patient, including name, admission date, address and birth date, emergency contact and closest relative, allergies, admitting diagnosis and attending physician.
Medical history and physical examination	The patient's initial medical examination and assessment data completed by the physician.
Initial nursing assessment form	Initial assessment.
Physician's orders	A record of a physician's medical orders.
Problem or nursing diagnosis list	List of nursing diagnoses.
Nursing plan of care	Plan for care of a patient.
Graphic sheet	A type of flow sheet showing graphic recording of the patient's temperature, pulse rate, blood pressure, and possibly daily weight.
Other flow sheets	Abbreviated progress notes, recording dates, times, changes in the patient's condition.
Medication administration record (MAR)	A recording of each medication the patient receives, including name, dosage, route, site, and date and time of administration.
Physician's progress notes	Physician's observations, notes on the patient's progress, and treatment data.
Nurses' progress notes	Patient care information, interventions, and patient's responses.
Consultation sheets	Reports of evaluations made by physicians and others called in for opinions and treatment recommendations.
Health care team records	Notes from other departments, including physical therapy and respiratory therapy.
X-rays, other diagnostic images, EKGs, etc.	
Diagnostic findings	Diagnostic and laboratory data—for example, hematology, pathology, radiology, and X-ray test results and transcriptions.
Consent forms	A patient's or patient's guardian's consent for treatment, special procedures or to release information.
Incident report	Information about a reportable event.

Advance directives	A legal, written document that specifies patient preferences regarding future health care or specifies another person to make medical decisions in the event that the patient is unable to do so.
Discharge plan and summary	A brief review of the patient's hospital stay and plans for care after discharge.

Admission to the hospital could be a result of a discharge from the emergency department (ED) or could be an "elective admission" pre-planned during a previous outpatient visit. Admission could take place in an admitting department, in the patient's room, or in the ED. Information for an elective admission could be entered ahead of time as a "pre-admission"; the pre-admission information would enable the admission to be completed quickly because most of the admission information would already have been collected and would allow diagnostic testing done prior to the admission to be identified as part of the hospital stay.

As a result of admission to the hospital, a *face sheet* is created, which includes the name, address, birth date, contact and other patient demographics information, and may include admitting diagnosis, admitting physician, attending physician, unit, room and bed location and assigned diagnostic related group. Other information may include patient allergies and an advance directive (instructions from a patient at admission informing medical personnel of the patient's wishes for treatments and care when the patient is incapacitated). The face sheet is usually put on the outside of the newly created or an existing paper inpatient chart.

Figure 4.2 identifies activities occurring in inpatient care involving physicians and nurses. The hypothetico-deductive approach described earlier for physicians in the outpatient process and shown in figure 4.1 is also applicable to inpatient care and forms part of figure 4.2. The physician's role in inpatient care shown in figure 4.2, to "(determine) diagnosis" possibly with the help of "diagnostic tests", to "(determine) treatment", to "observe results", and to "refine (a) hypothesis" is the equivalent of the same steps in the outpatient process shown in figure 4.1. In fact, the first iteration of this inpatient care process usually occurs in the outpatient patient setting, either in the ED immediately before the patient is admitted from the ED or during an outpatient visit occurring some time before a planned patient admission. During this ED or outpatient visit the admitting diagnosis, admitting physician, and often the attending physician, are determined. In the ED an H&P is produced that gathers as much of a history of past illnesses and conditions and of family history as possible as well as information on the current problem.

Once the patient is in the hospital, the physician re-examines the patient and may order diagnostic tests (X-rays, EKGs, etc.) receiving back *diagnostic findings*, possibly revising the diagnosis as a result. A treatment plan is determined, which may include orders for medications, radiation treatment, physical therapy, respiratory therapy, etc. Results of the treatment plan and patient care are observed, with possible further revisions of diagnosis or treatment. As in the outpatient setting, this information is recorded on the *H&P* and *physician progress notes*. The physician may ask for consultation advice from specialists requesting treatment recommendations, with the results of these consultations being put on *consultation sheets*.

Other steps in the diagram depicting the inpatient care process in figure 4.2 describe care activities of nurses and ancillary departments. The first step in the nursing process, occurring shortly after admission, is assessment. Assessment is the collection of a database of clinical information on the patient that may later be used in development of the nursing care plan. Upon admission, a nurse makes the *initial nursing assessment*. This usually includes the admitting diagnosis, a review of major body systems, medications taken, allergies, information on height and weight and other drug calculation information, psychosocial factors such as fears, anxieties, and support systems, potential for injury and self-care deficits, need for education of patient and family members to support care after discharge, and other needed post discharge information. The assessment is updated as necessary during the patient's stay.

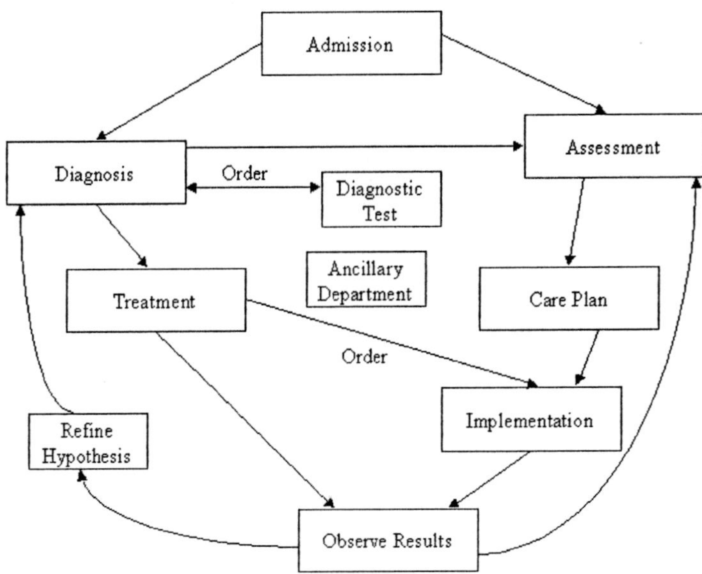

Figure 4.2 Inpatient Care by Physicians and Nurses

From the assessment, a nurse identifies a list of patient problems that can be resolved, diminished, or changed through nursing intervention and management, creating a *problem or nursing diagnosis list*. For each problem, a description of the problem is given, the probable cause is stated, and the signs and symptoms identifying that problem are stated. Based upon the nursing diagnoses, the nurse develops outcomes, or goals, for each diagnosis, that provide a mechanism for evaluating the patient's progress.

Note that a *nursing diagnosis* differs significantly from a medical diagnosis. A nursing diagnosis is any condition that relates to the patient's well being that can be resolved by patient care intervention. Examples are "impaired skin integrity related to prolonged bed rest" or "ineffective breathing patterns".

The nurse then develops a *nursing plan of care* that identifies prescribed nursing *interventions* for the various diagnoses required for achievement of the expected outcomes, where interventions are care activities to achieve or measure progress toward the outcomes. Note that recent trends have been to move away from detailed nursing care plans, and instead provide a basic plan of nursing care, which provides more flexibility in providing care.

Another trend is movement toward multidisciplinary care planning (Iyer and Camp 1995). Such a care plan may include physicians, ancillary department personnel, and other caregivers in the care plan, in addition to nurses. The multidisciplinary care plan may also include care activities outside the inpatient stay, possibly including diagnostic tests before admission and follow-up care after discharge, such as outpatient visits, and later care at sub-acute and skilled nursing facilities (SNFs). A case manager may be assigned to track follow-up care when it is likely to be of high risk or expensive; a clinical social worker may provide assistance for lower risk cases. A *clinical pathway*, a structured document to identify care activities and caregiver workflow needed to care for a patient, is one technique for multidisciplinary care planning.

Despite recent trends to move away from detailed nurse care planning for patients, there is the potential of making generation and maintenance of a complete and personalized nursing care plan for an inpatient stay much easier by computerization now that a standardized set of nursing diagnoses, interventions and outcomes have been developed (Johnson and Naas 1997). These standards have been developed in conjunction with the University of Iowa and include NANDA nursing diagnoses, NIC nursing intervention classifications and NOC nursing outcomes classifications (Johnson and Naas 1997). A nurse can select from the list of diagnoses, select applicable interventions and outcomes, producing the complete, personalized nursing care plan.

A number of documents are associated with *implementation* of the physician treatment plan and of his or her medication and orders, and with implementation of the nursing and other care plans. The physician's medication orders, which often include the patient current outpatient medications, are transferred over to a *medication administration record (MAR)*; upon administration of a medication the nurse records the date and time on medication administration record. Notes on therapy ordered by the physician with the orders implemented by ancillary departments are recorded on *health care team records* (e.g., radiation treatment, physical therapy, and respiratory therapy). Nurses document the interventions used to meet the patient's needs, which may include the type of intervention, the time of care and the identity of the nurse administering care; documenting of interventions is primarily accomplished using *flow sheets*. One type of intervention for insuring that a patient performs normal day to day functions, such as eating, bathing, tooth brushing and grooming; this is referred to as *activities of daily living*.

Nurses progress notes are used to record the patient's status and to track changes in the patient's condition. These progress notes describe in chronological order pertinent nursing observations, patient responses to interventions, progress toward expected outcomes, and need for reassessment.

Nursing and physician observations provide information for re-assessment of the patient and revision of diagnoses, treatments and care plans.

Although the nursing assessment identifies increased chances for incidents such as the patient falling, and possibly breaking bones, and the care plan may identify interventions to prevent these incidents, reportable incidents do occur. These are reported in *incident reports*.

For each nursing shift, the identity of the nurses caring for a patient changes. Because nursing care for a patient must continue as if there was no change in shift, it is important that there is significant communication about the patient and his care between the nurses on the different shifts. Two documents that are not part of the patient's chart that assist in this process, are the shift report and Kardex. The shift report for a patient is created to provide information on a patient for the following shift.

A Kardex is a trade-name for a card-filing system that allows quick reference to the particular need of an inpatient for certain aspects of nursing care (Loeb 1995). It is a type of document that this book calls an "inpatient clinical summary".

An "inpatient clinical summary" is a summarization document to quickly identify the current status of the patient, which, for example, might include the following:

- the patient's name, age, sex, marital status and religion
- medical diagnoses, usually by priority
- nursing diagnoses, usually by priority

- current physician orders for medications, treatments, diet, IV's, diagnostic tests, procedures, etc.
- consultations
- results of diagnostic tests and procedures
- permitted activities, functional limitations, assistance needed, and safety precautions
- care plan.

All information in an Inpatient Clinical comes from other documents in the patient's chart and thus does not become part of the chart.

Planning for discharge begins at the time of initial assessment and continues up to the time of discharge. Information is put on a *discharge plan and summary* document and may include the following information:

- family at home or other care support
- financial resources
- home environment, including barriers
- history of present illness
- history of compliance
- transportation availability
- impediments to self-care.

The discharge summary part of the document is usually completed immediately after discharge and may include

- all relevant diagnoses
- all operative procedures
- instructions specifying medications, level of physical activity, diet, follow-up care, and patient and family teaching.

An important document to control inpatient workflow is the *unit census*. It is a list of all patients in rooms in a hospital unit that identifies each patient in the unit, the patient's room location and the nurses and physicians assigned to care for the patient.

Emergency Department Clinical Information The emergency department (ED) is considered to be an outpatient department, but functions somewhat differently from other outpatient clinics.

The patient either "walks in" or comes in by ambulance. *Triage* is the assessment of patients' medical problems to determine urgency and priority of care to determine which patient is to be seen next, and is usually done by a nurse, called a *triage nurse*. The walk-in patient goes through a triage process whereas the patient who comes in by ambulance is usually immediately taken to an examining room.

Table 4.3 lists documents used in an ED.

Table 4.3 Possible Emergency Department Clinical Documents

Document	*Description*
Triage documentation	**This document, which may be a part of another document such as the** Nursing flow sheet, records information that determines how to triage the patient. Information may include mode of arrival, acuity, chief complaint, medications, allergies, nursing actions at triage.
Medical history and physical examination	The patient's initial medical examination and evaluation data. This document includes the following: chief complaint (CC), history of present illness (HPI), past medical history (PMH), family history (FH), social history (SH) and marital history, review of systems (ROS), physical exam (PE), assessment, diagnosis (Dx), impression, rule out (R/O), plan, prognosis (Px).
Progress notes	The physician's objective findings about improvement or stabilization of the condition.
Nursing flow sheet	Abbreviated progress notes, recording times, treatments, medications and diagnostic tests given, changes in the patient's condition, including vital signs.
Physician's orders	A record of a physician's medical orders.
Diagnostic findings	Diagnostic and laboratory data—for example, hematology, pathology, radiology, and X-ray test results and transcriptions.
Emergency room discharge instruction sheet	Lists discharge instructions for diet, treatments, medications, activities and follow-up visits.
Follow-up after discharge	Documentation of calls to patients following discharge from the ED.

The triage nurse examines and interviews the patient for information useful for triaging the patient and may provide care to the patient. Examples of information recorded are the following:

- mode of arrival
- priority
- chief complaint
- medications
- allergies
- nursing actions at triage.

The triage process may result in the patient

- waiting in the waiting room and later being escorted to an exam room in the ED
- being immediately escorted to an exam room in the ED
- being escorted to an outpatient clinic, outside the ED
- being told to come back to an outpatient clinic at a later date or time.

A nurse, physician or medical assistant may order the patient's chart. After being escorted to an exam room, the patient waits in the room for the nurse or physician. The nurse takes vital signs and may initiate diagnostic tests by protocol.

The physician comes into the exam room and follows a data collection and interpretation process as shown in figure 4.1. The principal difference from the standard outpatient clinic visit is that the patient usually stays in the room while diagnostic tests are done and perhaps while diagnoses and treatments are refined. This process is recorded on an H&P.

The physician and nurse may visit the patient a number of times, with the physician recording additional progress note information for the H&P and the nurse recording changes on a nursing flow sheet.

The H&P also is used to gather as much of a history of past illnesses and conditions and family history as is possible.

After a patient has been stabilized and is ready to be discharged or admitted to the hospital, the physician and nurse complete the documentation and the patient is discharged from the ED. The patient may be discharged to

- home
- the hospital (and thus admitted)
- some other place, such as a skilled nursing facility (SNF).

For those patients discharged to home or sometimes to other places, the patient is given a discharge instruction sheet, possibly identifying instructions for diet, treatments, medications, activities and follow-up visits. This sheet is important in documenting fulfillment of the professional responsibility to provide discharge instructions and to shift the responsibility for following these instructions to the patient.

In some cases, a call is made to the patient after discharge to evaluate his status. This call may be documented.

Important documents to control emergency department workflow that are not a part of the patient medical record are two lists of patients: (1) the *triage list*, the patients waiting to be triaged, and (2) the *emergency department census*, the patients in emergency department rooms.

Other than patients who come in by ambulance, all patients who come into the emergency department are seen by the triage nurse. The triage list is used by a triage nurse to list patients who have been seen by a triage nurse, listing the time the patient came in and the time he was seen by the triage nurse, and the priority of care determined by how ill the patient is. The times and priority of care is used to identify which patient should be seen next. Once the patient is escorted to a room, the patient is put on the emergency department census along with the physician(s) and nurse(s) caring for the patient.

Other Categories of Clinical Information There may be specialized documentation in the medical record, including in the following medical areas:

- oncology, chemotherapy
- psychiatry
- critical care
- respiratory therapy
- injection clinic
- obstetrical areas
- emergency medical services

- pre-surgery
- surgery
- surgery recovery room.

Documentation is also used by non-physicians who provide care, referred to collectively as *allied health professionals.* Medical environments where allied health professionals provide the bulk of care include the following

- *home health care*: skilled nursing and related care supplied to a patient at home
- *skilled nursing facilities (SNF)*: an establishment with a nursing staff that bridges the gap between hospital and home for elderly patients who need skilled nursing care or rehabilitation services.
- *hospice care*: care specifically given to terminally ill patients—generally those with six months or less to live.

4.5 REASONS FOR HAVING A PATIENT MEDICAL RECORD

Reasons for having a patient medical record are: (1) to record pertinent health information from the patient, (2) to record the caregiver's findings and treatments, (3) to communicate information to later caregivers who see the patient and to the patient, (4) to coordinate caregivers and organize their activities in the care to the patient, (5) to serve as a formal, in particular legal and financial, record of care, and (6) to provide information for public health, epidemiological studies, and clinical research.

4.5.1 Caregiver s Record of Information from the Patient

A caregiver records information from the patient interview, from a physical examination of the patient, from observations of the patient, and from direct measurements from the patient such a blood pressure, temperature, and other vital signs. This is the raw information before it is interpreted. Examples of documents to record this information are the history and physical (H&P) form and nursing flow sheets.

4.5.2 Caregivers Findings and Treatments

After talking to and observing the patient, possibly consulting with other caregivers and receiving the results back from tests, a caregiver will make and record an assessment of the patient's condition and problems (diagnoses), a treatment plan, and a prognosis. Results of consultations and diagnostic test results are recorded.

A physician makes an assessment of the patient's condition, develops a treatment plan, and determines a prognosis. For an inpatient, a nurse makes an initial assessment of the patient, establishes nursing diagnoses, and creates a nursing plan of care. A consulting specialist physician gets a referral letter from another physician and returns a consultation report. Ancillary departments such as physical therapy or respiratory therapy return health care team reports while departments such as clinical laboratories and radiology return diagnostic findings from tests administered to the patient.

4.5.3 Communication with Later Caregivers and with the Patient

Prior to and during a patient's visit, a caregiver needs to find clinical information on the patient recorded from previous visits, whether the patient saw the current caregiver or a different one. This enables the clinician to

- quickly evaluate the patient's overall health based upon current and past visits, social and family history
- identify what took place during any selected visit, especially the most recent ones (e.g., the treatments, test results, medications taken)
- find recorded diagnoses or problems to assist in current evaluations
- find patient complaints and information on previous observations to compare against present ones
- determine medications taken
- identify allergies, drug reactions, and immunizations.

This communication of chart information may also be with the patient. A patient is entitled to see his own chart and evaluate care given.

4.5.4 Coordinating and Organizing Caregivers in the Care of the Patient

Coordination of care is essential for quality and effective medical care for the patient and for a team approach to patient care. Currently, coordination of caregivers is most common in the inpatient setting. With the shifting of procedures from the inpatient to the outpatient setting and the large number of outpatient physicians who see the patient in managed care settings such as HMOs, caregiver coordination in the outpatient setting is becoming increasingly important. The patient chart is the primary vehicle for communication between caregivers and this coordination between caregivers.

"Demand management" also involves coordination of caregivers. *Demand management* (Schlier 1996) is an approach used in HMOs to lower medical care costs by educating the patient on self-care when it is appropriate, to insuring that a patient is seen by the most appropriate and cost-effective caregiver for the patient's medical condition, and by coordinating the caregivers giving care to the patient. Information in the chart may be useful in identifying when a member should be seen by one type of caregiver rather than another (e.g., a physician instead of a less-costly nurse practitioner because of the severity of the member's medical condition) or should be seen by a case manager in addition to a physician to insure that the best, most cost-effective, care decisions are made.

4.5.5 Creating a Formal Record of Patient Care

A formal record of patient care is required by law. Additionally, a formal record of care is required to record services so patients, the government or insurance companies can properly be charged for these services. A formal record of care is also required as the source for various forms of internal and external reports to be sent to the patient's employee, for example for workmen's compensation claims, and to government and industry regulatory agencies, to evaluate care within a healthcare organization.

If the patient sues a caregiver for malpractice, information to disprove the case must be found in the patient chart or other sources. Ideally, the total of information would be found in the patient chart.

4.5.6 Information for Public Health and Clinical Research

The patient medical record provides information for *public health* purposes, supporting community efforts to identify and prevent disease and to control communicable diseases. For example, a patient may come in because of food poisoning after having eaten at a number of different restaurants. A physician or epidemiologist could search for other patients with the same medical problem by looking through charts and contact those patients to determine where they had eaten and what they ate, so the restaurant where the problem occurred can be determined.

The patient medical record also provides information for *clinical research*, including research on safety and "efficacy" of treatment plans, procedures and drugs, where "efficacy" means the ability to produce the desired results. Various patient attributes also recorded in the chart must be taken into account during this clinical research, including the patients' current health, previous and current diagnoses, age, gender and current medications. Important for clinical studies is picking appropriately targeted patient populations for a clinical research project, which might be determinable from the chart.

4.6 OTHER ASPECTS OF THE CURRENT ENVIRONMENT

4.6.1 Special Characteristics of Patient Care in an HMO

Physicians have been increasingly banding together into "managed care" organizations to decrease costs. Such "managed care" organizations charge patients not for each service performed, but a certain amount per month independent of the services performed; this payment approach is referred to as "capitation". The primary types of managed care organizations are *Preferred Provider Organizations* or PPOs (where a healthcare organization contracts caregivers) and *Health Maintenance Organizations* or HMOs (where a healthcare organization primarily uses caregivers who only work in the HMO and work primarily in HMO facilities).

More traditional healthcare organizations, "fee for service" organizations, as the name implies charge a fee for each medical service provided, with patients most often having their medical fees paid in part or in total by their insurance companies.

Because of fixed payment for care, physicians in managed care organizations care about providing cost-effective patient care. For example, as compared to physicians in the fee for service setting, HMO physicians are less likely to order unnecessary diagnostic tests or expensive medications and less likely to perform non-cost-effective procedures.

In an HMO, one major way of cutting costs is referred to as *demand management* (Schlier 1996), a system to provide a patient with the most cost-effective care for the patient's medical complaint, by instructing a patient in self-care, by "triaging" the patient to the most cost-effective caregiver, and by coordinating the caregivers giving care to the patient.

Demand management might include the following:

- *advice nurse*: a nurse who accepts patient phone calls and advises the patient on medical care according to protocol; she advises the patient on when self-care is appropriate and when a patient needs to come in; if a patient needs to come in, she advises the patient on whether it is more appropriate for the patient to come in immediately to the emergency department, see a caregiver the same or next day (which is usually less costly than an emergency department visit), or come in at a later date
- *gatekeeper*: a primary care physician, usually in internal medicine, pediatrics or gynecology, who must be seen first before the patient is allowed to see more costly specialists
- *personal physician*: a physician who serves as the *primary caregiver* for assigned patients and who is responsible for coordinating the care of these patients, especially in the outpatient setting
- *non-physician primary caregiver*: a nurse practitioner and physician assistant, supervised by a physician, who serves in the place of a physician as the primary caregiver for a patient
- *hospitalist* (Moore 1997): a physician who is a specialist in in-patient medicine, who takes responsibility for a patient's care during the patient's entire hospital stay, and then returns responsibility to the primary caregiver when the patient leaves the hospital
- *case manager*: a healthcare professional who determines the most effective and least costly treatment programs and organizations for a patient who has a high cost and high risk disease and who insures that the patient receives that care
- *utilization manager*: a healthcare professional who determines a patient's eligibility and coverage for benefits (e.g., for durable medical equipment or for care in outside specialty facilities)
- *disease management caregiver or consultant*: a healthcare professional or consultant who provides care, advice, data or software for a particular disease area such as diabetes, cancer, coronary artery disease or asthma, with care given for the condition being measured against established treatment guidelines for the condition. (Whereas case management focuses on the sickest patients, disease management targets individuals at the earliest stages of known high-cost conditions (Mullahy 1998).)

Primarily to encourage the HMO member to only come in for care when necessary, rather than to make money for the HMO, HMOs often charge a co-payment for each outpatient visit. An HMO may not charge a co-payment for an inpatient visit, as a member would not come in for inpatient care without the approval of a physician.

Another part of demand management are wellness programs that attempt to decrease demand for health care services by screening patients for certain diseases or conditions and providing care before the disease or condition becomes costly to treat. Areas where wellness programs may be effective include the following: sigmoidoscopy (looking at the lower large intestine) or colonoscopy (looking at the whole large intestine) to screen for colon cancer, smoking cession programs to encourage members to stop smoking (and perhaps providing alternative means for weight control at the same time), and breast exams and mammography to screen for breast cancer

Patient education is an important part of demand management. A patient with a chronic disease, such as diabetes or asthma, could be educated about when self-care is appropriate and when it is absolutely necessary to come in to be seen. A new mother could be educated about childhood diseases and conditions and likewise could be told when at-home care for a child by the parent is appropriate and when it is not. This could be done through patient education programs or through distribution of a healthcare handbook to HMO members describing for various complaints when self-care can be administered and when it is important to come in for care (Wilson 1997).

Table 4.4 summarizes the way HMOs may be able to save money as compared to fee for service organizations.

Table 4.4 Cost Savings Approaches for Managed Care

Number	*Cost Savings*	*Assisted by Software Systems*
1	More efficient use of caregivers, because if one caregiver is not available then another caregiver in the same healthcare organization can see the patient.	scheduling and workflow systems
2	A larger number of patients per physician.	patient clinical systems; scheduling and workflow systems
3	Nurse practitioners, physician assistants or registered nurses may see patients in place of physicians.	scheduling system
4	Prescription of lower cost medications, either generic medications or those in the HMO drug formulary, or recommendation of over-the-counter medications (which most HMOs do not cover).	patient clinical systems, including pharmacy system
5	Greater chance of continuity of care because of greater chance of sharing of the patient's clinical information between caregivers in the same healthcare organization who see the patient than by caregivers in different healthcare organizations.	patient clinical systems
6	Because HMOs are more organized than fee for service organizations, computer systems, which make information more quickly available to caregivers and replace costly and time-consuming paperwork, are more common in HMOs.	all systems
7	Because of capitation, greater incentives to keep patients healthy, especially through preventive healthcare and patient education.	patient clinical systems; scheduling systems
8	Because of capitation, use of alternative delivery systems such as home, hospice and skilled nursing facilities instead care in hospitals.	patient clinical systems; financial systems
9	Because of capitation, outpatient surgeries sometimes replace more costly inpatient surgeries and inpatient stays.	patient clinical systems; scheduling and workflow systems
10	Because of capitation, lesser use of costly procedures and diagnostic tests and lesser use of expensive specialists.	patient clinical systems
11	Because of capitation, lesser use of purely defensive medicine, where the	patient clinical

	patient is given a large number of diagnostic tests to aid in the initial diagnosis and to protect against lawsuits.	systems
12	Efficient sharing of costly technology, where, for example, a CT scanner is used by physicians from all facilities in the healthcare organization.	scheduling and workflow systems
13	Demand management techniques (see section 3.6) such as advice nurses who advise patients on when self care is appropriate and when the patient should come in, and primary care physicians who serve as "gatekeepers" to determine if patients indeed need to see costly specialists. Drop in outpatients may be triaged.	patient clinical systems; scheduling and workflow systems
14	Lesser chance of unnecessary repeated tests or of need for multiple complete health histories because of sharing of clinical information between caregivers in the same healthcare organization.	patient clinical systems, including clinical laboratory system
15	Buying items in bulk for lower cost, for example, medications.	financial systems
16	Other efficiencies of scale including efficient collection of payments from employers (capitated payments), the government (e.g., Medicare payments) and insurance companies; efficient payment to drug and other external companies; and lower cost malpractice insurance because of having its own lawyers and sharing of liability among HMO caregivers.	financial systems
17	Attempts to substitute arbitration via the PPO or HMO contract to protect against costly malpractice suits.	
18	Telephone calls may substitute for outpatient visits, where applicable.	patient clinical systems, financial systems
19	The HMO would only pay for medical services outside the HMO that they could not provide and which they consider constitute standard patient care.	Financial systems
20	The HMO would scrutinize payments for medical services when the HMO member is outside the area covered by the HMO, and only pay for those services they consider reasonable and justified.	Financial systems
21	Least costly, most beneficial insurance reimbursements selected (e.g., care consistent with insurance company or Medicare payments or best insurance taken where both husband and wife have family coverage).	financial systems

A couple of trends are occurring within HMOs. First, many HMO members are willing to pay a greater capitation fee or pay co-payments for seeing providers outside the HMO; such healthcare policies are referred to as *point of service* policies. Also, some HMOs are contracting with outside healthcare organizations—called *alliance organizations*—to share hospital space and medical office facilities with the HMO.

4.6.2 Existing Automated Systems in the HMO

One of the advantages of managed care over the "fee for service" world is that, due to their usually larger size and tighter organization, they can better make use of computer software systems to decrease costs and also improve patient care.

These software systems fall into three areas:

1. systems to manage caregiver workflow such as scheduling systems
2. financial systems to collect and pay bills
3. patient clinical systems to provide information and capabilities to caregivers in the care of patients.

"Managed care" organizations have the potential to have lower costs than the "fee for service" institutions because of the types of cost saving measures previously listed in table 4.4. The types of software systems that can assist in each cost saving measure are also listed in table 4.4. Computerization, as can be seen, can play a major role in managed care organizations competing against the fee for service world and in managed care organizations competing against each other.

Existing automated systems that exist in many HMOs, and our example HMO, are the following:

- **outpatient appointment scheduling system:** A clinical / workflow system to schedule appointments for physicians, nurse practitioners, other caregivers, rooms and equipment
- **outpatient and emergency department registration system:** A clinical / financial system to register a patient, with or without an appointment, recording that the patient came in and recording any payments
- **inpatient admission, discharge and transfer (ADT) system:** A clinical / financial system to record a patient's admission to the hospital, discharge from the hospital or transfer from one room in the hospital to another or to another hospital, and to record payments
- **surgery scheduling system:** A clinical system to schedule surgery rooms for patients and to schedule all the surgeons, nurses, anesthesiologists and other personnel with the room, automatically ordering supplies for the surgery
- **HMO membership system:** a financial / clinical system to identify patients as members or not
- **patient demographics system:** a database to provide address, telephone and other basic contact information about the patient
- **billing system:** a financial system to bill insurance companies, employers of members or members, and to record services and other costs
- **clinical laboratory system:** a clinical system that records the results of clinical laboratory tests either by input from clinical laboratory personnel or directly from clinical laboratory instruments, and which usually allows input of clinical laboratory orders and displays results of tests
- **pharmacy system:** a clinical system for ordering and dispensing outpatient prescriptions or ordering and administration of inpatient medications, which may include drug interaction and other clinical checking
- **radiology system:** a clinical system to record diagnostic imaging tests and orders for these tests and return transcribed results

- **anatomic pathology system:** a clinical system to record anatomic pathology test results, where *anatomic pathology* is a department that determines if tissues are in fact abnormal or diseased
- **durable medical equipment (DME) system:** a financial / inventory system to order and control the inventory of durable medical equipment, where durable medical equipment is equipment leased or sold to patients for use in their homes (e.g., wheelchairs, walkers, canes)
- **paper chart ordering system:** a system to order paper patient medical records.

The systems listed above which are clinical systems fall into the following two categories:

- encounter systems (e.g., admissions, outpatient visits, emergency room visits, surgeries)
- ancillary systems that could receive orders and, if required, return results (clinical laboratory orders and results, medication orders, radiology orders and results).

Almost all these systems are also workflow systems, controlling the workflow of employees.

The basic question is "How are these systems related to an automated patient medical record?" Other questions are the following: Does the automated patient medical record replace these systems? Does it supplement these systems? Does it interface with these systems? How do you control redundancy of information? These are some of the questions that will be answered later in this book.

4.7 EXISTING BUSINESS PRACTICES TO PRESERVE

The following describe *essential business practices* dealing with patient care that HMO management and employees have decided should be preserved with an automated patient medical record system:

- support all caregivers listed in this chapter
- support caregiver workflows identified in this chapter, including providing lists of patients being seen by a caregiver or a group of caregivers: the outpatient schedule for outpatients, the unit census for inpatients, and the triage list and emergency department census for emergency department patients
- support recording and retrieval of care documentation in the patient medical record, including retrieval of types of documents that currently exist, including those listed in this chapter
- generate those documents that are derived from but are not included in the patient medical record: the inpatient clinical summary (similar to the "Kardex") and the medication administration record (MAR) for inpatients
- support ordering of diagnostic tests and of procedures, and support return and recording of results of orders
- support the purposes for the patient medical record listed in this chapter
- support demand management
- support the HMO cost saving methods listed in table 44 where appropriate
- support existing clinical systems, as listed this chapter.

Key Terms

activities of daily living
advance directive
ADT
adverse reactions to medications
allergy
allied health professional
assessment
ancillary services
board certified specialist
capitation
chief complaint
clinical laboratory
clinical social worker
consultation report
demand management
diagnostic findings
diagnosis (Dx)
discharge plan and summary
disease management
Doctor of Medicine (MD)
durable medical equipment (DME)
emergency department (ED)
emergency department census
encounter systems
essential business practices
family history (FH)
fee for service
flow sheet
gatekeeper
Health Maintenance Organization (HMO)
History and Physical (H&P)
history of present illness (HPI)
HMO member
home health care
hospice case
hospitalist
hypothetico-deductive approach
inpatient
Kardex
licensed practical nurse (LPN)
managed care
medical assistant
medical administration record (MAR)
medical researcher
medical transcriptionist
nurse
nursing plan of care
nursing diagnosis
nurse practitioner (NP)
objective
orders
outpatient
past medical history (PMH)
patient
patient demographics
personal physician
physical exam (PE)
physician
physician assistant (PA)
plan
Preferred Provider Organizations (PPOs)
primary care
prognosis (Px)
progress notes
quality manager
registered nurse (RN)
review of systems (ROS)
skilled nursing facility (SNF)
social history (SH)
subjective
triage
triage list
triage nurse
unit census
utilization manager
vital signs

Study Questions

1. Name some reasons to study the current environment first in a project.
2. Who are the principal players in the outpatient setting? In the emergency department? In the hospital? Who is the usual first point of contact in the emergency department?
3. Explain the hypothetico-deductive approach shown in figure 4.1.
4. Besides physicians, who else can diagnosis and treat illnesses in the outpatient setting? How does their role differ from that of the physician?
5. Name some the principal medical record documents. Name some primary documents that are not found inside the patient medical record, and explain why they can not be found in the patient medical record.
6. Name some the purposes of the patient medical record.
7. How do HMOs differ from fee for service healthcare organizations? How would an automated patient medical record be used differently in the two types of organizations?

CHAPTER 5

Reasons to Develop an Automated Patient Medical Record

CHAPTER OUTLINE

5.1 PROJECT CONTEXT: PROJECT OBJECTIVES SUPPORTING ORGANIZATIONAL OBJECTIVES

Projects are done to improve an organization. In order to justify spending a lot of money to do a costly project, an organization must identify the reasons for doing the project, comparing these reasons and resulting benefits against the costs. Further, the organization must choose between projects and pick the proper mix of projects to select a mix with the greatest overall benefits to the organization at the lowest overall cost.

One way an organization can evaluate, select and compare projects is to determine the reasons for doing each project, the *project objectives*, and compare these project objectives against *organizational objectives*—desired future positions of the organization—as projects must support organizational objectives.

Since all projects, and thus all project objectives, must support organizational objectives, a method for determining project objectives is to look at each organizational objective to determine if the project would positively impact the organizational objective. If so, a project objective can be determined from the organizational objective.

For example, one "organizational objective" may be to "decrease healthcare organization costs without impacting patient care". Two projects may each support this organizational objective: An automated patient medical record system will "reduce or eliminate the costs and time of finding, transporting, copying, storing, filing, and organizing the paper patient medical record", while a new membership system will "reduce the costs of collecting capitation fees". Another organizational objective might be to "improve patient care". Of the two projects, only the automated patient medical record project supports this second organizational objective; it improves patient care in many ways, including "making the patient medical record always available to authorized caregivers".

Once a project is completed, its project objectives can be used to measure its failure or success: a project can be considered successful if it meets its project objectives, enhancing the organizational objectives. Because a project objective is usually not directly measurable, a *goal* that can be measured should be set up to evaluate whether or not the project objective has been reached. For example, a project objective to "create an always available patient medical record" might have a measurable goal at the end of the project of "observing patient visits with physicians, an analyst must verify that for 99.5% of visits that the patient's medical record is immediately available on-line to the physician". This could be done statistically with the analyst visiting various medical locations and observing various physicians giving care, observing whether or not the patient's medical record is available on-line.

Because the project objectives are likely to take a long time to achieve, measurable goals may also be established at many different points during the project that can be used to measure the progress of the project towards the objective—An intermediate goal might be that "40% of HMO patient records will be automated after 3 years from the start of the project".

Table 5.2 lists project objectives for our project to automate the patient medical record derived from our HMO's organizational objectives. In the early stages of a project, project objectives can also be used to determine an initial set of *business requirements* for the project. A business requirement is a required characteristic of the organization at the end of the project. The total set of business requirements for the project, determined as the project progresses, describe the expected project effects upon the organization.

From these initial business requirements, an initial description of products of the project can be determined—In our case the product is an automated patient medical record. These initial products of the project can be described by a model of them, referred to here as a *conceptual view*. Section 5.5 presents an initial conceptual view of the automated patient medical record system based upon business requirements. More refined conceptual views can later be developed as the project is defined further, as additional business requirements are determined.

But again, before a project is started, it must be selected among many potential projects that might benefit the organization. The next section describes an approach that could be used by an organization to select and evaluate projects based upon organizational objectives.

5.2 SELECTION AND EVALUATION OF PROJECTS IN AN ORGANIZATION

An approach for selecting and evaluating projects within an organization is presented in reference (King 1988). It uses the following terminology, which is related to the overall organization rather than to a project:

- *Mission:* the business the organization is in.
- *Objectives:* desired future positions of an organization.
- *Strategies:* the general directions in which the objectives are to be pursued.
- *Goals:* specific targets to be sought at specified points in time.
- *Projects:* resource-consuming sets of activities through which strategies are implemented and goals are pursued.

Figure 5.1 shows the relationship between these elements together with an example for an HMO.

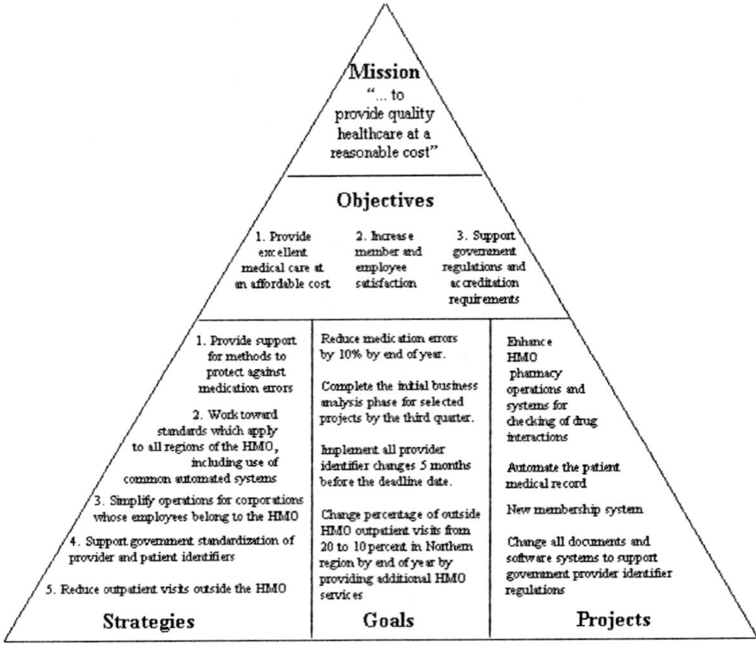

Figure 5.1 Relationships Between Organizational Mission, Objectives, Strategies, Goals, and Projects

The company has a specific mission. Based upon this mission and the market, the company defines objectives for the future for the company to enable the company to improve and advance. Strategies for achieving these objectives are determined. Goals, ways to measure the organizational objectives, are established.

Appropriate projects to fulfill the goals and objectives are picked. Projects themselves have project objectives. Projects are picked whose project objectives most closely match the organizational objectives taking into consideration constraints on the project, including availability of resources (money, time, people) necessary to do the project, the availability of technology to successfully accomplish the project, and other obstacles that might hinder accomplishment of the project.

But projects must not only be viewed singly, but together with other projects and existing business capabilities. Sometimes a project is picked over others even though it does not appear to promote organizational objectives because it is a critical in the functioning of a set of interrelated projects or business capabilities that together perform important functions in the organization: the project is one piece of a *business mosaic*—the set of interrelated business capabilities and projects that together define the present and future functioning of the organization.

After a project is picked, goals to measure project objectives during the course of the project are determined. Strategies for doing the project are later determined as part of the project plan.

The following are a set of organizational objectives of our example HMO that enhance the HMO's organizational mission of "providing quality healthcare at a reasonable cost":

1. Provide quality medical care
2. Promote HMO member satisfaction
3. Support healthcare workers and improve their efficiency
4. Make money
5. Fulfill the requirements of government and public health agencies and accreditation organizations.

The above describes the typical mission of an HMO and typical associated organizational objectives for an HMO.

5.3 DERIVING PROJECT OBJECTIVES: THE REASONS TO AUTOMATE THE PATIENT MEDICAL RECORD

Project objectives can be determined from organizational objectives as follows: (1) Each organizational objective must be evaluated as to how the project would cause it to happen. (2) If the project has a positive effect on the organizational objective, then some aspect of that HMO organizational objective should be a project objective. So let us consider these organizational objectives one by one and how they are positively affected by our project to automate the patient medical record. (The negative effects of the project will be considered in a later chapter.)

5.3.1 Provide Quality Medical Care

Automating the patient medical record would have a positive effect on patient care within an HMO and other healthcare organizations. This section identifies the ways that medical care could be improved by an automated patient medical record.

5.3.1.1 Reengineering to Improve the Quality of Patient Care

An automated patient medical record system affects the entire clinical workflow. Patient care is a joint effort of many people, including medical personnel and non-medical support personnel. Patient care is the result of interactions between many different departments inside and outside the HMO. The automated patient medical record system would support all these people and all departments that influence patient care.

Changing and improving the way an organization works is called *reengineering*. Reengineering involves looking at and possibly changing the workflows of employees in the

HMO to improve the workflows. Creation of an automated patient medical record system provides an excellent opportunity to make patient care better for both patients and employees through reengineering—improving patient care by changing caregiver workflows dealing with patient care.

5.3.1.2 A Complete, Immediately Available, Patient Medical Record

With automation of the patient medical record, there is the potential of having a complete patient medical record, containing information from both inside and outside the HMO (a *longitudinal* or *life time medical record*) that is available at any time to authorized caregivers both inside and outside the HMO. Whereas, the current (paper) patient chart may be only at one location at a time with transportation time between locations, and might even be temporarily misplaced, the automated patient medical record would be immediately available to all caregivers who needed it.

Over a patient's lifetime, a patient may be seen by many different physicians, nurse practitioners and other caregivers in many different healthcare organizations. The patient is therefore likely to have many separate paper charts in many different geographic locations.

Even when a patient has belonged to the HMO over his lifetime, the paper chart is likely to be fragmented. For example, figure 5.2 shows the many charts that may exist for a single patient within an HMO (e.g., separate charts in multiple HMO facilities and separate charts for inpatient, outpatient, psychiatry and genetics care). With the advent of "point of service" policies within HMOs, allowing members to see outside providers, and alliances with other healthcare organizations, HMO members are also likely to have charts outside the HMO. With automation of the patient medical record, the fragmentation shown in figure 5.2 should no longer occur.

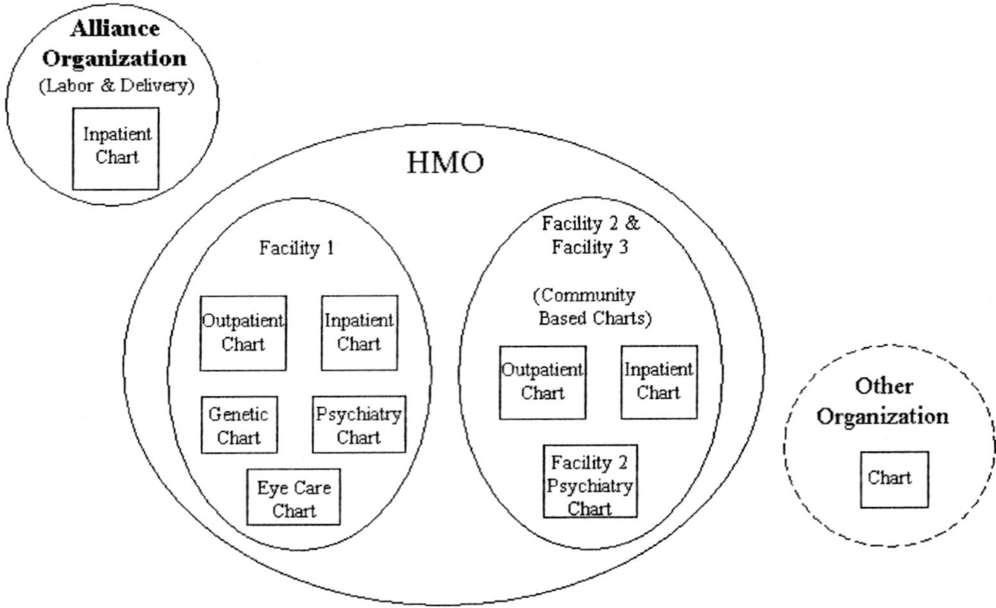

Figure 5.2 An example of the existing charts for an HMO patient.

Improvement of patient care would also occur in the following other ways:

1. Critical medical information, such as allergies to medications, advance directives, a complete list of medications the patient is taking, and an up-to-date patient and family history is likely to be immediately available. This information is especially important in the emergency department and the inpatient setting.
2. There would be fewer gaps in medical information.
3. There would be no delay between closely occurring visits to transport over the chart.
4. A caregiver can telephone a patient when needed instead of having to first wait for the arrival of the chart.
5. A patient can contact a physician by telephone and immediately receive informed advice because the physician will have the (automated) patient medical record in hand.
6. The patient medical record would now be available to advice nurses at the time a patient calls in for advice.
7. Multiple caregivers can view and/or update the patient medical record concurrently, even at two different geographic locations.

With simultaneous caregiver access to the patient medical record, *telemedicine*—the use of interactive audio and visual links to enable remote healthcare practitioners to consult in "real time" with specialists in distant locations—becomes more feasible. Telemedicine commonly involves an allied health professional co-located with the patient and a physician at a remote location or physicians at different locations working in consultation with each other.

5.3.1.3 Organization So Clinical Information can be Easily Found

If relevant information cannot be found in the patient medical record, then it is essentially equivalent to the information not being there. Patient care can be improved by making it easier to find clinical information in the patient medical record by organizing it.

Unlike the paper patient medical record which can be organized in a limited number of ways, the automated patient medical record can be electronically organized in an unlimited number of ways, for example by encounter, significant health problem, or type of caregiver.

An *encounter* will be used here to mean a face-to-face interaction between a patient and a healthcare provider or other direct communication that substitutes for a face-to-face interaction, such as some phone calls. Examples of encounters are an inpatient stay, outpatient visit, emergency department visit, advice nurse call, a phone call between a patient and a physician, a home health visit, or a skilled nursing facility (SNF) stay. A *significant health problem* is any significant medical condition or disease.

For example, methods that can be employed to organize the patient medical record and enable a caregiver to find relevant information are the following:

1. **Basic organization by encounter**: All documentation for a single encounter can be found, including progress notes, clinical laboratory reports, prescriptions, procedures, etc.
2. **Summaries**: Lists can be produced summarizing clinical information for a patient, including past encounters, current medications taken by the patient, significant health problems, allergies, and immunizations. Physicians could verify and revise the summary ensuring that it was accurate and up-to-date.
2. **Hypermedia and drill down**: Patient clinical information can be organized in a hierarchical fashion, including by encounter and significant health problem, so drill down is possible to relevant documents containing that information (e.g., drill down from an encounter selected from a list of encounters to a list of the medical record documents for the encounter).

3. **Organization by type of caregiver**: Categorize parts of the patient medical record so the parts relevant to a particular type of caregiver can be found (e.g., an ophthalmologist is interested in all eye problems, while a pharmacist may be interested in a patient's medical history and response to medications)
4. **Synopses**: Display a shortened, summarized, version of what happened during an encounter.

5.3.1.4 Continuity and Coordination of Patient Care Among Caregivers

Continuity of care is the coordination of care received by a patient over time possibly given by multiple caregivers. An automated patient medical record could assist caregivers in coordinating patient care in the following ways: (1) across encounters or (2) within an encounter.

Continuity of Care Across Encouters Continuity of care across encounters in an HMO is generally accomplished by having each HMO member pick a primary care physician or by assigning each member to a care team. When the patient comes in for care, the patient would be appointed with the primary care physician or a member of the care team. For continuing care with specialists (e.g., urologists, opthalmologists, or gynecologists) in an HMO, patients are most often appointed with the same specialist.

Independent of whether the patient primarily sees one caregiver, sees a care team, or sees many unaffiliated caregivers, patient care can be improved if there is better communication between the many or even the same caregiver as the caregivers treat the patient across many visits or hospital stays. The automated patient medical record is one vehicle for improving this communication.

To facilitate continuity of care across encounters, a caregiver should be able to identify only those encounters of interest to the caregiver. For example, a ophthalmologist may only be interested in encounters involving eye problems. A primary care physician in a patient's care team might be interested in all encounters within the care team.

To facilitate continuity of care across encounters, a caregiver should also be able to identify all encounters that are part of the same treatment plan. Such a series of encounters is called an *episode*. Possible ways of doing this are relating encounters in the patient medical record, for example by use of *case management* techniques or use of *clinical pathways*.

For high risk and costly medical conditions where tracking care is of importance, case management can be used with assignment of a case manager, either tracking a set of encounters (1) for a particular medical condition for a patient or (2) for all encounters.

A clinical pathway is a structured way to identify care activities and caregiver workflow needed to care for a patient with a particular condition or disease. Paths through a clinical pathway can be adjusted for the particular needs of an individual patient and updated as they change.

Through clinical pathways and cases, there is the potential to coordinate caregivers better within one outpatient visit, within one inpatient stay, or over any combination of inpatient stays and outpatient visits. Coordination of patient care can occur within one facility, a number of facilities, and potentially among care provided in multiple healthcare organizations. Care can be *multidisciplinary*, in other words, across multiple medical departments. This coordination promotes the team approach to providing patient care.

Continuity of Care within an Encounter Continuity of care within a stay in the hospital is clearly important as many different caregivers are involved. But continuity of care also applies to a single outpatient encounter.

If a patient talks to an advice nurse over the phone to seek advice and this sets up a subsequent outpatient visit with a physician or nurse practitioner, then the physician or nurse practitioner should know everything pertinent that occurred during the advice nurse phone call. This allows the physician or nurse to prepare for the visit and to spend her time more productively with the patient.

A diagnosis for an outpatient visit is often not completed until the results of a physician order come back, for example, the results of a clinical laboratory test, an interpretation of an x-ray, or the results of a procedure. Thus care extends beyond the time of the face-to-face meeting with the patient.

An automated patient medical record that associates all these care activities with the outpatient visit provides a more complete picture of the care given than one that does not.

5.3.1.5 Caregiver Ordering Through the Automated Patient Medical Record System

Caregivers, most often, physicians order tests or procedures from ancillary departments (e.g., blood tests or urine tests from the clinical laboratory, x-rays from radiology) with results being returned back from the ancillary department (e.g., blood or urine test values, or the analysis of the x-ray). With an automated patient medical record system, *orders* can be sent directly to the performing department through the system with *results* returned electronically, with automatic inclusion of both order and results in the automated patient medical record.

With automated ordering, tests can be ordered much more quickly than with a physician order sheet that is on paper. Orders and results could be automatically and immediately recorded in the patient medical record. The caregiver could be immediately informed of abnormal, STAT or panic results—*STAT* means needed immediately.

A caregiver ordering a treatment could be informed of costs, risks (e.g., side effects, interactions) and other factors in selection of treatments. The caregiver could immediately inform the patient, thus enabling the patient and caregiver to make wise joint decisions.

Clinical checking of medication orders can be done by the automated system as the order is input, including checking for wrong doses, wrong choices, wrong techniques, delays, known allergies, missed doses, wrong drugs, drug-drug interactions, wrong frequencies, and wrong routes. Body surface area, intravenous, pediatric, parenteral or other types of calculations for medication dosage determination can be provided, allowing these calculations to be documented (Pickar 1993). Prescriptions can be printed so mistakes due to poor handwriting and similarly named medications can be avoided. And ordered medications can be checked against the diagnosis—A report from the National Academy of Sciences' Institute of Medicine estimated that 44,000 to 98,000 people die annually due to mistakes by medical personnel, mainly in improper ordering and administration of medication (O'Conner 1999).

5.3.1.6 Evidence-Based Medicine

Treatments should be based upon the best medical evidence that they work. This is done by looking at treatments and the results of these treatments: their *outcomes*. Measuring outcomes based upon treatments is a way of evaluating treatments.

Use of the treatments and practices for diseases—*clinical practice guidelines*—that produce the best outcomes for the least cost as determined by the best scientific evidence is called *evidence-based medicine*. The automated patient medical record system could assist in two ways: (1) informing caregivers of the best treatments and practices for a disease, also called *best practice guidelines*, and (2) recording treatments and outcomes, thus enabling future evaluation of clinical practice guidelines.

The Agency for Health Care Policy and Research (AHCPR), a government agency, established a *National Guideline Database* of clinical practice guidelines for treatment of a number of medical conditions in association with private and public healthcare organizations based upon the best available scientific evidence (AHCPR 2004). This database has been superseded by the *National Guideline Clearinghouse*, a database that includes clinical guidelines from a number of medical organizations, including the Agency for Healthcare Policy and Research, the American Academy of Dermatology, the American Academy of Pediatrics, the American Cancer Society, the American College of Emergency Physicians, etc. (NGC 1998-2004).

HMOs might want to do their own determination of best practice guidelines. These HMO guidelines can provide additional guidelines to be used in the HMO together with the *National Guideline Clearinghouse* guidelines.

The automated patient medical record system could record actual outcomes to evaluate treatments for diseases. Some current outcome measures can be considered subjective while others are objective. Some groups consider outcomes to be related to the patient's perception of his or her health. A good outcome occurs for a disease (e.g., knee replacement or benign prostatic hypertrophy) if the patient's perception of his quality of life is good. A patient questionnaire—SF-36 (36-item short form) or HAQ (Health Assessment Questionnaire) (Fries and colleagues 2004) are existing ones—is used to measure such outcomes. Some outcomes are more directly measurable, such as a decrease in the patient's (systolic and diastolic) blood pressure, x-rays showing the healing of a broken arm or leg, the urinary flow rate or percentage of the bladder that is emptied upon urination to measure benign prostatic hypertrophy, or one year survival rate after a liver transplant.

5.3.1.7 Preventive Care

Preventive care are interventions directed toward preventing illness and promoting health. Automation of the patient medical record enables the HMO to establish preventive care programs (e.g., immunizations, cholesterol screening, blood pressure testing, weight control and stop smoking programs, flu shots, mammography, pap smears with human papillomavirus testing, breast exams, flex sigmoidoscopy, colonoscopy, tetanus shots, and diabetic retinal screening exams). A number of these preventive health measures have been shown to provide better medical care for the patient in that they catch diseases early on so they can be more easily be cured; also, many such preventive health measures have been shown to save an HMO money in the long run.

A clinical pathway covering the patient over the patient's life time (called a "life care path") can be set up to automatically send out "outreach" letters to a patient to come in to the HMO for a specific preventive care exam, with determination of which exams and how often to send out such letters being based upon the patient's sex, age, family history, social history and current health. Also as part of an outreach program, the automated patient medical record could identify pregnant women who came in for care, but who should be encouraged to come in for ongoing prenatal care.

Some preventive care can be supported by what I call trend documents. A *trend document* is a document that automatically records a value or values that a caregiver wants to track over time as the value(s) are input via other clinician documents—over time, caregivers could be reminded to capture this information. For example, a trend document could capture blood pressures, diagnostic images of a knee with degenerative osteoarthritis, the height for a child who is shorter than other children in her age group, and PSA values for detection of prostate cancer.

A trend document has the potential of being a valuable tool in preventive health care, diagnosing diseases early on and predicting the progress of diseases. It is also a valuable tool in patient education in demonstrating to the patient the progress of a disease. Dangerous health conditions can be potentially recognized by the automated system and automatically reported to the primary care physician, who could have the patient come in to be checked.

Currently, with a paper patient medical record, much of the information that could be in a trend document is lost for various reasons:

1. Older paper charts are archived or destroyed.
2. Charts may be fragmented such as shown in figure 5.2.
3. Diagnostic images, because of the space they consume, are often destroyed after a shorter period of time than the rest of the chart.

With an automated patient medical record, medical information referenced by a trend document can be kept immediately available, no matter how old.

5.3.1.8 Predicting Diseases and Individualized Treatments

According to the Journal of the American Medical Association (JAMA), "Individuals are born with a relatively fixed genetic status that in combination with environmental factors determines the propensities for a variety of disease states" (Kajii and Leiden 2001). According to IBM who is using computers to do gene research: DNA information for an individual, " . . . will probably become a key component of medical diagnostics and even individualized medical treatments, which tune a medical treatment or drug protocol to the genetic makeup of an individual and his or her medical condition (Swope 2001)."

Because identifying a patient's genetic make-up is a time consuming process, determining it and recording it only once would be the most cost-effective approach. If an individual allows recording of this information, then it makes sense to store it along the person's complete medical history. An automated patient medical record could contain both sets of information.

With the total of the patient's genetic information digitized and recorded in one place, then it would be available for any future genetic analysis based upon the future knowledge of the functions of particular genes. With a patient's genetic information, a complete medical and environmental history, and perhaps with trend documents tracking trends in indicators of disease, there will be a greater potential of predicting disease.

These indicators for disease are called biomarkers. *Biomarkers* for disease are "cellular, biochemical, molecular, or genetic characteristics or alterations by which a normal, abnormal, or simply biologic process can be recognized, or monitored (NIH 2004)." An individual's genome could provide permanent biomarkers while other biomarkers might change over time. Through biomarkers for various diseases, diseases could potentially be diagnosed or predicted. An automated patient medical record is a place where such biomarkers for an individual could be stored.

With disease prediction becoming more of a reality, a caregiver must be cognizant of the patient's values. A values questionnaire could collect this values information by asking questions of a patient such as the following: "If medical science was able to predict that you will develop a particular disease, would you like to know in advance? Would this depend upon the type of disease?" Such values questionnaires currently exist for end-of-life decisions—see section 5.3.2.4—and they should be available for other major medical decisions also.

5.3.1.9 Assistance in Clinical Research

Patient care can be improved by more thorough clinical research with larger patient populations. Clinical research can involve an investigation of a new method, medication, or procedure in the treatment of a particular disease or condition in comparison with a current, high-quality, standard method of care for that disease or condition.

With automation of the patient medical record there is likely to be much more medical information available to the researcher. This information could be made available without identifying the patients or caregivers, thus not compromising patient or caregiver privacy. This allows for very large-scale investigations. Removing information that identifies a patient from the patient medical record is called *de-identification*—see section 13.9.2.

Automation of the patient medical record also enables very long-term, longitudinal, studies, spanning from infancy to adulthood. For example, a longitudinal study enables determination of what in infancy or childhood is predictive of what happens in adulthood—For example, do temper tantrums in childhood have any relationship to bi-polar disorders later on in life? Doing such research with paper medical records would not be possible, as the volume of paper records over such a long time would swamp chart rooms, and finding the required information in these paper records would be very difficult. Large capacity storage devices and automated information searching methods make such longitudinal research feasible with automated patient medical records.

With an automated patient medical record, it is also easier to pick ideal target patient populations for research (e.g., patients with a targeted condition and no others, or patients who do not currently take medications which make it difficult to evaluate a new medication). This may increase the validity of the research.

Also, an automated system enables quick dissemination of the results of pertinent clinical research to caregivers.

5.3.2 Promote HMO Member Satisfaction

An automated patient medical record could promote HMO member and patient satisfaction in the following ways:

1. Provide personalized care and care tailored to the individual.
2. Provide patient-centered care for high-risk patients
3. Improve member access to care
4. Enable the patient and the patient's family to more fully participate in the care process.

5.3.2.1 Personalized Care

HMO member satisfaction can be improved by providing members with personalized care. Personalized care includes the following:

1. **Primary care physicians:** Having the patient select a primary care physician who knows the patient and records and keeps an up-to-date medical history of the patient and is responsible for overseeing care of the patient.
2. **Individualized treatments:** Providing treatment individualized to the patient.
3. **A personalized profile of the patient:** Providing information, a *personal profile*, to caregivers that enables them to more quickly and better serve an individual patient.

Primary Care Physicians When an HMO member first joins the HMO, he or she should select a *primary care physician* who meets with the patient to discuss and record the patient's health problems and concerns. *Primary care* is a department such as internal medicine, pediatrics for children, and sometimes obstetrics/gynecology for women, which would be the first point of contact in the HMO for a given episode of illness. The assigned primary care caregivers would be responsible for overseeing and coordinating all aspects of a patient's care; with an automated patient medical record, primary care caregivers would have the potential to oversee care no matter where it occurred, inside or outside the healthcare organization. Another term for such an assigned primary care phyisician is a *personal physician.*

Individualized Treatments Individualized treatment means that treatment is tailored to the individual. The automated patient medical record could insure the recording of information that could provide this individualized care, for example, care based upon:

- **The genetic makeup of the patient:** In the future, individualized medications and treatments for a patient can potentially be based upon the genetic makeup of the individual, providing more effective medications and treatments.
- **A patient s values:** The caregiver must consider the specific needs and values of the patient to determine the best treatment. For example, a medication prescribed to a terminally ill patient that keeps the patient alive but away from interacting with his relatives may not be appropriate.
- **Side effects of medications:** An ongoing record of a medication's side effects on a patient could help the caregiver and patient identify medications that could harm the patient. The replacement of one medication by another may have dramatic positive effects upon the patient's life (e.g., the new medication might no longer result in the patient being drowsy all of the time).

Personal Profile of the Patient Knowing what the patient considers important can also provide personalized care. What does the patient consider to be his or her most significant ongoing medical problem? Is she a mother and what are the names of her children? What is his or her wife or husband's name? What else is important to him or her? What ongoing specialty care is the patient being seen for? The HMO knowing this information enables caregivers in the HMO to more quickly identify ongoing medical problems, appoint the member's family members more quickly, and get the patient in for care more quickly.

5.3.2.2 Patient-Centered Care for High Risk Patients: Guardian Angel and Monitoring Systems

HMO member satisfaction with care can be improved by providing "patient-centered care" for patients with high-risk medical conditions. Such a patient could be given a computer system, perhaps a small computer using a pen for input (a *personal digital assistant* or *PDA*), for use outside the healthcare organization, at home or away from home, that can be used to monitor the patient's health either via patient input or instrumentation input. The PDA based system could give advice, health education and therapy plans to the patient, inform the patient of appointments or inform the patient to schedule appointments. The system could interface with the automated patient medical record to alarm physicians or other caregivers of critical situations. This approach has been used in the *Guardian Angel systems* at MIT (Szolovits et al. 1994) for patients with the following medical conditions: insulin-dependent diabetes, hypertension, angina, chronic anticoagulation, chronic renal disease, and pulmonary disease (COPD).

Similar patient-centered systems in the hospital are computerized equipment connected to patients in the coronary and respiratory ICU. These systems, like Guardian Angel systems, are *monitoring systems*. Such monitoring systems may collect a large amount of information from the patient. To feasibly store this information in the automated patient medical record, information, such as waveforms or input directly from patients, must be filtered, analyzed and selected for inclusion or not. As a result of the analysis, an alarm could be sent to a caregiver when a critical situation occurs. Enough additional information, besides the critical data, must be preserved to put the reasons for an alarm into context.

A less complicated version of a "Guardian Angel" system is a PDA that could be given to an elderly HMO member taking lots of medications, to inform the patient when a medication is to be taken. The member would need to respond, perhaps by a simple message box, when the medication was taken, with information on this sent to the automated patient medical record. If the member does not respond for a critical medication, he or she could be reminded by telephone. (It is estimated that 7-9% of admissions to hospitals are due to complications from medications.)

5.3.2.3 Improved Member Access to Care

HMO member satisfaction with care can be improved by removing bottlenecks or roadblocks to the member receiving care.

The most significant bottleneck removed by an automate patient medical record is the time taken by caregivers to receive the patient's medical record. The patient would no longer have to wait for receipt of the paper medical record before receiving care, especially in the emergency department or urgent care clinics. The caregiver would no longer have to wait for the patient's medical record in order to approve medication refills requested by phone.

An automated system could also cut down on paperwork and time to input medical information. With the availability of a medical history kept up-to-date by the previous caregivers who saw the patient, the medical history could be much more quickly updated. Insurance forms could be filled in based upon care recorded in the automated record.

Certain care activities could be pre-scheduled, either generically or for individual patients. Via a clinical pathway, events to handle a particular emerging medical condition could be pre-defined. For example, when a patient comes due to a stroke, activities to care for the stroke could be automately initiate, which may include scheduling of a CAT Scan or MRI.

Care activities can be pre-scheduled for members who come in for recurrent emergent care. For example, for a child with epilepsy, the patient's caregiver could inform the emergency department of the patient's arrival, identifying a particular predetermined care situation and an estimated time of arrival. This could be done by telephone and through the automated patient medical record system. This could initiate a clinical pathway that schedules all the necessary events to handle the emergency department visit. The clinical pathway could result in the patient's case manager being called and the initiation of care documentation; it could then keep an ongoing record of completed activities during the emergency department visit.

In creating and implementing the automated patient medical record, medical centers may have to be reengineered to accommodate automation and new caregiver workflows. In this process, further bottlenecks to patient access to care could be removed.

5.3.2.4 Greater Participation of the Patient and His Family in the Care Process

HMO member satisfaction with care could be improved by the greater participation of the patient and his family in his own care.

The patient should be given clear caregiver instructions on follow-up activities and care. The best quality medical care is useless if the patient does not comply with caregiver's instructions.

This can occur because the patient does not remember or understand the caregiver's instructions, because the information is not communicated clearly to the patient, or because the treatment does not fit into the life of the patient. If the patient does not follow his doctor's orders then he might as well have seen the doctor.

After a patient outpatient visit, the physician could complete his or her visit documentation and have orders and instructions for the patient and family printed out for a medical assistant or nurse, who could give it to the patient and review it with the patient or family members. Easy-to-read and understandable written instructions that the patient could keep with him or her would help with compliance. Where the patient and his family does not understand English, it may be appropriate for these instructions to be written in the language of the patient (e.g., Spanish, Chinese).

The printed document could explain the diagnosis, what the patient needs to do to get or keep healthy, and what medications have been prescribed or tests have been ordered. This is a document that is in the language the patient understands, matching the medical sophistication and interest level of the patient.

Also, after results of clinical laboratory tests came back, these results could be printed along with normal ranges of values and the meaning of the results. A physician can then either call the patient to discuss the results or send these results to the patient after possibly adding additional comments to the results.

Especially for patients taking multiple medications, help with scheduling of medications could be provided by the automated system. Where the required dosage of the medication has increased significantly and has made the taking of a medication possibly unmanageable, the caregiver could be informed by the automated system with alternative medication choices or dosages; for example, if the patient is taking several medications that are taken 2 times a day and the caregiver prescribes one to be taken 3 times a day, then the automated system could inform the caregiver of this potential conflict.

At the end of a hospital stay, a discharge summary is created. Although this is both for caregivers, and for the patient and the patient's family, a discharge summary should be generated for the patient which describes in clear language, restrictions and follow-up activities.

During a hospital stay or after an outpatient visit, the patient could be given an up-to-date FAQs sheet on each condition she or he is being treated for (e.g., pneumonia, pressure ulcers, etc.) printed through the automated system (FAQ stands for "frequently asked questions".) The sheet should be compatible with a *National Guideline Clearinghouse* guideline used for the condition.

Younger patients require the support of their family members in the care process. Other patients may also want the support of their family members. Information produced for the patient could be in a form useable by a patient's family, as well as the patient.

A patient or authorized family member should also have direct access to his actual medical record. Providing the patient with information from his medical record would enable the patient or family member to check for the accuracy of information and correct any inaccuracies. When the patient is verbally told information during a visit, a patient can insure that this is recorded in the chart. Accuracy of information in the patient medical record would facilitate later evaluation of clinical outcomes.

Full disclosure also opens up another possibility: that a patient could become significantly more involved in his own care and treatment. Patients may want to get a much better knowledge about the details of their medical conditions and treatments, as stated in their medical records, and have a stronger influence on how their care is handled.

This process is already occurring in many different ways. The gay community has had a big impact on new treatments for AIDS/HIV. Societies have sprung up for diseases as diverse as psoriasis and breast cancer; often, members of these societies know much more about research in the area of their medical interest than all but a few physicians. Lots of medical information, though not always accurate, is available on the Internet. Andy Grove, the CEO of Intel, has used his scientific research background to do an analysis of the treatments for prostate cancer, a disease he contracted (Grove 1996). Ideally, such societies, patients, laypersons, physicians and researchers can all support each other.

Through an automated system, up-to-date medical references of all kinds would be available. These could potentially include medical references for the patient to increase the patient's understanding of his medical conditions. On-line multi-media presentations to demonstrate medical conditions and procedures could potentially be available—These multi-media presentations could be made available at the patient's home through the Internet. The automated system could tell a caregiver when a patient education classes at the HMO might be beneficial for a patient.

An *advance directive* enables a patient to participate in his or her care when the patient is unconscious or otherwise incapacitated. Again, advance directives are written instructions a patient has prepared for medical personnel to inform them of the patient's wishes for treatments and care when the patient is incapacitated.

(Seriously ill patients and their families should be encouraged to discuss end of life decisions and the idea of assigning a *surrogate* or *proxy decision maker* for the patient via a *healthcare proxy*. A *values history questionnaire* eliciting a patient's own personal view of care at the end of life—such as appears in the book *Handbook for Mortals: Guidance for People Facing Serious Illness* (Lynn, Harrold, and University 1999)—can be used to assist family members in these discussions.)

5.3.3 Support Healthcare Workers and Improve Their Efficiency

The automated patient medical record system can make healthcare workers jobs easier and give them more time to care for patients. The automated patient medical record system can improve healthcare workers' efficiency in their care for patients and can improve a caregivers' satisfaction with their jobs.

5.3.3.1 HMO Caregiver Satisfaction

HMO caregiver satisfaction is a product of

- the caregiver receiving a decent salary
- the caregiver having a good working environment*
- the caregiver having an opportunity of making a difference in the healthcare organization*
- the caregiver's work activities matching the most productive and least stressful methods of providing care*.

Automation of the patient medical record can have a positive effect on those items with *'s. Reengineering of patient care with strong caregiver input, removing roadblocks and creating a less stressful atmosphere for caregivers, could greatly improve caregiver satisfaction.

With an automated patient medical record, strong support for provider workflow management could be provided. For example, it is known that providing a list of patients of interest to each caregiver that provides quick access to a patient's medical record provides enormous benefits to a caregiver in managing his workflow.

5.3.3.2 Automated Assistance to the Caregiver in Providing Care

The automated patient medical record system could improve the efficiency of caregivers by providing automated assistance with patient care.

With the automation of the patient medical record, information that is input to the patient medical record can be validated as it is input. Consistent terminology could be checked for and enforced as it is input by the caregiver. Legibility of information is guaranteed.

With ordering through the automated medical record system, orders could be made more quickly, with automatic return of results to the patient's medical record. Clinical checking of orders could be done to check for mistakes in orders.

The system could alert caregivers of patients with special needs or situations, for example,

- a paraplegic patient who needs extra time and someone to lift her out of her chair
- a patient who has a care or case manager
- a "drug jumper" who goes from one facility to another to try to get narcotics
- a potentially violent patient.

The system could inform a caregiver if an "at risk" patient is not complying with a drug regimen (e.g., by not picking up a prescribed medication or by not ordering refills within a specified time period) (Scott 1996). The system could inform the caregiver if the patient fails to keep important appointments or does not show up for an important diagnostic test.

Various other forms of assistance can be provided to the caregiver in the care of the patient. The system could automatically alert a caregiver of changes in a patient's health that are indicative of future health problems (e.g., changes in low-density lipoproteins, LDL, and high-density lipoproteins, HDL, for evaluation of serum cholesterol, blood pressure beyond normal age related values, clusters of a particular disease, etc.); for example, the system could inform a caregiver of trends in the patient's health based upon measurements taken over a period of time (e.g., increase in blood pressure over time). The automated system could assist the caregiver in making diagnoses. Duplication of tests can be immediately recognized. The automated patient medical record could inform the caregiver of *National Guideline Clearinghouse* best practice guidelines and additional HMO determined guidelines for care for various medical conditions.

On-line medical references, including those on the Internet, an Intranet or an Extranet (i.e., the Internet restricted to inside the HMO or inside the healthcare community), can be accessed during display of the automated patient medical record and during the input of information to the chart. Such on-line medical information may or may not be specific to the organization (e.g., the organizational drug formulary; organizational protocols and practice guidelines; DME formulary; poisons information; pre-travel vaccinations; CDC prevention guidelines for advising patients on how to prevent diseases such sexually transmitted diseases, hepatitis, bicycle injuries (Frieda et al. 1997), National Library of Medicine (NLM) database Medline (NIH 2004); or composite systems such as Micromedex). A physician or other caregiver should be able to subscribe to videos over the Internet to present new updates in treatments, diagnostic tests, or other aspects of patient care in the scope of care of the caregiver.

The automated patient medical record system would ideally tie together all existing clinical systems (the ADT system, the ordering system, the pharmacy system, the clinical laboratory system, etc.) and, over time, will require integration of additional non-clinical systems (e.g., inventory, financial) in order to completely automate the patient medical record. Entrance of information in one of the systems would flow to the others and may be recorded in the chart. As a result, the patient would not be asked for the same information over and over again and care of the patient could be completed much faster.

Automation of the patient medical record would allow the physician to communicate with a patient at any time regarding the patient's medical condition, emphasizing care decisions, and thus promoting greater compliance with these decisions. The physician would no longer have to wait for the patient medical record before communication with the patient over the telephone or via e-mail.

For significant procedure or test results, the physician can call the patient and have the automated patient record on-line to view. In all cases, results could be printed along with normal ranges of values and the meaning of the results (e.g., a high PSA value may be a result of prostate cancer, an enlarged prostate, or prostate infection); the results could be expressed in terminology understood by the patient and the physician could add his or her comments and send the results to the patient.

5.3.3.3 Reducing and Simplifying Documentation

Types of medical documents currently existing in a paper patient medical record are described in chapter 4 of this book. These would be replaced by automated documentation with simplified input of information, including by the following methods:

1. **Templates and abbreviations in progress notes:** During the time a caregiver enters a progress note, the problem can be selected from pick lists. A textual template for the identified problem (e.g., migraine headache) can be used, where the physician can fill in the blanks in the textual template or select from pick lists embedded in the template. Alternatively, when the caregiver enters textual information for the progress note, there is system assurance of use of a standardized medical vocabulary, and entrance of caregiver or organization determined abbreviations to expand to the full word (e.g., "AE" for "above elbow", "t.o." for "telephone order", "appy" for "appendectomy"). Caregivers can devise their own templates and abbreviation schemes, or organizations can devise templates and abbreviations for use in all caregiver notes.
2. **Entrance by exception :** Another method of simplifying documentation is to have information "entered by exception" by the system, with the user only entering information when it changes—This is call *entrance by exception*. For example, within a flow sheet entered every hour, an inpatient nurse might record inpatient status information including skin color (e.g., pale), heart rhythm (e.g., normal), pain? (e.g., yes), and nausea? (e.g., no), with the information for the current hour being assumed by the system to be the same as for the previous hour unless there was a change in status.

   "Entrance by exception" also applies to progress notes. A template describing a problem in detail might be used in a progress note that covers a large percentage of cases of that problem, where the caregiver would only need to make changes in small portions of the text that do not apply to the current problem.
3. **Automated clinical pathways:** A clinical pathway for a given medical condition identifies the care to be given over time for the medical condition based upon the outcomes of treatments given over time. Clinical pathways can include prewritten physicians' orders. Physician orders would be embedded in the clinical pathway describing normal treatment guidelines based upon outcomes. The clinical pathway would identify outcomes that are routine. Additional narrative documentation would only be required when there were variances from a normal expected outcome. Thus clinical pathways have the potential of significantly reducing the time to input information.

4. **Trend tracking:** By setting up automatic graphing of a measured variable over time (e.g., blood pressure, weight, height, serum cholesterol), perhaps together with a graph of normal age related values for these variables, any caregiver can quickly identify long term trends in a patient's health; this is what I have termed a *trend document*. For a caregiver to manually produce such a document would require much work.
5. **Automation of nursing diagnoses, interventions and outcomes:** At the start of an inpatient stay, nurses identify nursing diagnoses, patient problems identified through assessment findings in comparison with what is considered to be normal. For example, one nursing diagnosis might be "urinary retention". Nursing interventions that can be performed to alleviate or treat the diagnosis are identified (e.g., patient education on medication or catheterization) and expected outcomes of these interventions during the stay are identified (e.g., absence of urinary infection, recognition of urge to void). These interactions and outcomes could be made part of a nursing care plan for the stay identifying the timing of interventions and expected outcomes. The University of Iowa has identified a comprehensive set of nursing diagnoses, interventions, and outcomes (Johnson et al. 2000); additionally, they provide information on how these nursing diagnoses, interventions and outcomes all interrelate. Together, these classifications—referred to as *NANDA (North American Nursing Diagnosis Association) diagnoses*, *NIC (Nursing Intervention Classifications) interventions* and *NOC (Nursing Outcomes Classifications) outcomes*—could be computerized to automate the generation of nursing care plans as part of the automated patient medical record system.
6. **Patient tailoring:** Further ways to assist the caregiver in the documentation process is to have flow sheets, care plans, clinical pathways and other documents that could be tailored specifically for the patient. Non-applicable information for the patient could be excluded.
7. **Interfacing of systems to eliminate redundant entry of information:** An automated patient medical record system requires information that is also needed by other HMO clinical systems. This information includes proper patient identification information such as names, phone numbers and addresses; the start and end times of encounters; and orders and their results. As part of the automated patient medical record project, HMO clinical systems could be networked to share this information. As a result, caregivers would no longer be required to enter the same information multiple times in multiple HMO clinical systems. Inconsistent entrance of information would be eliminated.

5.3.3.4 Better Utilization of Caregiver Time

Automating paper-based systems would result in better use of personnel directly caring for the patient. Thirty percent of the time spent in the care of an inpatient is spent on filling out paperwork for the patient chart. As a result of less redundant entry of information and of use of "charting by exception" and other techniques, there will be significantly less time in such paperwork by nurses and unit assistants. Completely or partially automated coding and grouping of discharge diagnoses, procedures and supplies for inpatients and outpatients (ICD, CPT, DRG codes) is also potentially possible, substituting for the manual process.

Without an automated patient medical record and ordering system, there is significant paperwork involved in the care of a patient, especially in the ordering process. The physician writes the order on a paper order form, which is either given to the patient, a unit assistant, courier, or other employee and is transferred to the pharmacy, laboratory or other performing area. The performing area may then re-enter the order in its computers. For the clinical laboratory, radiology department or other performing area, results might later be printed and returned by courier to the physician, with the billing office sent a copy of the test to charge the patient or insurance company. Without an automated patient medical record and ordering system, inpatient medication orders are re-written on a paper medication administration record (MAR) in the unit, with a copy of the MAR later sent to the billing office; the billing office might then re-enter charges in their system.

With an automated patient medical record and ordering system, time and personnel costs of this paper flow would be greatly reduced. The physician's automated order would be sent in seconds to the pharmacy, laboratory, radiology or other performing area. Prior to sending, the order could be checked for drug interactions, allergic reactions, safe dosages, duplicate tests, etc., and the order could be corrected immediately, instead of later, making it unnecessary for later costly interactions between the performing department and the physician. Once a clinical laboratory test was completed, diagnostic image analyzed and transcribed, etc., results would be immediately sent back to the ordering caregiver, with charges sent automatically to the billing office. Inpatient medications could be immediately updated to the MAR automatically by the computerized system; when a nurse recorded a medication as taken on the MAR, the system would automatically send the charges to the billing office. If an outpatient did not have a test done, did not pick up a prescription, did not call in for a refill when an expected time period or did not have a procedure done, the ordering caregiver could be alerted of possible non-compliance with the order and call up the patient, possibly saving extra visits, avoiding future health complications and insuring against malpractice suits. With automated ordering, time spent by nurses, physicians, pharmacists, and others in verifying illegible orders would be saved.

Because the patient medical record would always be available, a physician would be able to authoritatively provide advice over the phone, possibly substituting a phone call for a more costly face-to-face meeting, consequently better using the physician's time.

The patient can be more quickly discharged, as the attending physician and other caregivers could be alerted that a discharge is pending, so a meeting with the patient for patient instructions can be scheduled and completed, discharge medications received, and follow-on procedures, tests, medications and appointments can be scheduled. Prior to discharge, caregivers can be informed of which discharge activities and documents are outstanding.

5.3.3.5 Special Assistance for Radiologists and Other Caregivers Doing Interpretations

Patient care can be improved by digitization of diagnostic images and digitization of test results that require interpretation so that these diagnostic images and test results can be quickly sent across networks to radiologists and other physicians who can interpret them, analyzing them for indications of abnormalities and possible disease. Examples include mammographies, fluorescein angiographies and pulmonary test results. Once completed, interpretations can immediately be sent back over the network directly to the automated patient medical record with the ordering physician being informed. Thus, the time lag between taking a diagnostic image or performing a test and receipt of the interpretation results can be greatly reduced for the ordering physician and for the patient.

Standards for transmission of diagnostic images are the DICOM (Digital Imaging and Communications) standards recognized by the American College of Radiology (NEMA 1993).

Digitization of diagnostic images also allows physicians doing interpretations to be assisted by computerized algorithms that would enable computer recognition of diseases, such as detection of cancers within mammographies.

Because diagnostic images take up a lot of space in chart rooms, they are kept for a shorter period of time than other parts of the patient medical record. Digitization enables efficient storage of diagnostic images, storing the diagnostic images on Picture Archiving and Communications

Systems (PACS). This makes it more cost effective to keep past diagnostic images around, thus promoting the ability to compare past diagnostic images with current ones, which can be useful in visually showing the progress of some diseases (e.g., degeneration of cartilage within the knee or the spread of cancer within the body).

5.3.4 Make and Save Money

An automated patient medical record could make and save money for the HMO.

5.3.4.1 Reengineering to Decrease the Cost of Patient Care

Chapter 11 discusses reengineering of the HMO, changing HMO employee workflows for greater efficiency and for cost savings. During the analysis of the changed workflows with an automated patient medical record, costly processes within the HMO can be identified, and eliminated or modified.

When discharge documentation is automated—or even when it is scanned in—then discharge processes can be done concurrently rather than all sequentially with passing around of the paper chart. This enables the patient to be discharged quicker and bills to outside insurance companies to be sent out quicker, both saving the HMO money. Figure 5.3 shows the discharge activities when a paper chart needs to be passed around and the discharge activities when there is an automated patient medical record or when documents have been scanned and are concurrently available (Yackel 2002).

5.3.4.2 Demand Management

In an HMO, one major way of cutting costs is referred to as *demand management* (Schlier 1996), a system to provide a patient with the most cost-effective care for the patient's medical complaint, by instructing a patient in self-care when appropriate, by "triaging" the patient to the most cost-effective caregiver for the medical condition, and by coordinating the care given when there are multiple caregivers. Demand management in an HMO was discussed in the previous chapter.

The following are examples of the ways an automated patient medical record could support demand management:

1. **Support for advice nurses:** The automated patient medical record could be available to advice nurses, providing summaries of the member's health problems, medications, past encounters, etc. This would assist the advice nurse in advising the patient on self-care, whether to come in or not, and whether to come in on an emergency basis or urgent basis.
2. **Support for caregiver direct communication with patients:** The automated patient medical record would be immediately available to physicians, nurse practitioners, physician's assistants and physicians' nurses, rather than having to be ordered, supporting direct communication with the patient over the telephone, which might save on the cost of a more costly face to face visit.
3. **Coordination of care for acute medical conditions:** It could support case management techniques to coordinate care between primary caregivers, specialists and others in care of a patient for an acute medical condition, clearly combining all documentation for the acute condition in one place and clearly identifying the overall treatment plan. This coordinates the care between caregivers and enables evaluation of the best, most cost effective, medical practices for a type of acute medical condition.
4. **Coordination of care for high risk patients:** It could support case management techniques to coordinate care for a high risk patient, for an elderly Medicare patient, for a

patient being treated for workman's compensation claims, for a pregnant woman, or for or a patient with a high impact medical condition (e.g., diabetes), with assignment of the case to a case manager. The case manager would coordinate care and insure that the most cost-effective care was given to the patient.

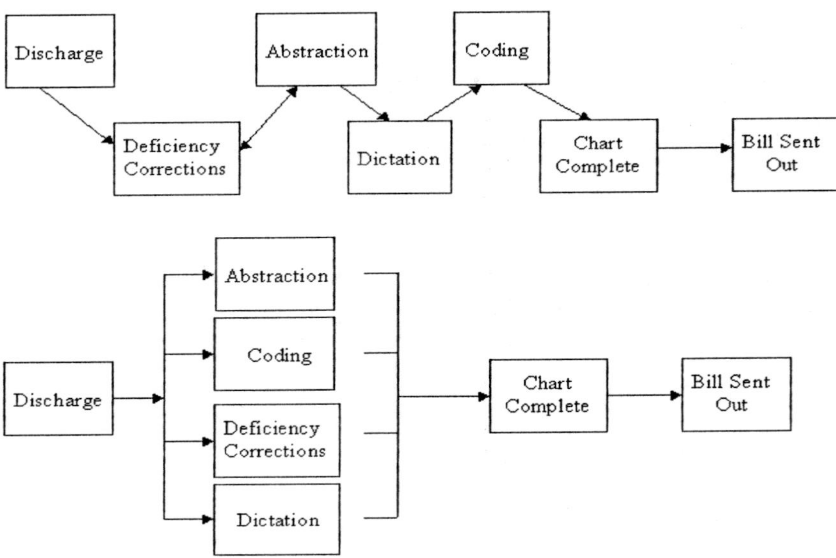

Figure 5.3 Serial and Parallel Workflow of Discharge Before and After Automation (Yackel 2002).

5. **Preventive care:** It could support wellness programs through clinical pathways based upon an individual's age, sex and medical condition that would automatically send out letters to individuals advising them to come in for preventive care. Examples of such tests are mammographies to test for breast cancer and sigmoidoscopies and colonoscopies for test for colon cancer. As a result of these tests, medical conditions could be identified before they become much more costly to treat.

5.3.4.3 Direct Savings to the HMO

It is estimated that there are costs of between $7 and $8 for each time a paper chart is retrieved (Moad 1996). Storage of diagnostic images digitally could save on the approximate cost of $40 per diagnostic image film. These costs alone could potentially pay for automation of the chart over time.

It is estimated that 11% of tests are reordered because the previous tests cannot be found. Complete automation of the chart will eliminate this. Not only would the HMO save money, but the patient would be spared the discomfort of taking additional unnecessary tests.

Transcription time and associated costs could be saved. Time and costs to do ordering could be cut, as well as costs of transporting paper orders and paper returned results. Communication between caregivers could be speeded, and the process of oversight of nurse practitioners and physician assistants by supervising physicians could be facilitated. All this could also potentially allow more patients to be seen, saving the healthcare organization costs on number of clinicians required.

It is estimated that *adverse drug events (ADEs)* occurring after hospitalizations cost hospitals $2 billion dollars per year. Checking during physician order entry could reduce serious medication errors by half (Bates et al. 1998). These errors include wrong doses, wrong choices, wrong techniques, delays, known allergies, missed doses, wrong drugs, drug-drug interactions, wrong frequencies, and wrong routes.

Automation of the chart can assist the HMO in identifying medical fraud. *Drug jumping*, where a patient may go from clinic to clinic to deliberately get the same drug, can be detected. Medicare and Medicaid fraud can be detected—It is estimated that fraudulent Medicare and Medicaid claims cost taxpayers as much as $30 billion annually for the many types of fraud (Methvin 1995). Excessive drug prescriptions and other unusual situations can be automatically identified. Suspicious charges can automatically be flagged by the system, in particular when this involves payments by the HMO for outside medical services.

5.3.4.4 Support for Billing and Electronic Commerce

Money can be saved in the HMO by electronic billing and electronic commerce supported by the automated patient medical record and by automatic recording of charges for medical services. As services are recorded in the automated patient medical record, charges for these services can be calculated and recorded for billing purposes.

An HMO, even one supported primarily by capitation, collects money for patient care from many sources, including from Medicare, Workman's compensation, and insurance companies. An HMO also pays out money for outside medical services. In these processes, there is a need for billing, collection and payment information, much of which can be captured by the automated patient medical record system, including diseases, procedures, providers, supplies and medications for a patient.

From this same information, medical supplies can be automatically re-ordered to replenish hospital units when necessary.

Electronic Data Interchange (EDI) is a standard (1) for payments for services sent and received automatically over electronic networks and (2) for ordering medical supplies and drugs without operator intervention. EDI is a standard for transmitting structured data using agreed upon message standards by "trading partners", from a sender to a recipient, from the sending computer to the receiving computer (Leyland 1993). This transmission can occur over private networks, referred to as *value added networks*, or *VANs*. EDI is increasingly being done over the Internet using industry agreed-upon formats in a language called XML, which is part of the same family of languages as HTML.

EDI can support automated billing and collection of medical payments from the government and outside insurance agencies based upon services recorded by the automated patient chart system. EDI can support automatic ordering of medical supplies based upon consumption of supplies recorded in conjunction with the automated patient chart system.

To support electronic healthcare claims to Medicare, the U.S. government, through the Health Insurance Portability and Accountability Act of 1996 (*HIPAA*) (CMS 2004), has mandated standards for electronic claim forms and for provider identifiers, and in the future patient identifiers.

A third financial capability related to the automated patient medical record is caregiver ordering of *durable medical equipment* for a patient through outside companies (equipment leased or sold to patients for use in their homes, e.g., wheelchairs, walkers, canes) through outside companies. Durable medical equipment can be supported by electronic commerce over the Internet.

5.3.4.5 Automated Advice on Lesser Cost Best Medical Practices and Medications

Through an automated patient medical record system, a caregiver can be provided with advice on least cost best medical practices as determined by the evidence. The caregiver can be provided with advice on medications with equal or better benefits for lower cost.

Because best practice guidelines identify treatments that work the best, over time such treatments should result in lower costs. Further, best medical practices take into account costs in that if there are multiple treatments of equal benefit, then the most cost effective one would be chosen.

A managed care organization controls drug costs by having a *drug formulary*. A drug formulary lists prescription medications that are preferred for use by the health plan. The drugs listed are determined by outcomes research, selected by clinical and cost effectiveness. On the formulary, generic drugs are preferred over more expensive brand-name drugs, where a *generic drug* is a chemically equivalent copy of a brand-name drug.

Formularies are *closed* or *open*. An *open formulary* allows a physician to select both formulary and non-formulary medications. A *closed formulary* limits coverage to drugs in the formulary.

Often managed care organizations do not cover drugs or treatments that they consider to be experimental, those undergoing clinical trials outside the organization.

The automated patient medical record system could provide references to caregivers on best medical practices. And when a caregiver orders a medication that is not in the formulary, the automated system could advise the caregiver on less expensive equally effective medications in the formulary.

5.3.4.6 Providing Information for Future Planning

According to reference (Lundy 1996), one problem of most managed care organizations is that they cannot accurately determine the true costs of patient care and they cannot predict future growth, or non-growth, of the HMO. As a result, information for future planning of the HMO is not available, e.g., for calculation of optimal capitation fees. The automated patient medical record facilitates capture of this cost and growth prediction information for future planning.

The automated patient medical record system and other systems can accurately record (1) services, tests and procedures given to patients, (2) costs of supplies and medications dispensed, (3) provider time caring for patients, (4) numbers and types of hospitalizations and visits, and (5) trends in membership growth and patient utilization. As a result, the actual costs of patient care can be better determined and trends in utilization can be determined.

This information facilitates future planning of personnel requirements and of budgets. It facilitates determination of optimal capitation fees, for example to cover actual HMO costs or to increase or decrease membership.

5.3.4.7 Decreasing Data Processing Costs Through Standardization

From the discussion so far, it is clear that the automated patient medical record system will be receiving information from many clinical and financial data processing systems in the HMO. These include

1. **Encounter systems:** Encounters (inpatient stays, outpatient visits, emergency department visits, advice nurse calls, phone calls between a patient and a physician, home health visits, skilled nursing facility stays, etc.) can be used to organize the automated patient medical record.
2. **Ordering and results systems:** The automated patient medical record system can be interfaced with ordering and results systems to receive orders made by caregivers through

the automated patient medical record system and send results back to the caregiver through the automated patient medical record.

3. **Billing and financial systems:** Billing and financial systems can be interfaced with the automated patient medical record system to collect medical charges to bill insurance companies, employers of patients, and patients.

Interfacing these systems with the automated patient medical record system is a huge initial expense to the HMO, but also has the potential for long term savings to the HMO, especially an HMO as large as ours with many different such clinical and financial systems, if this interfacing can at the same time result in standardization of clinical systems and software throughout the HMO.

The potential savings of standardized clinical systems is in future software and hardware *maintenance* costs for these systems. Maintenance is the process of updating and changing an automated system after it is in use. The National Bureau of Standards publication, "Guidance on Software Maintenance" (Martin and Osborne) estimates that 60 to 70 percent of total software resources are spent upon maintenance, as opposed to buying or developing it. Reference (Pressman 1992) estimates that as much as 80 percent of an information system's budget will be allocated to maintenance costs.

If a clinical system of a particular type was replaced by a company standard clinical system of that type at the time it was interfaced with the automated patient medical record system, then the following potential maintenance savings could result:

- **Less cost for installing systems:** Installation of a new system for a new user would be less costly, as there would be only one installation procedure instead of many.
- **Less help desk and system support staff:** If a computer or software system went down, standardized procedures could be followed to bring the system back up or to provide help for a user.
- **Less system maintenance staff:** With fewer total clinical systems to support, less system maintenance staff would be needed for adding new system features or correcting bugs in systems.
- **Less cost for upgrading a type of clinical system:** Replacement of a type of clinical system by a more powerful, improved one would be significantly less costly, as systems in the HMO could be all replaced at the same time.

In order to replace clinical systems within the HMO, they may have to first be *decoupled.* Consider figure 5.4 with shows interfaces that might occur between clinical systems in an HMO.

When the various clinical systems are interfaced with the automated patient medical record system to provide encounter information needed to organize the patient medical record, to send caregiver orders to the clinical systems, and to receive back results of orders, then the clinical systems could be decoupled. Proprietary connections between systems could be removed creating standard interfaces for each type of clinical system in the HMO, removing specialized connections between systems and creating ones where any system needing the information can get it. In such a setup, clinical systems become more independent (see figure 5.5). One of many possible ways of interfacing these clinical systems is through a computer referred to as an *interface engine* to which each of the clinical systems is connected.

In creating this independence of systems, care must be taken to not create (1) a *bottleneck* where all network traffic is concentrated into a single connection with resulting periodic overloads in the system nor to create (2) a *single point of failure* where a single failure in a software or hardware system could cause the entire network to cease functioning. Later chapters, 10 and 15, discuss these potential problems and ways to avoid them.

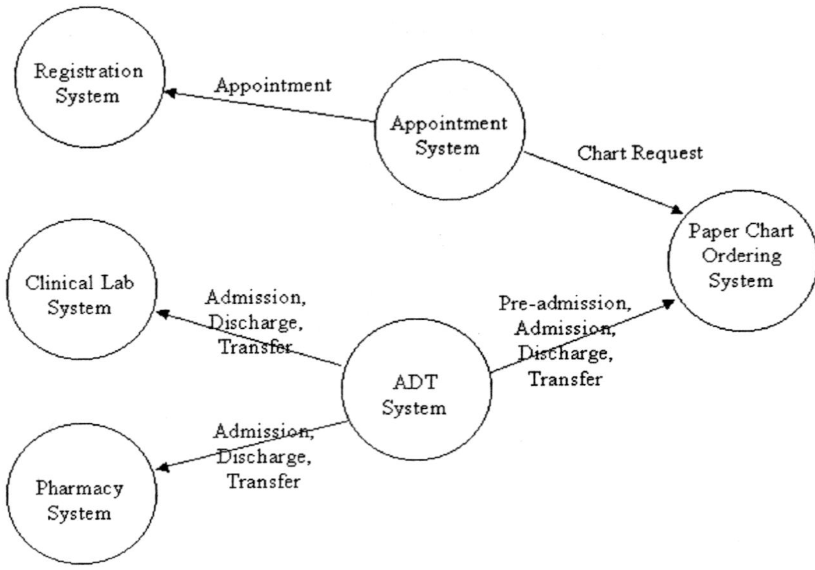

Figure 5.4 Example interfaces between HMO clinical systems.

An industry standard network protocol for healthcare system interfaces is HL7 (Health Level Seven 1997-2003). If this standard is used together with decoupling for each set of clinical systems in the healthcare organization, then there is the potential that any type of clinical system can be more easily replaced by another clinical system of the same type having the same interfacing scheme. Note that most commercial clinical systems have such HL7 interfaces. This concept of interchangeability of systems is referred to in this book as *component adaptability*, and is discussed later in this book—By the way, component adaptability means much more than just use of HL7.

Over time, proprietary and differing clinical systems could be replaced by common systems throughout the HMO.

All interfaces between clinical systems and with the automated patient chart system must be real-time interfaces unless the information is exceedingly static; otherwise, there is a great chance of information being out of synch. (This is both a cost and quality issue, although more a quality issue.)

Besides standardization of clinical systems, other types of standardization could also save the HMO money, such as organization-wide standards for computers and other hardware. Standardization of hardware in a healthcare organization, whether for clinical systems or the automated patient medical record system, could include standardization of brands and configurations, or alternatively different standards for different types of users, e.g., "power users" versus "non-power users". Such standardization could also save on help desk and support staff with standardized procedures in the organization for installing and fixing hardware.

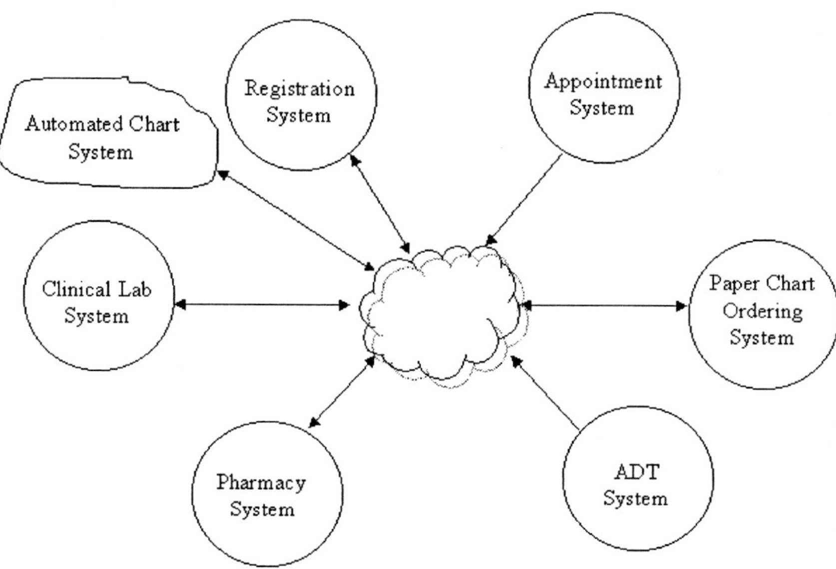

Figure 5.5 Proposed interfaces between HMO clinical systems.

5.3.4.8 Protection Against Costly Law Suits

Millions of dollars could be spent on malpractice suits in a large HMO in one year. With automation of the patient medical record, there would be one complete patient medical record available to all caregivers at all times, containing the patient's complete care history, instead of possibly many paper charts each showing only a small part of the patient's care. And, as stated earlier in this chapter, through organization of the chart for different types of caregivers, through information retrieval techniques, and through clinical summaries, caregivers would be able to quickly find relevant information. An automated patient medical record would thus decrease the chance of caregivers making mistakes due to lack of information or not finding information.

When care information is entered into the automated patient medical record by a caregiver, the system could verify that the information entered would be understandable by other caregivers, for example, that a standardized medical vocabulary was used (AHCPR 1994) and that abbreviations were either expanded and verified or were part of a standard set of abbreviations that could be understood in facilities in and outside the HMO (Leifer 1993). This would guarantee that the patient medical record was always readable, and never illegible.

Once a caregiver has completed the information on a patient's medical record for an encounter, the caregiver would sign off on the information, adding a digital signature (CMS 2004). The system would record the date and time and guarantee that the information could not be modified at a later date except through a clearly identified addendum. This removes the uncertainty that occurs in paper charts now that the caregiver could potentially modify the patient medical record after the fact.

Reference (Scott 2000), the book *Legal Aspects of Documenting Patient Care*, lists provider documentation errors that could be used against the caregiver in a malpractice suit. These errors are presented in table 5.1 along with an indication of whether automation of the patient medical record could potentially eliminate the error. Most, but not all, errors could be eliminated by automation of the patient medical record.

Table 5.1 Documentation Problems, Errors and Suggestions (Scott 2000).

Description	*Eliminated by Automation of the Patient Medical Record?*
Illegible notation	Yes
Failure to identify the patient being treated	Yes
Failure to identify the date (and time) of treatment	Yes
Use of multiple or inconsistent documentation formats by providers in a facility	Yes
Failure to use an indelible instrument to record treatment entry	Yes
Pen runs out of ink midway through a treatment entry	Yes
Provider editing chart removing the originally entered data	Yes
Not signing treatment entries	Yes
Not properly correcting errors in treatment entries	Yes
Unauthorized abbreviations	Yes
Improper spelling, grammar, and use of extraneous verbiage not affecting patient care	Yes
Physician orders: ambiguous orders, treating patients without written orders	Largely
Untimely documentation of patient care	No
Identifying the filing of an incident report in the patient record--it should not be mentioned	No
Delineating patient care rendered and clinical information supplied by another caregiver	No
Blaming or disparaging another provider in the patient treatment record	No
Expressing personal feelings about a patient in the treatment record	No

The 'O', 'A' and 'P' parts of the SOAP especially note must be written in objective, unambiguous and, where possible, quantifiable terms. Providers should avoid ambiguous conclusions such as "appears within normal limits".	Potentially
Not documenting with specificity	Potentially
Recording hearsay as fact	No
Special caution is not exercised when countersigning another provider's evaluation or treatment	No
Failure to document a patient's informed consent to treatment	Yes
Failure to thoroughly document discharge, home care, and follow-up instructions issued to patients and/or family members or significant others	To some extent
Failure to carefully document a patient's noncompliance with treatment orders	No
Failure to carefully document a patient's or family member or significant other's possible contributory negligence	No

An automated patient medical record could also promote HMO member satisfaction, as the member would no longer have to wait for the caregiver to receive the chart before the caregiver could take action, such as refilling a prescription. A satisfied HMO member is less likely to bring a lawsuit and also tends to be more compliant to treatment regimes, also reducing the chance of a lawsuit (Hughes 1991).

HMO strategies for handling lawsuits could change significantly with changing laws. For example, some HMOs are protected from lawsuits by requiring members to accept contracts that require arbitration to resolve disputes. If this changed and lawsuits did become a significant problem in the future, for example as a result of changes in the law such as a "Patient Bill of Rights", then the HMO might potentially have to change its practices to more strongly protect against these lawsuits. Caregivers in the HMO might be encouraged to perform more clinical tests as a form of defensive medicine; this would increase costs to the HMO and subject the patient to possibly unnecessary tests.

Another possibility would be that physicians would be required to follow only "best practice guidelines". One possibility is using *National Guideline Clearinghouse* guidelines whenever possible. This could be facilitated by an automated patient medical record system in that quick access to the guidelines would be available and that carepaths could be set up for the guidelines. If best medical practices are strictly followed, then there is little basis for a lawsuit.

5.3.4.9 Reduction of Healthcare Personnel Costs

With automation of the patient medical record, the cost of HMO staff can be reduced in a number of very different ways:

- Some caregiver services could be consolidated and outsourced, thus saving the HMO money.
- Chart room staff and couriers transporting charts and orders could be decreased, reducing costs.

Outsourcing and Consolidation of Services Done Independently from the Patient Outsourcing or consolidating medical services done independently from the patient would be much easier with automation of the patient medical record. For example, a group of radiologists could interpret diagnostic images and transcribe results for multiple health care organization locations or for multiple health care organizations. The automated diagnostic images would remain available to the caregiver caring for the patient during its interpretation. The ordering caregiver could be immediately alerted when results came back.

The Changing Nature of Chart Rooms Even though the chart room will be needed until the patient chart is fully automated, there will be less ordering of patient charts because sufficient chart information will often be available on-line. This will result in a decrease in the chart room staff. Also, there will be less time spent in tracking down a misplaced paper chart.

A decrease in chart room staff could also result from off-site storage of chart information. At one time, the former Pacific Bell Company (now SBC) was trying to establish a service to store diagnostic images of California health care organizations at Pacific Bell; Pacific Bell estimated that such storage of diagnostic image information at Pacific Bell or other outside institution could save a health care organization about 30%-40% of the current dollar costs of storage of diagnostic images (Kohli 1996). The outside organization, and not the HMO, would have responsibility for storing back-up data off-site, and responsibility for the costs of insurance for possible destruction of the chart information.

5.3.5 Fulfill the Requirements of Government and Public Health Agencies, Accreditation Organizations, Laws, and Industry Standards.

Many groups look at overall patient care, not just care for an individual patient. These groups include accreditation and government agencies, public health agencies, and agencies that keep information—called *disease registries*—on specific diseases and medical conditions. The automated patient medical record system could be designed to look at patient care from these many different perspectives and could report on information of interest to these organizations. The automated patient medical record could (1) automate quality control checks, (2) automate the recognition of infectious outbreaks, both inside and outside the medical organization, and (3) automate the recognition that relevant patient information needs to be sent to disease registries.

The automated patient medical record system could potentially automatically collect the information required by accreditation and government agencies (e.g., JCAHO, OSHA). It could then alert management when it identifies that care is not up to the standards set by these agencies.

The automated patient medical record system could also be designed to identify infection outbreaks, cases where multiple patients have the same communicable disease. This information could be sent to the HMO department of infection control and *epidemiology* groups (groups that study diseases and their causes). Automated notification of incidents of communicable diseases will allow the infection control department to quickly report such incidents to the public health department, to identify *nosocomial infections* (i.e., infections acquired by patients during their hospital stays), and to insure that proper isolation procedures are followed. Healthcare personnel should also be trained to recognize outbreaks and epidemics.

Voluntary and government mandated disease registries have been established for various disease and health problems, including cancer, AIDS, birth defects, diabetes, implants, organ transplants, measles, trauma and hazardous substances (Abdelhak et al. 2001). Some HMOs have their own disease registries (e.g., Kaiser Permanente has a confidential registry to track patients with the BRCA1 gene that predisposes a patient to breast or ovarian cancer). The automated medical record system could automatically collect disease registry information or, alternatively, alert a caregiver when disease registry information should be collected based upon the diagnosis for the patient.

The automated patient medical record system can be designed so it automates reports for accreditation organizations and disease registries, which now are most often done manually: Reports based upon patient care can be automatically generated and information can be transferred over networks to outside organizations rather than be compiled by hand. This information may include information for the *NCQA (National Committee for Quality Assurance)* database (NCQA 2004), a national database for evaluating HMOs, and include information for generation of the HEDIS report, an HMO "report card". It can include information for the *JCAHO (Joint Committee on Accreditation of Healthcare Organizations),* the primary healthcare accreditation organization for hospitals and other health care facilities. Upon entrance into the automated patient medical record system, disease registry information can be automatically transmitted outside the organization to the appropriate registry.

The automated patient medical record system must satisfy the requirements of the *Health Insurance Portability and Accountability Act of 1996 (HIPAA),* which mandates standards for healthcare organizations dealing with Medicare. And the system must incorporate healthcare industry standards. For both these, see the appendix.

Further, the automated patient medical record system must also be designed to satisfy all federal and state laws, and with a potentially international system, laws of other nations and international agreements.

5.4 SUMMARY OF PROJECT OBJECTIVES DERIVED FROM ORGANIZATIONAL OBJECTIVES

In section 5.3, objectives for the project were derived from objectives for the organization. Clearly, the automated patient medical record project furthers each of the organizational objectives. Table 5.2 summarizes the results of section 5.3, identifying the organizational objectives and derived project objectives.

The last column in table 5.2 identifies, for each project objective, a way of measuring the project objective, a measurement that can be used to set goals to determine whether or not a project objective has been fulfilled. At the end of the project, or sometimes earlier, fulfillment of the project objective can be determined by whether a predetermined final goal has occurred. At other times during the project, a preliminary goal can be set up to determine if the project is progressing toward the corresponding project objective. Measurement of goals should also be done at the beginning of the project to set a baseline for the later measurements.

Some of the measurements of the goals can be answered by yes/no answers—"Is such and such provided or not?" These are used for *functional goals.*

Some of the measurements of goals can be answered via quantitative measures—"What quantity of this is provided?" These are used for *attribute goals.* In such a case, acceptable quantities must be supplied to describe the goal.

For example, to measure the objective that "there will be a complete and always available patient medical record", an evaluator could observe encounters to determine how often a patient's medical record is unavailable. A measurable goal determining if a final objective has been achieved might be to have the patient medical record with all HMO medical information for the past 2 years available at 98% of the patient encounters. A measurable intermediate goal for 3 years from now might be to have an automated patient medical record with all HMO medical information for the past year available at 90% of encounters. These are attribute goals.

Table 5.2 Project Objectives Derived from Organizational Objectives

Number	*Organizational Objective*	*Number*	*Project Objective*	*Metrics for Goals*
1	Provide quality medical care	1	Re-evaluate the entire clinical workflow of the HMO to completely eliminate unnecessary steps and restructure non-productive steps while incorporating the automated patient medical record system.	Count unnecessary steps in caregiver workflow of representative categories of caregivers. Measure times of defined activities.
		2	Create a complete and always available patient medical record.	Observe encounters to determine the percentage of time the patient's medical record is unavailable during an encounter. What percentage of time is the caregiver missing parts of the chart generated within a given time period (e.g., the last year)?
		3	Allow simultaneous viewing and update of the patient medical record.	Can automated patient medical record be simultaneously viewed and updated? Evaluate for various categories of updaters and viewers at both local and remove locations.
		4	Enable a caregiver to quickly find relevant information in the patient medical record by methods such as providing summarization information, organization, information retrieval and tailoring of information related to the type of caregiver.	Observe how quickly caregivers can find information. Interview caregivers to determine how often they give up on looking for appropriate information.

5	Provide methods to track a treatment for a particular condition across multiple encounters, possibly with multiple different caregivers, potentially in different departments and in different geographic locations.	Are there approaches to track a treatment across encounters. Survey caregivers to determine if they feel that the approaches are successful.
6	Automate caregiver ordering and results reporting to make ordering easier, quicker and more accurate and integrate it with the automated patient medical record system.	Measure the time between orders and results. Identify paperwork used.
7	Do automated clinical checking of medications, such as drug/drug interactions and patient allergy checking. Reduce errors including reordered tests, adverse drug reactions, billing errors, etc.	Determine the percentage of applicable orders for which clinical checking was done. Was it done correctly in each case? Count reordered tests, adverse drug reactions, billing errors, etc. before and after automation.
6	Provide information to caregivers on best practice guidelines using NGC and/or local guidelines; provide medical reference information.	Compare guideline compliance in non-automated versus automated chart by reviewing patient medical records. Identify percentage of caregivers who use the medical references and guidelines.
7	Collect clinical outcomes information to further evidence-based medicine (identifying best treatments and practices for diseases which produce the best outcomes as determined by the best scientific evidence).	Determine how much time on average it takes to collect information for evidence-based medicine from non-automated versus automated patient medical records.

8	Automate the recording of biomarkers for diagnosis and prediction of diseases. Combine this with identification of trends in the patient's health through trend documents, especially in cases where there is an emerging health problem (e.g., an increase in the patient's blood pressure).	Does the automate patient medical record break out the identification of important biomarkers for the predication and diagnosis of disease? Is there an approach to track trends? Survey caregivers to determine if they feel the approach is successful in helping predict disease, as opposed to non-automated methods.
9	Generate letters to HMO members to come in for preventative health exams (e.g., colonoscopies) based upon age, sex, family history and other factors.	Determine percentage of HMO members for whom preventative health letters are being sent out. Determine how often they respond to these letters.
10	Provide the ability to record a detailed social, family, environmental and genetic history of HMO members who agree to provide this information. Identify family members of these HMO members and their relationships to the HMO member, especially family members who are themselves HMO members.	This is a new area that should be researched and thus goals would be set later after that research.
11	Explore predicting diseases from information in the automated patient medical record, including from risk factors and biomarkers.	This is a new area that should be researched and thus goals would be set later after that research. Are risk factors and biomarkers for disease being recorded?
12	For medical research purposes, enable useful access to clinical information without providing the identities of patients.	Is access to clinical information without identifying the patient provided? What is the level of researcher satisfaction with this process?

		13	For medical research purposes, enable controlled access to clinical information to identify patients who are appropriate for specific clinical trials and other medical studies.	Is the capability to identify clinically appropriate patients provided? Is the security adequate? What is the level of researcher satisfaction with the process?
2	Promote HMO Member Satisfaction	1	Have each HMO member chose a primary care physician. Have the automated system identify a patient's primary care physician(s) and associated caregivers.	What percentage of HMO members have assigned primary care physicians?
		2	For members who approve, store genetic and other information to enable individualized treatments and medications in the future.	This is a research area.
		3	Personalize care for the patient through personal profiles.	What percentage of patients have personal profiles?
		4	Evaluate the feasibility of the automated patient medical record system receiving input from monitoring systems, including "Guardian Angel" systems.	Is the automated patient medical record system integrated with monitoring systems? Are outcomes improved in comparison to non-use of "Guardian Angel" systems or non-integration of monitoring systems?
		5	Reengineer the care process to eliminate roadblocks that inhibit the patient from receiving prompt care.	Survey patients to measure patient satisfaction and patient identification of roadblocks to patient care.
		6	Pre-schedule activities, both generically and for individual patients, and, where possible, pre-fill paperwork or fill in paperwork when care is given, such as insurance forms.	Survey patients and their caregivers to determine if these measures are indeed removing bottlenecks to care.

		7	After an outpatient visit, provide the patient and the patient's family information on clinician orders and other encounter information to promote compliance with physician instructions and orders. After clinical laboratory results are returned, enable physicians to print and annotate results, sending them to the patient; terminology used sgiykd be understood by the patient.	Determine the percentage of time patients are provided this information after a visit. Follow up with interviews of patients to determine patient compliance with instructions and satisfaction with this service.
		8	Where appropriate, provide the patient with automated scheduling of medications and determination of alternative medicines or dosage choices.	Survey patients to determine if their taking of drugs is being simplified or not.
		9	Generate a discharge summary for the patient which describes in clear language, restrictions and follow-up activities.	Survey patients to determine how clear the discharge summary is.
		10	Incorporate patient education information in the automated system for the patient.	Survey patients to determine their satisfaction with patient education materials.
		11	Get patients and their families more involved in the patient care process.	Does the automated system provide mechanisms to get patient and family more involved in the care process? Survey patients to determine if they feel they are sufficiently involved in their own care.
		12	Record advance directives in the automated system.	For what percentage of patients are advance directives recorded?
3	Support healthcare workers and improve their efficiency	1	To reengineer the care process based upon input from employees so that employees' work activities match the most productive and least stressful methods of providing care.	Survey employees to determine if they feel they are providing quality care, are productive or are under stress.

2	Check for or insure consistent terminology in the medical record.	Review medical records to insure that medical records use consistent terminology.
3	Automate the process of identifying situations where patients are not complying with orders that seriously affect the patient's health.	Is patient non-compliance checking done in the automated system? Review charts to determine if it occurs at the appropriate times.
4	Provide other automated assistance to the caregiver in providing care, including the following: alerts, trends, assistance in diagnosis, conformance to best practice guidelines, identifying inconsistencies.	These areas require more research.
5	Provide on-line medical references for the caregiver to use when providing care.	Survey caregivers to identify the usefulness of these on-line medical references.
6	Eliminate redundant entrance of information in clinical systems, eliminating possible contradictory information.	Identify and count situations where the same information is collected more than once.
7	A member's medical record will be available to authorized physicians at any time.	Verify that the medical record for any identified member is available at random times at various locations within the HMO.
8	Use techniques to simplify documentation listed in section 5.3.3.3.	Are these techniques being used? Survey caregivers to determine if they consider them to be useful?
9	Support automated care documentation for inpatient nurses, including computerized generation of nursing care plans.	Is automated generation of nursing plans supported and used? What percentage of care plans are on paper?
10	Automate coding of diagnoses, procedures, and supplies (such as ICD, CDT, DRG codes). and unit census.	Measure the time to code diagnoses and procedures.

		11	Automate non-chart documentation done manually, such as the Inpatient Clinical Summary, MAR, emergency room census.	Survey caregivers to determine if automation has saved caregivers time.
		12	Cut down on paperwork during the care process, instead, transferring information quickly via networks rather than by costly, slow, and error-prone manual transport.	Record the paperwork required during an identified number of outpatient visits and inpatient stays.
		13	Alert attending physician when discharge is pending so discharge procedures can be quickly accomplished. Enable post-discharge activities to be accomplished concurrently.	Measure the time from identification of patient discharge to when the patient is discharged. Measure time from discharge until all post-discharge activities are completed.
		14	Evaluate the feasibility of using digitized diagnostic images with the automated patient medical record system. Enable quick transmission of images to medical professionals who can interpret them.	Are PACS systems implemented? Survey radiologists to determine whether PACS systems are being used and whether they perceive it adds value.
4	Make and Save Money	1	Re-evaluate the entire clinical workflow of the HMO to eliminate or revise costly processes while incorporating the automated patient medical record system.	Count costly steps in caregiver workflows of representative categories of caregivers.
		2	Support demand management in all its forms.	Compare the non-automated and automated patient medical record to determine the percentage of time demand management documents are found in the patient medical record. Survey users on how useful the automated record is in supporting demand management.
		3	Reduce errors including reordered tests, adverse drug reactions, billing errors, etc.	Count reordered tests, adverse drug reactions, billing errors, etc. before and after automation.

4	Identify and report on potential patient abuse such as "drug jumping", going from facility to facility for narcotics orders.	Identify cases of drug jumping in old and new systems. For what percentage of cases does system catch drug jumping before it is recognized manually.
5	Identify suspicious charges for medications and services when payments are to be made to outside healthcare organizations.	Identify cases of suspicious charges to outside agencies. Count when system catches these charges.
6	Support automated collection of payments for medical services from the government and insurance companies via EDI. Support automated payment for medical services. Support automated collection of Medicare payments using HIPAA standards.	Do more medical payments occur via EDI? How many? Are there systems remaining which should use EDI? Is EDI for Medicare payments for Medicare supported?
7	Support electronic commerce, in particular DME ordering such as over the Internet.	Does DME ordering occur through the system through electronic commerce? Do users use this capability?
8	Provide automated advice on least cost best practices, including lower cost medications that provide equal or better benefits, including advice to use generic medications rather than brand name ones.	Is this capability implemented? Observe a representative sample of encounters to determine the percentage of encounters where best practices are being followed.
9	Record information for prediction of HMO costs in the future: services, tests and procedures given to patients, supplies and medications, provider time caring for patients, hospitalizations and visits, and trends in membership growth and patient utilization.	Are future financial predications more accurate? Does the automated system produce the necessary financial information? Measure financial employee satisfaction with this information.

		10	Interface the automated medical record system with encounter systems, ordering and results systems, and billing and financial systems to share information.	Does the automated medical record system directly interface with all these systems to share information?
		11	Where possible, standardize hardware, system software and clinical systems within the organization.	What are the numbers and percentages of common hardware, system software and clinical systems? Which of these common systems use national standards?
		12	Standardize clinical system interfaces using industry standards (such as HL7).	Do all interfaces between the automated system and other clinical systems use HL7? How many and what percentage?
		13	Design the automated patient medical record system to eliminate documentation errors identified in table 5.1 to protect against costly lawsuits.	Are the checks in table 5.1 performed?
		14	Support consolidation, and possible outsourcing, of medical services where the patient is not seen, such as interpretation of diagnostic images.	Does the patient medical record system support these services? Is money saved?
		15	Evaluate the possibility, feasibility and cost-effectiveness of off-site storage of automated patient medical record information.	Is the automated patient medical record information being stored off-site? What percentage of the patient medical records?
5	Fulfill the Requirements of Government and Public Health Agencies, Accreditation Organizations, Laws, and Industry Standards	1	Automatically collect registry information based upon patient diagnoses and alert a caregiver when registry information should be collected.	When a diagnosis occurs that should be reported to a registry, is it recorded? Determine for each registry.

2	Provide automated recognition of infection outbreaks, in particular infections occurring within HMO hospitals. Healthcare personnel should also be trained to recognize outbreaks and epidemics.	Determine time of recognition of each infection outbreak. Did automated patient medical record system identify each outbreak? Did the automated system recognize the outbreak before it would have been otherwise recognized?
3	Automate quality control checks that insure that clinical information complies with accreditation agency (e.g., JCAHO) and government standards and which generates proof of compliance.	Is this capability provided? Ask JCAHO and government agencies if they receive the information they require?
4	For reporting based upon medical-related information (e.g., HEDIS), set up automatic generation of these reports and transmission to outside agencies (e.g., the NCQA).	Are these reports being generated? Are the applicable agencies satisfied with the content and timeliness of the reports?

With the many project objectives identified in table 5.2, it is surely not feasible to implement them all at once. These objectives should be prioritized, perhaps as those that are absolutely essential, those that are very important, and those that are less important. Also, project objectives that require further study or research would be identified.

However, some project objectives can logically be included with others or included with little extra cost. Some project objectives are logically done before others. In these cases, it might benefit the project to logically order the project objectives and to not base the order solely on the priority of the project objective.

5.5 AN INITIAL CONCEPTUAL VIEW OF THE AUTOMATED PATIENT MEDICAL RECORD

As can be seen from the list of project objectives in table 5.2, a project objective is basically a high-level business requirement. As more and more project objectives and business requirements are created for a project, systems and workflows become more and more defined. At some stage it is useful to develop basic models of systems or workflows, which I will referred to as *conceptual views*, and which might also be called "straw man" models. They are views of the system used for communication, with the idea that these conceptual views can be quickly changed if they don't agree with the business requirements or with added business requirements.

Combining current essential business practices that the HMO wishes to preserve as identified in section 4.7 with the added project objectives, we derive a conceptual view of the automated patient medical record system. See figure 5.6.

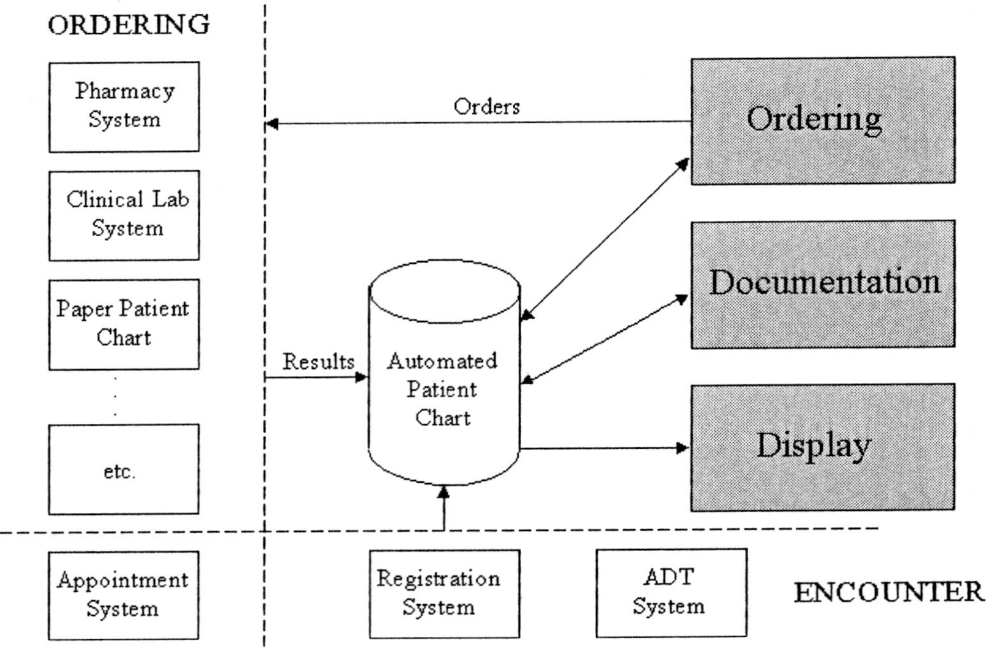

Figure 5.6 A Conceptual View of the Automated Patient Medical Record System.

The basic functions of an automated patient medical record system within a healthcare organization are (1) a part to **display** the patient medical record, (2) a part to enable caregivers to **document** all aspects of patient care, and (3) a part to enable caregivers to **order** medications, clinical lab tests, paper charts, appointments, etc. and to receive **results** back from the clinical systems within the healthcare organization.

In order to organize clinical information by encounter, information on encounters and when they begin and end must be received by the automated patient medical record system from healthcare organization encounter systems. Encounters include hospital admissions, transfers and discharges from the ADT (hospital) system, outpatient visits from the registration system, and booked, canceled and completed appointments from the appointment and resource scheduling system.

Order and result information must also be organized by encounter. The automated patient medical record system would send orders entered by caregivers to other healthcare organization clinical systems that handle these orders—including the pharmacy system for medications, the clinical laboratory system for clinical laboratory orders, the radiology system for x-ray and other diagnostic imaging orders, saving the order to the patient medical record. When the caregiver issues an order, the caregiver must associate it with the encounter. Results of orders could be received back from these clinical systems and stored within the automated patient medical record system with the order, and thus also would be organized by encounter.

The automated patient medical system thus ties together all clinical systems in the HMO, including encounter systems and systems through which orders could be made and results received. As a result, patient clinical information would no longer need to be redundantly entered in these systems. Orders could be accomplished electronically instead of on paper; and results would be received back electronically and thus more quickly. A list of patient encounters could be created electronically for each caregiver, inpatient unit, and the emergency department to guide caregiver workflow.

The interfaces of other clinical systems with the patient medical record system are likely to occur through network interfaces. To maximize the benefits of tying together all these healthcare organization clinical systems with the patient medical record system, network interfaces should use standard healthcare applications level network protocol, HL7 (Health Level Seven 1997-2003).

This model identifies a basic automated patient medical record system that incorporates the project objectives above and preserves the current essential business practices identified in section 4.7

5.6 PROJECT STRATEGIES

A *project strategy* is a change in direction of the organization that is part of a project that is presumed to result in an objective or objectives of the organization being fulfilled. Although project strategies can be determined at this stage, project strategies are most often deferred until the time of breakup of the project into phases, as project strategies commonly determine what phases and product sets are to be done first and which are to be done later.

For example, strategies for our automated patient medical record project might include the following:

- Standardize clinical system interfaces of existing systems using HL7 and component adaptability, so that they can be easily integrated with the automated patient medical record system.
- Standardize patient care within the HMO.
- Reengineer patient healthcare based upon interviews with caregivers in the various regions of the HMO.
- Integrate financial systems, including billing, with the automated patient medical record system early on in the project.
- Implement the automated patient medical record system in one region initially.
- Use national standards for the formats of clinical information, including those for identification of patients, providers and health care plans, and those for coding diagnoses and procedures.
- Develop parts of the system with high payback first.

5.7 PROJECT GOALS

Project goals are measurable quantities to determine (1) if a project objective has been achieved or (2) whether progress is being made toward a project objective. Goals are most easily determined after the project is broken up into phases, so goals can be measured after a phase is complete, or, alternatively, after the whole project is complete.

5.7.1 Measurability of Goals

Goals should always be measurable. Goals are either *functional goals* or *attribute goals* (Gilb 1988). *Functional goals* are absolute goals that have only one of two values: true or false. *Attribute goals* are goals that can be expressed on scales of measurement. Attribute goals either refer to qualities or resources. Qualities are good things that you want as much as possible (e.g., return on investment). Resources are what you use or consume; resources are always limited (e.g., number of resources you have to do the project or time you have to do the project).

5.7.2 Return on Investment

For most projects, a financial goal is "return on investment". *Return on investment (ROI)* is a standard way of determining if a project is cost justified and a standard way of comparing the project on a monetary basis with other projects. ROI are the dollar returns so far as a result of implementation of the project divided by the summation of the investments made so far to implement the project. ROI can be both estimated based upon the project plan and calculated as the project is in progress. Ideally this ratio should (eventually) be greater than 1, unless the project has nothing to do with making or saving money for the HMO (e.g., implementation of a set of government regulations).

ROI over time, say year to year, can be estimated or calculated. Initially ROI may be small or non-existent as money is spent on the project without revenue benefits. Projects can be compared according to their ROI's to the healthcare organization and by the duration of the project and length of time until the ROI is greater than 1 called the *payback period*, the period of the time from the start of the project where the project pays back for itself.

The automated patient medical record system "project" can probably be better described as a *program*, rather than a project, as it is probably best done by breaking it down into component subprojects, or phases. One potential subproject or phase within the program, at least for a large HMO, is standardizing interfaces between the automated patient medical record system and its database and the HMO clinical systems; doing so allows the clinical systems to be later standardized throughout the HMO, saving the HMO a lot of money. Such a subproject is likely to have a much quicker payback period than the automated patient medical record system and therefore it is very useful to break it out from other parts of the automated patient medical record program, so the benefits of the automated patient medical record program can be perceived to occur early on in the program.

Mathematically, ROI (Sounder 1988) can be estimated as follows:
$ROI_n = (\Sigma (R_i / (1+r)^i)) / (\Sigma (I_i / (1+r)^i))$,
where ROI_n is the return on investment for the nth year, Σ is the summation from the first up to the nth year, R_i is the net dollar returns of the project in the ith year, I_i is the investment expected to be made in the ith year, and r is an interest rate to correct for inflation. The numerator is the worth of all revenues generated by the project, and the denominator is the worth cost of all investments.

One set of costs that must be estimated are costs if particular risks occur and costs for contingency planning to insure the risks do not occur or resolve these risks if they do occur. These costs can best be calculated based upon the probability that they will occur. For example, if a risk has a 50% chance of occurring the cost is C if the risk does occur, then the expected cost of the risk is (0.5 * C) or if the time delay is T if the risk occurs, then the expected time delay of the risk is (0.5 * T).

It is not easy to estimate ROI. For example, one HMO who is automating the patient medical record made money one year and lost substantial money the next. This loss was not due to creation of the automated patient medical record system. However, if they had started the project earlier and used the ROI as a measure, they would have gotten a very deceptive measure of the project.

The HMO lost money because of a combination of other factors, including the following:

- because of a nursing shortage, having to pay higher wages for nurses than expected
- more members were hospitalized than expected
- more members joined the HMO than expected thus requiring more costly care outside the HMO
- a jump in prices of medications
- previous agreements with large union organizations whose members were HMO members kept capitation rates low.

5.7.3 The Balanced Scorecard: Goals in Combination to Measure Success

Table 5.2 shows project objectives together with how measurable goals could be developed for each of these project objectives. However, using each goal independently and equally to determine the progress of the project may not be appropriate, as this assumes that all the project objectives are independent of each other and of equal importance. Consider the following:

1. Project objectives must be properly weighted according to how important each is to the success of the project; otherwise, some project objectives will be treated as more, or less, important and than they really are.
2. Some project objectives may be redundant with other project objectives.
3. Meeting a project objective and an associated goal entails a cost; thus, for some goals, the expense of meeting the goal may negate the benefits of meeting the goal.

Let's consider points 1 and 2, proper weighting and redundancy of project objectives: Assume there are 5 equally important factors for the success of a project, and that every project objective and associated goal could be put into a factor category. If there were 100 project objectives for the first factor, 20 for the second, 1 for the third, 45 for the fourth and 2 for the fifth, and each goal was treated equally without regard to category, then the importance of meeting the goals under project objectives 3 and 5 may not be recognized.

Let's consider point 3 that project objectives or goals may not be worthwhile to meet. One project objective might be to speed ordering and return of results of diagnostic images via digitization and PACS systems. A PACS system may be of benefit to the healthcare organization, but the benefits, and a goal of implementing PACS systems organization wide, might not cover the high cost.

The *Balanced Scorecard* is a management technique for measuring the future financial health of an organization based upon the impacts of strategic objectives for the organization. It does this by using financial figures to determine the current financial health of the organization, and predicts the future financial health of the organization based on positive aspects of an organization that affect the strategic objectives of an organization. Robert Kaplan and David Norton of the Harvard Business school introduced this concept in 1992 (Kaplan and Norton 1996).

The Balanced Scorecard puts strategic organization objectives into 4 important categories for measuring the success of an organization. These categories are

1. **Financial perspective**: How do we look to the financial world?
2. **Member perspective:** How do health care organization members and patients see us?
3. **Internal perspective:** Do we excel in the important things?
4. **Learning and growth perspective:** Can we continue to improve and create value?

The theory behind the Balanced Scorecard is that not only must the financial condition of the organization be measured in terms of revenue and spending, but also factors that can promote and sustain the future financial health of the company must be measured (customers' views of the company, ways the company excels, and efforts being made to improve the company).

Measurable goals are created for the 4 categories. Goals can be leading indicators measuring the different financial perspectives in the short term, and lagging indicators measuring the financial perspectives in the long term. The goals can be used to measure how successful the company is in answering the questions above.

The Balanced Scorecard can also be used to measure and predict the financial benefits of a single project rather than the entire organization. Project objectives replace strategic organizational objectives. Goals for the project objectives and associated categories are identified as leading indicators for measurement as the project progresses and as lagging indicators as the project is completed, with leading indicators measuring short term success of the project, and the lagging indicators measuring long term success of the project. Besides being of use to measure the financial benefits of a project, **the Balanced Scorecard resolves our goal-weighting problem**. A weight can be assigned to each category as determined by the organization, with, for example, each category being weighted as to its importance to the organization or each category weighted as to how much the project impacts that category. Each goal within a category can then be apportioned as to its effect upon the category. When a project is weak in a category, then the project could potentially be redesigned to include changes in that category.

Table 5.3 shows information for a simplified Balanced Scorecard for our project.

Table 5.3 Example of a Balanced Scorecard

Perspective	*Project Objectives*	*Goals (Measures)*	
		Lagging Indicators	*Lead Indicators*
Financial	Reengineer the care process to get rid of low value costly processes.	The healthcare organization saves money. Positive return on investment for the project.	The healthcare organization saves money.
Member	Get patients and their families more involved in the patient care process. Reengineer the care process to get rid of roadblocks to care and low value costly processes.	Member retention. Improved medical care. Lower capitation fees to members.	Patient satisfaction survey.
Internal	Create a complete automated patient medical record. Automate and integrate ordering and result processing.	Improved outcomes. The medical record is always available to a caregiver.	The ordering process is speeded up and the time to return results is reduced.

Learning and Growth	Provide on-line medical references. Provide automated advice on least cost best practices. Reengineer and continue to enhance caregiver workflow based on caregiver input. Adapt the training and capabilities of the automated patient medical record system.	Improved outcomes. Caregiver retention.	Information availability. Caregiver satisfaction.

5.8 PROJECT CONSTRAINTS

For large-scale complex systems, there commonly is not enough money to implement all the identified business requirements. Finding enough qualified people to do the project may be a problem, especially because it is especially hard to find people with a combination of experience in the medical field and technical expertise. The organization may require that the project be done by a particular date to keep up or surpass the competition.

These factors do not define the desired product of the project—They constrain the project. They are the factors that cause one to buy a "Ford" when one would rather have a "Mercedes".

These *constraints* on the project usually deal with resources: money, time, and available people to do the project.

Key Terms

advance directive
attribute goal
Balanced Scorecard
best practice guidelines
biomarkers
bottleneck
case management
clinical checking
clinical pathway.
clinical practice guidelines
closed formulary
component adaptability
constraints
continuity of care
de-identification
demand management
disease registry
drug formulary.
durable medical equipment
Electronic Data Interchange (EDI)
encounter
entrance by exception
epidemiology
episode
evidence-based medicine
functional goal
goal
Guardian Angel systems
Health Insurance Portability and Accountability Act of 1996 (HIPAA)
healthcare proxy
HIPAA
interface engine
Joint Committee on Accreditation of Healthcare Organizations (JCAHO)
life time medical record
longitudinal medical record
maintenance
mission
monitoring systems
multidisciplinary
North American Nursing Diagnosis Association diagnoses (NANDA)
National Committee for Quality Assurance (NCQA)
National Guideline Clearinghouse
NIC (Nursing Intervention Classifications) interventions
NOC (Nursing Outcomes Classifications) outcomes
nosocomial infection
objective
open formulary
orders
organizational objective
preventive care
primary care
primary care physician
program
project
project objective
project strategy
reengineering
results
return on investment (ROI)
significant health problem
single point of failure
strategy
trend document
value added network (VAN)
values history questionnaire

Study Questions

1. Why do organizations do projects? Describe ways an organization picks one project over another? How can the success of a project be measured?
2. Name some advantages of a single complete patient medical record.
3. This chapter lists ways to organize the patient medical record. What does this book consider the most basic way to organize the medical record?
4. What is evidence-based medicine?
5. What are advance directives?
6. What is a monitoring system? Why is it difficult to record information from a monitoring system in any medical record?
7. What is a Guardian Angel system? How is it like a
10. How can an automated patient medical record save time and money at discharge?
11. What is EDI? What is a VAN?
12. What is a system interface? What is the industry standard network protocol for healthcare system interfaces?
13. What are the reasons for interfacing clinical systems with the automated patient medical record system?
14. What are standards? In automating the patient medical record, what types of standards are important?
15. What is HIPAA? What is the NCQA? What is JCAHO?
16. What are goals? What are functional goals? What

monitoring system?

8. Name some ways input of medical record information can be made quicker?
9. What is demand management? What is a drug formulary? What is an open and a closed formulary?

are attribute goals? What is Return on Investment? How does a Balanced Scorecard assist in evaluating a project?

17. What is a conceptual view?
18. What are project strategies? What are project constraints?

CHAPTER 6

Steps Toward a Universal Patient Medical Record

CHAPTER OUTLINE

6.1 PROJECT CONTEXT: A VISION ANTICIPATING THE FUTURE

Vision is "anticipating the future". Vision is required when an organization plans any project that takes a long time to complete. And vision is especially needed when management needs to evaluate and compare many different projects, selecting those that, together, would best benefit the organization in the future.

Because a large-scale complex project, such as the automated patient medical record system, takes a long time to complete, vision, anticipating the future, is required. Vision is required to identify at the beginning of the project business requirements that apply at the end of the project; otherwise, the products of the project could be obsolete by the time the project is complete.

But any single project cannot be viewed in isolation. Management must also look beyond a single project and look at all of its projects. It must pick the best mix of projects to meet the future needs of the organization. It must predict how all its projects will work together to change the organization—this may be especially difficult when projects are completed at different times and when projects depend upon each other for information or interact in other ways.

It is very difficult for any individual or organization to have vision—Predicting the future entails a significant risk that the predicator is wrong. There are, however, two ways for an organization to have some control over the future:

1. Firstly, management can guide the organization to follow a particular direction.
2. Secondly, management can insure that members of the organization follow industry standards and, if the organization is large enough, can provide representatives to standard organizations where the standards could benefit the organization. Following standards and creating beneficial standards is especially important when a project will extend beyond the organization and include other organizations in the same industry—in the case of an automated patient medical record system, the industry is the healthcare industry.

Even using these ways to "control the future", there is significant risks of wrong decisions being made. Such risks can be ameliorated by *risk management:* planning alternative measures if a prediction turns out to be wrong. See chapter 16.

One vision, a prediction of the author of this book, is that there will be a universal patient record. A large healthcare organization that develops an automated patient medical record system could have a significant influence over standards for such a universal patient record, insuring that the universal patient record is compatible with the needs of the healthcare organization and compatible with its automated patient medical record system.

6.2 ASSUMED ATTRIBUTES OF A UNIVERSAL PATIENT RECORD

The following are assumed attributes of a universal patient record:

1. To allow communication between differing healthcare institutions, the universal patient record must have a commonality of information.
2. However, to support the different needs of healthcare organizations, the universal patient medical record must also allow for a diversity of formats for medical record documentation.
3. The universal patient record must use agreed-upon healthcare industry data standards.
4. The universal patient record may be stored anywhere and retrievable from anywhere and thus requires a common secure network shared by healthcare organizations.
5. The universal patient record must be able to employ security measures to control the visibility and availability of information. Authorized parties can request permission to copy documents, and the owner or creator of a document can grant permission to an authorized party to copy the document, perhaps with certain categories of permissions granted by policy.
6. The universal patient record must be able to accommodate information in any language that care is given in.
7. The universal patient record must be judiciously introduced so that it is used in situations where a caregiver can have confidence that, for a particular patient, the patient record is complete or largely complete; for example, until the universal patient record becomes widely used, its use is better suited for a large HMO that can enforce its use throughout the HMO and where there are few member visits outside the HMO.

Based upon these assumed attributes, this section surmises what a future universal patient record would look like and describes how it could be incorporated into an automated patient medical record system.

Paper patient medical records currently differ from one healthcare organization to another. To create a common automated record, healthcare organizations must first agree upon common standards for the patient medical record.

A *Computer-based Patient Record (CPR) repository* that can be used by many healthcare and other organizations should be developed to store patient chart information in a format using national or international data standards. An example of such a format is the ASTM (American Society for Testing and Materials) E1384 standard for content and structure of automated patient health records (ASTM 2002). Such a CPR repository would not contain all the information in a patient's chart, but a significant summary of this information. The ASTM E1384 standard, for example, includes patient identification information, a patient problem list, patient practitioners, patient encounters (i.e., inpatient stays, outpatient visits, Emergency Department visits, etc.), services (including medications, diagnostic tests, immunizations, procedures and therapies), assessments/exams, and care plans.

At each healthcare organization, there would be automated documents making up the medical record, which I will refer to as *source documents,* together with paper medical records. Such source documents and paper medical records are those discussed in chapter 4 of this book. These documents are likely to differ in format and structure, and even in kind, from one healthcare organization to another. At least one information organization, the former Pacific Bell in California (now part of SBC), has attempted to set up a data base for storage of these source documents—in Pacific Bell's case, this was storage of diagnostic images for all Northern California healthcare organizations (Kohli 1996).

In addition to storing summary clinic information on patients in CPR repositories, I predict that many healthcare organizations will eventually choose to store their source documents externally from the healthcare organization, as they could save money on chart room space, chart room personnel and couriers and, more importantly, they could instantaneously transmit the source documents to wherever they are needed rather than have them physically transferred.

Such source documents would then either be electronically stored outside the healthcare organization in a *source document repository*, within the healthcare organization in a source document repository, or still be stored on paper and be in a chart room. In order to associate source documents and paper medical documents with encounters, I propose that each patient encounter identified in a CPR repository include the storage locations of all the medical documents generated during the encounter. See figure 6.1. (The E1384 standard currently provides for storage of one location.)

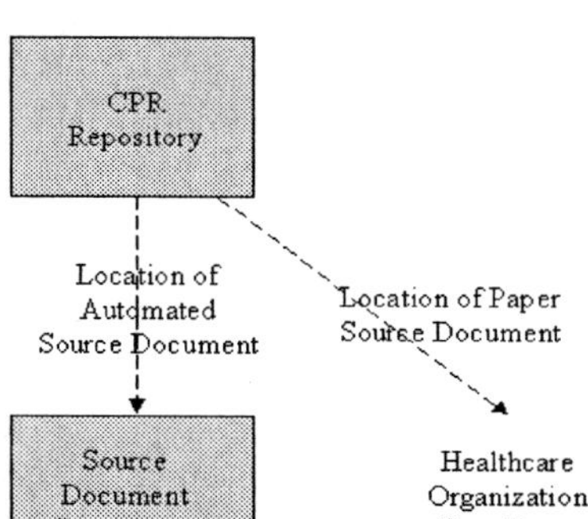

Figure 6.1 CPR Repository and Source Document Repository

From this information in the CPR repository and source document information, each healthcare organization could display a summary of clinical information for the patient with drill down to more detailed CPR and source document information. This summary, which I refer to as a *Patient Clinical Summary*, would include patient description information, a list of encounters, significant health problems, medications, orders, etc. See figure 6.2. More detailed patient clinical information could be available by selecting and "drill down" to this information and to source documents.

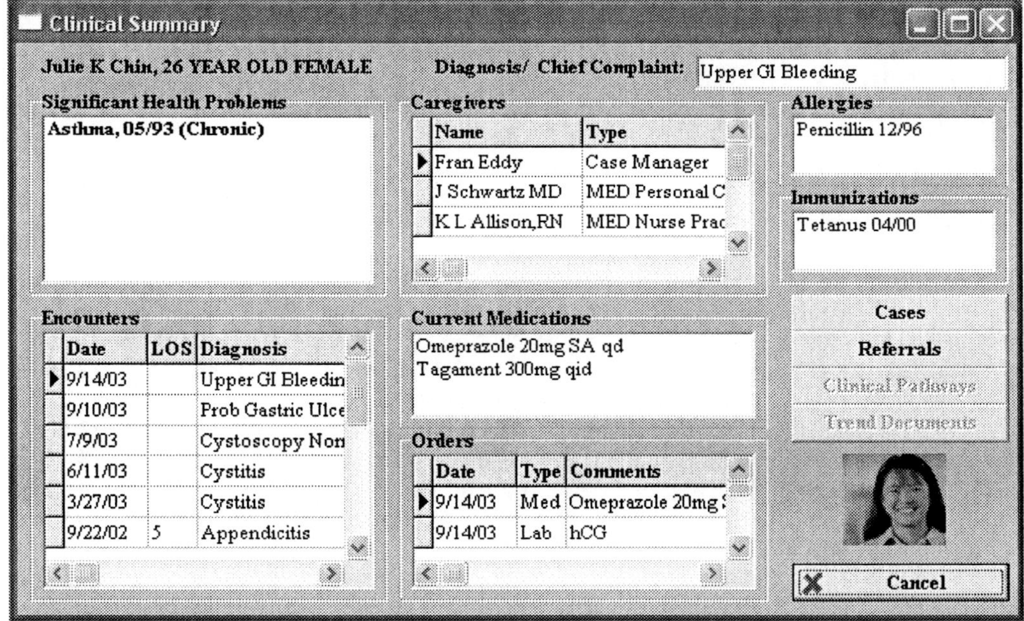

Figure 6.2 Patient Clinical Summary

A CPR repository or source document repository could exist within a healthcare organization, as part of a regional, national or international database, or within a private organization, such as SBC.

This book views a patient's universal patient record as the total of clinical information for a patient available within CPR repositories, source document repositories and on paper in chart rooms. In order to produce the universal patient record information needed by the CPR and source document repositories, a healthcare organization needs to do the following during an encounter:

1. as source documents are being created (e.g., H&P, vital signs documents, orders, Progress Notes), summary information would be generated for the CPR repository
2. medical documents that are electronically stored would be archived to a source document repository, or included in the paper chart
3. after an encounter, the summary information would be sent to the CPR repository along with the location of the source documents and paper medical documents.

It is proposed that the CPR not only be updated from source documents, but by direct caregiver and patient input to keep information, such as current medications and significant health problems, up-to-date.

A different philosophy on developing a document similar to the CPR and to the Patient Clinical Summary—see figure 6.2—is to rely on patients to enter the medical information rather than the information primarily being generated from source documents. This is called a *Personal Health Record.* The patient would have responsibility of keeping the information up-to-date. The Personal Health Record would provide information for emergency medical care. (NZ 0800 MEDBOOK 2001)

6.3 POSSIBLE EVOLUTION

Automation of the patient medical record is likely to occur first in the most organized and automated of healthcare organizations, large HMOs, like the one for our example project. If these ideas for a universal patient record, consisting of CPR repositories and source document repositories, are followed, the likely way the universal patient record would evolve is as follows:

Initially, an HMO and alliance healthcare organizations, or different regions of an HMO, will band together to set up a CPR repository, so they could share patient medical record information. The HMO might also start to store medical documents electronically in a source document repository to save on costs of its chart rooms. See figure 6.1.

In such a setup, an HMO or HMO region would know about the encounters in its own organization or region, so what the HMO or region would want to be informed about are encounters outside the HMO or HMO region for HMO patients. See figure 6.3. The CPR repository might be set up to inform the HMO when any such outside encounter occurs, or when there is a change in CPR encounter information for such patients. The HMO could then pick up the new CPR information and may choose to also pick up any associated source document information in the source document repository or alternatively order paper medical documents from chart rooms (e.g., paper chart documents stored physically in the outside organization). Also, whenever there is a new HMO member or whenever there is a non-member visiting the HMO, the HMO might query the CPR repository for any outside organization CPR information and pick up that CPR information and any associated source documents for that patient. (The alliance organizations or other HMO regions could follow the same procedures to get encounter information for its members and patients.)

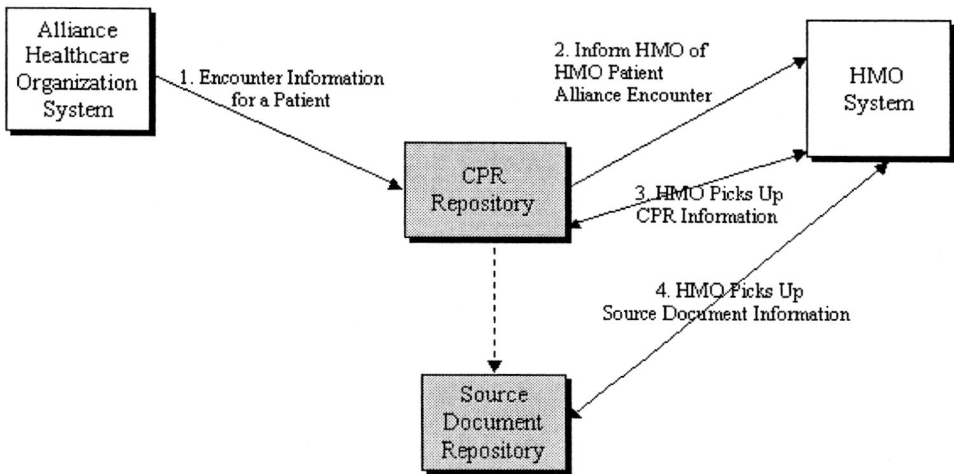

Figure 6.3 Functioning of the Repositories

Over time, further healthcare organizations might want their own CPR repositories and source document repositories, possibly shared with other healthcare organizations. A healthcare organization might then want to receive any encounters for a patient of interest from these other outside healthcare organizations.

A likely possibility at this stage would be that third party organizations would set up CPR repositories or source document repositories. Such a third party organization could charge a fee per transaction, operating as an application service provider, where an *application service provider (ASP)* is a company that offers individuals or enterprises access over the Internet to application and related services that would otherwise have to be located in their own personal or enterprise computers. Sometimes referred to as "apps-on-tap," ASP services are expected to become an important alternative, especially for smaller companies with low budgets for information technology . . . "on a rental, pay-as-you-use basis" (searchWebServices.com 2003). An ASP could provide a small healthcare organization with an automated patient medical record system that could store information on a CPR repository and source document repository.

Eventually, with greater use of source document repositories by healthcare organizations, the source document repository organization could take over the responsibility to update the CPR repository information from source document information, sending the CPR repository only information to be stored in the CPR repository and no other. The healthcare organization would then no longer have to send information directly to the CPR repository.

In order to link up all the CPR repositories, a *patient registry* could be set up to identify all patients in the CPR repositories and to identify the (subscribing) healthcare and other organizations, such as insurance companies, who are interested in each patient. See figure 6.4. Whenever a patient encounter was identified within a CPR repository, or CPR encounter information changed, then the patient registry would be informed by the CPR repository. The patient registry could then in turn inform any (subscribing) healthcare organization (or an insurance company) that had an interest in that patient of the encounter and send it the location of the CPR information for that encounter. An organization that was informed of the new encounter information could then optionally pick up the patient encounter information from its own CPR repository (for an alliance organization or HMO region) via a high bandwidth connection; or could pick up the patient encounter information from any other CPR repository (a non-aligned organization) perhaps via a lower bandwidth, say an Internet-like, TCP/IP, connection. Source documents could optionally be ordered or electronically requested from the outside healthcare organization or from a source document repository.

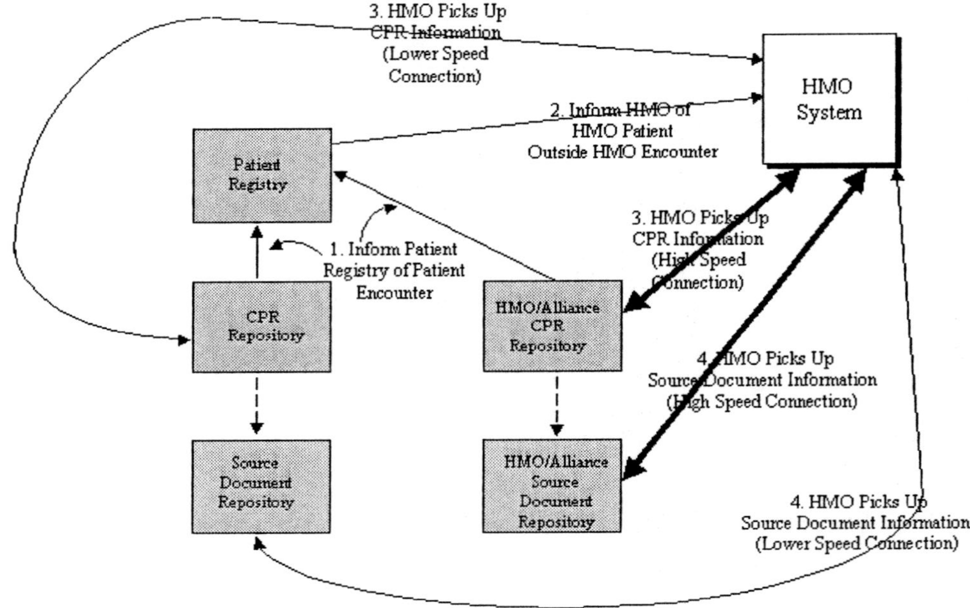

Figure 6.4 Later Repositories and Registry

For each new HMO or healthcare organization member and for each visit by a non-HMO member, the healthcare organization could query the patient registry and find all the CPR repository locations where the patient had encounter information. The healthcare organization could then go to each of the CPR repositories to pick up this CPR information and pickup or order associated information from each of the source document locations or chart rooms.

By these procedures, healthcare organizations would have a complete universal patient record for every patient of interest to them (every HMO patient and patient visiting the HMO). The approach is *scalable*, in that more CPR repositories could be connected to a patient registry, and CPR and source document repositories could be combined or partitioned. Changes in CPR and source document repositories structures may be required due to changing healthcare organization alliances or management reorganizations or to take advantage of lower cost or higher speed networks.

Some periodic synchronization (auditing) of CPR repository information with clinical information may have to be done to verify that information was up-to-date and consistent in all databases.

6.4 REQUIRED CHANGES WITHIN A HEALTHCARE ORGANIZATION

In order to (1) provide information for a universal patient record and (2) make use of this information to improve patient care, a healthcare organization must automate the patient medical record within its organization. Automation of the patient medical record within the healthcare organization along with creation of a complete, automated, universal patient record would enable caregivers to get a more complete picture of a patient's health and of the patient's present and past care.

The basic functions of an automated patient medical record system within a healthcare organization, as presented in the previous chapter in figure 5.6, are (1) a part to **display** the universal patient record, including Clinical Summaries and source documents, (2) a part to enable caregivers to **document** all aspects of patient care, e.g., producing source documents, and (3) a part to enable caregivers to **order** medications, clinical lab tests, paper charts, appointments, etc. and to receive **results** back from the clinical systems within the healthcare organization.

During the documentation step and order/results steps, information for the CPR repository would be created. After an encounter, this CPR information would be sent to the CPR repository. Documents (including orders and results of orders) would be sent out to a source document repository if there was one, with the locations of these source documents sent to the CPR repository. Clinical information would be organized by encounter in both the CPR repository and source document repository.

In order to organize clinical information by encounter, information on encounters and when they begin and end must be received by the automated patient medical record system from healthcare organization encounter systems, including ADT (for hospital admissions, discharges and transfers), the outpatient registration system, and the appointment system.

Order and result information must also be organized by encounter. The automated patient medical record system would send orders to other healthcare organization clinical systems that handle these orders—including the pharmacy system for medications, the clinical laboratory system for clinical laboratory orders, the radiology system for x-ray and other diagnostic imaging orders—and save each order, associating it with the encounter. Results of orders could be received back from the clinical systems and stored within the automated patient medical record system with the order, and thus also would be organized by encounter. This automation of the patient medical record, besides organizing patient clinical information by encounter for a universal patient record, would also result in the organization of all patient clinical information within the healthcare organization by encounter, whether the information was part of the universal patient record or not.

Automation of the patient medical record in the healthcare organization, would have the additional benefit that it would tie together all healthcare organization clinical systems, including encounter systems and systems through which orders could be made and results received. As a result, patient clinical information would no longer need to be redundantly entered in these systems. Orders could be accomplished electronically instead of on paper; and results would be received back electronically and thus more quickly. A list of patient encounters could be created electronically for each caregiver, inpatient unit, and the emergency department to guide caregiver workflow.

To maximize the benefits of tying together all these healthcare organization clinical systems, it is recommended that each organization clinical system, where feasible, communicate with the automated patient medical record system using the standard healthcare applications level network protocol, HL7 (Health Level Seven 1997-2003). This (theoretically) would enable a healthcare organization clinical system (e.g., a clinical laboratory system) to be replaced with an improved equivalent clinical system that used the same communications protocol without changing the existing interface between the existing clinical system and automated patient medical record system; this would also enable a large healthcare organization with different clinical systems at different geographic locations to standardize on the "best-of-breed" of each type of clinical system by substituting one clinical system for another of the same type.

The existence of a universal patient record through the CPR repository, source document repositories and patient registry would enable the healthcare organization to get a complete view of care of the patient in all the healthcare organizations where the patient was seen. As a result of the CPR repositories, a *Patient Clinical Summary* could be available that would show all patient encounters, medications, clinical laboratory tests, etc. Detailed information on each encounter would be available by drill down. An example of such a Clinical Summary appears in figure 6.2.

The location of any source document or papter medical document could be identified through the CPR repository; the source document could then be retrieved from source document repositories or the paper medical document could be electronically ordered, whether the source document was located within or outside the healthcare organization.

6.5 A UNIVERSAL PATIENT RECORD IN CONTEXT

How would a universal patient record affect patient care? Let's consider the universal patient record from several points of view:

1. the patient
2. society as a whole
3. an HMO, where automation of the patient medical record is likely to occur first.

6.5.1 Effect on Patients

What are the benefits of a universal patient record from a patient's point of view?

Wherever the patient goes for health care he will have a complete, rather than partial, history of his health problems and past medical care. For example, if the patient shows up in an Emergency Department, then the patient will have a complete chart and medical history immediately available. Any delays in treatment due to the need to record previous patient medical problems, allergies, patient family history, advance directives, can be avoided. As seen by figure 5.2, a complete chart may not otherwise be available even if the patient's medical care was in a single healthcare organization.

Another way a universal patient record would improve care for a patient is that communications between the caregiver and patient would be improved. During any phone call with a patient, a caregiver would now always have the patient's medical record. The caregiver would not have to wait until the patient's medical record is ordered.

An always-available automated patient medical record would also improve caregiver collaborations in the care of a patient. During a primary care physician's consultations with a specialist or with a person from an ancillary care department, both would have the patient's medical record, no matter where they were physically located. At the time a physician receives a consultation request from an advice nurse after a patient phone call, the physician would no longer have to order, and wait for, the patient medical record. A nurse practitioner, or a physician assistant, often consults with supervising physicians in the care of her patients; during their conversations, both could now be viewing the patient medical record whether they were in the same room or not.

Insurance and Medicare payments can be accomplished quicker so the patient would have a shorter time to worry about a medical bill being paid or not. Evaluation of injuries and illnesses for worker's compensation payments by the federal government and states could be done quicker.

6.5.2 Effect on Society as a Whole

A universal patient record would also benefit society as a whole.

Because of the patient medical record, there would be a greater knowledge base of clinical information. As a result, care given to patients could be evaluated more easily, including better determination of best treatment guidelines and of which treatments work best. There would be better selection of patients as subjects for research, for example, patients with only the subject disease, and no other diseases, could be identified.

Public health activities and epidemiological studies could be accomplished more quickly. Outbreaks of particular diseases could be recognized more quickly and more quickly controlled, within a hospital, the country, or the world. Where a patient gives his consent, a patient's genetics can be recorded along with the patient's medical history; thereafter, through anonymous medical studies, genetic markers can be associated with diseases, advancing the ability to diagnose and treat diseases.

Actual costs of medical care could be evaluated. Studies on how medicine could be made more cost-effective could more easily be done.

Medical fraud could be more easily detected. An insurance company or the government, once being informed of an encounter for a patient via the patient registry, could pick up medical service and other information from the healthcare organization where care occurred to help determine whether charges are legitimate.

6.5.3 Effect on a Healthcare Organization

When we are looking at a universal patient record from the point of view of the patient or society, we are viewing the universal patient record mainly with respect to its humanitarian aspects. Although an HMO, or other healthcare organization, in certain aspects, is a humanitarian organization, the HMO has also been set up to survive and prosper by being better than its competition and by making money. In this sense, it is no longer just a humanitarian organization. As competitors with other healthcare organizations, why should an HMO then want to have a universal patient record that not only benefits itself but also all other healthcare organizations?

Clearly, an HMO would benefit from the universal patient record. At the very least, this would combine together the entire healthcare organization's charts—see figure 5.2. But this could also be done by a proprietary approach decided upon solely by the HMO, potentially locking out other competitors. At first glance, agreement with other health care organizations on standards for a universal patient record seems contradictory to an HMO trying to get a competitive advantage—but let us consider further whether there would be such a competitive advantage.

Consider three typical categories of HMO patients and the effects of a universal patient record on each: (1) patients who almost always see a single primary care physician, or alternatively a team of caregivers within the same facility, for any health problem, (2) patients who go to multiple HMO facilities but do not go outside the HMO, and (3) patients who may be seen either within the HMO or outside the HMO.

For a patient in category (1), who primarily sees a single caregiver, a single patient chart in the facility of the primary care physician would probably suffice to provide adequate care. A universal patient record system may not enhance care all that much, although it would create greater organization of information in the chart and make the information easier to find, as this could be done by computerized searching or other techniques.

For a patient in category (2), who goes only to HMO facilities, a universal patient record would essentially combine all the charts in figure 5.2 and make them available to all caregivers in the HMO, but also would an HMO-only automated patient medical record system, whether proprietary or not.

For a patient in category (3), who goes both inside and outside the HMO for care, a universal patient record would combine patient medical records of both the HMO and outside healthcare organizations. Category (3), through "point of service" plans in HMOs, is fast becoming the majority case in many HMOs. Other healthcare organizations seeing HMO patients will most certainly not be using a proprietary HMO automated patient medical record system. The best, and cheapest, hope for category (3) patients then is for the whole healthcare industry to agree upon a standard universal patient record, in particular a standard for the CPR repository, the part that would contain an agreed-upon standard summary of patient clinical information. Such CPR repository information would be accessible by all healthcare organizations. Each healthcare organization would pay for its own interfaces to CPR repositories, but each would benefit from the combined information for the patient contained in it.

Through such a universal patient record, the HMO could also track care and treatments over a number of encounters both inside and outside the HMO. Best practice models could be enforced across healthcare organizations, ensuring a continuum of care even though the patient is seen both inside and outside the HMO.

An HMO developing an automated patient medical record system is thus best off if it works with other healthcare organizations in developing standards for a universal patient record prior to automating the patient medical record, even though this approach may appear to cause the healthcare organization to lose its competitive advantage in the short run.

Further, a large HMO that first develops an automated patient medical record system using an industry agreed-upon universal patient record can have a large influence on the direction of standards for such a universal patient record, and thus can insure that the standards for it entirely fit the needs of the healthcare organization. This could provide a significant competitive advantage to the HMO.

As stated earlier, a universal patient record is not possible without automation of the patient medical record within the healthcare organizations that provide the information for the universal patient record. **This book proposes that in anticipation of a universal patient record that an HMO when developing an automated patient medical record system plan for the design of a CPR repository structure to store patient clinical summary information using healthcare industry standards, for example the ASTM E1384 standard for electronic health records. This would make the future transition to a healthcare industry-wide system easier. The next section and the next chapter propose how this could be done.**

6.6. XML AS A BASIC STANDARD

XML is quickly becoming a standard for electronic storage of source documents, serving as a base for other standards. For example, the E31 committee of the ASTM is studying using XML together with the E1384 standard for electronic health care records (ASTM 2001). The HL7 committee in charge of the HL7 healthcare standard for network communications between healthcare computers is studying an XML implementation of a "Clinical Document Architecture", merging HL7 in with the XML description of medical record documents (HL7-Australia 2003). The Clinical Document Architecture, which was previously known as the Patient Record Architecture, will provide models for various types of clinical documents (e.g., discharge summaries and progress notes) so they can be transmitted between organizations.

Although a proposed CPR repository might not use XML in the storage of information, it could use the XML source documents as the source of information to be added to the CPR, translating information in H&P's, patient consultations and other source documents to the CPR structure. The E1384 structure of the CPR is described in the E-R diagram in figure 6.5 taken from reference (ASTM 2002), where E-R diagrams are described in section 13.7; this E-R diagram of an E1384 version of the CPR is described in more detail in section 6.6.3.

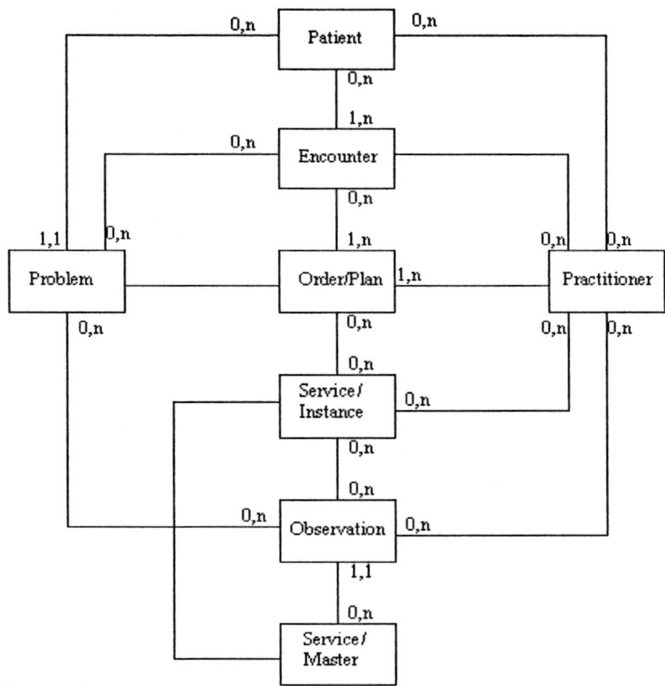

Figure 6.5 Patient Record Object Model (ASTM 2002).

6.6.1 What is XML?

XML and its various components (e.g., XML DTDs, XML Schemas, and XSL) are important because they allow data to be kept separate from a description of the formats of the data and kept separate from how the data is rendered (e.g., how it is presented on a form, in a voice message or on a computer screen). XML is used to identify data values, while XML DTDs or XML Schemas identify the format of this data (e.g., an integer), while XSL is used to identify how the data is to be displayed, printed, or spoken.

XML is a text-based tag language from the same family of languages as HTML. *HTML*, short for **H**yperText **M**arkup **L**anguage, is a text-based tag language used to create pages on the Web. HTML defines the structure and layout of a Web document by using a variety of tags and attributes. An HTML document starts with <HTML><HEAD><TITLE>, followed by the title of the Web page, followed by </TITLE></HEAD><BODY> and ends with </BODY></HTML>. Most of the information making up the Web document appears between the <BODY> and </BODY> tags. For example, within <H1> (Put Large Heading Here) </H1> would be headings, within <H2> (Put Smaller Heading or Text Here) </H2> would be smaller headings or text, and within <H3> would be even smaller headings or smaller text, etc. Within an <IMG . . . > or "image" tag would be a file identifying a picture to be displayed; such a tag could also identify another Web page that could be selected by the user clicking the picture. These are a very few of the many tags available in HTML. Reference (Raggett 2002) gives the URL of a Web site that presents an example of how HTML code translates to a Web page.

XML, eXtensible Markup Language, is a text-based tag language like HTML for defining documents. But, unlike HTML, which describes how data is displayed, XML states what the data is. XML is defined and standardized by the World Wide Web Consortium (W3C) (Bray et al. 2000), the group who controls standards on the Web.

To display an XML document, another language, XSL (eXtensible Stylesheet Language), is used together with XML—for example, XSL can generate HTML from the XML document. Because XML treats a document as data and does not format it for display, the same XML document can be used to display or otherwise "render" the data on different types of devices, including on a PC screen, PDA screen, over a telephone or over another type of voice device. XML can be used to present the data on different formats on the same screen—All that is needed is a different XSL document to translate the XML document to the wanted format.

Additionally, to describe the formats of data elements making up an XML document in detail, an XML DTD (Document Type Definition) can be created, which can either be included in or separate from the XML document. For example, the DTD can describe the data elements and formats of data elements making up a History and Physical document, Patient Consultation document, Patient Referral document, or Physician's Medication Order document, although it does not identify the layout of anyof these documents.

For example, figure 6.6 shows XML for a Patient Referral document identifying the data making up the particular patient referral.

```
<?xml version="1.0" encoding="UTF-8"?>
<patientreferral >

 <Header>
  <TransmissionFrom>...TRANSMISSION-FROM Information ...</TransmissionFrom>
  <TransmissionTo>...TRANSMISSION-TO Information ...</TransmissionTo>
  <DateIssued>2001-01-10</DateIssued>
 </Header>

 <Patient>
  <IdList>
```

```
    <Id type="universal">
     <IdMnemonic>0912873456</IdMnemonic>
     <AssigningAuthority>U.S. Assignment Authority</AssigningAuthority>
    </Id>
    <Id>
     <IdMnemonic>38933845</IdMnemonic>
     <AssigningAuthority>Lytton HMO</AssigningAuthority>
    </Id>
   </IdList>
   <PersonName>Jane Louise Doe</PersonName>
   <Sex Sex.HL70001="F" >Female</Sex>
   <BirthDate>1960-02-29</BirthDate>
  </Patient>

  <DiseaseList>
   <Disease>
    <DiseaseString>Lump or mass in breast</DiseaseString>
    <DiseaseCode>611.72</DiseaseCode>
    <DiseaseCodeSystem>ICD-9</DiseaseCodeSystem>
   </Disease>
  </DiseaseList>

  <ReferralPurpose>Evaluation of mammogram.</ReferralPurpose>

  <OtherDocumentList>
   <OtherDocument>Mammogram</OtherDocument>
  </OtherDocumentList>

</patientreferral>
```

Figure 6.6 XML for a Patient Referral Document

Figure 6.7 shows an XML DTD for the Patient Referral document, in this case stored externally from the XML, describing the data elements used within the XML document. Such "data describing data" is called *metadata.*

Symbols within a DTD mean the following:

- ',' between data elements means they must appear in the order shown within the document
- '|' between data elements means that only one of the data elements may appear
- Nothing following a data element name means it must appear once and only once
- '+' following a data element means it must appear once, and possibly many more times
- '*' following a data element means it may appear any number of times (including zero)
- '?' following a data element means it is optional, but it may only appear once.

XML DTDs provide the following methods to identify the format of data elements:

- #PCDATA is "parsable data", text that is to be parsed by an XML parser.
- #CDATA is text that is not to be parsed by an XML parser.

```
<?xml version = "1.0" encoding="UTF-8"?>
<!DOCTYPE  patientreferral [
  <!ELEMENT patientreferral (Header,Patient,DiseaseList,ReferralPurpose,
                            Comments?,OtherDocumentList?) >
  <!ELEMENT Header (TransmissionFrom,TransmissionTo,DateIssued) >
  <!ELEMENT TransmissionFrom (#PCDATA) >
  <!ELEMENT TransmissionTo (#PCDATA) >
  <!ELEMENT DateIssued (#PCDATA) >
  <!ELEMENT Patient (IdList,PersonName,Sex,BirthDate) >
  <!ELEMENT IdList (Id+) >
  <!ELEMENT Id (IdMnemonic,AssigningAuthority) >
  <!ATTLIST   Id  type (local|national|universal) "local" >
  <!ELEMENT IdMnemonic (#PCDATA) >
  <!ELEMENT AssigningAuthority (#PCDATA) >
  <!ELEMENT PersonName (#PCDATA) >
  <!ELEMENT Sex (#PCDATA) >
  <!ATTLIST   Sex Sex.HL70001 CDATA #IMPLIED >
  <!ELEMENT BirthDate (#PCDATA) >
  <!ELEMENT DiseaseList (Disease+) >
  <!ELEMENT Disease (DiseaseString,DiseaseCode,DiseaseCodeSystem) >
  <!ELEMENT DiseaseString (#PCDATA) >
  <!ELEMENT DiseaseCode (#PCDATA) >
  <!ELEMENT DiseaseCodeSystem (#PCDATA) >
  <!ELEMENT ReferralPurpose (#PCDATA) >
  <!ELEMENT Comments (#PCDATA) >
  <!ELEMENT OtherDocumentList (OtherDocument+ ) >
  <!ELEMENT OtherDocument (#PCDATA) >
]>
```

Figure 6.7 XML DTD Document for the Patient Referral Document

Because this description of XML data elements with XML DTDs does not match the element description capabilities in databases, a replacement for DTDs has been created: XML Schema. XML Schema is a W3C-sponsered effort to define an alternative to DTDs for defining the structure of XML documents. Within XML Schemas, data elements can be described at a lower level (byte, date, integer, user-defined, and others) and the exact number of occurrences of each data item can be identified; and unlike the DTD, an XML Schema is itself an XML document (W3C 2000-2003). Figure 6.8 shows an XML Schema for the patient referral.

```
<?xml version="1.0" encoding="UTF-8"?>
<xsd:schema xmlns:xsd="http://www.w3.org/2001/XMLSchema">

  <xsd:annotation>
    <xsd:documentation xml:lang="en">
      Patient referral document
    </xsd:documentation>
  </xsd:annotation>

  <xsd:element name="patientreferral" type="PatientReferralType" />

  <xsd:complexType name="PatientReferralType">
    <xsd:sequence>
```

```
    <xsd:element name="Header" type="HeaderType" />
    <xsd:element name="Patient" type="PatientType"/>
    <xsd:element name="DiseaseList" type="DiseaseListType" />
    <xsd:element name="ReferralPurpose" type="xsd:string" />
    <xsd:element name="Comments" type="xsd:string"
                 minOccurs="0" maxOccurs="1" />
    <xsd:element name="OtherDocumentList" type="OtherDocumentListType"
                 minOccurs="0" maxOccurs="1" />
  </xsd:sequence>
</xsd:complexType>

<xsd:complexType name="HeaderType">
  <xsd:sequence>
    <xsd:element name="TransmissionFrom" type="xsd:string" />
    <xsd:element name="TransmissionTo" type="xsd:string" />
    <xsd:element name="DateIssued" type="xsd:date" />
  </xsd:sequence>
</xsd:complexType>

<xsd:complexType name="PatientType">
  <xsd:sequence>
    <xsd:element name="IdList" type="IdListType" />
    <xsd:element name="PersonName" type="xsd:string" />
    <xsd:element name="Sex" type="SexType" />
    <xsd:element name="BirthDate" type="xsd:date" />
  </xsd:sequence>
</xsd:complexType>

<xsd:complexType name="DiseaseListType" >
  <xsd:sequence>
    <xsd:element name="Disease" type="DiseaseType"
                 minOccurs="1" maxOccurs="unbounded" />
  </xsd:sequence>
</xsd:complexType>

<xsd:complexType name="DiseaseType">
  <xsd:sequence>
    <xsd:element name="DiseaseString" type="xsd:string" />
    <xsd:element name="DiseaseCode" type="xsd:string" />
    <xsd:element name="DiseaseCodeSystem" type="xsd:string" />
  </xsd:sequence>
</xsd:complexType>

<xsd:complexType name="OtherDocumentListType" >
  <xsd:sequence>
    <xsd:element name="OtherDocument" type="xsd:string"
                 minOccurs="1" maxOccurs="unbounded" />
  </xsd:sequence>
</xsd:complexType>

<xsd:complexType name="IdListType">
  <xsd:sequence>
    <xsd:element name="Id" type="IdType"
                 minOccurs="1" maxOccurs="unbounded" />
  </xsd:sequence>
```

```
</xsd:complexType>

<xsd:complexType name="IdType">
  <xsd:sequence>
    <xsd:element name="IdMnemonic" type="xsd:string" />
    <xsd:element name="AssigningAuthority" type="xsd:string" />
  </xsd:sequence>
  <xsd:attribute name="type" type="conversionCategory" default="local" />
</xsd:complexType>

<xsd:complexType name="SexType" >
  <xsd:simpleContent>
    <xsd:extension base="xsd:string" >
      <xsd:attribute name="Sex.HL70001" type="xsd:string"/>
    </xsd:extension>
  </xsd:simpleContent>
</xsd:complexType>

<xsd:simpleType name="conversionCategory">
  <xsd:restriction base="xsd:string">
    <xsd:enumeration value="universal" />
    <xsd:enumeration value="national" />
    <xsd:enumeration value="local" />
  </xsd:restriction>
</xsd:simpleType>

</xsd:schema>
```

Figure 6.8 XML Schema for the Patient Referral Document

A XML DTD or XML Schema is equivalent to a structure chart, such as in figure 6.9, describing the data in the document. In programs using XMLs, a generic XML parser can be used to break out the individual data elements and data values from the XML document into a tree structure (similar to that in figure 6.9) based upon the XML DTD or XML Schema. The data and data elements can then be used in the program, for example, to output to a database.

6.6.2 Sharing the Medical Record

Patient medical records are a series of single documents. Some of these documents are similar throughout the United States and the world. Common documents include the following:

- **History and Physical:** The patient's initial medical examination and evaluation data.
- **Patient Referral:** A request from one physician to another for specialty care or advice.
- **Patient Consultation:** A request from one physician to another for specialty advice.
- **Progress Note:** Documentation for a follow-up visit.
- **Physician s Order:** Prescription, laboratory test order, etc.
- **Consultation Report:** Response to a referral.
- **Discharge Summary:** Report on a patient on discharge from a hospital.

If a common structure can be agreed upon for such documents, then there could be increased sharing of patient medical records between healthcare institutions, with transfer of the medical records over the Internet or healthcare network from one medical institution to another.

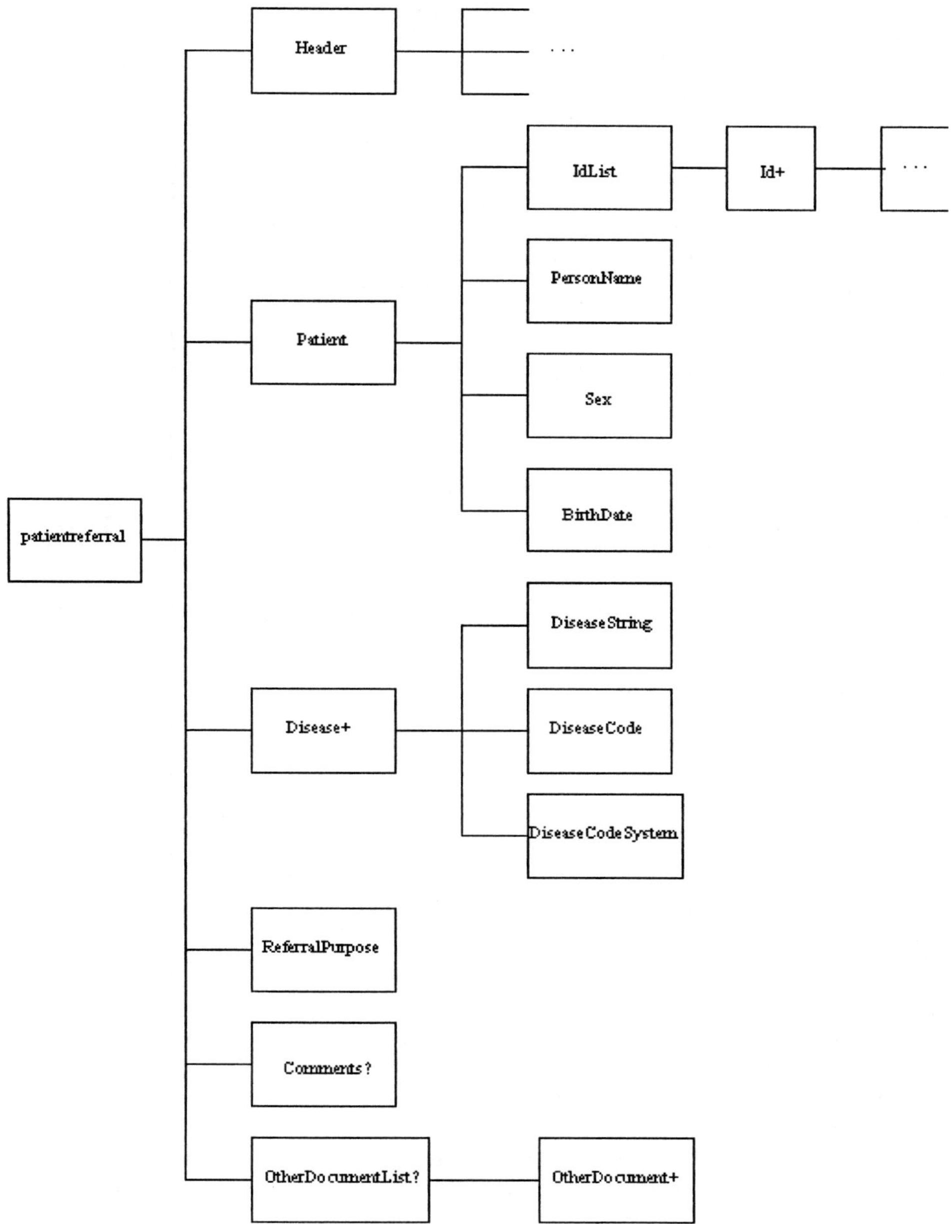

Figure 6.9 Structure Chart Equivalent of DTD Document

Clinical Document Architecture is a way of passing medical documents in terms of data values and data element formats to other healthcare institutions. Another proposal is presented here that also passes the rendering in the form of a local form to other healthcare institutions and data to convert local data values to healthcare industry standard data values.

6.6.3 Use of Standardized Data

Source documents can potentially be used to produce the CPR repository database that is defined by the E-R diagram in figure 6.5. Using data in source documents, the CPR repository system can identify encounters for the patient, the practitioners involved in the encounter, and orders, procedures (services) and results (observations) for each encounter. Encounters could be organized by the problem.

For a source document to be displayed at the facility where it was created, it must preserve local data values. However, for the data in the CPR repository or for source documents to also be useful at other healthcare organizations, it must translate these local values into standardized ones whose formats are agreed upon by the healthcare industry. Two potential universal standards are HL7 and ASTM E1384 for communication of clinical information and data in the CPR repository, with ASTM E1384 based upon HL7.

For many years, a standard for network communication of clinical information between healthcare computer systems has been "Health Level 7", or HL7 in short. Seven refers to the seventh level (the applications level) of the OSI seven level network model.

HL7 enables communication of clinical information such as the following:

- patient identification (see figure 6.10)
- physician identification
- queries
- admissions, discharges and transfers (hospital care)
- outpatient visits
- physician orders
- financial transactions
- order results.

PID|2||987654321^^^AZ||JONES^JOHN^RICHARD||19900607|M^MALE^HL70001<CR>

Figure 6.10 HL7 Patient Identification Network Message

Since some of the same information can occur within patient medical records, HL7 can potentially be used within XML for patient medical records. This could be done by use of XML attributes that identify HL7 tables. For example, the Sex.HL70001 attribute in the XML document in figure 6.6 identifies to use the HL70001 table to interpret values for the sex of a patient. The corresponding HL70001 table values are displayed in table 6.1.

The ASTM also has standards for the patient medical record—these standards are compatible with the HL7 standards: the ASTM E1384 standard for the electronic health record (ASTM 2002), ASTM E1633 standard for coded values in the electronic health record, (ASTM 2002), and ASTM E1714 standard for properties of a universal healthcare identifier (ASTM 1995).

Table 6.1 HL70001 Sex Table

Value	*Description*
F	Female
M	Male
O	Other
U	Unknown

It is the author's opinion that each source document must preserve the original values entered and should have the ability to also include national or universal standard values. The example in figure 6.6 shows the local data element for <SEX> as being "Female" and the HL7 standardized value as being "F" as an attribute. The HL7 sex value comes from the domain of values in the HL70001 table. Note that using data elements with attributes is only one approach to including both the local and standard values in the same source document.

A second approach for storing both standardized and local data elements at the same time is to have an element occurring more than once. This approach is also shown in the XML document in figure 6.6 for the IdList with contains multiple Id elements. The element, in this case "Id", occurs twice, once for the standard patient identifier (type="universal" meaning a standard and universal value) and once for the corresponding local patient identifier (a missing type attribute implies a "local" value). The first "Id" indicates that the standard patient identifier was assigned by a national assigning authority, while the second "Id" identifies that the local patient identifier was assigned by the HMO.

A way of identifying XML elements and attributes as belonging to a certain markup vocabulary, perhaps such as being standard parts of a standard patient referral document or as HL7 elements, is using *namespaces* (ASTM 1999). This involves preceding the elements or attributes with a prefix with a colon, and then associating the prefix with a URL location of documentation associated with the markup vocabulary. For example, figure 6.8 shows use of an arbitrary prefix "xsd:" and associating it with the URL location of XML Schema documentation, thus identifying the elements and attributes using the prefix as part of the XML Schema markup vocabulary.

6.6.4 Clinical Document Architecture

The group who created HL7 is working on standards for clinical source documents (such as discharge summaries and consultation notes) using XML within an architecture referred to as the *Clinical Document Architecture* (HL7-Australia 2003). Example documents could include those listed in section 6.6.2 and all others. Each XML document would have an architecture consisting of three parts: (1) a header, (2) a DTD structure for the document, and (3) XML content.

The header would contain the document type, authentication details, encounter, patient, and practitioner. There would be a separate DTD structure for each specialty/domain/document. Perhaps, the DTDs would be replaced by XML Schemas in the future.

The Clinical Document Architecture deals with content rather than rendering, where *rendering* is identifying how the data is to be presented on a device (e.g., within a display, such as on a PC or PDA screen, or over the telephone).

The Clinical Document Architecture is based upon *HL7 Reference Information Model (RIM)*. The RIM is HL7's object-oriented information model of the healthcare domain; all future HL7 message and document specifications will be derived from the RIM.

Using the Clinical Document Architecture (CDA), the content of a clinical source document can be recorded and then sent within an HL7 message to another healthcare location (Dolin et al. 2001). Data within the CDA document can be defined based upon the RIM, based upon other standards (e.g., LOINC, codes for clinical laboratory observations), or based upon local standards.

6.6.5 Outline of a Proposal for Use of XML with the Universal Patient Record

XML documents store data in structured form, also giving a name to each data element. XML DTDs or Schemas contain metadata describing the structure and format of each data element within the XML. And XSL enables rendering of the XML using the XML DTD or Schema, identifying how to display the information on a PC or PDA screen, how to output the XML information via voice to a wireless phone, how to output it to a printed form, or how to output it in another format.

XSL also has the capability to transform one XML document to another XML document. This capability exists through a major subset of XSL that has been standardized by the W3C (W3C 1999): XSLT, Extensible Stylesheet Language Transformations.

An *XML parser* is software that enables data values and data element names to be broken out from an XML document, for example, for storage on a database. A validating XML parser further validates the format of information on the XML document to be in the format identified by an XML DTD or Schema associated with the XML document.

My proposal for use of XML for the universal patient record is as follows:

Data in each source document would include local data values as they were entered at a healthcare organization for that source document. For each local value **where possible**, the associated healthcare industry standard value would also be stored.

Each source document must have a patient identifier. For the patient identifier, the associated healthcare industry standard value **is required**, as this would be used to associate the document with the correct patient in the CPR repository and source document repository. For documents that are to be associated with encounters or orders, healthcare industry values to identify encounters or orders should also be included.

For a limited number of industry agreed-upon types of source documents, perhaps such as listed in section 6.6.2 (e.g., the H&P), the documents **must** have specific data elements required by that source document, including both local and healthcare industry standard values (though the values may be missing or "null"). Additional data elements can be added by a healthcare organization as needed, with the additional values either only including a local value or the local value and the healthcare industry standard value.

For any source document, data values—local or local and health industry standard values—would be stored in an XML document. Metadata describing the data elements and their formats both for the local and healthcare industry standard data as the data appears in the XML document would be stored in a XML Schema (or XML DTD) document. XSL would identify how to render (display) the local data on a computer screen in the format of a paper form that would be used at the healthcare organization where care was given, with optional display of any associated healthcare industry value, perhaps by the user putting the mouse over a local value when it is displayed.

See figure 6.11. The XML document, XML Schema (or XML DTD) Document, and XSL document would be stored on the source document repository by the healthcare organization automated patient medical record system and provide all the information needed to display each source document with local values as if were entered at the healthcare organization in the format of a form, and also, where feasible, enable translation of a local value to its healthcare industry standard value.

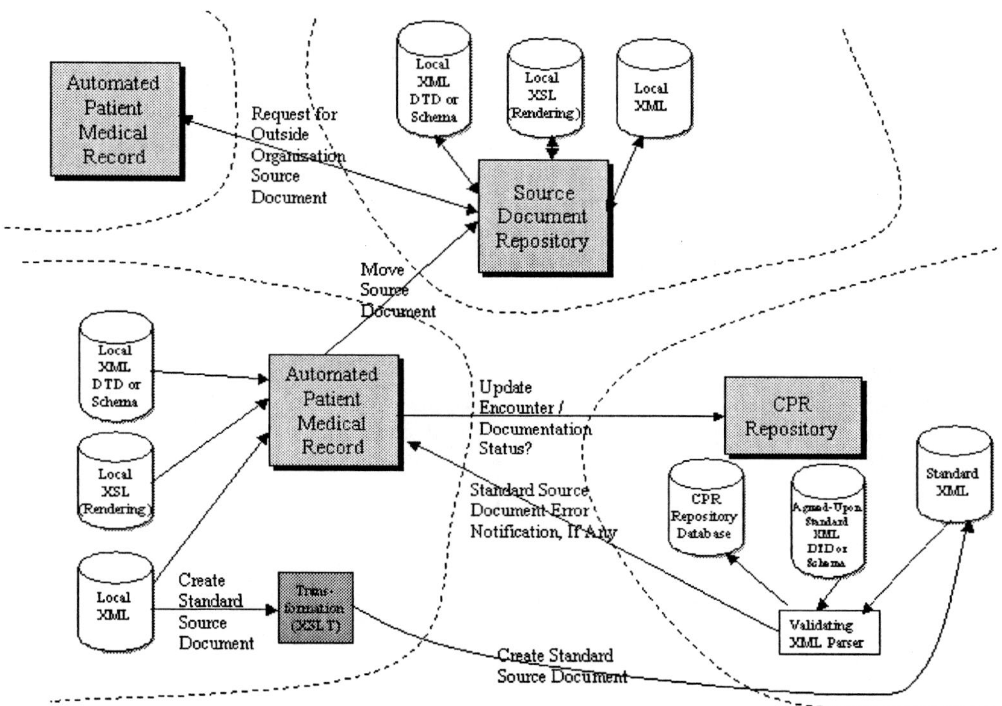

Figure 6.11 Storage and Retrieval of Source Documents from the Source Document Respository and Creation of the Information on the CPR Repository for the Associated Encounter, Order and Patient.

If the source document was one of the agreed-upon types, then additional XSL (in this case XSLT) would identify how to strip out from the XML document those data elements required by that type of document together with the healthcare industry standard values for these data elements—excluding local values—to produce a pared-down XML document. The collection of these standard versions of the agreed-upon documents could be used to collectively create the CPR repository.

Before agreed-upon standard source documents are sent to the CPR repository, the CPR repository could first be notified of a new patient encounter occurring so it could organize data it receives from these source documents by encounter in the CPR repository. The end of an encounter or the end of documentation for an encounter could also be sent. A agreed-upon standard source document could be for an order, encounter and patient; for an encounter and patient; or just for a patient, and the CPR would organize information from the source document accordingly. The CPR repository, perhaps as shown in the E-R diagram in figure 6.5, could result.

The CPR repository would then contain all the data needed to create a patient clinical summary as shown in figure 6.2 and described in section 7.7.4.1.

The CPR repository software could use an XML parser to split out database values and data element names from the standard XML documents using the agreed-upon XML DTD or Schema for that type of source document, populating the CPR repository database. For a CPR repository database in E1384 format, such a database's structure is described by the E-R diagram in figure 6.5.

When a healthcare organization asks the source document repository for a document generated by another healthcare organization, the local XML, XML DTD or Schema and XSL for display at the healthcare organization that created the document should be sent to that healthcare organization. When the document is rendered, it could then be rendered as entered by the originating healthcare organization when such informaiton is input on a form; when the user places the mouse over a local value, the standardized value could be displayed, similar to display of text that occurs when you place the mouse over an image in many Web documents.

Because of security reasons, the network for transmission of XML documents between large medical institutions should probably be a private medical network, but to enable communication with smaller medical organizations, use of the Web is probably necessary. There are standards for communication of XML documents over the Web.

Certain data elements in a source document, such as free format text, could be identified as "translatable" to other languages. Automated translation between languages is a possibility.

Other potentially useful XML capabilities are the following (Wilde and Lowe 2002): *XML Namespaces (*which allows you to avoid namespace collisions when defining XML elements and attributes, especially combining information from two different sources that may have the same basic data element names), *XPath* (which allows you to use patterns to identify sections of an XML document), *XPointer* (which extends XPath to allow you to address points in the document and ranges between points), and *XLink* (which enables you to create links within XML documents).

6.7 THE SOURCE DOCUMENT REPOSITORY AS A CONTENT MANAGEMENT SYSTEM

Therefore it is proposed that the Source Document Repository be composed of XML, XML Schema and XSL documents. Furthermore, XML can itself contain voice, pictures and videos and links to other documents (through XLink). Also source documents themselves should be able to be text, fax, voice, graphics, picture, video, or scanned images as long as each is in a standard format (e.g., JPEG for pictures, MP3 for sound, TIFF for images, office documents, PDFs). XML contains Unicode, a character set for text that enables that text to be in many languages (Unicode Consortium 1991-2004),.

Storage of such a set of information can be accomplished through *content management systems,* also known as *document management systems*. A content management system is a system for storing different types of unstructured content (such as Web content, office documents, scanned images and faxes, e-mail and rich media) and semi-structured content (such as printed reports) as well as structured content (XML and associated documents) (Moore and Markham 2002).

Documents in document management systems can have attached textual values such as medical record number, provider id, encounter date, etc. to order the documents and to enable their retrieval. This is especially important for storage of scanned images, which otherwise would not have items that would enable retrieval of them. Scanning paper medical records and including indexes is a way of including these documents in the automated patient medical record.

FileNET™, Documentum™, IBM™, and OpenText™ are examples of companies that provide document management systems / content management systems.

6.8 OTHER CONSIDERATIONS

Four other considerations for a universal patient record are

1. security and privacy
2. granting/requesting permission to receive copies of source documents and paper medical records
3. language for recording information, and
4. correctness and accuracy of information.

A universal patient record must provide security measures that disallow unauthorized use of the information and protect the patient's privacy. These security measures must conform to any applicable security rules and laws. Security laws and rules may vary by country or region of the world. For example, in the United States, security of patient medical records is governed by state and federal laws and by rules from the US Department of Health and Human Services referred to as HIPAA—see section 13.9 and the appendix. What rules and laws apply when care is given across countries? And what happens if such rules and laws hinder medical care?

Authorized parties can request permission to copy source or paper documents, and the caregiver who created a source or paper document or his healthcare organization together with the patient can grant permission to an authorized party to copy the document. Perhaps, certain categories of permissions can be granted by policy and/or pre-approval of a patient. For example, an HMO might automatically, by policy, be granted the authority to copy source or paper documents of patients who are HMO members, and insurance companies might automatically be granted authority to copy financial information from source or paper documents for patients who they insure. The government, healthcare organization, caregiver, or patient might establish general policies for sharing medical information and also information requiring special security (e.g., genetic or mental health information). Standards for the relationship of these grants and requests with the CPR and source document repositories, and for the communication paths of these grants and requests with people and systems need to be developed.

A universal patient record must be able to record care in any language in which care is given. View of records by a caregiver who speaks another language may require translation. Translation with the help of the recording caregiver may or may not be possible or practical.

The universal patient record should be correct and accurate. The mere fact that information is recorded for all to see is a risk to a caregiver recording the information, especially in nations such as the United States where misinformation may result in lawsuits. Translation from one language may also introduce errors.

Privacy and absolute accuracy of medical information is viewed to be of utmost importance in some developed nations, whereas just having some medical care is more important in many developing countries. If a specialty physician located somewhere else in the world could assist a family practice physician in the care of a patient in a developing nation, or if a physician could assist a non-physician healthcare worker, would security rules or laws, or fear of lawsuits, disallow or hinder this care?

Good medical care is a necessity for people to live well. Perfect care—perfect privacy and absolute correctness and accuracy of information—is a luxury, and probably will never be a reality nor a necessity. Could this quest for perfection hinder introduction of a universal patient record, a method to improve medical care? Or could it hinder caregivers from giving good medical care, as inaccuracy could also potentially cause harm?

In any case, storage of the universal patient record in a CPR and source document repository and chart rooms must account for the various security and privacy laws of the world and protect view or transfer of information to unauthorized people. Storage of the universal patient record must be allowed in any language in which care can be given, with the capability to support translation to the languages of other caregivers. Medical information should be accurate, but more importantly, it should be based upon providing well-reasoned care.

Key Terms

application service provider (ASP)
ASTM E1384
Clinical Document Architecture
Computer-based Patient Record (CPR) repository
content management system
document management system
HL7 (Health Level 7)
HL7 Reference Information Model (RIM)
HTML
metadata
namespaces
Patient Clinical Summary
patient registry
Personal Health Record
rendering
risk management
scalable
source document
source document repository
vision
XLink
XML
XML DTD
XML Namespace
XML Schema
XPath
XPointer
XSL
XSLT

Study Questions

1. Why is it hard for an organization to have "vision"? How can an organization protect against being wrong?
2. Section 6.2 lists 7 assumptions about a universal patient record. Discuss the contradictions between assumptions 1 and 2. Why is the security assumption in 5 problematic? Discuss assumption 6 and potential problems with it. Why, as stated in assumption 7, is there the possibility that a caregiver could lack confidence in a universal patient record?
3. Critique the author's vision of the future? What is this book's view of the CPR. Of a source document repository.
4. What is the relationship of the CPR repository and the Patient Clinical Summary.
5. How does the *Personal Health Record* idea differ from what is presented in this chapter?
6. At what point would a patient repository be needed?
7. This book predicts how small healthcare organizations could use the universal patient record. What is this approach?
8. What effects would a universal patient record have on patients? On society as a whole? On a healthcare organization?
9. What is the ASTM standard for electronic health records that might be used to for the CPR? Explain the E-R diagram in figure 6.5.
10. What is XML? What are XML DTDs and XML Schemas? What is XSLT? Which of these XML documents contain data, format information, rendering information?
11. HL7 has proposed use of the Clinical Document Architecture (CDA) to describe source documents—There would be no standard format for documents. How are this book's ideas for source documents the same? How do they differ?
12. This book proposes that information for an encounter and associated encounter summary information in the CPR repository be built using the source documents—How would this be done?
13. What other XML constructs exist that could be of use for source documents? What is "rendering"?—Explain how XML constructs can be used to separate data from format from rendering information.
14. What are content management systems (aka document management systems)? How do they relate to source document repositories?
15. How could security potentially make the universal patient record unfeasible?
16. What is the danger of translating source documents?

CHAPTER 7

Business Requirements for an Automated Patient Medical Record

CHAPTER OUTLINE

7.1 PROJECT CONTEXT: DERIVING BUSINESS REQUIREMENTS

Business requirements are required characteristics of an organization at the end of a project. Business requirements are primarily derived from the following sources: (1) from identification of current automated systems and business practices to be preserved, (2) from project objectives,

(3) from a vision of the future, (4) from improvements suggested by employees and others, (5) from projecting how the future environment and systems will function, (6) from identification of obstacles to the project.

A conceptual view of the automated patient medical record system so far—including a universal patient record—is presented in figure 7.1. At the end of this chapter in section 7.9, a new conceptual view of our project is presented that incorporates the business requirements in this chapter.

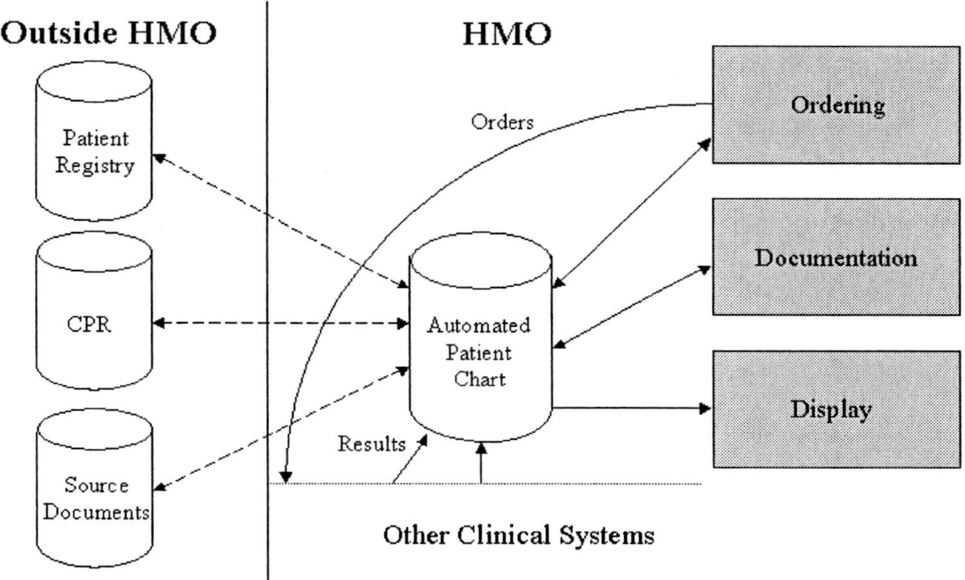

Figure 7.1 A Conceptual View of the Automated Patient Medical Record So Far

Since a business requirement, like a project objective, may not, as stated, be measurable, it is also useful to identify a goal for each business requirement. A total list of business requirements for the automated patient medical record together with a goal for each business requirement appears later in this book in section 10.16 after business requirements are added that are identified as a result of looking at obstacles.

7.2 MEDICAL DOCUMENTS: SOURCE DOCUMENTS AND THOSE ON PAPER

The basic medical information included in the automated patient medical record will continue to be medical documents making up the medical record such as are identified in section 4.4, whether these documents are stored as automated source documents or are paper medical documents. *Source documents* are automated medical record documents and can be in the form of text, fax, voice, graphics, picture or video, or any combination of these, with embedding of graphics or pictures within the text. Links to other source documents can appear anywhere within the text.

7.3 ORGANIZATION

One project objective listed in table 5.2 for an automated patient medical record project is to "enable a caregiver to quickly find relevant information in the patient medical record by methods such as providing summarization information, organization, information retrieval, and tailoring of information related to the type of caregiver".

The following are proposed methods for providing organization to the automated patient medical record:

1. **encounters:** Each document in the medical record is associated with the encounter (e.g., outpatient visit, inpatient stay) in which it was created
2. **significant health problems:** An encounter is associated with a significant health problem, so selection of the health problem identifies all the encounters where care for the health problem occurred.

7.3.1 Encounters

A natural and seemingly straightforward way of organizing documents making up the patient chart is to categorize medical documents and other patient clinical information as to whether they apply to an

- inpatient stay, including hospice, SNF, sub-acute care facility, etc.
- outpatient visit
- emergency department (ED) visit
- surgery
- phone call consult that takes the place of an outpatient visit
- e-mail consult (Spielberg 1998)
- observation visit (for a possible impending birth)
- home health care visit.

Each of the above is an *encounter*. The ASTM (American Society for Testing and Materials), which develops and publishes standards on a wide variety of topics in health care informatics through the ASTM E31 committee, defines an encounter as "an instance of direct (usually face-to-face) interaction, regardless of setting, between a patient and a practitioner vested with primary responsibility for diagnosing, evaluating or treating the patient's condition, or both, or providing social work services. (Encounters do not include ancillary services visits or telephone contacts.)" (ASTM 2002). (The ASTM definition would thus not include phone call consults, and also would probably not include e-mail consults, as encounters. This book—like reference (Richards and Rathbun 1999)–considers a telephone contact to be an encounter if the telephone contact is significant enough to take the place of an outpatient visit and if either a physician-patient relationship has already been established or one will be established in the future.)

Associating each medical document with an encounter would enable a caregiver to select all patient clinical information associated with a particular encounter. Although the use of an encounter to categorize a document is useful, there could be some possible complications in doing this tying of documents to an encounter, although I think all these complications can be overcome.

Consider an inpatient visit. Sometimes diagnostic tests are done prior to admission, in particular prior to an admission to the hospital for a surgery. If it is deemed desirable to associate the diagnostic tests done prior to the admission with the inpatient stay, then these tests must be temporarily associated with some data item other than the admission, perhaps with a pre-admission, and then later tied to the admission. A further complication is that the admission may never occur.

Another possible complication occurring with an inpatient stay is the chance of a temporary transfer of a patient to another location while the patient remains admitted in the first location. An example is the transfer of a patient for a cardiac catheterization in a second facility, while still being considered admitted to the first facility.

There are also possible complications with tying documents with an outpatient visit. During an outpatient visit, there may be orders for diagnostic tests and for treatments. Usually these tests and treatments take place after the outpatient visit is complete. These tests and treatments even could occur at a different facility and prescriptions could be filled at a non-HMO pharmacy. Thus tying together documentation of a test result, treatment, or the dispensing of a medication with the outpatient visit may require some sophistication in the computer systems involved and possible computer network communication between facilities.

Also, outpatient diagnostic tests could be done prior to the outpatient visit. Such tests might have to first be associated with an appointment and then with the outpatient visit. Again, as with the inpatient situation, the outpatient visit could fail to take place.

There are a number of types of documents that cannot always be tied uniquely to one encounter, including *phone messages* and *e-mail messages*. Phone messages and e-mail messages dealing with patient clinical information can occur prior to encounters and independent of encounters. Documents listed in the next section, section 7.4, cross encounters and also cannot be tied to a single encounter.

The identification of encounters as well as the start date/time and end date/time of an encounter usually comes from other HMO computerized clinical systems independent from the automated patient medical record system. Another value that could come from these systems is an *encounter status*, an event that may logically precede, occur during or be a result of an encounter or potential encounter, or event that is a result of a situation causing the encounter not to occur.

Types of encounters and associated encounter statuses are the following:

- *inpatient stay* (with status pre-admitted, admitted, admitted—newborn, transferred to another location or facility, scheduled for discharge, discharged, transferred while retaining admission, case abstract after discharge creating codes for the diagnoses, admission reversal, etc.—and also post hospital outpatient visit). This information would come from the ADT system for hospital stays or from other systems for other types of inpatient stays (e.g., admission to a SNF)
- *outpatient visit* (with status wait-listed, appointed, appointment canceled, appointment no show, patient registered, in the examination room, visit completed, diagnoses and procedures identified). This information would come from the appointment system, from the registration system (to collect co-payments and record the patient has come in for a visit) or from other clinical systems
- *ED visit* (with status patient registered, in the examination room, discharged from ED to home, discharged from ED to hospital, diagnoses and procedures identified) from the ED system and registration system
- *surgery* (with status scheduled, in progress, completed, canceled, case abstracted) from the surgery system

- *telephone call* (with status pending, completion of a non-encounter, completion of an encounter) potentially from the appointment or registration systems, but, as stated earlier, in this section, the ASTM E31 committee does not consider telephone contacts to be encounters (ASTM 2002)
- *observation visit* entrance to a medical facility for observation (with status recorded, returned to home, admitted to hospital) from the ADT system (e.g., a pregnant woman in the early stages of labor may be brought in for an observation visit after which she may be sent to labor and delivery or go home)
- *home care visit* (with status care at home, termination of care at home).

Sometimes the associated encounter information is unavailable to the automated patient medical record system before a document is entered. This might be due to the encounter clinical system (e.g., ADT, the appointment system or registration system) being down, its network connection with the automated system being down, or due to the encounter not yet being entered into the encounter system. In such cases, the tying of the document to an encounter might have to occur later, after the encounter is later received.

Some events could occur a long time after the encounter, and, if it is necessary to record them in the automated patient medical record, it may be difficult to associate them with the encounter. For example, a physician could review the automated patient medical record to determine whether a medication should be reordered. The encounter where the medication was ordered could have occurred a long time ago.

At the beginning of automation of the chart, especially with an HMO with point of service contracts, some facilities or associated healthcare institutions may not be part of the automated system, and associating documents and orders with encounters in these facilities or outside health institutions may not be possible, at least not until there is a universal patient record.

Despite possible complications with doing so, associating each patient medical record document with an encounter appears to be a useful and necessary first step in organizing the patient chart.

7.3.2 Significant, Persistent, and Long Lasting, Health Problems

Often a patient comes in many times for a significant health problem (hypertension, an allergy, asthma, urinary incontinence, a prostate problem). A *significant health problem* is a current, permanent or long-lasting disease or medical condition. For a caregiver to have a list of these significant health problems is extremely useful to quickly identify the patient's significant health history.

But in addition, identification of such significant health problems could also help organize the patient medical record so that all encounters associated with that problem could be easily found, so that patients who would benefit from health education on a problem could be identified, and so that similar but more severe problems can be anticipated (e.g., obesity may be associated with diabetes, BPH symptoms may be similar to symptoms for prostate cancer). A previous attempt at organizing the patient chart by significant health problems is the Problem-Oriented Medical Record (POMR) (Loeb 1995).

The automated system could identify or help identify a patient's significant health problems, and caregivers could be trained to identify a patient's significant health problems.

7.4 DOCUMENTS TO TRACK CARE ACROSS ENCOUNTERS

Some project objectives listed in table 5.2 deal with "tracking care across multiple encounters". For purposes of continuity of care, it is important to track care that may occur across encounters, possibly with different caregivers, in different medical facilities, and in different healthcare organizations.

A model for patient care, both for inpatient and outpatient care, was presented in figure 4.1 (Shortliffe and Barnett 2001). As shown by this figure, the process of care is as follows: The patient is identified and the problem (referred to as the "chief complaint") is recorded. Through various means, the caregiver hypothesizes on the diagnosis. Based upon a selected diagnosis, the caregiver develops a treatment plan for the patient, observes the results and may refine his or her hypotheses and diagnosis. After the caregiver observes the results, the diagnosis or treatment may be changed. This process often occurs over many encounters.

Types of documents to record care across multiple encounters are the following:

1. *Case management document*: A document that associates encounters for a named patient for some reason—to track care for a condition until an expected final outcome (defined outcome) is reached; to track care for a condition that is expected to be ongoing (e.g., for a chronic condition); to track care across conditions (e.g., a high risk patient or a worker's compensation case).
2. *Trend document*: A document recording a clinical value for a patient collected over various encounters.
3. *Clinical pathway document:* A document generically describing a "standard of care" given over multiple encounters, based upon a particular medical condition, which may be applied to a patient with this condition.
4. *Care notes*: A caregiver or care team may provide continuing care for a patient over a long period of time but the care is not so significant that it requires constant tracking, such as by a chronic care management case. Instead, the caregiver can create care notes for a patient that can be associated with types of encounters of the patient that are within the scope of care of the caregiver or care team.

In order to accurately record the care process in the patient chart when there are many encounters for the same treatment, I propose that a case management approach be used, with a case referencing the encounters spanning the treatment of the patient for the medical condition. A case to track a treatment for a particular patient and usually non-chronic medical condition over a number of encounters where the condition is not likely to require long term continuing care, I will refer to as a *defined outcome case*, as the expected, and finally the actual, outcome needs to be identified along with the treatment in order to evaluate the treatment. A case to track a patient who is being treated for a chronic condition over many encounters where there is likely to be long term continuing care, will be referred to as a *chronic care management case*. Defined outcome cases differ from chronic care management cases in that the former are expected to have a concluding outcome (e.g., the condition is relieved, goes away or is cured), while the latter would have periodic outcomes (e.g., the number of hospital stays during the period). An important care activity in a chronic care management case are patient education visits where the member is educated on when it is appropriate for the member to administer self-care for his chronic condition and when it is mandatory that the member come in for care.

Also, I propose that there be a type of case, a *patient case*, which can be used for management of high-risk and high-cost patients by case managers. Such a case can be created independently from any specific medical condition or as part of a defined outcome case or chronic care management case. A patient case could be useful for Worker's Compensation patients and frail and elderly Medicare patients to track patients and reduce costs.

The entity-relationship (E-R) diagram in figure 7.2 proposes a structure for a case—section 13.8 describes how to interpret E-R diagrams. *Defined outcome cases* and *chronic care management cases* would consist of a list of case managers; a description of the treatment plan with any later changes to it, including treatment notes for each encounter; expected outcomes of the treatment, may include references to documents describing the treatment plan in detail such as clinical pathway documents and treatment guidelines (e.g., *National Guideline Clearinghouse* clinical practice guidelines (NGC 1998-2004)); and may include a document I call a "trend document". The case document would identify encounters associated with the case and might also include case notes and other documents entered and used by an overall case manager, who together with a physician might oversee the case. Eventually, the actual outcomes of the treatment would be associated with the case, so the treatment could be evaluated; three types of outcomes need be considered: financial, clinical and patient satisfaction.

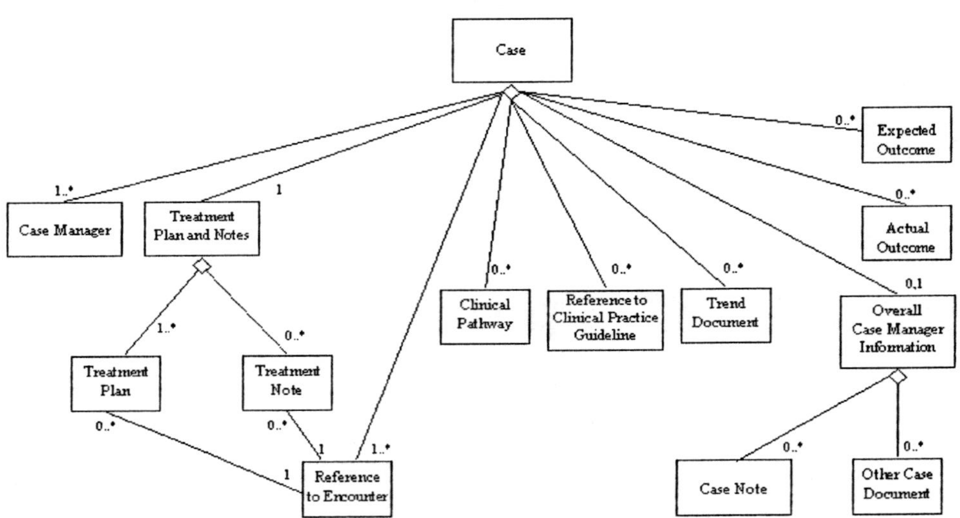

Figure 7.2 Case Documentation

A *patient case* allows a case manager to track a patient over multiple encounters, whether or not the encounters are for a specific medical condition. It would consist of case notes and other case documents, as part of overall case management information.

Defined outcome cases and chronic care management cases tie together all the documents and encounters associated with care of a patient for a particular condition, whether the encounters are inpatient, outpatient, Emergency Department or other type of visits. Defined outcome cases and chronic care management cases should clearly identify treatments given, care plans followed and patient characteristics (e.g., the condition of the patient at the start of treatment). And defined outcome cases and chronic care management cases should record expected and actual outcomes of these treatments.

After defined outcome cases for similar medical conditions and similar patients have been completed, various treatment plans for the same health problem can be evaluated for the most favorable outcomes and thus the best treatments, supporting what has been called "evidence-based medicine" (Sackett et al. 1996). Results of such studies could produce treatment plans that result in best medical practices, those with the greatest chance of success at the least cost and the greatest benefit to the patient as determined by the best scientific evidence.

Outcomes of chronic care management cases for chronic conditions could involve comparing costs, quality and patient satisfaction results for patients being tracked by chronic care management cases with patients with the same chronic disease who are not being tracked to see if there is a measurable impact of the care plan. Alternative successful care plans can be compared. Through this process, care plans can be chosen that best improve the care of patients for these chronic conditions. Defined outcome cases and chronic care management cases thus provide a means to evaluate and improve medical care.

The case management approach can also be used for automated evaluation of care, with system determination that care being given may be inconsistent with a treatment plan or best practice guidelines, or that inappropriate medications or treatments were being given. The case manager could be notified by the system, who then could consult with practitioners to verify that proper care was being given. Also, practitioners who need to be retrained could be identified.

A chronic care management case, and possibly a defined outcome case, can be associated with a significant patient health problem. The list of significant health problems for a patient could then identify which problems have associated case(s).

Ideally, defined outcome cases, chronic care management cases, and patient cases will become part of the CPR repository so that cases can be tracked, and possibly managed, across health care organizations. Supporting documentation, such as clinical pathway documents, should also being captured, e.g., in the source document repository.

Defined outcome cases and chronic care management cases require a new discipline of care. A treatment plan in a defined outcome case or chronic care management case may be set up by one caregiver and generally needs to be followed by later caregivers who see the patient, even if the later caregiver has a different style or philosophy in providing care. If the same caregiver continues to see the patient, change in care philosophy is not a problem and thus is usually the preferred situation; assignment of a patient with a limited number of physician(s), nurse practitioners and other caregivers, a *care team*, who oversee the patient's care and understand each others' care philosophy is an alternative approach that may work well.

Some analysis has to be done to determine what should happen if a physician sees the patient for a second opinion on a disease, condition or treatment. For example, should the physician providing the second opinion review a defined outcome case or completely ignore the defined outcome case so he isn't biased by the treatment given by the other caregiver(s)?

Use of defined outcome cases and chronic care management cases require discipline and some extra work by physicians and other caregivers, but could provide tremendous benefits to patients, to healthcare organizations, and to society as a whole.

7.4.1 A Defined Outcome Case

Another useful concept is an *episode*. The ASTM defines an episode as "one or more healthcare services received by an individual during a period of relatively continuous care by healthcare practitioners in relation to a particular clinical problem or situation" (ASTM 2002).

As evidenced by discussions of outpatient and inpatient care in chapter 4, the treatment of a particular health problem is an iterative process, possibly extending over many outpatient and inpatient visits. This is true of almost all significant health problems.

Automation of the chart allows for the possibility of clear communication of a treatment extending over many encounters with expected outcomes of the treatment, and eventually the final outcome of the treatment. By HMO personnel **consciously identifying these encounters as part of a treatment** and tracking the treatment, long term patient treatment plans could be better managed, evaluated and be more successful, resulting in much improved patient care. A proposed set of documents to document such a treatment for an acute (i.e., short duration) condition will be referred to as a "defined outcome case" because the treatment can be best managed by case management techniques and can be evaluated by identifying the final outcomes of the treatment, comparing them again the expected (defined) outcome.

The following describes the characteristics of a defined outcome case:

- when a treatment for acute care extends over more than one encounter, a defined outcome case can be developed with *treatment plans* and *treatment notes* explaining the treatment and follow-up notes being attached by later caregivers to identify continuation or change of the treatment
- the defined outcome case can optionally reference national or HMO clinical practice guidelines (e.g., from the *National Guideline Clearinghouse* database)
- for a defined outcome case, an optional *clinical pathway* document based upon the patient condition can be attached, guiding the treatment
- for a defined outcome case, an optional *trend document* can be used, that automates collection of particular data values, such a blood pressure over the various encounter, growth charts (height and weight), etc.
- each encounter associated with the defined outcome case will be identified.

A defined outcome case should be assigned to a case manager to enable the case manager to track the treatment. The case manager may be the patient's principal primary care provider or other caregiver. Through the defined outcome case, assigned caregivers and/or the case manager could optionally be notified if critical events in the defined outcome case fail to occur.

7.4.2 Chronic Care Management Case

According to a reference on the Internet (Marks 2003), chronic diseases account for about 70% of all U.S. deaths and about 75% of health care costs each year. Management of chronic diseases often requires long-term treatment management controlling costs and patient accessibility to services. The assignment of a case manager could assist the patient in accessibility to services. Such a case will be referred to here as a "chronic care management case".

Examples of diseases possibly requiring long-term management are the following:

- HIV/AIDS
- asthma
- diabetes
- severe depression
- seizure disorders
- renal disease.

A number of health organizations provide disease management advice or services, including (NDDIC 2003) and (ACAAI 1998) and (CMI 2003). For example, Kaiser Permanente (CMI 2003) provides disease management services for asthma, cancer, chronic pain, coronary artery disease, depression, diabetes, elder care, heart failure, obesity, and self-care/shared decision making, and have shown there can be significant cost savings.

As part of a chronic care management case, a clinical pathway could be developed that combines case manager activities together with physician, nurse, pharmacist and other caregiver activities. With the use of a clinical pathway, caregivers and the patient would be assured that the correct medication or treatment was given at the right time according to clinical practice guidelines. Any national or HMO clinical practice guidelines that are being followed could also be referenced.

Patient compliance with showing up for treatments and following prescribed drug therapies in the chronic care management case could be tracked. For example, through the automated patient medical record system, caregivers could be notified when a patient misses an appointment (and thus misses a treatment) and when medications are not picked up from the pharmacy. In the future, chronic care management case tracking of patients could be supported by "Guardian Angel" computer systems in the patient's possession to track patient compliance with treatments (see section 5.3.2.2).

7.4.3 Patient Case

It is often useful to assign a high-cost or high-risk patient (for example, an elderly, frail Medicare patient or a patient paid for by workers' compensation) to a *case manager* whose job is to guide the patient through the system, determining the most appropriate treatments or health care entities (SNF's, hospices, etc.). Such a case will be termed a *patient case*, as case management of the patient may occur across many patient encounters that may not be related to the same treatment or medical condition.

Documents necessary to support this tracking of high cost, high risk, patients should be stored by the automated patient medical record systems as a patient case. At the very least, these documents should include *case notes* for recording of notes by the case manager, which can optionally be associated with patient encounters.

Chronic care management cases or defined outcome cases can also have a patient case containing case manager case notes independent from treatment notes.

7.4.4 Clinical Pathway

A structured approach to patient care is a *clinical pathway* (sometimes called a "critical pathway" or a "life care path"). A clinical pathway encapsulates a care or treatment plan for a specific condition or encapsulates preventative care for patients in a particular category, in particular based upon best medical practices as determined by the best available evidence ("evidence-based medicine").

A clinical pathway identifies care activities and caregiver workflow needed to provide care for a category of person for preventive care or for a patient with a particular condition or disease. Paths through a clinical pathway can be adjusted for the particular needs of an individual patient.

A clinical pathway document may stand-alone or be part of a defined outcome case, chronic care management case, or a patient case. It describes a series of care activities that may be conditionally performed either as part of a treatment (e.g., for Alzheimer's, kidney stones) or as part of a strategy for preventative care (e.g., preventative health activities to be performed on the patient of such a sex and age such as mammography). The latter type of clinical pathway identifying preventative care for a member is termed a "life care path", as it exists over the life time of the patient, not just during a specific treatment.

A *clinical pathway* identifies a *standard of care* for caregivers for a particular *patient problem or condition* with consideration of *risk adjustments* which may be based upon patient psychological, health and social factors, family/genetic history, patient age, race and sex. A clinical pathway may exist for outpatients, inpatients or both—see (Dowsey et al. 1999) and (PCCM 2003). A clinical pathway may be used for treating illnesses or for managing health and wellness (and may then be known as *health paths* or *life care paths*). For example there might be a clinical pathway for all female patients over 50.

A clinical pathway consists of the following elements:

- *Clinical pathway template*: a network structure diagram identifying all recommended alternative paths of care based upon intermediate goals and outcomes. A clinical pathway template consists of a series of *care activities*, *paths* between care activities, and optionally **times** between care activities in a path as identified by fixed time values or by *probability density functions (pdf)* identifying likely time values, with one time or pdf for the organization and one for the health care industry as a whole. From one care activity there may be one or many paths leading to other care activities. A number of care activities could lead to the same care activity. Network diagram paths eventually may lead to *final outcomes* that identify the conclusion of the care path (e.g., discharge from the hospital), or paths may be ongoing. A care activity may consist of text identifying care to be given, a goal, an order or appointment to be automatically scheduled, a protocol defined elsewhere in the system (e.g., "Implement 'anticoag' protocol"), or another clinical pathway; for example, there may be a clinical pathway template identifying all likely paths for care activities for women over 50, including paths identifying that the patient has been confirmed as having breast cancer and thereafter treating the patient, with a care activity consisting of a different clinical pathway specifically for the treatment of breast cancer. There would be another path identifying that the patient is healthy. One possible final outcome in the breast cancer clinical pathway may be total remission of the cancer.
- *Selected path*: one of the paths through the clinical pathway template selected by caregiver(s) upon intermediate outcomes, goals, and final outcomes, identifying care to be given to the patient as determined by the clinical pathway template. During an encounter between the patient and a caregiver, the caregiver can select the next path to take in the clinical pathway template based upon a goal or an intermediate patient outcome. For example, a clinical pathway may include a care activity that consists of giving the patient a mammogram, with the intermediate outcome that the patient has a normal mammogram, and thus the patient would be scheduled for the next care activity, a mammogram a year later.
- *Actual path*: a path identifying actual care activities given to the patient, which tracks the outcome-directed "selected path" except that actual times, if applicable, may be assigned to paths, care activities may be added or skipped, additional intermediate and final outcomes may result. The actual path identifies what actually happened; it may consist of the same path as the outcome-directed path but with actual times between activities or additional care activities within the path.
- *Variances*: each variance between an actual path and a selected (projected) path; variance between expected and actual times, variance in care activities; variance in costs; variance

between actual and projected immediate outcomes; and the variance between the actual final outcome and the initially projected final outcome.

During an encounter of a patient with a caregiver, the caregiver can identify the next path to take, adding to the selected path. The next care activity in a selected path may be an encounter and optionally include *automatic scheduling of the encounter* or may put the encounter on a *wait list* for later scheduling of the encounter. A care activity in a selected path may also optionally *automatically schedule an order*. The caregiver may be informed if a care activity is not performed within the required time (e.g., a patient with a critical condition does not show up for his appointment and does not reschedule the appointment in the required time). The caregiver can add or skip care activities changing the selected path, and creating an actual path different than the selected path.

After assignment of a clinical pathway to a patient, a clinical pathway can be discontinued, merged with other clinical pathways or identified as completed by a caregiver. Merging of clinical pathways would take into account *co-morbidity*, i.e., interaction of the care activities in multiple clinical pathways. Care activities in different clinical pathways that are merged could be color coded by the clinical pathway the care activity came from and highlighted for co-morbidity. As paths through the clinical pathway are completed, times for actual paths would be included in with the pdf's for the organization in the clinical pathway template.

As stated earlier, a clinical pathway could be used to pre-schedule activities for members who come in to the emergency department often for recurrent emergent care. For a child with epilepsy, the patient's parent could inform the emergency department of the patient's arrival, identifying a particular predetermined care situation and an estimated time of arrival. This would initiate a clinical pathway that initiates care activities including necessary care documentation.

A clinical pathway structure could also include care activities that a patient himself or herself is advised to follow (e.g., a drug therapy program for the patient).

7.4.5 Scope of Care and Care Notes

Often in an HMO, a patient receives continuing care over a long period of time from a single primary care physician, a single specialty physician, or a care team. Such a caregiver or care team may be always interested in all of a patient's encounters or may be primarily interested in a subset of encounters (e.g., encounters in a specialty area, encounters with the care team, or encounters with the physician). It is proposed that a caregiver or care team be able to identify encounters within the *scope of care* of the caregiver or care team, and, over time, associate care notes with the set of such encounters for this patient.

For example, a patient may be routinely seeing a urologist for continuing care for a prostate-related problem. The problem is troubling and is likely to worsen, eventually even requiring surgery, but problem is not serious enough to track with a chronic care management case. Care notes for the patient, associated with urology encounters for the patient, would be a way for the urologist to remind him- or herself of ideas for future treatments and other care decisions for the patient.

Thus the automated patient medical record can combine together a patient's total medical record, but it can also enable the medical record to be partitioned in any way that promotes medical care. Within encounters within a scope of care, the caregiver or care team could also include cases—defined outcome cases, chronic care management cases—and clinical pathways.

7.4.6 Care Management Versus Case Management Versus Disease Management

It is useful to distinguish between care management, case management, and disease management, although these types of management of patients and patient care overlap. The following are definitions:

- *case management*: An organized system for delivering health care to an individual that includes assessment and development of a plan of care, coordination of services, referrals and follow-ups.
- *care management*: Aggregates encounters and other events into episodes for a particular occurrence of a medical condition, possibly across care settings, rather than just focusing on a single encounter or event of an illness or injury.
- *disease management*: Identifies populations (patients) with particular acute and chronic diseases, such as diabetes, cancer, coronary artery disease or asthma, and introduces interventions throughout the life cycle of the disease that would both improve the patient's quality of life and lower the costs associated with the disease process.

These categories of care are not mutually exclusive of each other. Care management and disease management are encompassed by case management.

Defined outcome case documents, chronic care management case documents and patient case documents are documents that can be used for case management. Defined outcome case documents apply to care management, as they are intended for episodes for a single occurrence of a medical condition. Patient case documents are intended for case management of high-risk patients, where case management is done independently of the medical conditions being treated. Since disease management generally tracks chronic diseases and potentially chronic diseases, chronic care management case documents are most useful for disease management.

7.4.7 Trend Document

A *trend document* automatically records a value that a caregiver wants to track over time as they are input via other source documents. Examples are blood pressure readings, blood glucose readings, and the patient's height and weight. A trend document may either stand-alone or be part of a defined outcome case or chronic care management case.

Whenever the patient comes in, the automated patient medical record system could prompt the caregiver to record that required value. Additionally, patients could call into the healthcare organization to have recorded their own blood pressure readings, blood glucose readings, etc. See figure 7.3 for an example of a trend document for blood pressure. Trend documents may also stand alone, independent of defined outcome cases or chronic care management cases.

Trend documents, like in figure 7.3, could also record mean, maximum and minimum expected values for what is being measured, for example mean, maximum and minimum systolic and diastolic values for males varying by age. They could be set up to be *actionable*, i.e., to automatically inform identified caregivers when a measured value is out of range. A trend document as described is a *control chart* in the field of statistical process control.

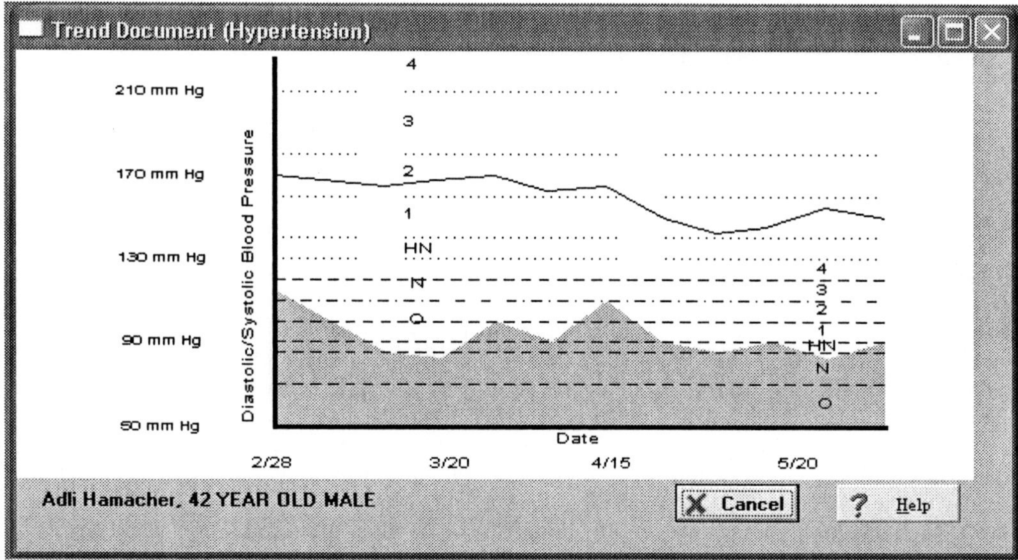

Figure 7.3 Trend Document

7.4.8 Recording of Biomarkers

The NIH has defined *biomarkers* as "cellular, biochemical, molecular, or genetic characteristics or alterations by which a normal, abnormal, or simply biologic process can be recognized, or monitored." Biomarkers can be used in disease diagnosis and prediction in four general ways:

1. to identify the presence of an organism in the patient (e.g., by microbiology),
2. to estimate the patient's prior exposure to an organism or other environmental factor
3. to identify current changes or effects within the patient (e.g., toxicological effects or disease symptoms)
4. to assess the patient's underlying susceptibility to a disease (e.g., through genetics).

Biomarkers are information of long-lasting interest to caregivers. The automated patient medical record can record permanent biomarkers or record the values of changing biomarkers over time in trend documents. Currently existing biomarkers are :

- Positive results for the Pap (Papanicolaou) smear and the presence of some strains of the human papillomavirus (HPV) to test for cervical cancer (Solomon and Nayar 2004)
- The prostate specific antigen (PSA) to test for prostate cancer
- Systolic and diastolic blood pressure values as a test for heart disease and stroke.

In the future, it is expected that many more biomarkers will be used in the prediction and diagnosis of disease, including genes to measure susceptibility to developing diseases and gene expression of proteins and RNAs to diagnose diseases. See section 17.5.

Biomarkers could be expensive and difficult to obtain, critically important to medical care, and be highly sensitive information. Therefore, biomarkers should be easily available to physicians who are providing direct care to the patient and who have a need to know the information, but should be protected health information, with a patient's name unavailable to those who could misuse the information. See section 13.9.2 for security of protected health information.

The automated patient medical record could provide researchers with biomarker values together with diagnosed diseases, hiding the names of patients. This would enable researchers to identify the effectiveness of these biomarkers in predicting disease.

7.5 A DISTRIBUTED PATIENT MEDICAL RECORD

One project objective listed in table 5.2 is "to create a complete and always available patient medical record". There are lots of possible ways of storing an automated patient medical record.

With automation of the patient medical record, an HMO can eventually consolidate all their chart information in a single data repository in the HMO, if they so choose. Thus, the example of the many charts for a patient in an HMO as previously shown in figure 5.2—and shown now in figure 7.4—could change so that this clinical information could be combined into a centrally located computerized patient medical record, a patient medical record completely outside the HMO, or something in between. With complete automation of the chart in the healthcare organization and alliance organizations, where the automated patient medical record is actually stored could be transparent and irrelevant to the user as long as the technology to retrieve it is fast enough.

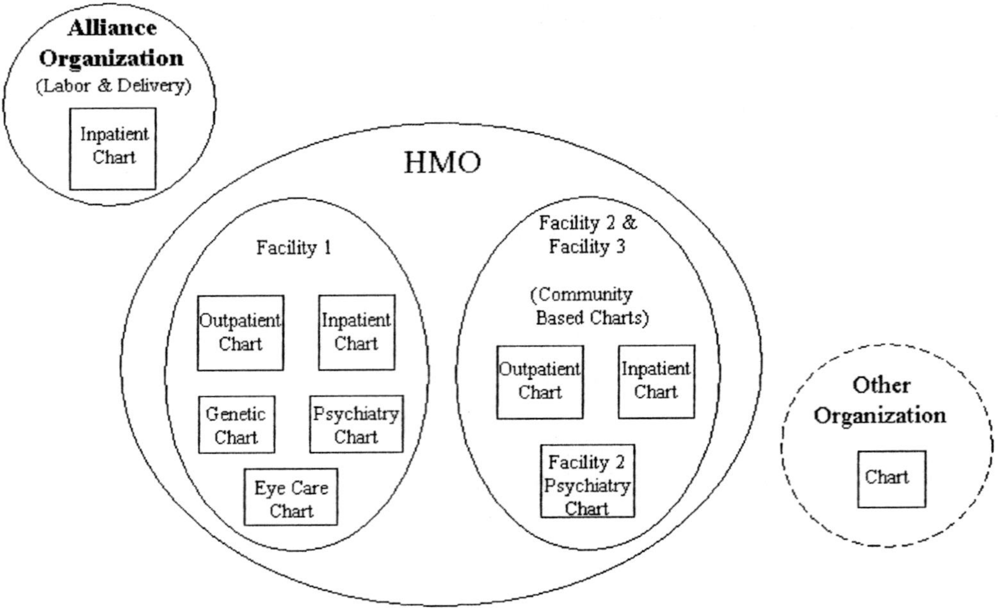

Figure 7.4 An example of the existing charts for an HMO patient.

But patient medical record information outside the HMO is likely to be, at first, on paper. And during the interim phases of automation of the HMO's own patient medical record, HMO clinical information is likely to be both automated and on paper.

So, in summary, with an automated patient medical record:

- as long the technology is fast enough to retrieve the parts of the automated patient medical record, it doesn't matter whether the automated part of the chart is stored, in many locations or only one, as the user would not notice any difference
- however, part of a patient's medical record is likely to be on paper.

7.5.1 A Prediction of the Future

At this point, the author will reiterate and expand upon some predictions made in the last chapter about the storage of automated patient medical records in the future. See figure 7.5.

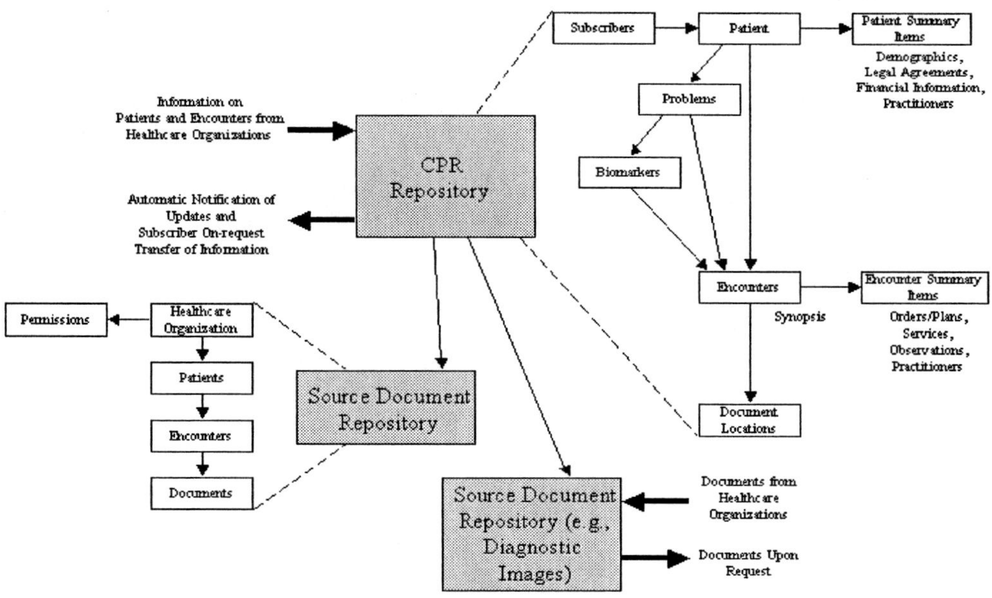

Figure 7.5 Remote storage of clinic information in the patient medical record.

In the future, there will be a computer-based patient record (CPR) repository to store a summary of patient chart information nation-wide developed from source documents for the patient. Additionally, medical documents as input by caregivers will be increasingly computerized with healthcare organizations storing these patient records electronically on source document repositories.

Source document repositories in the future could even be located outside of healthcare organizations, in other organizations. (Pacific Bell, for example, proposed building a repository to store diagnostic images for California healthcare organizations (Kohli 1996).) The source document repository organization would take over responsibility for storage of clinical information, duplicate storage of clinical information at a second off-site location, and the costs of insurance for accidental destruction of the chart information.

The CPR repository could also store the location of the medical documents, whether on paper in a chart room or in a source document repository wherever the source document repository is located. A healthcare organization could be informed of member medical record information added to the CPR repository for encounters occurring outside the healthcare organization and of changes in locations of source documents where the locations are outside the healthcare organization.

Whenever a healthcare organization was informed in a change to the CPR, the healthcare organization could retrieve the CPR information from the CPR repository and the associated source documents from the source document repository or other locations as identified in the CPR repository.

The CPR repository and source document repositories could be organized by patient and patient encounter. Upon completion of an encounter in the healthcare organization, the healthcare organization could send a summary of the encounter to the CPR repository. This information could include encounter summary items, together with current patient demographics information. Further, the healthcare organization could identify a list of patient health problems and associate encounters with these health problems. Periodically, the source documents could be sent to the source document repository, sending the changed location to the CPR repository.

If it turns out that there are multiple CPR repositories, then it would be useful to have a patient registry that receives information from CPR repositories on additions to the CPR repositories. The patient registry, rather than the CPR repositories, would then inform the healthcare organization of updates to the CPR repositories. Such CPR and source document repositories and patient registry could be structured as pictured in figure 6.4.

There are a number of standards for the structure and content of the CPR—see the appendix. As a representative standard, this book will assume the ASTM E1384 standard for the CPR (ASTM 2002). This includes the following information:

- patient demographics
- patient legal agreements
- patient financial information
- practitioners
- patient problems
- immunizations
- health history
- assessments
- patient reported data
- clinical orders
- diagnostic tests
- medications
- scheduled appointments/events
- encounters
- chief complaints/diagnoses
- clinical courses
- therapies/procedures.

Although **not part of the ASTM E1384 standard**, as stated here, it is proposed that each CPR repository also keep the locations of all medical documents associated with the encounter. Medical documents could be located (1) within a non-healthcare organization source document repository, (2) within a healthcare organization source document repository or (3) on paper within a healthcare organization. (The ASTM E1384 standard does, however, include a single location for the paper or automated patient medical record for each encounter.)

It is also proposed that a synopsis of each patient encounter be kept in the CPR repository, although, again, this is not part of the ASTM E1384 standard. For healthcare organizations that have not yet computerized the patient chart and thus cannot send any other information to the CPR, this synopsis could be sent to the CPR repository by e-mail together with an indication that the associated chart is located on paper at the healthcare organization.

Subscribers to the patient registry (see figure 7.5 again) would pay to receive notification of new encounters of interest, identifying the patients and conditions under which the subscriber would be notified. For example, an insurance company subscriber could get information on any patient encounter where the patient owns insurance issued by that company and where that insurance applies for that encounter. An HMO subscriber could get information on any encounter for a current HMO member that occurs outside the HMO so the HMO could have a complete record of the patient's encounters and of the locations of associated documents; additionally, an HMO subscriber could pick up all patient clinical information for a patient who is a new member of the HMO and could pick up information for non-members scheduled to visit the HMO. Upon identifying the location of encounter documents from the CPR, the subscriber could later retrieve or make a request to receive the medical documents from the source document repositories or from chart rooms outside the healthcare organization.

Some source documents could cross multiple encounters. Defined outcome cases and chronic care management cases could cross multiple encounters. A clinical pathway is a document that provides a care plan for a patient that may cross multiple encounters. A trend document could collect and display information, possibly graphically, from values collected during multiple encounters and from values called in by the patient to an appointment clerk or advice nurse (see figure 7.3). Trend documents identify trends in the patient health based upon a defining patient condition, a significant health problem or a potential problem (a concern) to be studied. Examples are a growth chart showing age versus height for a child being studied for small stature in an endocrinology clinic, or charts showing blood pressure, LDL and HDL levels for serum cholesterol versus time for a patient with cardiac problems. Clinical pathways, trend documents and references to clinical practice guidelines can be included within a defined outcome case or chronic care management case, identifying a treatment for the patient.

A referenced clinical practice guideline should be available on-line. Because a clinical practice guideline may be used by many patients in many different cases, there should be some repository for storing a clinical practice guideline one time. Also, since a clinical practice guideline might change over time, a history of these changes should also be kept (for example, with a version number for each set of changes). CPR repositories could reference these clinical practice guidelines.

As stated in section 7.4, I think that defined outcome cases and chronic care management cases (including treatment plans and notes, case notes, and references to clinical pathways, trend documents and clinical practice guidelines) should be made part of the CPR repositories. This would enable a defined outcome case or chronic care management case to be used across many healthcare institutions.

Biomarkers could be associated with health problems or diseases and the encounters where the biomarker was identified or changed.

The patient registry, CPR repositories and source document repositories are the constituent parts of an automated patient medical record. If this prediction of repositories and registries is correct, many standards for repositories and registries need to be developed.

CPR repositories should store information using agreed upon format standards. Source document repositories should store documents in the format of the healthcare institution of the document in order to preserve the appearance of the document; however, stored with each source document in the source document repository, ideally, should be information to translate proprietary health institution data elements to standard data elements, so other healthcare institutions could also make use of the documents. (For example, an outside healthcare institution may receive the source document in the form it appears at the originating healthcare institution with proprietary data elements highlighted; pressing a right mouse button over the highlighted data element might display a caption with the standard, translated, information.)

Although CPR repositories would store information using agreed upon standards and source document repositories might need to have information to translate clinical information based upon data standards, these standards might change or be expanded to include additional data over time. A mechanism to coordinate these changes in standards and communicate these changes to healthcare institutions needs to be established.

It is expected that some standard data elements appearing in the CPR will require a mechanism for immediate assignment at a healthcare organization, such as patient identifiers. For example, if there is a new patient to the HMO, the HMO should have the ability to do an inquiry through a remote organization who assigns such identifiers to determine if the patient already has a patient identifier and either return a newly assigned identifier or return the existing identifier. Other standard data elements not requiring immediate update might be handled via tapes listing the values for these data elements, periodically sent to the healthcare organization from the assigning organizations.

7.5.2 Existing Standards for a Distributed Patient Record

There have been many standards groups meeting to determine healthcare standards for an automated patient medical record. Healthcare standards have been discussed for the following:

- patient identifier
- provider identifier
- care site identifier
- product and supply identifier
- computer to computer communication message formats
- clinical data representation
- patient chart content and structure
- therapies/procedures.

See the appendix of this book for more information.

An indisputable standard for communication of healthcare information across networks is HL7. This is discussed in more detail in section 13.11.6.

7.6 INCORPORATING HEALTHCARE ORGANIZATION BUSINESS POLICIES

An HMO or other organization has business policies governing the way it works. Further, business policies may differ for different parts of the organization. For example, in an HMO, each HMO facility and each department in a facility may work differently. Departments of a particular type (e.g., dermatology, medicine, and pediatrics) might each have their own set of rules. And each provider may sometimes be able to override a business policy.

Organizational business policies are implemented through organizational procedures and automated systems. This involves determining what parts of the business policy are implemented through employee workflows, through code and internal tables, through databases, through user interfaces, and through interfaces between systems.

A major failing of computer system design and maintenance is that companies entrust computer people to properly incorporate business policies into a system, rather than the people in the groups who are responsible for these policies. Further, incorporation of these policies into the system may involve changes to code in many different parts of systems; thus, no matter how competent the computer people are in incorporating the business policies, maintenance of, and especially documentation of, these business policies may be extremely difficult.

It is proposed that the automated system provide a means by which such business policies can be easily implemented within the automated system by the people controlling these policies rather than computer people, with easy re-implementation when a change in business policy occurs. Thus the people responsible for enforcing a business policy should be involved in the design of all aspects of the business policy. An *agent* is defined in this book as a way of categorizing and separating out a set of independent business rules incorporating a business policy—possibly embedded in code or tables, databases, interfaces between systems, and user interfaces through a number of different computer systems, as well as administrative rules followed by employees—so that the business policy can be easily changed without effecting the other code in the system.

These business policies can be business policies related to the organization, a particular job category within the organization (e.g., physicians or nurses), a region of the organization, a particular job category within the region of an organization, a group of facilities, a particular job category within a group of facilities, a facility, a particular job category within a facility, a department type, a particular outpatient department or hospital unit, a particular job category within a department or unit, or an individual caregiver, with differing business policies for each level. Table 7.1 shows a proposal for a hierarchy of agents within an HMO, with agents with a lower priority number overriding an agent with a higher priority number. Thus a set of business rules may be defined at one level, say for the whole HMO, but be overridden at a lower level, say by caregivers within a particular job category, such as for inpatient nurses, and be overridden at yet a lower level, say by an individual named caregiver; thus, even though Nurse Jones is an inpatient nurse, she uses an agent for her individually, while other inpatient nurses use a lower level organizational job category agent for inpatient nurses.

In order to perform its task, an agent may perform its work in any computer within the distributed system. Further, the code to execute the agent might be stored anywhere on the network, possibly shipped down to be executed. Such techniques would enable, say, a regional agent to be compiled and implemented only once, within the regional computer for the entire organization and not every computer, but still allow it to be used anywhere, e.g., within a local system for a particular healthcare facility.

Table 7.1 Priority of Agents

Priority	*Agent Type*
1	Personal Agent
2	Unit / Department Job Category Agent
3	Unit / Department Agent
4	Unit / Department Type Agent
5	Facility Job Category Agent
6	Facility Agent
7	Facility Group Job Category Agent
8	Facility Group Agent
9	Regional Job Category Agent
10	Regional Agent
11	Organizational Job Category Agent
12	Organizational Agent

Examples of business policies that might be implemented in the automated medical record system by agents, through code and tables, databases, user interfaces, interfaces between computers, and work flows are the following:

- **A Policy for Assigning Personal Care Providers with HMO Members:** A consistent policy for the entire healthcare organization could be implemented both for the automated patient medical record system and other HMO clinical systems.
- **A Policy for Tailoring the System by Caregiver Type:** Various types of caregivers need different types of access to the system. Each caregiver should be able to select all encounters within the caregiver's scope of care. Inpatient physicians, outpatient physicians, inpatient nurses, inpatient nurses probably all require different types of patient lists. A "patient list" is a list of patients of interest to a caregiver stored within the automated patient medical record system, usually automatically built from encounters and encounter statuses from other clinical systems. See section 7.7.5 for a discussion of patient lists. An inpatient nurse needs a unit census and an outpatient physician needs quick access to his schedule. These are two, of many different types of, patient lists. An organizational job category agent could be set up based upon job category of the caregiver (nurse, outpatient physician, inpatient physician, etc.) to display the required "patient lists" for the caregiver in the format required by the particular type of caregiver. A particular caregiver could define a personal agent to present a set of patient lists different than the standard set, with the personal agent overriding the organization job category agent. Besides patient lists, other information is appropriate for tailorability by job category (e.g., patient clinical summaries—see section 7.7.4.1).
- **A Policy for Archiving Radiology Images:** A radiology image should be archived after X years; an organizational agent, say within the regional system, could implement this automatic archiving and destruction of electronic radiology images within the organization.

- **A Policy for Collecting CPR and Source Document Information on an Appointment:** For each appointment the physician sees, an outpatient physician needs to find all information in the automated patient medical record related to the chief complaint. An agent is created to be executed the night before an outpatient appointment that automatically does a search through the automated patient medical record for clinical information related to the chief complaint so an index to this information can be presented to the caregiver.
- **A Policy for Collecting CPR and Source Document Information on an Preadmission, Dependent Upon the Hospital Unit:** A Med/Surg inpatient unit needs all chart information on the patient for the last 5 years during the inpatient stay. Previous to a scheduled inpatient admission, an agent could automatically order copies of all paper charts and retrieve automated patient medical record information from remote sites for encounters within the last 5 years.
- **A Policy for Collecting Hypertension Information Set up by a Facility:** Clinical research needs to be done on the effectiveness of hypertensive medications given in a facility in Bakersfield for the next half year; a facility agent could be set up to automatically record data for this research whenever a caregiver entered information on such a patient via SOAP notes.
- **A Policy for Profiling a Provider at a Facility by Provider Category:** A caregiver's activities could be automatically profiled (i.e., tracked) for a group of related facilities via a facility group job category agent.
- **A Policy for Organizational Security:** An organization agent could control access to department-related information and specific documents. The agent could provide security against unauthorized access and disclosure, maintain the integrity of the data, and confirm the identities of the originators and requesters of the data.
- **A Policy for Collecting Information on Regional Public Health:** A regional agent could alert the HMO region and public health officials of usual increases in the incidence of influenza, specific bacterial infections or other public health problems.
- **A Policy for Collecting Information for a Registry:** A regional agent to recognize when a medical condition should be recorded to a Registry and automatically record it or inform the caregiver.
- **A Policy for Collecting QA / Costing Information:** An agent to inform the caregiver of lower cost equally effective procedures or medications and possible drug interactions based upon previous medications and patient medical history. The agent could also check for other quality assurance issues such as compliance with recommendations from JCAHO or other professional organizations, with state or federal regulations, or for possible duplication of orders.

7.7 TYING EVERYTHING TOGETHER TO CREATE A USEFUL SYSTEM FOR CAREGIVERS

This section presents further requirements for an automated patient medical record system. This section is based upon automation of some of the current manual processes in the HMO (see section 4.7) and additional capabilities to implement project objectives listed in table 5.2 that tie together the automated patient medical record.

The automated patient medical record system would substitute for paper patient charts, but also allow paper charts to exist: It would provide for enhanced access to patient chart information, whether automated or on paper. Additionally, it would provide other capabilities such as functions for ordering, communication between caregivers and clinical research. These capabilities are as follows:

- document patient care
- issue medical orders and receive results
- display the clinical information that makes up the patient medical record
- create and display summary information from the patient medical record
- search for and select clinical information for display
- identify trends in the patient's health
- identify patients of interest to a caregiver (e.g., patients in a provider's schedule, inpatient nursing census, ED census)
- provide communication between caregivers
- incorporate healthcare organization business policies
- enable clinical research.

7.7.1 Documenting Patient Care

This section on documenting patient care assumes the existence of repositories for source documents and a repository for the Computer-based Patient Record (CPR) as described in chapter 6, and describes how source documents could be displayed, entered, and stored.

Medical documents are created in the care of patients. Through these documents, vital signs, progress notes and other clinical information such as identified in section 4.4 are created and added to the patient medical record. A document for a patient can be created by a caregiver (e.g., H&P or progress notes) or can be created by transfer of information from another system to the automated patient medical record system (e.g., test results being returned from the clinical laboratory system). Before sending a completed document to the patient medical record that the caregiver creates, a caregiver must sign, or for an automated patient medical record "electronically sign" (CMS 2004), the document verifying the identity of the caregiver.

Documents can include various forms of information: text, graphs, voice, video, pictures, drawings, scanned images, or waveforms. Waveforms come from medical instruments and can be voluminous; thus there must be algorithms for selecting and filtering of waveform information, or caregivers to select the information, so only the most significant waveforms would be stored on the document database. Textual documents may have embedded graphs, pictures, drawings, scanned images or waveforms and may be paired with a diagnostic image (e.g., an x-ray and a transcription of results), a waveform document (an ECG and an interpretation of results), or other documents.

The format of a document on the screen (e.g., an H&P SOAP note) can be different from the equivalent printed document (see figure 7.6). For example, an on-screen document (e.g., a SOAP note) can often be combined with on-screen display and entrance of other clinical information (e.g., a list of the patient's health problems, medications or allergies). Proposed is that there be a "document description database" that defines both screen displays of source documents and the printed forms of the source documents. The printed form can also be displayed on a screen and provide an alternate means of entrance of information, e.g., recording patient examination and interview information; this printed form on the screen would ideally have the same format as a printed form that was used when the patient chart was on paper and could be used both for routine use and for times when the automated system was down. With source documents and the Source Document repository being in XML, it is appropriate for the document description database to be in XSL, and the format of the data being in the form of an XML Schema.

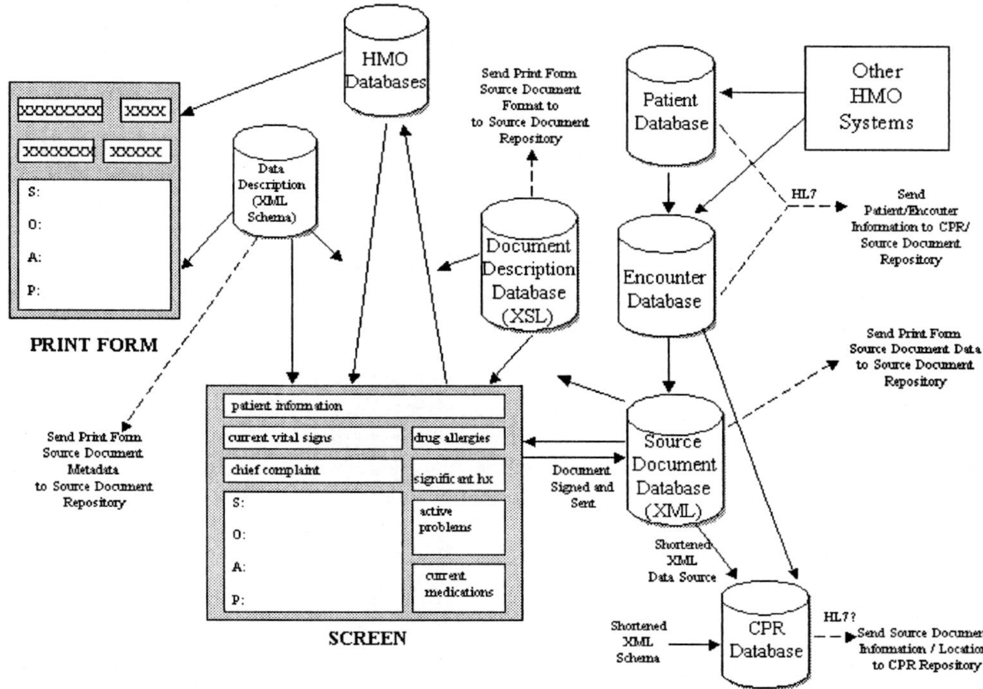

Figure 7.6 Documentation.

The document description for the screen would describe the document in terms of fields for display or entrance of data, while the document description for the printed form would describe the document in terms of fields as they would appear on printed forms. These fields can be as simple as displaying or allowing entrance of a patient identifier, a patient name, a patient date of birth, a provider identifier or a provider name and can be as complicated as a section for word processing that uses semi-structured elements such as provider-generated templates to facilitate entrance of information on the screen (e.g., generic text for abdominal pain in the subjective portion of a progress note).

To enable communication of information with outside organizations, documents should use standardized data elements including universal patient identifiers, and industry standard provider and location identifiers, and other elements (see the appendix for a discussion of healthcare standards). Standardized patient identifiers are required to associate documents with the correct patient; ideally, standard data for encounter and ordering identifiers would be included where appropriate to associate documents with the correct encounter and order. These same standards would also be used by registries and repositories. (There is no agreed-upon universal patient identifier as of yet.)

The "document description" database would identify titles and other static information and would identify the following for each document field: the field type, domain, field length, font, borders, security level and screen or print location. For the screen document description, each field would be identified as display only or enterable. Additionally, for each field, the HMO data base and database data item currently containing the field data, or which will contain the field data, would be identified.

When a document is to be displayed on a screen or printed on a printer, the document description database would be used to identify how the document is structured and data from the HMO databases and data element standards file would be merged in to produce the document on the screen or printed form. Data elements that the user does not have security to view would be excluded. When data is entered for a document on the screen and the document is signed and sent, the document would be moved to the HMO data bases with data element locations for the entered fields as identified in the document description file. The document would also be stored in the document database and related to the patient encounter.

After completion of the encounter, the printed form version of the source documents during the encounter consisting of XML elements (XML, XML DTD or Schemas, and XSL) that includes standard data elements with the local data elements within each XML document would be sent to the source document repository. The storage locations of these source documents or of paper documents created during the encounter (the identified source document repository or chart room for a paper document) would be sent to the CPR repository.

Since source documents sent to a source document repository could vary in format from one healthcare institution to another and a particular health institution might use non-standard data elements, it would be useful to have information sent along with the source document to the source document repository that translates information into standard data elements. This would facilitate interpretation by an outside healthcare institution and facilitate retrieval of the source documents based upon caregiver entered search criteria based upon standard data elements. A technique might be provided to enable users at other healthcare institutions to interpret non-standard data elements (e.g., pressing a right mouse key over a data element might show a caption with the interpreted standard data element value).

Before the encounter documents are sent to the source document repository and medical document locations are sent to the CPR repository, associated patient and encounter information must first be received by both CPR and source document repositories so the document or document locations can be associated with the patient encounter. Patient and encounter information may come from systems other than the automated patient medical record system, which may be the ADT system, visit registration system, or resource scheduling and appointment system.

As a document is being created, CPR information, summarizing the encounter could be created. At the end of the encounter, patient and CPR information in E1384 format could be collected and sent to the CPR repository using HL7 network protocol. (What constitutes the end of an encounter and when it is the appropriate time to send encounter information to the CPR requires further study; for example, sometimes diagnostic tests connected with the encounter are not completed well after the encounter—should the transfer to the CPR wait until after these are complete?)

Many documents used during the patient care process will not provide information that is sent to the CPR repository (e.g., flow sheets during an inpatient stay). All documents that are currently part of a paper patient chart would be saved as source documents (e.g., flow sheets). Documents generated during an encounter that are not currently stored as part of a paper patient chart will not be saved as source documents (e.g., the Kardex and equivalent Inpatient Clinical Summary during an inpatient stay). Nevertheless, an automated patient medical record system could provide support for all these documents.

It is also proposed that each encounter should be summarized after the encounter, either directly by the caregiver or by the system from caregiver input to documents. This is referred to as an "encounter synopsis". The encounter synopsis would enable caregivers to quickly evaluate encounters and facilitate future caregiver finding of information in the automated patient medical record by searching for the specific medical information. This encounter synopsis could be sent to the CPR repository to be stored with the encounter information in the CPR repository. For healthcare organizations who have not automated the patient medical record, this encounter synopsis information could be sent to the CPR repository by e-mail and perhaps would be the only information sent to the CPR for a patient encounter.

As source documents are being entered in the HMO, techniques for facilitating input of source documentation could be used. These techniques include

- re-use of previously entered information

  (e.g., patient age, height, phone number entered on one document or from data from another HMO system would be available for other documents)
- templates generated by organizations, departments or individual physicians

  (e.g., templates—see figure 7.7—could be created by physicians for various chief complaints, such as for "abdominal pain", displaying text and pick lists and areas to enter text; when interviewing the patient, the physician would pick selections from pick lists and fill in the text)
- abbreviations and symbols

  (e.g., an approved set of abbreviations and symbols for Hospital XYZ for all SOAP notes, with expansion of the abbreviation or symbol upon caregiver request)
- pick lists—drop down lists

  (e.g., selecting "nature" via a pointing device in figure 7.8, might display a drop down list showing "burning, sharp, dull, cramping, crushing, constant, or intermittent")
- documentation tailored for the patient encounter

  (e.g., a nurse could use a flow sheet tailored to the patient's diagnoses, rather then a generic one)
- automatic ordering within a clinical pathway

  (e.g., a clinical pathway for prenatal care could automatically set up a series of appointments and schedule various procedures associated with prenatal care)
- entrance of information by exception

  (e.g., a flow sheet allowing an inpatient nurse to record the patient's status every hour could be structured such that the nurse would only have to input information when the patient's condition changes)
- generation and maintenance of complete, personalized, patient care documents based upon the patient's diagnoses, such as nursing care plans or critical path documents

  (e.g., a nursing care plan generated by a program such as Davis's Electronic Care Plan Maker (Doenges, Moorhouse, and Geissler-Murr 2002)).

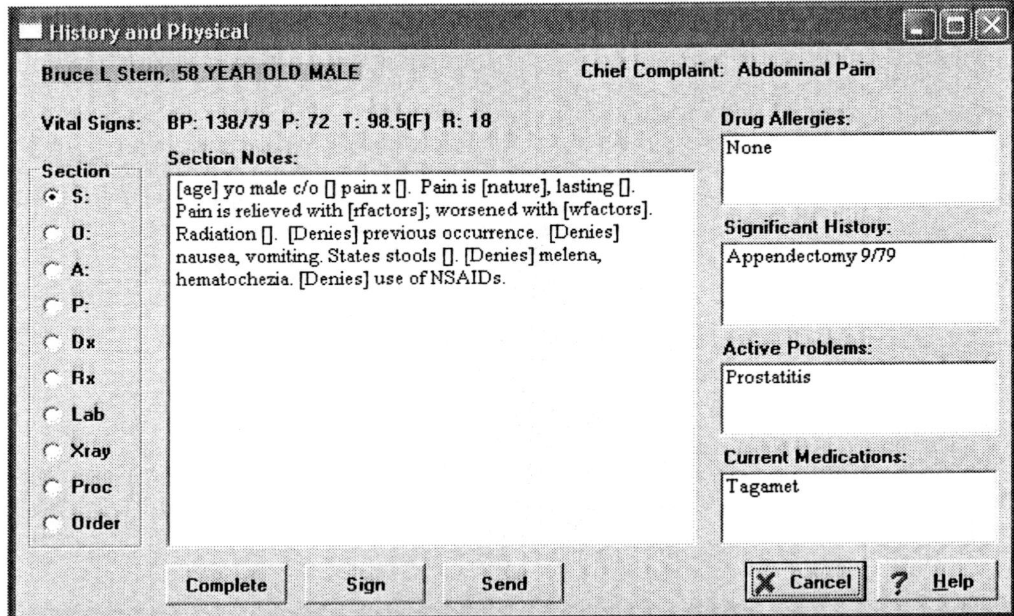

Figure 7.7 History and Physical Using Templates and Pick Lists.

The following is an example of use of a template: A template for the subjective section of a progress note for abdominal pain might look as follows (see figure 7.7): "**age** yo male c/o [] pain x []. Pain is [**nature**], lasting []. Pain is relieved with [**rfactors**]; worsened with [**wfactors**]. Radiation []. [Denies] previous occurrence. [Denies] nausea, vomiting. States stools []. [Denies] melena, hematochezia. [Denies] use of NSAIDs. []".

age is filled in by the system. [**nature**] can be defined as a multi-item pick list of values of "burning, sharp, dull, cramping, crushing, constant, and intermittent". [**rfactors**] can be defined as a multi-item pick list of values of "antacids, food, and rest". [**wfactors**] can be defined a multi-item pick list of values of "coffee, activity, lying down, bending, alcohol, meals, and fatty foods".

The template might be used as follows:

As a physician interviews the patient and comes to the subjective section of the progress note, the physician selects the disease, (1) selecting from a pick list of body area, with abdomen picked. (2) from a pick list of organ systems with gastrointestinal picked, and (3) from a pick list of diseases dealing with the body area and organ system, with abdominal pain picked. The template for abdominal pain is shown to the physician. The physician then either fills in the blank fields of the template or selects from a pick list for a field in the template; the NEXT key goes to the next field, while the PREVIOUS key goes to the previous field. At each jump point the physician enters the following: ...(types) epigastric ... (types) 1 mo. S/p appy x 3 mos... (selects) burning, intermittent... (types) 20-30 minutes... (selects) antacids, food... (selects) coffee, bending... (types) -none... (skips)... (skips)... (types) well-formed... (skips)... (stops). The abbreviation "appy" expands to "appendectomy" upon entrance.

The resulting text would then show the following (see figure 7.8): "69 yo male c/o [epigastric] pain x [1 mo. S/p appendectomy x 3 mos]. Pain is [burning, intermittent], lasting [20-30 minutes]. Pain is relieved with [antacids, foods]; worsened with [coffee, bending]. Radiation [-none]. [] previous occurrence. [Denies] nausea, vomiting. States stools [well-formed]. [Denies] melena, hematochezia. [Denies] use of NSAIDs. []", with the system automatically filling in the age from previous recording of birth date.

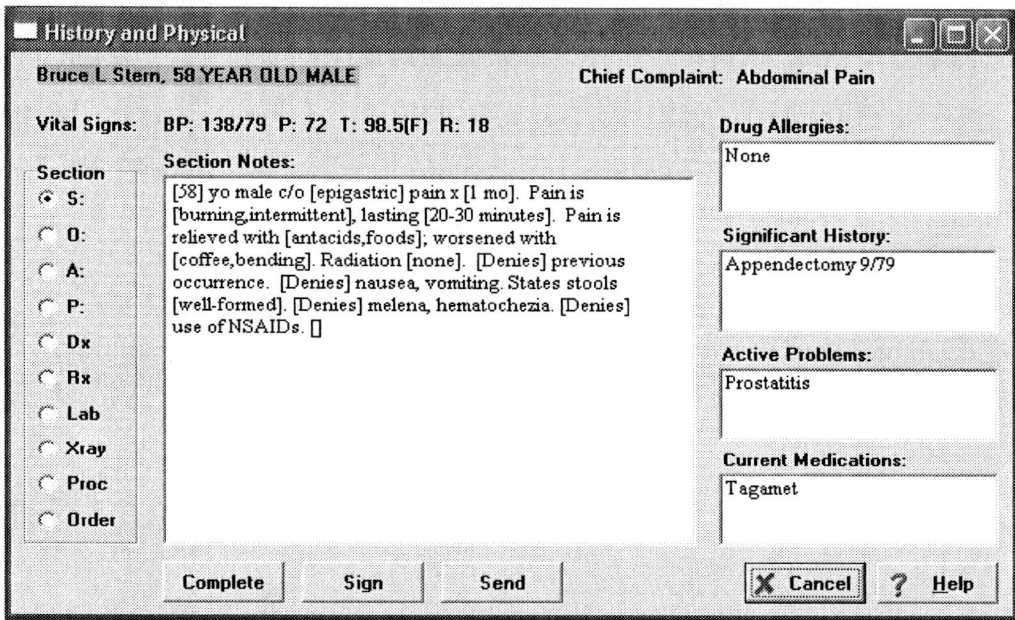

Figure 7.8 History and Physical Using Templates and Pick Lists After Picking Items.

When the input was accepted in figure 7.8 and the Complete button was accepted, the text would display "69 yo male c/o epigastric pain x 1 mo. S/p appendectomy x 3 mos. Pain is burning, intermittent, lasting 20-30 minutes. Pain is relieved with antacids, foods; worsened with coffee, bending. Radiation -none. Previous occurrence. Denies nausea, vomiting. States stools well-formed. Denies melena, hematochezia. Denies use of NSAIDs." See figure 7.9. The physician would then press the Sign button and enter information to verify his/her identity. The caregiver would then press the Send button.

As stated earlier in this chapter, it is the author's opinion that when a caregiver inputs information while examining or interviewing the patient (referred to as "point of care" computing), the caregiver should use a non-intrusive computer, such as a (wireless handheld) tablet computer. Much source documentation is initially created when examining and interviewing the patient.

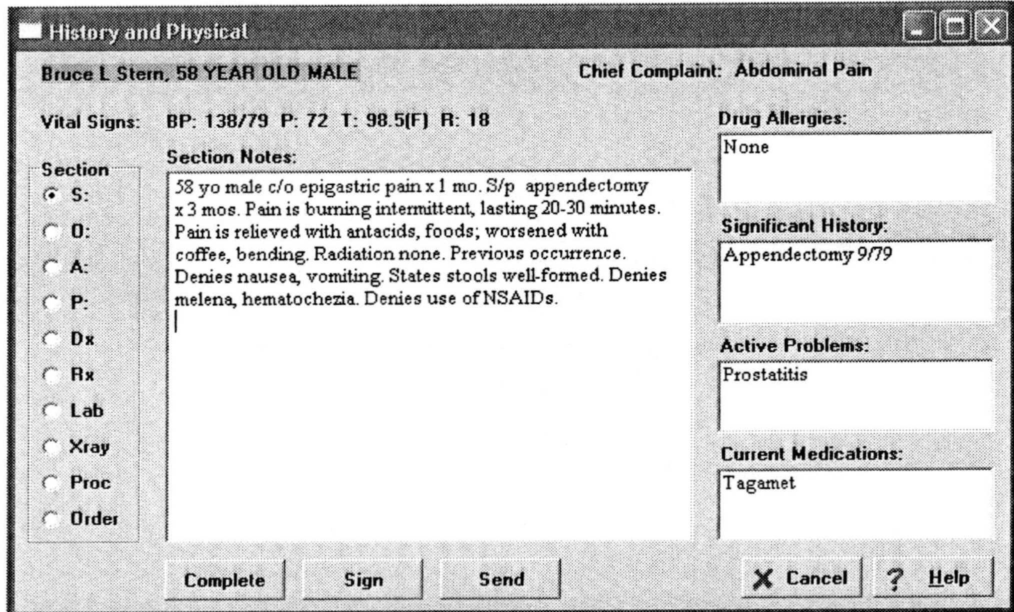

Figure 7.9 History and Physical Using Templates and Pick Lists After Caregiver Accepts Results.

Use of a tablet computer while interviewing the patient would probably involve pen, rather than keyboard input. Pen input of SOAP notes on a tablet computer is facilitated by caregiver use of templates, pick lists and textual input using abbreviations. Abbreviations could later be expanded to the full text by the computer.

7.7.2 Medical Orders and Results

Automated ordering and return of results, which may be part of an automated patient medical record system, is referred to as *computerized provider order entry (CPOE)*. We will assume that it is part of our automated patient medical record system. See figure 7.10.

The automated patient medical record system would enable orders to be entered by a caregiver with transmission directly to the computer system of the performing ancillary department providing ancillary services. Such ancillary department computer systems include the clinical laboratory system, pharmacy system, radiology system and pathology system. The healthcare industry standard for an application level network protocol for sending orders between computer systems is HL7.

Results and order status changes may be returned from the ancillary computer system to the ordering caregiver or other users at the automated system. The caregiver could receive an alarm for a panic result or when a result is returned for a STAT order, an order requiring immediate attention. The network protocol for return of results is also HL7.

The ordering system/ancillary system must handle simple individual orders as well as complex orders, multiple orders being generated from a single order and/or an order with frequency and timing requirements or conditions. For example,

- "Give 75 milligrams of Demoral intramuscularly every 4 hours when necessary for pain"

- A single caregiver order of "Complete blood count (CBC)" might result in a series of tests being done on a blood sample in the clinical laboratory—an order based upon an "order set": hemoglobin concentration, hematocrit, red and white counts, differential white cell count, and stained smear for red cell and platelet examination.

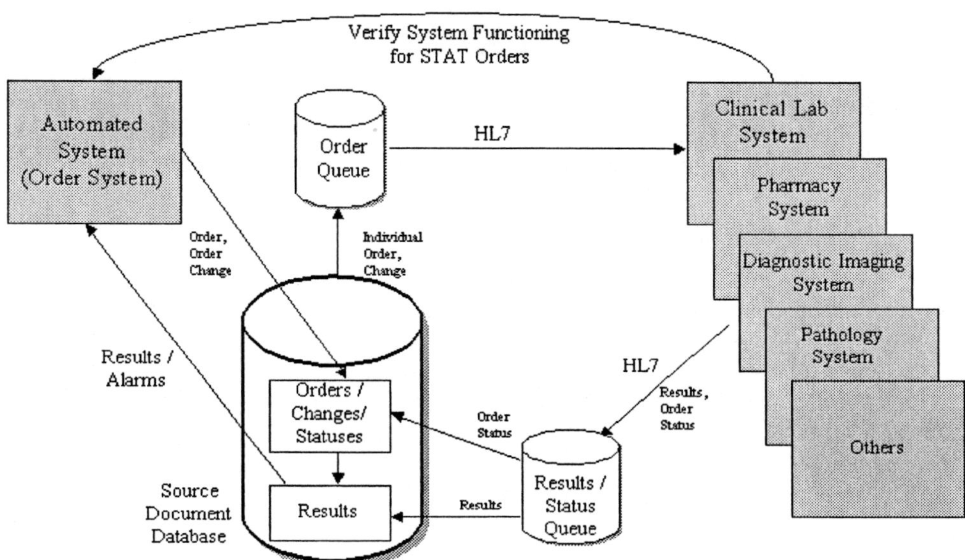

Figure 7.10 Orders and Results.

For complex orders such as a CBC, the ordering system might generate multiple orders from a single order (e.g., WBC, Hct, etc. from the CBC) and send them to the clinical laboratory computer system or alternatively the ordering system might create a single order (e.g., CBC) ot have the order interpreted by the clinical laboratory system.

Common parameters in all orders would include (a) identity of the patient, (b) date and time order was written, (c) priority or urgency of the order (STAT, routine, rush), (d) identification of the associated encounter, and (e) electronic signature of person who wrote the order (CMS 2004). Other parameters vary according to the ancillary system. For example,

- an inpatient medication order to the pharmacy system might include (a) the identity of the drug to be administered, (b) dosage of the drug, (c) route by which the drug is to be administered. (d) time and/or frequency of administration, (e) registration number and address for a controlled substance. Types of medications orders are *standing orders* (carried out until the physician cancels it) and *repeating orders* (carried out at prescribed intervals), *prn* orders (as needed) or other *conditional orders* (based upon a condition), *single (one-time) order* (an order given only once) or *STAT order* (given immediately and only once).
- a prescription for an outpatient medication might include (a) drug name, strength and dosage, (b) the number of tablets or amount to be dispensed, (c) information to be written on the label (e.g., directions to the patient, directions for refilling and whether the drug

name should be put on the label), (d) DEA registration number and address for a controlled substance, where the DEA is the Drug Enforcement Administration, a U. S. **Government agency to enforce the distribution of controlled substances, (e) optional identification of the pharmacy where the medication will be dispensed (either inside or** outside the HMO). (When a generic drug is ordered its name is usually in lower case, whereas brand-name drugs are capitalized.)

- a clinical laboratory test, diagnostic imaging, skin test, mycology, microbiology, EKG or other diagnostic test, an immunization, physical therapy, chemotherapy, or other therapy, might include (a) known full name or abbreviation of test or therapy, (b) optional performing area for test or therapy, (c) optional instructions, (d) optional information for scheduling test or therapy, either an appointment date, an indication that the patient will be put on a wait list or that the patient has the responsibility for dropping in for the test or therapy.

The ordering system must recognize the authority level of the caregiver and appropriately control ordering. In general,

- a physician can order any service, but needs a *DEA license* to authorize administration of controlled substances
- a nurse practitioner, physician assistant, registered nurse or registered respiratory therapist can order certain services in accordance with standardized procedures and protocols approved by a supervising physician
- based upon healthcare organization protocols, certain caregivers (e.g., registered nurses, physician assistants, pharmacists, respiratory therapists) may be able to enter the verbal orders of a physician, with the later co-signing of the order by the physician (e.g., within 24 hours)
- some categories of nurses are allowed to administer certain types of medications while others can not
- a medical assistant cannot order services.

In addition to placing an order, a caregiver can suspend or restart orders, modify an order, or delete, cancel, discontinue or renew an order. Additionally, a caregiver making an order should be informed of repeating orders about to expire and upon ordering, of a possible duplicate order. Orders can be for a future date and time. For a repeating medication order, there can be a "one off order", meaning an extra dose is given this one time. Outpatient medication prescriptions have the additional dimension of the ordering of refills.

HMO pharmacy systems include a *drug compendium* listing all the drugs a caregiver can order. Normally, an HMO also identifies which of these drugs it recommends, supposedly the most effective and least cost ones; these recommendations form the HMO "drug formulary". The drug compendium may include drug costs and information for clinical checking (i.e., drug interaction checking). Such a drug compendium/formulary could be made available or be duplicated for the automated patient medical record/ order entry system. For medication orders, either the ordering system or the pharmacy system could do immediate clinical checking of the order along with other stored patient clinical information, including checking of drug/allergy, drug/drug, drug/food and drug/laboratory interactions. Such clinical checking could be done by the computer while the caregiver is entering the order. The ordered drug could be checked as being in the HMO formulary, with the system informing the caregiver if it isn't and suggesting alternative less costly or more effective drugs.

Kaiser Permanente's Care Management Institute has identified drugs that could be harmful for elderly patients because the elderly often have multiple medical conditions, slower metabolism, or greater sensitivity to side effects of drugs. For example, drugs that could cause confusion or falls could be especially harmful for the elderly. They identified drugs as those to "always avoid" or those that should only be used in the short-term. (*Testimony of Francis J. Crosson, MD, Executive Director, The Permanente Federation, Kaiser Permanente* 2004)

When its discovered that a patient is allergic to a medication, this allergy should be entered either into the pharmacy system or automated patient medical record and transferred to the other. Also, the medication allergy should be sent to the CPR and reported to registries recording drug allergies.

Some allergies may not be clear cut—for example, a patient may be allergic to a medication but the patient may still want to use it because the benefit exceeds the side effects (e.g., Prednisone for severe asthma), some allergies occur inconsistently, for example, only when the patient takes the medication over a long period of time, and some allergies are assumed to be allergies and are not yet confirmed. Such not so clear-cut allergies will be referred to as "ambiguous allergies". An ambiguous allergy should be recorded also for a patient and identified as such, recording the reason for the ambiguity.

Dietary orders could also do clinical checking for drug/food interactions. Clinical laboratory orders could also check for drug/laboratory interactions.

The Controlled Substances Act of 1970 puts special restrictions on the ordering and dispensing of certain drugs, including narcotics, some stimulants and depressants, hallucinogens and steroids, and of chemicals used in the illicit production of controlled substances. Controlled substances are divided into five classes called *schedule I through schedule V*. Schedule I drugs are experimental and can be dispensed by a very limited number of institutions or are drugs that, on an emergency or temporary basis, have been determined to pose an imminent hazard to the public safety. Prescriptions for schedule II drugs must be written and may not be refilled; schedule II drugs have a "high potential of abuse" (PDR-Staff and Physicians 2003). Prescriptions for schedule III and IV drugs may be written or oral but may only be refilled up to five times within 6 months; schedule III drugs have "some potential for abuse" while schedule IV drugs have a "low potential for abuse"(PDR-Staff and Physicians 2003). Schedule V drugs are less restricted but can be dispensed only to patients at least 18 years old; a patient must offer identification and have his or her name entered into a log maintained by the pharmacist; schedule V drugs may be "subject to state and local regulation" (PDR-Staff and Physicians 2003). Schedule I drugs include street drugs of no medical use (e.g., heroin, LSD and marijuana currently); schedule II drugs include street drugs of some medical use (e.g., cocaine, methamphetamine) (NIDA 2001). Physicians who order controlled substances must have a DEA number.

The FDA also rates drugs as to their risk in being used during pregnancy (PDR-Staff and Physicians 2003). Categories of such drugs are category A, "controlled studies show no risk"; category B, "no evidence of risk in humans"; category C, "risk cannot be ruled out"; category D, "positive evidence of risk"; and category X, "contraindicated in pregnancy".

The HMO clinical laboratory system would include a test directory used to validate laboratory test requisitions, containing information such as test name, test measurement units, and normal reference range and low and high crisis (panic) values that may be calibrated for a specific clinical instrument. The automated patient medical record / order entry system needs the same information for clinical laboratory order validation and to provide information to the ordering caregiver, especially when the results are out of range. Other ancillary systems require additional test directories available to the ordering system for order checking.

Ordering of certain urinary and blood clinical laboratory tests for street drugs (e.g., cocaine, heroin and marijuana), for alcohol and for HIV (AIDS), and view of their results may be controlled by health care organization policies, regulatory commission regulations, and federal and state laws.

Upon entrance of a STAT order, the ordering system, if possible, should check to see if the clinical system receiving the order is up and network connections are up. If not, the caregiver could be informed so he/she could consider taking alternative actions in getting the order through (e.g., through telephone communication with the clinical laboratory).

Once an order is input by the ordering caregiver, then the ancillary system or ordering system could assist other caregivers in the performance of the order. For example, a clinical laboratory or other diagnostic test system could print out test preparation instructions for the technician or nurse to execute the test (e.g., take a blood specimen), precautions, normal test values and crisis values, implications of results and post-test care. A pharmacy system could automatically record inpatient medications that were ordered on an automated medication administration records (MAR) within the unit where the patient is located so a unit nurse could record on the system when the medication was administered. Calculations could be done to assist in the performance of an order, for example, body surface area calculations to determine the proper dosage of a medication.

Ancillary departments that perform tests or handle changes in order status, could record and return the result or order status back to the automated patient medical record / caregiver ordering system. HL7 also is the standard applications level network protocol for this.

In order to enable the automated patient medical record system to match up the order with the performing system and to match up returning results or order status with the original order, HL7 provides match up mechanisms. When an order is created, the automated patient medical record system / order system (the system placing the order) adds a *placer* application identifier to the order identifying the automated patient medical record system / order system as the system through which the order was placed; a unique placer order number is also assigned to the order to uniquely identify the order within the system placing the order. Along with the order would also be an identifier of the system filling the order (e.g., the clinical laboratory system, the pharmacy system); this *filler* application identifier would be used to route the order to the correct performing application system. The placer application identifier would be used by the system filling the order to determine the system to which results or order status should be sent; once the result or order status is received by the ordering system, the placer order number would be used to match up the returned results with the original order.

Results could be identified as normal, abnormal, or panic (crisis) value by the ancillary system. The ordering system could periodically check for returning results and *alarm* the caregiver of an abnormal or panic value result or of a result for a STAT order. As part of the order, the ordering caregiver could identify the conditions under which he would be alarmed (e.g., for a patient with a known condition, the caregiver could include a larger reference range so the caregiver would not be alarmed when the test result is abnormal but an expected value, or, on the other hand, the caregiver could indicate to be alarmed when a particular set of results come back, independent of their values). Normal ranges could be based upon age and race. Caregiver teams for the ordering caregiver could be set up so that a caregiver in that team could be notified of the alarm if the ordering caregiver is unavailable.

Order statuses would also be returned. Order statuses might include the following: open statuses (order held or suspended with resume criteria, order scheduled, specimen collected, specimen received, service performed, results transcribed, medication dispensed, medication administered), historical statuses (order completed, canceled or discontinued).

Where the ancillary department is not yet automated, then orders and results could be communicated to the ancillary department via e-mail and put on a work list. Results could be returned via e-mail for storage with the automated patient medical record.

In some cases there can be orders coming from the ancillary system, bypassing the ordering system (e.g., lab requisitions and results initiated through the clinical laboratory system). Some clinical laboratory systems automatically generate an order if a test is out of range, usually to verify that the result is actual rather than due to equipment problems; this is referred to as "reflex testing".

When an order is made within the automated patient medical record system by a caregiver, the order must be tied to the associated encounter so it can be associated with the encounter within the automated patient medical record. If the system cannot accurately identify the encounter, then the system might have to request the caregiver to select the encounter from a pick list of encounters. When the order originates outside the automated system (e.g., a "reflex order") information from the ancillary system might have to be passed to the automated patient medical record system to identify the encounter.

Before sending an order to an ancillary department or performing area and recording it on the automated patient medical record, a caregiver must "electronically sign" the document verifying the identity of the caregiver. At that point, the system could verify that the caregiver has the authority to make the order.

Some results of tests or other orders require interpretation by experts, producing diagnostic findings. Diagnostic images may require interpretation by radiologists. Anatomic pathology specimens require interpretation by specialized experts, as do pulmonary function tests to test respiratory function.

Anatomic pathology deals with wet specimens, tissues, anything out of the body (a piece of bone, skin tissue, muscle, blood vessel, bullet). Anatomic pathology includes surgical pathology, cytology (study of cells), histology (microscopic structure of tissues) and autopsy (multiple body parts). Cytology deals with smears: vaginal, sputum, semen—fluids with cellular material.

An addendum is an appendage to an existing diagnostic finding document that contains supplemental information. The parent document remains in place and its content is altered by the addendum. For example, a clarification or correction to a diagnostic finding for an anatomic pathology specimen might produce an addendum.

An addendum could occur after any order is complete to amend the order, results or diagnostic findings. Once received, this must be stored with the original order.

See figure 7.6. Orders, results, diagnostic findings, and addendums are recorded on the HMO source document database; these are matched up with encounters in the HMO CPR database, or new encounters are added to the HMO CPR database.

Information on the encounter should eventually be sent to outside source document and CPR repositories. Ideally, these transmissions should occur after all encounter documentation has been completed and after all associated orders, results, interpretations and addendums are complete, so a complete description of the encounter would be available.

7.7.3 Communication Between Caregivers and with Patients

Patient medical record documentation is the primary way for one caregiver to communicate clinical information about a patient to a future caregiver seeing the patient. Word of mouth is the primary method for communication between caregivers currently seeing the patient, whether this communication is face to face, on the telephone or over pager or a loud speaker. Electronic communication, e-mail, and more generally "messaging", is becoming a more and more important method of communication between caregivers.

7.7.3.1 E-mail, Messaging, Alerts and Reminders

E-mail from one caregiver to another or other caregivers can be formatted and non-formatted messages with optional saving of the e-mail in the automated patient medical record. Types of e-mail include the following: (1) formal memos between caregivers, (2) communication of patient phone messages from one caregiver, especially an advice nurse, to a physician, and responses from the physician to the originating caregiver, (3) communication of patient requests of drug refills from an automated drug refill phone system to the ordering caregiver or to a surrogate, (4) when there is no other direct on-line connection between the ordering system and an ancillary system associated with a diagnostic test, communication of the order to a performing area, with possible display of orders on a performing area work list, and optional communication of results back to the ordering caregiver, and (5) for small healthcare institutions, communication of a summary of a patient encounter for storage in the CPR, which might have to substitute for the more detailed CPR information that could be provided by a larger healthcare institution.

Electronic communication here will be separated out into two systems: *standard e-mail* and *caregiver messaging*. Beyond normal e-mail capabilities, there should be a capability to (1) associate an e-mail with a patient and (2) optionally include it in the patient medical record.

A *caregiver messaging system* to allow communication between caregivers for care of the patient should have additional capabilities beyond e-mail, including the ability to identify a patient and optionally include the message in the patient medical record. Usually such phone calls originate as a result of phone calls from patients to one caregiver (often an advice nurse), with the message going to another caregiver (usually a physician), with a response coming back to the originating caregiver and/or to the patient. The following are some capabilities suggested:

- enable messages required by the HMO to be pre-formatted with a "fill-in the blanks" capability
- enable a forwarding capability that enables (1) the first caregiver (e.g., an advice nurse or appointment clerk) to send the message, (2) a receiving caregiver to receive and respond to the message, optionally sending it to the originating or another caregiver to convey the information to the patient
- enable the receiving caregiver or the caregiver responding to the patient to "close out" the message, indicating it has be taken care of
- enable assignment of an "importance level" that a receiving or responding caregiver could use to determine what messages to handle first; this importance level could be associated with a "close out time period" (e.g., must be closed out within 2 hours)
- enable identification to the initiating caregiver, receiving caregiver or responding caregiver of messages that have been closed out and that have not; enable identification of messages that are past due or are close to reaching the end of the close out period
- enable association of a care team with a receiving caregiver or with a responding caregiver to receive the message if it is not handled within a given period of time
- enable the care team to redirect messages to other receiving or responding caregivers when the referenced one is not available; enable the setting up of system controlled redirection based upon the unavailability of the caregiver, e.g., based upon the dates and times the caregiver is out-of-clinic or on vacation, perhaps based upon the caregiver's schedule

- enable the initial and responding caregivers to document their conversations with the patient
- keep a telephone call history of telephone calls, especially from patients, that initiate message, and an audit trail for the subsequent messages to the various caregivers and care teams
- keep messages, orders and results, and e-mails in an "in-box" for later retrieval, either for a particular caregiver, a care team, or a nursing unit
- enable display of a message, order, order and result and/or addendum, order pending a result, or e-mail upon selection from the in-box
- upon selection of a message for a patient from an "in-box", enable the associated patient medical record to be retrieved
- enable messages to be recorded in the patient medical record along with documentation for encounters and telephone calls with the patient
- enable reminder and to-do messages for a caregiver to send to himself at a later date or time
- support *unified messaging*, allowing messages to be text, fax, voice, graphics, picture, Internet page, or video, or any combination of these by embedding non-text within the text or linking to an item within the text
- enable sorting or filtering of messages by type, importance level, recipient
- enable messages to be in many different languages.

Telephone communication to caregivers from patients can be supported by computer telephony integration (CTI), computer supported directing of calls. This enables telephone calls from patients to an HMO to be directed to a category of caregivers (e.g., an advice nurse for advice or an appointment clerk for an appointment). Other communication could be re-fill requests sent to the pharmacy or to the appropriate physician.

The standard methodology (Webopedia 2002) to exchange messages between originators and recipients is X.400 external to the Internet; this standard is implemented globally. The standard methodology for e-mail within the Internet is RPC 832 or Simple Mail Transport Protocol (SMTP). Commercial e-mail and other messaging systems generally use these standards. For a universal patient record, e-mail must not only support English, but other languages as well, and thus must use a character set such as Unicode rather than ASCII that directly supports many languages besides English. Also e-mail addresses through the Internet, unlike currently, must support non-English language characters—this is a major concern in Europe and Asia (Marsan 2003).

Another form of communication between caregivers, which does not involve e-mail or messaging, is recording of *alerts* (more urgent) and *reminders* (less urgent) identifying notification messages describing patients put in by one caregiver to later inform other caregivers. These alerts and reminders might be recorded permanently or could be in effect only for a defined time period. These may be allergies, notification of sight, hearing, speech or mobility impairment, notification of problems such as violent patient or of drug concerns, notification of existence of advance directives, or notification that a patient who calls in should be transferred over to a particular provider. These alerts and reminders should be shown to caregivers based upon their security and "need to know".

E-mails from patients should also be supported, with the same capabilities as CTI. For example, a patient might send an e-mail with a health question to an advice nurse that could be answered by any available advice nurse. A re-fill request could be automatically send to the pharmacy or the appropriate physician. Such e-mails are most easily handled through the Internet, which would tack on the correct recipient, rather than having a patient do this him or herself.

7.7.3.2 Written Communication and Medical Vocabularies

Medical vocabularies are medical terms, including diseases, diagnoses, procedures, and codes for them. *Controlled medical vocabularies* are the codes (e.g., ICD-9, CPT-4 or SNOMED). *Medical terminology* in this book are free text medical terms.

Large healthcare organizations have found that there is a large variety of different medical terminology in the free text medical vocabulary found in medical charts, making it hard for one caregiver to understand another caregiver's chart. As a result, there have been a number of efforts to standardize medical technology used in the medical record—see the appendix, section A.8. Standardization of medical terminology for caregivers may have the additional benefits of enabling an automated translation of the free text into controlled vocabularies (e.g., ICD-9 or CPT-4), and make searching for free text information more accurate.

This book also advocates that the patient medical record be a communications vehicle between caregivers and patients. After an outpatient visit, a patient and the patient's family could be provided information on clinician orders and other encounter information to promote compliance with physician instructions and orders; after outpatient test results have been returned to a caregiver, these could be sent to the patient via mail in clearly understandable language. After an inpatient visit, a patient and the patient's family could be provided a discharge summary that describes in clear language, restrictions and follow-up activities. All these may require standardization of a different kind of medical terminology, one for the patient rather than for other caregivers, although a sophisticated patient may prefer the caregiver's version so the patient could do research on the illness.

7.7.4 Proposed Summarizations

The current paper patient chart is composed of the documents such as is listed in section 4.4. It is proposed that an automated patient medical record, besides including the same information and additional information suggested in this chapter, also include summarizations of information in the patient's medical record that could be derived either automatically by the system from the information in the documents or by additional input by caregivers:

- patient clinical summaries
- past encounter synopses
- encounter document lists.

This information summarizes or indexes information in the patient medical record.

7.7.4.1 Patient Clinical Summaries

A *patient clinical summary* could be generated from patient medical record document information (e.g., medications prescribed from medication orders) with additional information added by caregivers (e.g., medications currently being taken, whether prescribed or over the counter). It is suggested that there be two categories of patient clinical summaries:

- *overall clinical summary,* available all the time
- *inpatient clinical summary,* available during the current inpatient stay only.

For all patients there would be an *overall clinical summary* that could consist of any of the elements in the summary information in the CPR repository. This overall clinical summary could, for example, follow the ASTM E1384 standard for the CPR and contain the information listed in section 7.5.1. On the computer screen, the overall clinical summary could be tailored for the caregiver.

Selection of a data element from the screen could drill down to other patient medical record information. For example, one aspect of a patient clinical summary could be a list of significant health problems; upon selection of a problem, associated summary information would be displayed, such as encounters dealing with that problem.

The ideal patient clinical summary would consist of data elements available in universal CPR repositories that follow strict data standards. This would enable the clinical summary to display patient clinical information from outside healthcare institutions as well as from the HMO. A capability to translate the universal standard data elements to local data elements might be accomplished by a caption produced by right clicking a pointer device over a national standard data element (e.g., clicking a universal patient identifier might display the local identifier of the patient, such as a medical record number)—this would be the reverse of a source document from the source document repository that would be stored in the format of a healthcare organization and where right clicking a data element might display the data in the format of a universal standard data element.

An example overall clinical summary was presented in the last chapter and appears again here in figure 7.11. Such an overall clinical summary could be built by selecting from the following information:

- shortened patient demographics
- a list of encounters (inpatient stays, outpatient clinical visits, ED visits, phone call encounters, surgeries), including diagnoses
- a list of significant health problems / current medical conditions / concerns as entered and updated by healthcare practitioners
- a list of risk factors and biomarkers for diseases
- a list of medications ordered and dispensed through pharmacy systems
- a list of those medications that the patient currently takes. This would include all prescribed, over-the-counter and herbal medications currently being taken by the patient. (Clearly this list is more pertinent to the patient's current health than the previous list)
- a list of clinical orders and results, including all procedures for the patient
- a list of allergies and adverse reactions, as recorded in ancillary systems, such as the pharmacy system. Note that some allergies may not be clear cut allergies--for example, a patient may be allergic to a medication but the patient may still want to use it because the benefit exceeds the side effects (e.g., Prednisone for sever asthma), some allergies occur inconsistently, for example, only when the patient takes the medication over a long period of time, and some allergies are assumed to be allergies and are not yet confirmed. Such allergies will be referred to as "ambiguous allergies"
- a list of allergies and adverse reactions as recorded and updated by healthcare practitioners *Ambiguous allergies* may be identified as such, where an ambiguous allergy is an allergy that is not clear cut (e.g., the allergy is not confirmed, the benefit of the substance causing the allergy outweighs its allergic side effects, or the substance causing the allergic reaction only causes the reaction some of the time).

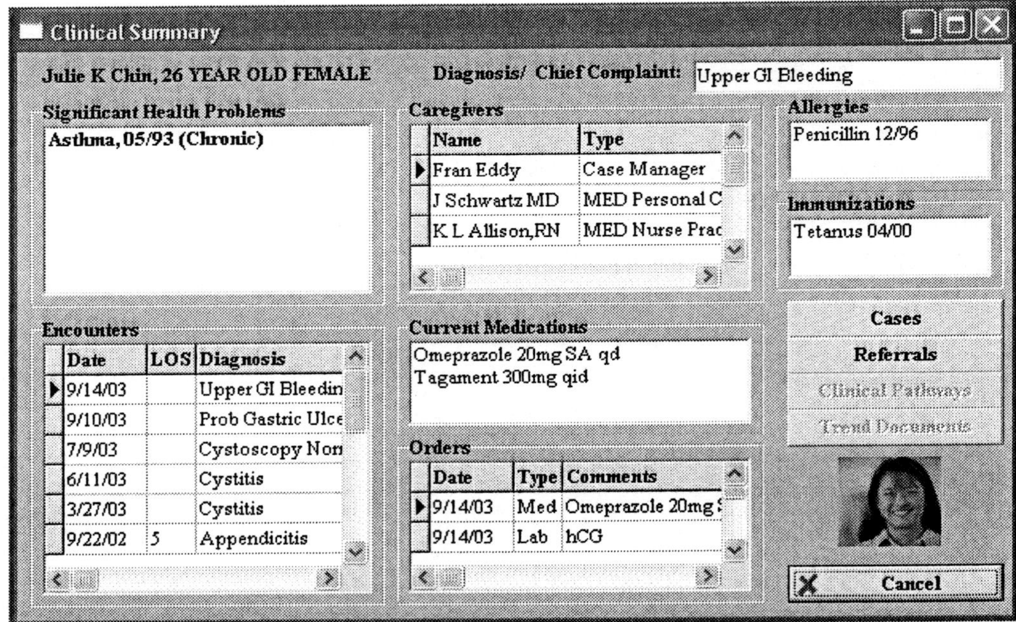

Figure 7.11 Overall Clinical Summary.

- a list of immunizations, skin tests and reactions, recorded by the immunization system with updates by the healthcare practitioners
- a list of appointments
- a list of assigned caregivers, including any assigned principal primary care provider and case manager, if any
- active cases
- referrals
- active critical pathway documents / trend documents
- alerts and reminders (e.g., violent patient, court injunction against patient, drug seeking behavior)
- a picture of the patient—This may be important to insure against fraudulent use of an HMO identification card and resultant inaccuracy of information in the patient's medical history.

an inpatient stay, there could be an *inpatient clinical summary* that is similar to the Kardex that is generated at the start of the inpatient stay based upon patient medical record information and disappears after discharge. For possible information in such an inpatient clinical summary, see section 4.4.1.3.

The information in a clinical summary would come from other clinical systems, through other parts of the automated patient medical record system (e.g., through orders, progress notes, etc.), or through caregiver direct entrance of information as a result of caregiver interviews of the patient or other sources (e.g., current medications, allergies. and significant health problems).

Often the patient clinical summary information would be enough to give a caregiver a good overall picture of the patient's health without the need for the caregiver to look further at documents in the patient medical record.

7.7.4.2 Past Encounter Synopses

What would greatly assist a caregiver in identifying what happened during a particular encounter, in the process of evaluating encounters of interest, would be a synopsis of each encounter. This synopsis could be specifically created by a caregiver after an encounter or it could potentially be generated by the automated system automatically after an encounter. Perhaps the HMO could require that a synopsis be created for every encounter. A caregiver might then, for example, ask to select all encounters related to urinary incontinence and get the synopsis of each such encounter.

7.7.4.3 Encounter Document List

Selection of an encounter from a patient clinical summary could list all documents for the encounter. From a *document list*, a caregiver could select and display a document.

7.7.5 Identifying Patients

Although the automated patient medical record is patient-oriented, each caregiver works with many patients. Therefore each caregiver needs a list of patients he or she is caring for and a way to select a particular patient from such a *patient list*, without having to specifically enter a patient identifier.

The list of patients required by a caregiver depends upon the job category and location of interest of the caregiver. Patient lists could include the following:

- *patient panel* for a particular caregiver that lists all patients for whom the caregiver is an assigned physician or nurse practitioner.
- *unit census* that shows all admitted patients in a nursing unit.
- *inpatient physician list* that lists all admissions for which a physician is either the attending or admitting physician, a consultant, or attending resident.
- *outpatient list* (or *schedule*) that consists of a complete schedule for a caregiver in all outpatient clinics he/she works in for a particular date in a healthcare organization and a less detailed schedule of the caregiver when he/she is outside the outpatient setting. Each patient with an appointment or registration in the healthcare organization is shown along with the type of appointment or registration. Other times where there is no appointment or registration are identified as to purpose and may be (1) time where the caregiver is outside outpatient clinics or outside the healthcare organization, (2) time where the caregiver can see outpatients but where patients normally cannot be appointed (e.g., a drop-in clinic) and (3) time where an outpatient can be appointed but there is no appointment yet. Other times identified independent of whether there are appointments and registrations or not are the following: time that is in transition from appointment time to non-appointment time whose future purpose is identified and either (1) current appointments are kept or (2) current appointments are canceled.
- *emergency department list* that includes all patients registered in the Emergency Department.
- An *outpatient clinic*, *inpatient unit* or *emergency department room map* that is a diagram of all rooms in an outpatient clinic, in an inpatient unit or in the ED that identifies the

patient, if any, currently in the room and the room status. Room statuses can be "room to be cleaned," "room available", "patient in room", "patient ready to see nurse", "patient ready to see physician", "patient seeing physician" and/or "patient seeing nurse". When the room is to be cleaned, housekeeping could be notified and when the patient enters the room, a caregiver may be notified. Note that the outpatient clinic room map is also the easiest mechanism for identifying the end of a patient outpatient visit, when the patient is identified as leaving the room. Physicians and nurses could wear electronic trackers that could identify the rooms they are in. (Combined with the time of a visit registration, room status changes can be used to measure waiting times in the wait room and time to see various caregivers.)

- *surgery list* listing surgeries for the attending caregivers (primary surgeon, assisting surgeon, co-surgeon, consulting surgeon, anesthesiologist, nurse anesthetist, or nurse midwife).
- *work list* that lists orders to be performed by an ancillary department (e.g., blood to be collected), together with details on the order, where an ancillary department is a department providing services for patients or for other medical departments that provide direct patient care.
- *caregiver-defined patient list* that is a list created by a caregiver from selecting patients from other Patient Lists. A caregiver may "attach" a label to a Caregiver-defined Patient List. Caregiver-defined Patient Lists may be date oriented or not.

Selection of a patient on a patient list would identify the patient and might drill down to clinical information for the patient, for example, to patient demographics, a patient clinical summary or the document list. Alternatively, the patient identifier could be entered to individually identify the patient, with optional drill down to the patient clinical information.

Patient panel lists should be primarily generated from member selection of primary care physicians. The patients on each patient panel should be equally distributed among primary care physicians in the HMO according to each physician's working schedule. The automated system might use past visit information and factors such as age and sex to predict how often patients are likely to come in for an outpatient visit in the next year and use this information to equitably assign patients to patient panels. For example, assignment of a healthy teenager to a caregiver's panel is certainly not equivalent to assigning an octogenarian.

A unit census or inpatient unit room map could be used by inpatient nurses and unit assistants. The automated system might provide a means to interface with a nurse assignment system to assign nurses with patients, taking into account patient acuity.

A unit census and inpatient physician list could be used by inpatient physicians. An outpatient list (schedule) and outpatient clinic room map could be used by outpatient physicians, outpatient nurses, in-clinic medical assistants and advice nurses. An emergency department list and an emergency department room map could be used ED physicians and nurses, including triage nurses. Surgery lists could be used by all caregivers involved in surgeries.

A caregiver-defined patient list, created by selecting patients off other lists or by individually identifying patients, could be used by physicians, nurses, advice nurses and all other caregivers. A capability to allow the caregiver to input a patient identifier to identify the patient would be provided.

When the patient identifier is not available and the patient is not on a patient list, then it is useful to have a search by patient name to find the patient identifier. The telephone number, address, sex and date of birth can then be used to verify that the patient information found indeed belongs to the patient. In the healthcare industry, a common search is a "Soundex Search". The user enters the first and last names of the patient, sometimes the sex and birth year. The system comes back with all possible matches, including the telephone number, address, sex and date of birth to determine the correct selection, and the patient identifier.

In general, patient lists can be created automatically by the automated patient medical record system from encounter and related information sent to it by other clinical systems (e.g., from the ADT system, outpatient scheduling system, registration system, etc.) In some cases, however, the automated patient medical record system might have to initiate an encounter or an encounter status change itself because the automated patient medical record system might learn about the encounter or encounter status change ahead of the clinical system: For example, adding a patient to an unit census or inpatient unit room map is a possible way to do a quick admission , with the sending of information on the admission to the ADT system so the admission could be completed by the ADT system. Removing a patient from a room in an outpatient clinic room map could be used as a way to identify the end of an outpatient encounter, which otherwise could not be known.

7.7.6 Organization, Selection and Information Retrieval

In order for a caregiver to find clinical information of interest for a given patient, the system should provide

- **Organization:** Organize clinical information so that the information of interest to a particular caregiver can be easily found.
- **Selection Based on Established Relationships:** Select clinical information based upon previously established relationships of information.
- **Information Retrieval:** Find clinical information where there are no previously established relationships of information.

7.7.6.1 Organization

The automated patient medical record could be organized so that information could be easily found by a caregiver. This organization could include summaries of clinical information. It could include categorization of clinical information such as putting it into categories relevant to a caregiver. The organization of information could be tailored for a particular type of caregiver.

Examples of summaries are the "overall clinical summary", summarizing all patient clinical information, and the "inpatient clinical summary", summarizing clinical information while the member is an inpatient. An example of categorization is creating chart tabs categorizing the patient medical record into categories relevant to the caregiver (e.g., a chart tab for medication-related documents when a pharmacist views a patient's medical record).

7.7.6.2 Selection Based Upon Previously Established Relationships

Relationships could be set up during the creation of the automated patient medical record that could later be used for selection of display of related information, for example by "drill down".

Figure 7.12 shows example relationships between a patient's problems, conditions, or concerns and other elements in an automated patient medical record. For example, selection of a patient's health problem could go to the cases associated with that health problem, trend documents associated with a condition, or clinical pathways associated with the condition.

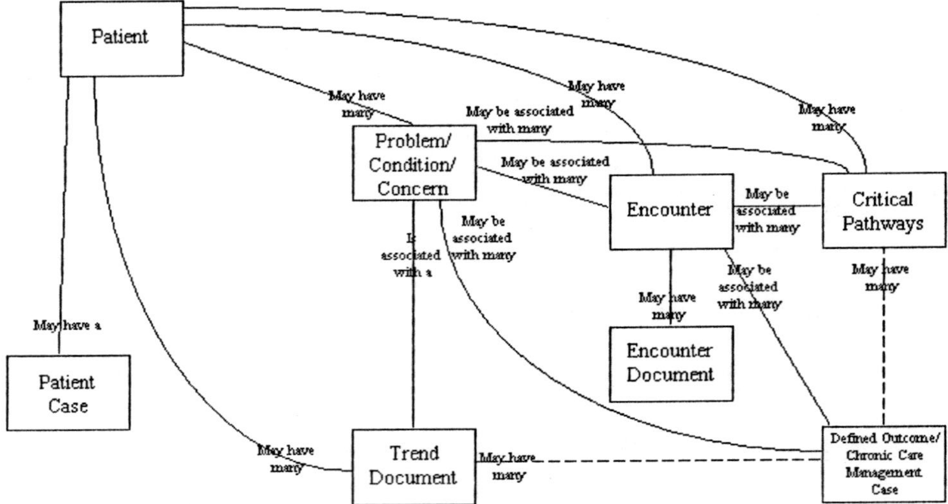

Figure 7.12 Example Relations for Problems/Conditions/Concerns.

Establishing this type of relationship requires an effort from caregivers, but is worth the effort because it enables a caregiver to quickly find clinical information on the patient dealing with a specific problem. After or during an encounter, a caregiver could associate the encounter with one or more problems. Based upon a specific problem, the caregiver could set up a clinical pathway of clinical practice guidelines identifying patient care to be given, possibly across multiple encounters (e.g., for a pregnancy, from pre-natal care through the birth of the baby). With a suspected problem (a concern) the caregiver could identify an associated trend document to automatically track an item that measures the concern (e.g., a growth chart or a blood pressure, HDL and LDL graphed over time). Later, the caregiver could select for display the encounters associated with a particular problem; the caregiver could also identify that a clinical pathway, trend document or follow-up message is associated with a particular problem.

When a provider defines a defined outcome case to track a treatment, a caregiver must associate the defined outcome case with a problem. A defined outcome case could include a treatment plan and notes, clinical pathway or clinical practice guidelines to define the treatment plan, or a trend document.

Figure 7.13 identifies possible relationships between items in the overall clinical summary and other clinical information in the automated patient medical record. Selection of an item in the overall clinical summary could go to more detailed information on the selection; for example, selection of an encounter could display a list of documents created during the encounter. Such relationships could be tailored by use of agents.

A basic organization described in section 7.4.5 is to allow a caregiver to select only those patient counters for a patient within the scope of care of the caregiver (e.g., all eye-related encounters for an opthalmologist).

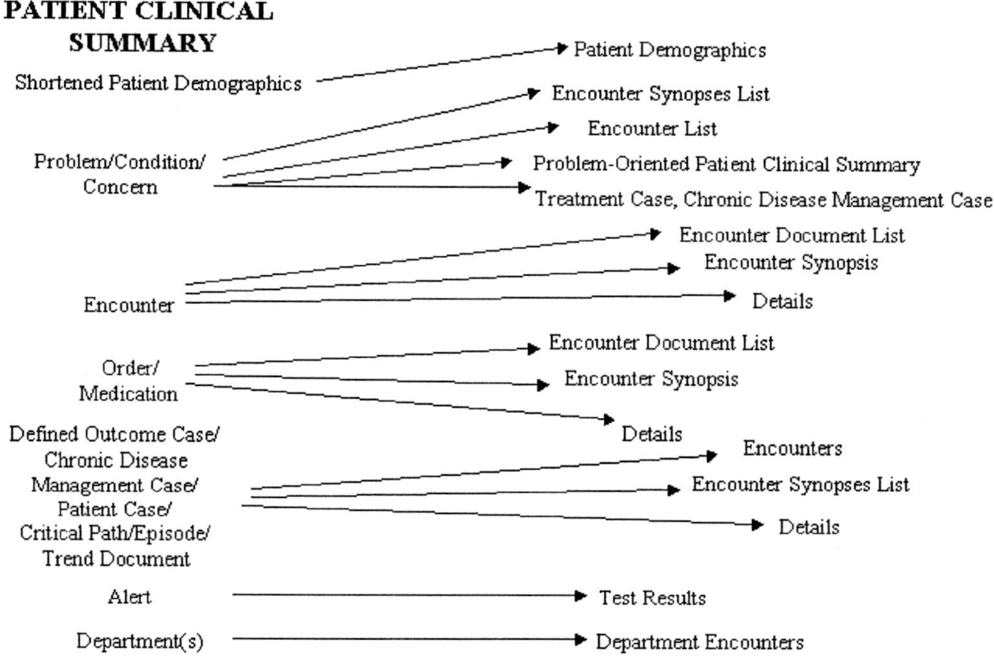

Figure 7.13 Example Relationships for the Overall Clinical Summary.

7.7.6.3 Information Retrieval

Information retrieval is a field of computer science that deals with the automated storage, searching through, and retrieval of textual documents. Textual documents can either be structured so searching and retrieval is very quick or it can remain unstructured, in which case searching and retrieval is slower. The automated patient medical system and also medical references require powerful information retrieval capabilities to find the appropriate document or information.

References (Jones and Willett 1997) and (Hersh 1995) respectively discuss information retrieval in general and information retrieval in healthcare. The book *Information Retrieval: A Health Care Perspective* (Hersh 1995) covers both patient specific searching, as discussed here, but also knowledge-based searching (e.g., medical research journals, summaries of medical information, etc.)

Searches can be done to find all encounters with a particular diagnosis or chief complaint, picking up associated documents, can be done for particular clinical tests with a specified range of values for results, etc. Searches can be done within one database or across many distributed databases, possibly in different healthcare organizations, in CPR repositories and source document repositories. Searching can be done by searching for particular data values in identified fields, by searching text that is pre-indexed or by searching through the words in free text, where "free text" is unstructured, uncoded, text.

Two words describe the ideal search: "precision" and "recall". *Precision* means retrieving only exactly what you need, limiting the number of items retrieved. *Recall* means retrieving everything you need, possibly broadening the number of items you retrieve. Clearly these two concepts can be at odds with each other.

Within the automated patient medical record may be the following types of fields that can be searched:

- fields (ideally using agreed-upon healthcare standards) with a small number of possible values (e.g., male, female, unknown for sex)
- fields with numeric information (e.g., the results of a clinical laboratory test)
- fields with a very large, but finite, number of values (e.g., ICD-9 diagnosis codes)
- free text fields (e.g., SOAP notes).

For fields with a small number of values, **searches for exact matches** are useful (e.g., find "myocardial infarction"). For fields with numeric values, **searches using numeric conditions** are useful (find "urine calcium > 275 mg/24 hours").

As far as searching for clinical information within fields with a large number of values or within free text is concerned, I think there are two other types of searching that are useful. One type of searching is to search for exact matches but to also search for all synonyms (e.g., a search for "myocardial infarction" would also find occurrences of "heart attack"). Because this type of searching excludes searching for related items that are not matches, I will refer to it as *exclusive searching.*

A second type of searching that I think is useful for free text and fields with a large number of values is to search for exact matches and synonyms but also to search also for related clinical information. Say any exact match or synonym is given a "match" value, *m*, of 1.00, but when related information is found, then a partial match is found with a "match" value of less than 1.00, identifying how close the match is.

Consider figure 7.14. Say the user searches for "BPH" in encounter documents. If "enlarged prostate", "prostate hypertrophy", "benign prostatic hypertrophy", "BPH", or a disease code such as an ICD-9 code for this disease, 222.2, is found in a document, then the document contains a perfect match with *m*=1.00. If "prostate" or "prostatis" is found in a document then the document contains a partial match with *m* being high but less than 1.00. If "urogenital" is found in a document, then *m* might be a low value indicating a partial match that is less specific. Perhaps a document with "bladder" in it might get an *m* greater than 0 but an even lower value.

Such a search, I will refer to as *inclusive searching*, because it includes searching for related items as well as the item entered. Reference (Wong, Kan, and Young 1996) identifies one information retrieval algorithm that identifies how to do an "inclusive search". This approach falls under the category of "thesaurus construction" discussed in references (Jones and Willett 1997) and (Frakes and Baeza-Yates 1992).

Whether using an exact match, numeric condition, exclusive or inclusive search, searching in the automated patient medical record system could be described as follows: "Search through field W in item X for strings Y, selecting Z where strings Y is found". For example, field W might be SOAP notes fields, item X might be encounter documents and Z might be encounters. Y might be a single string or some logical combination of strings, using logical operations; for example, search documents for "urinary infection" **or** "bladder infection", or search documents for "pain" **and not** "denies pain".

The results of the search that are returned—the documents with the matches or potential matches—could be primarily ordered by most recent document first to least recent document, or primarily ordered by the document with the closeness match to the lease closest match.

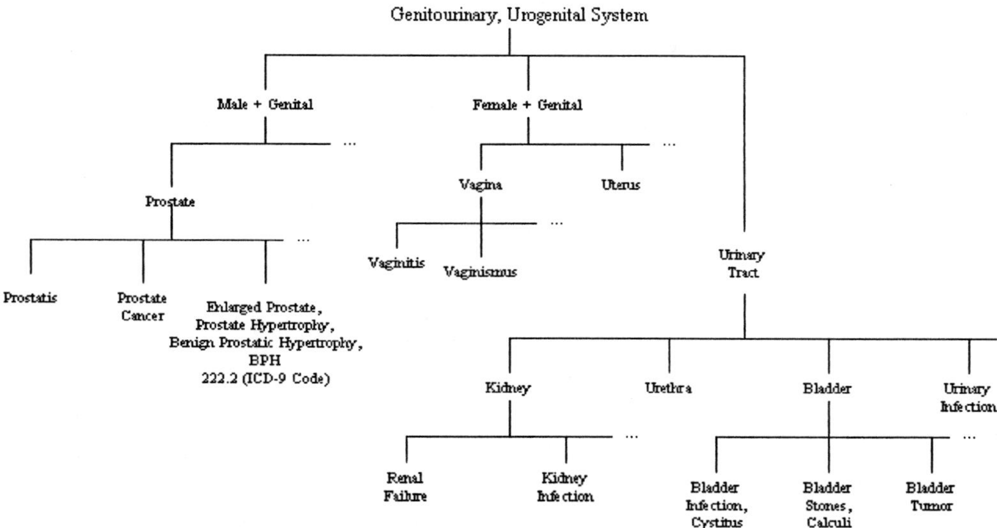

Figure 7.14 Relationships that could be Used for Inclusive Searching.

Searching through multiple fields within multiple items to select items, such as encounters, is also possible. Such complex searches if done over and over again are better done through agents (see section 7.6), set up previously, than for ad hoc searches. For example, an agent could be set up that runs the day before the appointment to search the automated patient medical record for items related to the chief complaint, producing a problem-oriented patient clinical summary.

With the popularity of the Internet, many companies use information retrieval from many different Web sites on the Internet based upon user entered free-form text (e.g., Yahoo (Yahoo 2004), Google (Google 2004), etc.). Expertise from these companies might be used for methods to search through the automated patient medical record. Reference (Barlow 1996-2002) describes how many of these "search engines" work.

7.7.6.4 Feature Analysis, Extraction, and Selection

One form of information retrieval is analysis of images and waveforms for "features" selecting them based upon the existence of these features. Diagnostic images, waveform information (e.g., EKGs) and other graphic or image information should be in a form where, in the future, they can be analyzed by an automated system to do automated diagnostic interpretation and thus assist caregivers in doing clinical interpretation of these images and graphics. Additionally, the automated system should provide support to caregivers in selecting information from *monitoring systems* (e.g., ICU, Guardian Angel systems) for inclusion in the automated patient medical record, as usually such information is too voluminous to store permanently in the patient medical record. These are forms of *feature analysis* and extraction that could supplement an automated patient medical record system.

7.7.7 Medical References Outside and Inside the Healthcare Organization

Medical references should be available on the Internet, via CD or on hard disk storage. Prominent medical references currently available via computer include the following:

- medical information on the Internet, some reliable, some not reliable
- MEDLINE, medical databases that include information from various medical journals produced by the National Library of Medicine
- Micromedex , reference libraries produced by the Denver-based MICROMEDEX, Inc., with comprehensive reference libraries for toxicology, pharmacology (including drug interactions), emergency and acute care, occupational medicine, chemical safety, and industrial regulatory compliance
- on-line PDR (*Physicians Desk Reference*) or equivalent, providing physicians with information on prescription drugs
- for many healthcare organizations, local healthcare organization databases including the healthcare organization drug formulary, DME (durable medical equipment, such as wheelchairs, crutches, etc.) formulary, policy and procedure manuals, clinical practice guidelines and protocols, best practice alternatives.

An appropriate mechanism to display such textual material is the Internet or a locally created or enterprise wide *Intranet* or multiple healthcare organization *Extranet*. Such documents could include hyperlinks to other documents and include pictures, graphs, Java programs, spreadsheets, movies, sounds and any other images that can be contained on a computer file. Documents could be viewed by browsers such as Netscape Navigator or Microsoft Explorer.

Rather than on paper, enterprise-wide on-line documentation is becoming an increasingly important part of many major businesses, as is evidenced by the many companies going into the on-line documentation business, such as Documentum™, IBM™ and FileNET™. Such documentation is largely handled through Intranets. These documentation systems enable enterprise-wide creation, controlled access, review and update, routing and management of documents. A current standard for describing such documents is use of XML to describe the data and HTML to present the data for display. Such systems are called document management systems or enterprise content management systems and are proposed in this paper for the Source Document Repository (see section 6.7).

Both XML and HTML were derived from another markup language, SGML (Standard Generalized Markup Language). SGML has been used to publish very large documents, but has been superseded by XML and HTML for documentation because of their simplicity as compared to SGML. A standards body that controls both the structure of HTML and XML on the Internet is the World Wide Web Consortium (W3C) (Bray et al. 2000). (XML and associated components, such as XSL and XML Schema, were discussed in the previous chapter.)

Enterprise wide policy and procedure manuals, clinical practice guidelines and protocols could be created, controlled and distributed via an Intranet using XML, SGML or HTML. XML, HTML and SGML are languages of "tags" used to format text. Tags usually come in sets, such as <B> ahead of the text and </B> after the text in order to bold the text on the screen. Tags are used to structure the text (e.g., define headings); for presentation formatting (e.g., to define the fonts); for links to other document pages often at other completely independent sites; for graphics, dividers, backgrounds and colors, special characters, forms and tables within the text.

Even programs can be embedded in the script or be initiated in the script to return another Web page. Such programs can produce sound or animations, retrieve information from databases for display, or generate forms that collect information from the viewer and return a response. Such programs are written in the computer languages of Java (which can be embedded in HTML script or separate), JavaScript (embedded in script), or follow an interfacing standard CGI (for common gateway interface).

Web servers handle requests from browsers on PCs to produce web pages on request for the PC users. CGI is a standard for passing a web user's request to an application program and to receive data back to forward to the user; CGI could consist of C++, Perl, Visual Basic, Java, or other languages.

(Besides being used for medical references, a Web server within the Internet, an Intranet or Extranet could potentially be used to create parts of the automated patient medical system. The appropriateness of this is explored in section 12.4.)

7.7.8 Supporting Clinical Research

Supporting clinical research entails three parts:

- searching for candidate patients to participate in the clinical research
- recording results of the research with selected patients who agree to participate in a research project
- recording the results of research while protecting the identify of patients and providers.

Searching for candidate patients would involve the searching techniques of section 7.7.6.3, but where what is being searched for are patients with certain characteristics. For example, for research on a drug for a particular medical condition, ideal candidates for such research may be patients with the targeted medical condition and no others and who do not take other drugs conflicting with the targeted drug.

Agents could be used to collect clinical research information on-line for patients as care is being given, or alternatively, information could be collected afterward from the patient medical record after it is complete. Research could potentially be done anonymously, with the identity of the patient removed, which would potentially allow research to be done without the consent of the patients; this could be done by putting out medical record information on a research database (a data warehouse) excluding the identity of patients. Identities of providers could also be removed.

When clinical research is done with many patients, then it is much easier for a system or caregiver to do searches on encoded information rather than textual information. For example, a caregiver can search patient medical records for patients with cardiovascular disease by searching for instances of words associated with cardiovascular disease, but the caregiver would have to do some additional analysis of the clinical information to determine if the patient did indeed have cardiovascular disease or just have symptoms of the disease. On the other hand, if patient diagnoses were encoded (e.g., into ICD-9 codes), then patients who have cardiovascular disease could be found with certainty by searching for all ICD-9 codes associated with cardiovascular disease. For clinical research of a large number of patients, encoded information is thus far preferable to textual information.

7.7.9 Supporting Patient Safety

As many as 98,000 patients die a year due to medical mistakes, and ten times as many are injured each year (Kohn et al. 2000).

Many of these errors are medication errors, with 2 out of 3 of these errors due to misinterpretation of handwriting on prescriptions or medication orders. The automated patient medical record, with on-line ordering, would eliminate these handwriting errors.

Research on what causes medical errors could be supported by an automated system by allowing caregivers to record these errors and the reasons they occurred, anonymously sending this information to state or federal government organizations, a central location in the healthcare organization, or to other healthcare organizations, with the automated system protecting the confidentiality of caregivers, patients and the healthcare organization by removing their identities.

7.7.10 Contextual Framework

This paper views an automated patient medical record system as separate from other clinical systems such as the hospital admission, discharge and transfer (ADT) system; the appointment and resource scheduling system; and the clinical laboratory system; and separate from non-clinical business systems such as billing and inventory. In reality these systems are quite dependent upon each other. Section 10.5 discusses needed interfaces between the automated patient medical record system and other systems.

Automation of the patient medical record could support electronic commerce with regard to on-line ordering of durable medical equipment, such as wheelchairs and crutches for patients, automatic ordering of other medical supplies whenever they are needed, collection of medical payments from the government and outside insurance companies, and payments for member medical services outside the HMO. Automatic ordering and billing is possible because automation of the patient medical record would result in collection of detailed information on all orders, medical supplies, and medical services. As medical supplies are used, requests for new supplies could be periodically sent to suppliers over computer networks. When a patient encounter ends, billing of medical services could automatically occur, sending the bills to insurance companies or government agencies for payment, such as to HCFA (Health Care Financing Association) for Medicare payments. Notification of a member encounter outside the health care organization together with a recording of medical services provided could trigger automated calculation of reasonable charges for this services; when the HMO is billed, these estimated charges can be compared against billed charges with automatic payment of reasonable charges and review of other changes.

A current standard for electronic commerce is Electronic Data Interchange (EDI), a standard for structured data, using agreed upon message standards by the sender and recipient, from the sending computer to the receiving computer. The Health Insurance Portability and Accountability Act of 1996 (HIPAA) (CMS 2004) under the control of HCFA mandates standards for EDI communications for Medicare payments. The United Nations is also developing standards that are now being used in Europe. See the appendix.

Another possibility with an automated patient medical record, that could conceivably replace EDI in the future, is for the government agencies and insurance companies to be subscribers to the CPR repository or patient registry for patients of interest so they can pick up all medical service and order information from the CPR repository for such patients as encounters for these patients are completed. In such a case, agreements between the healthcare organization and insurer must be made to account for cases where the patient is multiply insured. The ASTM 1384 standard for the CPR also includes financial information besides clinical information.

7.7.11 Financial Aspects

Some members in HMOs have the bulk of their care paid by capitation payments, payment of a monthly fee by a member or his or her employer for care. These may be combined with the requirement that the member pay a co-payment for each visit. However, medical costs are still an issue in medical care in an HMO.

HMOs often do not pay for treatments they consider to be "experimental". Further, they often restrict drugs to those in the HMO's formulary, requiring the patient to pay more or the whole amount for drugs not in the formulary; this is often part of a three tier system where "tier one" drugs (in the formulary) are entirely paid for by the HMO, "tier two" drugs are partially paid for by the patient, and "tier three" drugs are entirely paid for by the patient. Additionally, HMOs sometimes restrict the number of visits of particular types (e.g., psychiatry visits) and require co-pays for some types of treatments, diagnostic tests, or medications.

As a result, caregivers devising treatment plans, making orders for diagnostic tests or prescribing medications, now have to consider the financial impact of their decisions on the patient. Thus, information on the patient's benefits should be available to physicians, appointment clerks and advice nurses, among others.

It is proposed that each HMO member be assigned a healthcare services representative who would serve as an ombudsman for the patient. The healthcare services representative would be the person in the HMO who could thoroughly discuss patient benefits with the patient, in particular on what services the HMO covers and does not cover for the patient.

7.8 ACTIONABLE INFORMATION

Information that is so important that it should be immediately sent to a caregiver for action is referred to as *actionable information.* Actionable information should be sent by the automated patient medical record system to a caregiver or care team associated with the patient, either for display or printing. Actionable information could include the following:

- when a trend document indicates a value (e.g., a blood pressure, blood glucose level, etc.) is significantly out of range (see section 7.4.7)
- when clinical checking of a medication with other prescribed medications determines that there is a drug/drug interaction (see section 7.7.2)
- when the ordering caregiver is given an alarm that clinical laboratory results are out of range or are returned as a result of a STAT order (see section 7.7.2)
- when a message is received by a caregiver to which the caregiver or care team must respond (see section 7.7.3)
- when a clinical decision support system identifies that there is a choice of a less expensive medication than the one ordered, that there is a duplicate order, or that a practice guideline is not being followed (see section 17.4.11).

7.9 ANOTHER CONCEPTUAL VIEW

This section presents another conceptual view of the automated patient medical record based upon business requirements so far.

The automated patient medical record system should be patient-oriented like the current paper chart. In order to select a patient of interest to the caregiver, each caregiver should have lists of his/her patients. Selection of a patient on a caregiver's patient list or identification of the patient in other ways would provide access to the patient's medical record. The basic elements of this proposed automated patient medical record system are presented in figure 7.15

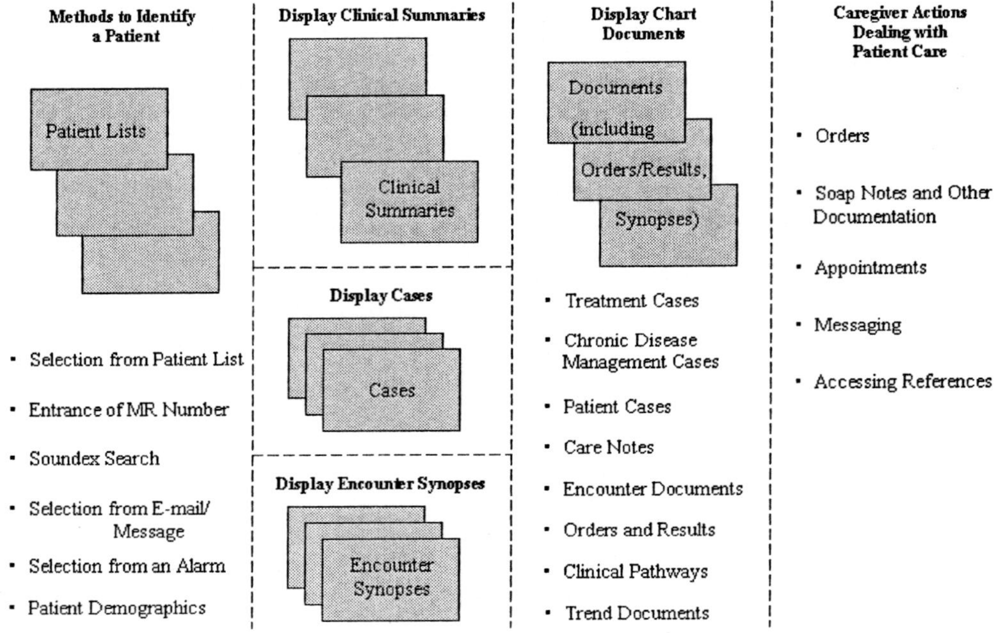

Figure 7.15 New Conceptual View.

These basic elements are as follows:

- **methods to identify patients of interest to a caregiver:** methods to select a patient and verify that the correct selection has been made, including methods to select patients tailored to a caregiver
- **a quick overview of clinical information for a patient:** summaries of patient clinical information some of which may be tailored to the caregiver (e.g., current medications, past encounters, immunizations, etc.)
- **synopses of past encounters for a patient:** a list of caregiver or automated system generated summaries of each encounter; synopses could also exist for a case and a clinical pathway

- **defined outcome cases, chronic care management cases, and patient cases for a patient:** a list of cases tracking treatments for a patient (identifying treatment plans and related information) and patient cases (identifying case notes for a case manager)
- **care notes:** a caregiver's notes to him- or herself with encounters for a patient within the scope of care of a caregiver or care team
- **documents making up a patient medical record:** the set of documents making up the patient medical record, with documents organized by encounter, defined outcome case, chronic care management case, patient case, or clinical pathway or organized as required by the caregiver
- **the ability to perform and record actions dealing with the patient s care:** this covers all activities to schedule or perform services and record care, including the following: (1) ordering clinical lab test, medications, diagnostic images, etc., and receiving back results, including alarms of abnormal results; (2) documenting patient care, producing documents in the patient medical record; (3) messaging between caregivers; (4) making patient appointments; (5) viewing medical and HMO reference information, including HMO guidelines and drug formulary.

The proposed automated patient medical record system would be tailorable, such as by job category or individual caregiver via agents. Tailoring could identify the scope of information available to a caregiver (i.e., the total of the information a caregiver has available to bring up for display) and how the information is connected (e.g., how selection of an item, such as an encounter, drills down to other information, such as a document list).

7.10 TRACING ESSENTIAL BUSINESS PRACTICES AND PROJECT OBJECTIVES TO BUSINESS REQUIREMENTS

Current essential business practices in our HMO that the HMO wants to preserve were identified in chapter 4. Objectives for the project were identified in chapter 5. This chapter identified business requirements that preserve these business practices and fulfill project objectives.

Table 7.2 cross references current business practices to preserve with the business requirements. Table 7.3 cross references project objectives with business requirements.

Table 7.2 Current HMO Business Practices to Preserve From Chapter 4

Number	*Essential Business Practice*	*Addressed in this Chapter?*	*Business Requirements*
1	Support all caregivers listed in section 4.2	Partially	The automated patient medical record system provides capabilities for multiple types of caregivers (see all sections in this chapter) and can be tailored by type of caregiver via agents (see section 7.6). See chapter 11for re-engineering and 12 for user interfaces for various caregivers.

2	Support caregiver workflows as identified in section 4.3, including providing lists of patients being seen by a caregiver or a group of caregivers.	Partially	See section 7.7.5 for various types of lists identifying patients of interest to various caregivers, supporting caregiver workflow. See chapter 11for re-engineering and 12 for user interfaces for various caregivers.
3	Support recording and retrieval of care documentation in the patient medical record, including retrieval of source documents that currently exist, as listed in section 4.4.	Yes	Proposed care documentation is described in sections 7.2, 7.3, 7.5 and 7.7.1.
4	Generate the documents listed in section 4.4 which are derived from, but are not included in the patient medical record.	Yes	See section 7.7.2 for the medication administration record (MAR) for inpatients, and section 7.7.4 for an overall clinical summary and an inpatient clinical summary (similar to the "Kardex").
5	Support ordering of diagnostic tests and of procedures, and support return and recording of results of orders. See sections 4.3 and 4.4.	Yes	See section 7.7.2 for ordering and return of results.
6	Support the principal purposes for the patient medical record listed in section 4.5.	Partially	See section 7.4 for tracking of care across encounters and other sections, especially section 7.7, for support for other purposes of the patient medical record.
7	Support demand management and other HMO cost-saving methods in section 4.6.1.	Partially	See sections 7.4 for tracking of care across encounter, sections 7.7.3 and 7.8 for messaging between caregivers. See chapter 11 for re-engineering and 12 for user interfaces for various caregivers.
8	Support existing HMO clinical systems as listed in section 4.6.2.	Yes	See section 7.3.1 for encounters from encounter systems, section 7.7.2 for orders and results from ancillary systems, and 7.8 for actionable information from other clinical systems.

Table 7.3 Project Objectives from Chapter 5

Number	*Organizational Objective*	*Project Objective*	*Project Objective Addressed in this Chapter?*	*Business Requirement*
1	Provide quality medical care	Re-evaluate the entire clinical workflow of the HMO to completely eliminate unnecessary steps and restructure non-productive steps while incorporating the automated patient medical record system.	No	See chapter 11 on reengineering.
		Create a complete and always available patient medical record.	Yes	Store the patient medical record electronically, making it available to caregivers both inside the HMO and within other healthcare organizations. See section 7.5.
		Allow simultaneous viewing and update of the patient medical record.	No	A research area—see the chapter 17.
		Enable a caregiver to quickly find relevant information in the patient medical record by methods such as providing summarization information, organization, information retrieval and tailoring of information related to the type of caregiver.	Yes	Electronically organize the patient medical record for various types of caregivers, provide a summary of the patient's health history, enable searching for relevant information, and enable tailoring of the presentation of information based upon user characteristics. See sections 7.3, 7.4, 7.5, 7.7.4, and 7.7.6.
		Provide methods to track a treatment for a particular condition across multiple encounters, possibly with multiple different caregivers, potentially in different departments and in different geographic locations.	Yes	Provide case management techniques to track treatments across multiple encounters. See 7.4.

Automate caregiver ordering and results reporting to make ordering easier, quicker and more accurate and integrate it with the automated patient medical record system.	Yes	Enable ordering and results reporting through integration of the automated patient medical record system with other HMO clinical systems. See section 7.7.2.
Do automated clinical checking of medications, such as drug/drug interactions and patient allergy checking. Reduce errors including reordered tests, adverse drug reactions, billing errors, etc.	Yes	In the process of entrance of medication orders, do clinical checking of medications. See section 7.7.2.
Provide information to caregivers on best practice guidelines using NGC and/or local guidelines; provide medical reference information.	Yes	Provide medical references, including NGC clinical practice guidelines. Provide clinical pathways that encapsulate evidence-based care. See sections 7.4.6 and 7.7.7.
Collect clinical outcomes information to further evidence-based medicine (identifying best treatments and practices for diseases which produce the best outcomes as determined by the best scientific evidence).	Yes	Provide case management techniques to track treatments across multiple encounters to make it easier to evaluate treatments, procedures, medications, etc. Provide research database (data warehouse) to support evaluation of medical care. See sections 7.4.6 and 7.7.8.
Automate the recording of biomarkers for diagnosis and prediction of diseases. Combine this with identification of trends in the patient's health through trend documents, especially in cases where there is an emerging health problem (e.g., an increase in the patient's blood pressure).	Yes	Provide "trend documents" that, once set up, automatically record specified values entered in documents (e.g., blood pressure) and report on situations of concern. See sections 7.4.2 and 7.4.5.
Generate letters to patients to come in for preventative health exams (e.g., colonoscopies) based upon age, sex, family history and other factors.	No	

		Provide the ability to record a detailed social, family, environmental and genetic history of HMO members who agree to provide this information. Identify family members of these HMO members and their relationships to the HMO member, especially family members who are themselves HMO members.	Partially	Develop a database (data warehouse) for HMO member use to predict potential future diseases and for research. For an individual, store that person's genome or the equivalent if the member consents. This is a research area. See chapter 17 and section 7.7.8.
		Explore predicting diseases from information in the automated patient medical record, including from risk factors and biomarkers.	No.	This is a research area—see chapter 17.
		For medical research purposes, enable useful access to clinical information without providing the identities of patients.	Yes	Develop database (data warehouse) for research and reporting. See 7.7.8.
		For medical research purposes, enable controlled access to clinical information to identify patients who are appropriate for specific clinical trials and other medical studies.	Yes	Develop database (data warehouse) for research and reporting. See 7.7.8.
2	Promote HMO Member Satisfaction	Have each HMO member chose a primary care physician. Have the automated system identify a patient's primary care physician(s) and associated caregivers.	Partially	One patient list displays the patients on a primary care physician's panel.
		For members who approve, store genetic and other information to enable individualized treatments and medications in the future.	No	In the future, record a member's genome if the member agrees in order to predict disease. This is a research area. See chapter 17.
		Personalize care for the patient through personal profiles.	No	See section 8.2.1.5.

Evaluate the feasibility of the automated patient medical record system receiving input from monitoring systems, including "Guardian Angel" systems.	Partially	A research area. See section 7.4.2.
Reengineer the care process to eliminate roadblocks that inhibit the patient from receiving prompt care.	Partially	Being automated, the patient chart will be immediately available to all HMO caregivers, eliminating delays in care. See chapter 11.
Pre-schedule activities, both generically and for specific individual patients, and, where possible, pre-fill paperwork or fill in paperwork when care is given, such as care documentation and insurance forms.	Yes	See section 7.4.4.
After an outpatient visit, provide the patient and the patient's family information on clinician orders and other encounter information to promote compliance with physician instructions and orders. After clinical laboratory results are returned, enable physicians to print and annotate results, sending them to the patient; terminology used should be understood by the patient.	Partially	Medical terminology specific to the patient may be needed. See section 7.7.3.2.
Where appropriate, provide the patient with automated scheduling of medications and determination of alternative medicines or dosage choices.	No	See section 8.3.3.
Generate a discharge summary for the patient which describes in clear language, restrictions and follow-up activities.	Partially	Medical terminology specific to the patient may be needed. See section 7.7.3.2.
Incorporate patient education information in the automated system for the patient.	No	See section 8.3.4.

		Get patients and their families more involved in the patient care process.	No	
		Record advance directives in the automated system.	Yes	See section 7.7.3.
3	Support healthcare workers and improve their efficiency	To reengineer the care process based upon input from employees so that employees' work activities match the most productive and least stressful methods of providing care.	No	See chapter 11 on reengineering.
		Check for or insure consistent terminology in the medical record.	No	
		Automate the process of identifying situations where patients are not complying with orders that seriously affect the patient's health.	No	A research area.
		Provide other automated assistance to the caregiver in providing care, including the following: alerts, trends, assistance in diagnosis, conformance to best practice guidelines, identifying inconsistencies.	Partially	Alerts are discussed in section 7.7.3.1. Trend documents in are discussed section 7.4.5. And medical references for best practice guidelines are discussed in section 7.7.7.
		Provide on-line medical references for the caregiver to use when providing care.	Yes	Provide medical references, including NGC clinical practice guidelines. See section 7.7.7.
		Eliminate redundant entrance of information in clinical systems, eliminating possible contradictory information.	Partially	Interface the automated patient medical record system with other clinical systems to gather information on demographics, encounters and orders and results. Other information may be redundant. See sections 7.3.1 and 7.7.2.

A member's medical record will be available to authorized physicians at any time.	Yes	Store the patient medical record electronically, making it available to caregivers both inside the HMO and within other healthcare organizations. See section 7.5.
Use techniques to simplify documentation listed in section 5.3.3.3.	Yes	See section 7.7.1.
Support automated care documentation for inpatient nurses, including computerized generation of nursing care plans.	Yes	Record documents in source document repositories and summarize in the computer-based patient record (CPR) repositories. Provide various techniques for input of document information. See sections 7.4 and 7.7.
Automate coding of diagnoses, procedures, and supplies (such as ICD, CDT, DRG codes). and unit census.	Partially	See section 7.7.3.2 for consistent medical vocabularies that may make automated coding more feasible.
Automate non-chart documentation done manually, such as the Inpatient Clinical Summary, MAR, emergency room census.	Yes	See section 7.7.2 for the medication administration record (MAR) for inpatients, and section 7.7.4 for an overall clinical summary and an Inpatient Clinical Summary.
Cut down on paperwork during the care process, instead, transferring information quickly via networks rather than by costly, slow, and error-prone manual transport.	Yes	See section 7.5, putting together a distributed patient chart.
Alert attending physician when discharge is pending so discharge procedures can be quickly accomplished. Enable post-discharge activities to be accomplished concurrently.	No	See section 5.3.4.1.

		Evaluate the feasibility of using digitized diagnostic images with the automated patient medical record system. Enable quick transmission of images to medical professionals who can interpret them.	No	
4	Making and Saving Money	Re-evaluate the entire clinical workflow of the HMO to eliminate or revise costly processes while incorporating the automated patient medical record system.	No	See chapter 11 on reengineering.
		Support demand management in all its forms.	Yes	See section 7.4 and 7.7.
		Reduce errors including reordered tests, adverse drug reactions, billing errors, etc.	Yes	Do error checking during ordering. See section 7.7.2.
		Identify and report on potential patient abuse such as "drug jumping", going from facility to facility for narcotics orders.	No	Requires analysis of cost-effectiveness of doing so.
		Identify suspicious charges for medications and services when payments are to be made to outside healthcare organizations.	No	Requires further research and analysis.
		Support automated collection of payments for medical services from the government and insurance companies via EDI. Support automated payment for medical services. Support automated collection of Medicare payments using HIPAA standards.	Yes	Support automated collection of payments for medical services from the government and insurance companies via EDI. Support automated payment for medical services. See section 7.7.9.
		Support electronic commerce, in particular DME ordering such as over the Internet.	Yes	Support electronic commerce, in particular DME ordering such as over the Internet. See section 7.7.9.

Provide automated advice on least cost best practices, including lower cost medications that provide equal or better benefits, including advice to use generic medications rather than brand name ones.	Yes	This could be actionable information; see section 7.8. Develop agent code to recognize that best practices are not being followed and make recommendations on low cost treatments, medications and procedures. See section 7.6. See section 7.4 for defined outcome cases that can be used to evaluate treatments.
Record information for prediction of HMO costs in the future: services, tests and procedures given to patients, supplies and medications, provider time caring for patients, hospitalizations and visits, and trends in membership growth and patient utilization.	No	See section 13.8.3 for a financial database (data warehouse) for research and reporting for identification of true costs. See section 7.7.10 for recording costs.
Interface the automated medical record system with encounter systems, ordering and results systems, and billing and financial systems to share information.	Yes	See sections 7.3.1, 7.7.2, and 7.7.10.
Where possible, standardize hardware, system software and clinical systems within the organization.	No	
Standardize clinical system interfaces using industry standards (such as HL7).	Yes	Interface the automated patient medical record system with other clinical systems to gather information on encounters and enable ordering and results reporting using HL7. See section 7.3.1, 7.5.2 and 7.7.2.
Design the automated patient medical record system to eliminate documentation errors identified in table 5.1 to protect against costly lawsuits.	Partially	Validate orders and clinical information entered into documents. See 7.7.1 and 7.7.2.

		Support consolidation, and possible outsourcing, of medical services where the patient is not seen, such as interpretation of diagnostic images.	No	
		Evaluate the possibility, feasibility and cost-effectiveness of off-site storage of automated patient medical record information.	No	
5	Fulfill the Requirements of Government and Public Health Agencies, Accreditation Organizations, Laws, and Industry Standards	Automatically collect registry information based upon patient diagnoses and alert a caregiver when registry information should be collected (e.g., cancer; SARS and other infectious diseases).	Yes	Develop agent code to recognize and record Registry items. Develop for each kind of registry. See section 7.6.
		Provide automated recognition of infection outbreaks, in particular infections occurring within HMO hospitals. Healthcare personnel should also be trained to recognize outbreaks and epidemics.	Yes	Develop agent code to recognize documentation of infection outbreaks. See section 7.6.
		Automate quality control checks that insure that clinical information complies with accreditation agency (e.g., JCAHO) and government standards and which generates proof of compliance.	Yes	Develop agent code to recognize where JCAHO rules are not being followed. See section 7.6.
		For reporting based upon medical-related information (e.g., HEDIS), set up automatic generation of these reports and transmission to outside agencies (e.g., the NCQA).	Yes	Develop database (data warehouse) for research and reporting from which reports can be generated and transmitted to outside agencies, e.g., via agents. See sections 5.3.5 and 7.6.

Key Terms

automated patient medical record
computer-based patient record (CPR)
actionable information
agent
alarm
alert
biomarker
care activity
care management
care notes
care team
caregiver messaging
caregiver messaging system
caregiver-defined patient list
case management
case manager
case notes
chronic care management case
clinical pathway
conditional orders
control chart
controlled medical vocabulary
defined outcome case
disease management
document list
drug compendium
ED visit
e-mail
electronic health record
electronic medical record
electronic patient record
e-mail messages
emergency department list
emergency department room map
encounter
encounter status
episode
exclusive searching
Extranet
feature analysis
filler
home care visit
inclusive searching
information retrieval
inpatient clinical summary
inpatient stay
inpatient unit room map
Intranet
medical references
medical vocabulary
observation visit
outcomes
outpatient clinic room map
outpatient visit
overall clinical summary
patient case
patient clinical summary
patient list
patient panel
phone messages
Physicians' Desk Reference
placer
prn
probability density functions (pdf)
reminder
repeating orders
schedule
schedule I through schedule V
scope of care
significant health problem
single (one-time) order
source document
standing orders
STAT order
surgery
Surgery List
telephone call
treatment notes
treatment plans
trend document
unified messaging
unit census
variance
wait list
work list

Study Questions

1. What are business requirements? Name some ways to derive business requirements.
2. What are source documents?
3. Name two major ways of organizing the automated patient medical record. What is the POMR?
4. Name some types of encounters and encounter statuses for each. Is a telephone call an encounter?—Discuss.
5. Name some types of documents to track care

11. What does the author feel is a current failing with many organization business policies incorporated within automated systems, and what is the author's solution to this?
12. Name some ways that source documents can be made easier to enter using an automated system?
13. What is the standard network protocol for communicating encounters, orders and results between healthcare systems?

across encounters.

6. What is more appropriate for a fragile elderly Medicare patient, case management, care management or disease management? If you wished to provide specialized care for all patients with type II diabetes which approach would you use? If you would like to track a patient with asthma over time, which approach would you use?
7. What is a biomarker? Give an example of non-changing biomarker. What document would allow a healthcare organization to track a biomarker over time?
8. With an automated patient medical record, where can source documents be stored? Devise at least two architectures where a source document would still be available if the previous network connection to it went down.
9. For the CPR repository, what do I suggest be included that the ASTM E1384 standard does not provide?
10. What are existing healthcare standards that could be used with an automated patient medical record?
14. Which caregivers can normally make orders? What are schedule I, II, III, IV, and V drugs?—What must a caregiver have to order or dispense such drugs? What's a STAT order? Standing order? Prn order? What's the MAR?
15. What does a caregiver messaging system provide that a pure e-mail system does not provide? What is unified messaging?
16. When is a medical vocabulary a closed medical vocabulary?
17. What are patient clinical summaries? Patient lists? Document lists?
18. Identify approaches to allow information in automated patient medical records to be found? What is exclusive searching, and what is inclusive searching?—How does this relate to precision and recall? How does feature analysis relate to monitoring systems?
19. Name some types of medical references.
20. What areas outside of direct patient care can the automated patient medical record support?
21. What is actionable information?

CHAPTER 8

Anticipated Future Use of the Automated Patient Medical Record

CHAPTER OUTLINE

8.1 PROJECT CONTEXT: DESCRIBING THE FUTURE ENVIRONMENT AND SYSTEMS

There are a number of purposes for anticipating the future organization after the project is complete: (1) It enables upper management to provide input into the future environment. (2) It could be used to generate additional business requirements for the project that insure that the future environment can be achieved. (3) It could be used to identify additional automated systems or automated systems that need change. (4) It could provide information for the reengineering of the organization and definition of user interfaces.

This chapter gives an example of the results of determining the future environment and systems for the automated patient medical record system. Additional business requirements derived from the projection of the future environment and systems are listed in section 8.8.

Although the automated patient medical record helps physicians, nurses and other caregiver do their jobs, the real context should be on how the automated patient medical record helps HMO members.

8.2 PROJECTED FUTURE USE

The following identifies one approach to use of an automated patient medical record, where the approach might be defined after discussions between HMO management, HMO staff and industry experts with the facilitation of business analysts, based upon business requirements determined so far. From this analysis, additional business requirements for the project, and user interfaces and employee workflows, could be determined.

8.2.1 Overview of Changes to Patient Care

The automated patient medical record system presents a complete record of clinical information for patients in the HMO available at any time to all caregivers in the HMO. A properly structured automated patient medical record has the potential of evolving into a universal patient health record.

The automated patient medical record system enables

- selection of a patient
- presentation of a quick overview of the patient's health problems, current medication and previous encounters
- display and information retrieval of all the documents in the patient's chart
- quick caregiver ordering, electronically sending of the order to an ancillary department and quick return of results
- appointment making
- input of documentation to be included in the chart, from current chart documents to e-mail.

Just introducing automation to these activities will require significant changes in the way caregivers currently work.

The following additional features are provided if HMO caregivers make an effort to input information that is not collected in the current system. These features would be more difficult to implement because they not only introduce new automation, but also new approaches to giving care. The new approaches to care are tailored specifically to the health problems of the individual and thus is care centered around the individual. *(patient-centered care),* with caregiver *team care* for the patient's significant long-term medical conditions and *preventive care* over the individual's life time.:

- Through defined outcome cases and chronic care management cases, allow those caring for the patient to quickly track the patient's current treatments that span over multiple visits.
- Through use of a case document, allow a case manager to record, evaluate, and manage care given to a high-risk patient (e.g., the frail elderly, patients with severe kidney disease, etc.)
- Allow those caring for a patient to quickly access all the clinical information related to a particular health problem of a patient (e.g., all patient clinical information for diabetes).
- Allow all those caring for a patient to get a quick summary of each patient encounter.
- Through a complete social, family, environmental and genetic history developed for members, allow the automated patient medical record to identify for caregivers and researchers those members who have the greatest propensity for diseases for which preventative care would be appropriate
- Through "life care paths" for members based upon age, sex, and medical chart information, allow the automated patient medical record system to a schedule preventive care appointments when most advantageous for the member.
- Allow caregivers to call on compliance managers to provide assistance to members in making life style changes and in complying with treatments prescribed by physicians.
- Allow caregivers giving continuing care for a patient to associate care notes with the patient to record care information to be carried over to future encounters within the caregiver's scope of care.

The following sections propose a list of duties of all caregivers that would organize the automated patient medical record and enable these additional features. See figure 8.1.

8.2.1.1 Extra Information Collected for New HMO Members

Soon after a new member joins the HMO, the member can be contacted. The member can either be invited in for an interview where a health questionnaire can be filled out, or the member can be sent the health questionnaire, which the member can fill out and return.

From the questionnaire, information for a summarization of the patient's health, a *patient clinical summary* referred to in this book as the *overall clinical summary* could be created. When a member is new to the HMO or is a *low-utilizer* (a health organization member who seldom comes in for care.), this information in the patient's overall clinical summary might be the only clinical information available. This information would be particularly significant for an unconscious or uncommunicative patient in the emergency department and could then provide some of the same information as the health history part of a *history and physical (H&P)* document.

The questionnaire could also be used to start an ongoing social, family, environment and genetic history that could be added to and updated over time. In the future, the member's genome could be recorded—A *genome* is the whole of the genetic information for an individual.

Based upon sex, age and health factors determined from the questionnaire, all new members could be assigned a *life care path* identifying preventive health care to be automatically scheduled for the patient by the automated system for the patient. This would send out letters requesting that the patient come in for an appointment for a specific type of preventive health care (e.g., blood pressure check, sigmoid, etc.) The letter could be sent out in coordination with the appointment system to insure availability of appointment time. Determination of which patients to send letters to first—like by which patient is the most likely to get the associated disease—could be based upon health information recorded in the automated patient medical record.

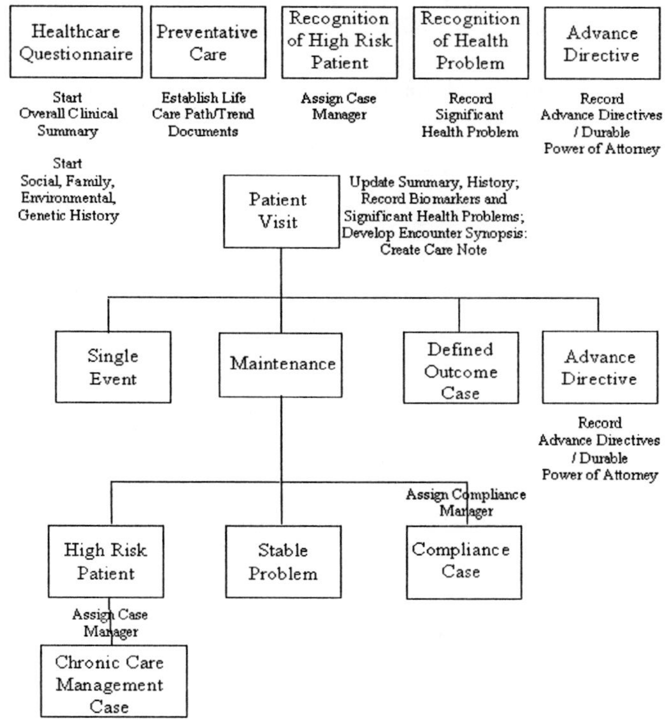

Figure 8.1 A Model for Patient-Centered Healthcare Within an HMO

From the questionnaire, *high-risk patients* (e.g., needs custodial care, has life threatening diabetes, etc.) could be identified. Such a patient could be assigned a case manager, significant health problems could be recorded, and case documentation could be started. If the patient has lower risk but significant and reoccurring health problems—the significant health problem could simply be recorded (and thus be available within the clinical summary) and identified as stable, not requiring a case manager.

8.2.1.2 Extra Information Collected During Patient Visits

Whenever a member comes in for a visit due to a health complaint, the visit may involve a problem that could be handled in a single visit, it may involve a treatment over a number of visits, perhaps including inpatient stays, or it may involve a chronic disease that requires continuing long-term care.

New *significant health problems* can be identified and recorded during visits.

As the patient comes in for care, *biomarkers* for prediction and diagnosis of diseases could be collected, with determination of what biomarkers to choose determined by factors such as age, sex, symptoms, and previous measurement of other biomarkers. The automated patient medical record could provide assistance in monitoring of a biomarker through a trend document. A "trend document" could be set up that records biomarkers over time, requesting physicians to record the biomarker during successive visits. For example, a member with borderline high blood pressure may be assigned a trend document for tracking blood pressure.

Biomarkers are cellular, biochemical, molecular, or genetic characteristics or alterations in an individual by which a normal, abnormal, or simply biologic process can be recognized, or monitored. An individual's genome could provide permanent biomarkers while other biomarkers would change over time. Blood pressure is a biomarker for heart disease. Biomarkers for diseases should be recorded and monitored to diagnosis and predict diseases, especially biomarkers that do not require invasive procedures to determine; additional more invasive biomarkers could be added when other biomarkers suggest the possibility of the presence of the disease. The increased recognition and use of biomarkers for diseases could produce a more "science-based medicine" and enable patient care to be more proactive.

After a visit, the caregiver could create a synopsis summarizing the encounter or the automated system could create this summary. This could be used to provide easy-to-read information for later caregivers.

Defined Outcome Cases As part of the outpatient appointment or inpatient stay, it would be determined if care for the problem needs to be tracked beyond the single appointment or inpatient stay; if so, a defined outcome case based upon the health problem could be established possibly along with a clinical pathway to guide the care for the particular health problem. If the treatment was completed, the case would be removed as a active defined outcome case. Over time, the defined outcome case could involve multiple outpatient or inpatient encounters, or both, and involve care both inside and outside the healthcare organization. Treatment notes could be recorded as part of the defined outcome case. Trend documents could also be started, which could be terminated at the end of a defined outcome case or could continue thereafter.

Caregivers should make a significant effort to identify when care for the problem no longer needs to be tracked and the defined outcome case could be made inactive. The automated system could also employ automated approaches to doing this inactivation of defined outcome cases.

High Risk Patients and Chronic Care Management Cases Upon a visit to the HMO, a patient could be assigned a ongoing case manager if it is deemed that the patient is a high-risk patient.For example, the patient could be high-risk because of being frail and elderly, or the patient could be identified as high risk due to a specific chronic condition, in which case the patient may be assigned a "chronic care management case", tracking care for the chronic condition. *Predictive modeling* is a technique using mathematical and statistical algorithms based upon visit and patient medical record information to identify which HMO members would benefit the most from disease and other case management.(Baldwin 2004)

Biomarkers for Prediction and Diagnosis of Diseases When a patient comes in for care, measurement and collection of biomarkers for various diseases could be collected and recorded (e.g., Pap smears and presense of HPV for cervical cancer and PSA for prostate cancer). Some of these biomarkers, such as information from an individual's genome are fixed. Other biomarkers would change over time. Diseases could be predicted or diagnosed from combinations of biomarkers, and treatments and medications could be more individualized.

A trend document could be set up for a changeable biomarker, in which case the automated patient medical record system could remind a caregiver to measure and record a biomarker when the patient comes in for care.

Encounter Synopsis After an encounter, a summary of the encounter could be created by the caregiver or by the automated patient medical record system. This would enable later caregivers to more easily search through encounters in the chart and review the results of information retrieval of encounter information.

Care Notes A caregiver can generate notes for him- or herself or a care team about ideas for the future care of the patient within the scope of care of the caregiver or care team (e.g., eye care, urology, oncology).

8.2.1.3 Improvements in Care from this Extra Information

Collection of this additional information for new HMO members and additional information during a patient visit for all members does the following:

- It provides a summary of the health of each HMO member, including those who will seldom come in, thus insuring that health information is always available (e.g., available in the emergency department)
- It establishes a defined outcome case to track a treatment and a chronic care management case for a high risk patient with a chronic condition, making the current treatment clear to all caregivers seeing the patient
- It assigns case managers to high risk patients so case managers could assist such patients
- It enables all caregivers, including advice nurses, to be aware of current cases and to be aware of case managers and of caregivers who are seeing the patient for these cases
- It allows caregivers to identify persistent and reoccurring health problems of a patient
- It organizes encounters by significant health problems, allowing encounters to be associated with a particular health problem, thus allowing the encounters to later be easily found upon caregiver selection of the health problem
- It allows a caregiver, through encounter synopses, to quickly review the patient's previous encounters
- It enables an automated system to automatically schedule patients for preventive care
- It allows recording of biomarkers used to diagnosis disease, and individualize treatments and medications
- Through a complete social, family, environmental and genetic history, together with the tracking of biomarkers, it may enable probabilistic determinations of diseases that a patient might develop.

8.2.1.4 Change in Access to the Patient Medical Record

The paper medical record is available to only one practitioner at a time and can get lost. An automated patient medical record does not face these same restrictions.

An automated patient medical record cannot get lost. It can be available to multiple caregivers at the same time. Because of this, the automated patient medical record could now potentially be available to a much wider variety of caregivers without the fear that it would get lost or that it would be unavailable when needed.

This availability of the patient medical record has the potential of improving medical care for a patient, but makes greater the risk of unauthorized access to sensitive patient information.

Access to the automated patient medical record still is governed by the same laws and restrictions of the paper medical record. These include federal and state laws, rules of regulatory bodies, and HMO rules and protocols.

Currently, the paper patient medical record is singularly available to practitioners: physicians, or nurse practitioners, physician assistants and nurses with the supervision of a physician. With the automated patient medical record, availability could be extended to new types of caregivers and to multiple caregivers at the same time. These new types of caregivers who might now have the patient medical record could include advice nurses talking to the patient on the telephone, pharmacists reviewing dispensed medications, case managers, those caregivers interpreting results of tests or procedures (for example, x-rays or pulmonary function tests), and others.

Dependent upon government and HMO security requirements, physicians caring for a patient may not have total access to a patient's medical record. For example, depending upon HMO rules and protocols, psychiatric and genetic medical information may not be available to physicians outside these respective departments. Emergency department physicians would make a case that the total of patient medical information should be available to them.

Rules and restrictions on access to the patient medical record must be established for each of these types of caregivers. Rules and restrictions must also be established on concurrent access and concurrent updating of the automated patient medical record by multiple caregivers.

8.2.1.5 Greater Patient-Centered Care

Care should be personalized for the patient. Provider instructions should be in the patient's language and patients should be encouraged to have family members participate in the patient's care, as both these things foster greater compliance of the patient with a physician's instructions. A *post visit report* in the language of the patient after an outpatient visit is proposed. This is described further in section 8.3.2.

Family participation in the care of a patient applies both for inpatients and outpatients. As an outpatient, if the patient desires, family members could be involved in receipt of the outpatient physician's instructions to the patient, thereafter supporting the patient in following the instructions. For inpatients, a close family member may be able to stay at the hospital to assist and provide emotional support for the patient and provide medical staff with information that the patient may find it difficult to convey because of his or her medical condition. For all inpatients, including a patient without a family, a Patient Representative or Clinical Social Worker could be assigned to assist the patient, in particular advising the patient on available patient services within the hospital or upon discharge.

The patient should be recognized as an individual, different from other patients. A *personal profile* is proposed, which identifies the patient's description of herself or himself (e.g., a mother, having diabetes, with 3 children, Carol, John and Susan) together with a description of special care being given (e.g., assigned to case manager of Ellie Nelsen, CSW). A personal profile could provide caregivers with quick useful information about the patient.

For a patient with one or more major medical conditions, this might include the patient's major ailments also within the patient's medical record, but it would also need to include other patient information.

For example, the patient's personal profile might also include the following:

- patient's name
- where the name is difficult to pronounce, a phonetic version of the name in parentheses
- whether the patient is male or female
- age (derived from date of birth)
- the major relatives (e.g., children, wife's name, husband's name)—pointing to another patient (member) profile.

But to be most useful, the profile should be constantly changing to fit changes in the life and health of the patient. One possibility is to have the HMO member create his own personal profile and have the member periodically update it.

Examples of personal profiles are the following:

Jay Leeds
53 year-old male
Wife Sally Leeds, a paraplegic
No children
Prostate problems, BPH
Seeing a urologist
Old left leg fracture
Sulfa allergy

and

Lynne Spencer
Prefers to be called "Mrs. Spencer"
42 year-old female
Husband John has diabetes
2 Children
    Jane
    Kelly
No significant medical problems.

A personal profile could enable transfer over to another personal profile or a telephone transfer to a clinical department. For example, the personal profile for a husband (John), wife (Sally) or child of a patient (Kelly) could be accessible from the personal profile of the patient by selecting the husband, wife or child name line respectively. Selecting a specialist (e.g., urologist) could do a telephone transfer over to the department of urology.

When a patient calls in to an appointment clerk and wanted to get an appointment for her daughter, this personal profile transfer capability would allow the booking operation to be quickly switched over to the patient's daughter. When a patient calls in to an appointment clerk and is being seen in a specialty department (e.g., urology), this personal profile transfer capability would allow the patient phone call to be transferred quickly over to the specialty department.

8.2.2 New HMO Members

When there is a new HMO member, the member will be asked to come into the HMO facility that he expects to visit most often. When arriving at the HMO the member will be directed to a new member's area. There, the following will happen:

- The member will be assigned a healthcare services representative, who the patient can call to serve as an ombudsman and inform the member above his benefits.
- The member will be assigned a life care path, identifying preventive care appointments, based upon his age, sex and current health.

- The member will be given the choice of physicians and nurse practitioners in primary care who would be assigned as the patient's principal primary care provider(s), either in family practice, internal medicine, or pediatrics, based upon his age.
- A woman will be given the choice of a physician or nurse practitioner who would be assigned to provide the bulk of any future care for the patient in family practice or Gynecology.
- The member will be asked "What do you want known about you, which should include your name, age, children, husband/wife, and may include major problems, etc.—anything brief and substantive?" This would be used to create an initial *personal profile*. This information will be used locally only and will not be given to anyone outside the HMO.
- A picture will be taken to be included in the patient clinical summary to insure against fraudulent use of an HMO identification card and resultant inaccuracy of information in the patient's medical record.

The new member will be interviewed by a medical professional to evaluate the member's existing health problems. Significant health problems will be recorded for input into the automated patient medical record system for the Clinical Summary. If it is determined that the member would be a *high-risk patient*, then the member would be assigned a case manager.

Note that the automated patient medical record system upon identifying that there is a new member will request that all patient medical record information from outside the HMO be transferred to the HMO from outside CPR repositories and source document repositories.

Based upon the patient's existing medical conditions and interest in medical information, a new member can pick the various ways in which she may wish to receive medical information:

- **doctor s opinions only:** The member is only interested in receiving medical information from the doctor during the time of the visit.
- **conditions and risk factors that increase the probabilities of a future condition occurring, and preventives for the future condition:** The member is interested in the probabilities of certain diseases, conditions or situations occurring based upon preceding conditions and risk factors. For example, preceding conditions for knee replacements may be a severe knee injury, crepitus and cartilage tears. A risk factor increasing the chance of lung cancer is smoking; a preventative is to stop smoking.
- **health education classes:** The member may be interested in health education courses in the future.
- **mentor program:** The member may be interested in talking to other members with particular medical conditions who have had a particular treatment or procedure who will discuss the positives and negatives of the treatment or procedure (e.g., knee or hip replacement) with the member. See section 8.3.4.
- **medical research:** The member may be interested in talking to employees of the HMO doing medical research on particular conditions or procedures (e.g., psoriasis).

After any visit, the member can update this information.

8.2.3 Choice of a Primary Care Physician

New members and members without an assigned *primary care physician* would be able to choose a primary care physician. Additionally, members with an assigned primary care physician would be able to select a different one. Such an assigned primary care physician is sometimes said to be the member's *personal physician.*

Primary care is the first contact in a given episode of illness that leads to a decision regarding a course of action to resolve the health problem. *Primary care departments* are internal medicine, pediatrics, family practice and obstetrics/gynecology. Other departments are *specialty departments*, normally departments receiving referrals from primary care physicians.

For members 18 or over the personal physician would be in internal medicine. For members under 18, the personal physician would be in pediatrics. Females over 12 could also have a second personal physician in obstetrics/gynecology. Having one primary care physician in medicine or pediatrics helps insure that care is not fragmented.

Upon the visit of a new member to the HMO as described in section 8.2.2 or at any other time, a member would be able to chose a primary care physician based upon criteria such as gender, how recently the physician graduated from medical school, subspecialties, medical school name, etc.

Upon choice of a primary care physician, the member would be appointed for an introduction appointment. At this introduction appointment, the primary care physician could review and update clinical summary for the member and the member's current medications. The member could be treated for current ailments, referred to specialty care providers, or assigned a case manager.

See section 8.2.7 for further discussion on member-chosen primary care physicians.

8.2.4 Internet Access to Members, Employers and Caregivers

The Internet will provide access to members, employers who pay for premiums for employees who are HMO members, and HMO caregivers. In order to access information, the member, employer or caregiver must enter his PIN number.

HMO members will be able to get the following information, and perform the following activities through the Internet:

- get information on benefits
- get information on the patient's healthcare services representative, assigned providers or case manager
- make appointments
- get a list of health care facilities and providers based upon entered zip code
- get information on providers who could potentially be assigned with the patient (e.g., biographies)
- select primary care and other providers to be assigned to the patient based upon characteristics (e.g., locations, sex, subspecialties, works on Saturday or Sunday, minimum and maximum years of experience, languages, affiliations, etc.) with identification of the most important characteristics
- send comments to the HMO
- enter periodic patient clinical values for trend documents (e.g., the patient's blood pressure, blood glucose levels, height or weight)
- get information on preventive care recommendations by sex and age
- get information on the latest treatments, including alternative medical care provided by the HMO

- get multi-media explanations of health problems (e.g., the University of Virginia used to have a Web tutorial on asthma, showing animated diagrams of breathing, showing the constriction of breathing and build of mucous associated with asthma and showing how the lungs function normally and with asthma.)
- start chat rooms with psychiatrists and other medical providers and send e-mail for medical advice to nurse practitioners
- get information on the medical center layouts.

8.2.5 Healthcare Services Representatives

At any time, the member will be able to contact via telephone a healthcare services representative. During the day, the patient should normally be able to directly contact the healthcare services representative assigned to him. The healthcare services representative will provide the member with guidance through the health care system, especially as related to the member's normal facility. She will be able to contact physicians, nurses and other HMO personal directly. She will be able to give advice on benefits, treatment options, providers to be assigned to the patient, and any other information that is also available to the patient through the Internet as mentioned in section 8.2.4. The healthcare services representative will also have all the capabilities of an appointment clerk as identified below, although she should normally have the patient call an appointment clerk to perform this function.

In areas of the nation where an HMO has a significant number of members from a non-English speaking community, the assigned healthcare services representative should be able to speak the preferred language of such a member.

The healthcare services representative will have available to her through the automated patient medical record system, the ability to identify providers who could be assigned to the patient, to identify referrals and active cases for the patient. She will be able to create and add to "Patient Lists", callback lists with comments about the member.

Healthcare services representatives from one facility should work closely with healthcare services representatives in other facilities. The member should be introduced to and transferred to a specific healthcare services representative in another facility when the patient also uses the other facility regularly (e.g., a facility near work, whereas the member's normal facility is near home) or when the member wants to get information on caregivers in the other facility who could see the member to give a second opinion on a health concern.

8.2.6 Call Centers: Appointment Clerks, Advice Nurses and Call Center Physicians

An important first point of contact for a member with a health problem is the *appointment clerk* or *advice nurse*, usually located in a *call center*. The advice nurse and physicians in the call center are probable users of the automated patient medical record.

A *call center* is a bank of telephones in a managed care healthcare organization with appointment clerks and advice nurses who together (1) make appointments for the member, (2) give the member advice on medical care based upon protocols, including when self care is appropriate and when the patient should come in, and (3) connect the member with medical resources, including physicians and patient education.

At any time, the member will be able to call a phone number that advises the member to call 911 for emergencies, asks the patient for his/her patient identifier, and allows touch-tone or voice access to the following choices via a Interactive Voice Response (IVR), a software application that accepts a combination of voice telephone input and touch-tone keypad selection and provides appropriate responses for each:

- an appointment clerk to make an appointment
- an advice nurse to get medical advice
- an automated prescription number to refill prescriptions
- an automated cancellation number to cancel appointments
- an automated system to book some categories of appointments, and cancel and reschedule previously scheduled appointments.

For the first two selections an *automated call distribution (ACD)* system routes the call to the next available agent (appointment clerk or advice nurse).

There will be the capability to record on audio a telephone call from a patient and include it in the patient's automated medical record. Where the telephone call leads to an encounter, there will be the ability to associate the telephone call with the encounter.

For a patient with a high priority defined outcome case or chronic care management case, the automated system will automatically transfer over the call to an advice nurse, with potential of transferring over calls for some patient's to the member's case manager if the case manager is available.

Any member who feels intimidated by the touch-tone phone system could be given the option to call his or her healthcare services representative rather than go through the touch-tone or voice system. This is particularly important for frail and elderly members who may not be sick enough to be assigned a full time case manager but who might sometimes need immediate service or need more explanation than a touch-tone system could provide.

A further analysis will be done to determine whether appointment clerks, advice nurses or both should be located in call centers or in HMO facilities. Putting advice nurses in local facilities would simplify messaging between the advice nurses and local physicians, and make use of facility knowledge, such as the current unavailability of a physician. On the other hand, putting advice and appointment clerks in a call center would potentially decrease telephone call wait times and queue sizes.

Computer telephony integration (CTI), hardware and software that enables a computer to support a call center, provides capabilities for touch-tone and other control of incoming phone calls, for directing of calls (say to the longest waiting appointment clerk or advice nurse, or to a case manager), and for possible member input of a member's patient identifier or desired facility or department (e.g., Pediatrics, Medicine, Gynecology). Additionally, the transfer of the call to the appointment clerk, advice nurse or case manager could include the popping up of a computer screen containing member-entered information.

The HMO appointment clerk and advice nurse will function following HMO established protocols for each.

The call center appointment clerk will

- through the automated patient medical record system, identify case managers, providers assigned to the patient, referrals and active defined outcome cases and chronic care management cases for the patient; receive any alerts or alarms for the patient that are relevant to the appointment clerk

- help the patient choose or change assigned primary care and other providers, if the patient wants one and does not have one
- identify the reason or chief complaint related to the appointment
- transfer the patient's call to the refill phone if a patient prefers to refill appointments this way; otherwise, transfers refills to an advice nurse or pharmacist
- transfer a patient over to his/her case manager
- transfer the patient's call on a priority basis to an advice nurse if there is detected a medical urgency to the call, in particular if there is a "red flag" word such as "chest pain"; the HMO could establish protocols for doing so related to the chief complaint
- transfer the patient's call to an advice nurse if the member expressed any question at all about the medical need for an appointment and wants to talk to the advice nurse
- transfer the patient's call to a healthcare services representative if there is a question about the benefits coverage for the patient and the patient is concerned about possibly paying an extra amount or if the patient needs guidance through the healthcare system, especially as related to the facility where the patient normally comes for medical care
- book an appointment for health education or initiate a tape on a specific medical area that the patient wants to learn more about (e.g., menopause, hypertension, mammography, sore throat, smoking cessation, etc.)
- book a same day or next day urgent care appointment as long as there is time within a schedule, ideally with a patient's assigned provider; if none is available, follow protocol for booking or transfer the patient over to an advice nurse
- transfer the patient over to the correct facility department upon a referral; using a list of displayed patient referrals, the automated system should allow selection of the referral to transfer the call to the correct department's appointment phone
- for a follow-on appointment associated with an active defined outcome case or chronic care management case, the automated system would provide a list of such cases for the patient from which the appointment clerk could select (see figure 12.20); from the case document selected, the appointment clerk could transfer the patient to the appointment phone for that case by a click of a "transfer" button (see figure 12.21); if the appointment clerk is unable to determine the case, the call should be transferred to an advice nurse
- cancel, and reschedule, appointments when requested; if an appointment is marked as part of a defined outcome case or chronic care management case and is thus a type of appointment that requires special consideration when canceling, transfer the patient to an advice nurse
- book a future routine appointment, especially one related to preventive health care generated by a life care path or an appointment in alternative medicine
- transfer the patient's telephone call to an advice nurse, sending her a message, for advice, allowed member-initiated lab tests, etc., perhaps generated from a pre-formatted message
- view a call history for the member
- schedule allowed member initiated lab tests (for example, as allowed by California law, such as pregnancy, glucose, cholesterol and occult blood colorectal cancer tests) or just inform the member to drop in to the appropriate clinic
- accept pre-agreed-upon patient input of a blood pressure reading or a blood sugar reading, with the automated system verifying the validity of the inputs and recommending transfer to an advice nurse if the values are out of range (note that such

inputs could automatically be transferred to a previously set up "trend document" by the automated patient medical record system)

- through a *personal profile* for the patient available from patient demographics, the appointment clerk can transfer to information for the patient's husband, wife, or children and transfer the patient to any identified specialty department where the patient is receiving care (see section 8.2.1.5).

The appointment clerk, based upon her conversations with the patient, should advise the patient of services that are available (e.g., assignment of a principal primary care or other provider with the patient, healthcare services representative conveyance of member benefits, health education classes and health tapes, member initiated lab tests). The appointment clerk will not deal with medical decisions other than to evaluate the member's certainty of needing an appointment and determining if the patient has immediate medical concerns. Any such uncertainty or concerns should result in the appointment clerk advising the member to talk to an advice nurse. Otherwise, in general, if the patient wants an appointment, the appointment clerk should attempt to find an appointment for the patient.

The call center advice nurse will be able to do the following:

- do anything the appointment clerk can do
- have controlled access to the automated patient medical record which may include the overall clinical summary (including assigned providers, active defined outcome cases and chronic care management cases, referrals, current medications, and lab test results) and the documents in the patient medical record; and through the automated patient medical record system, document all conversations with the member for inclusion in the automated patient medical record
- create personal Patient Lists, in particular to list patients to later call back
- give the patient medical advice based upon HMO protocols for the patient's complaint
- view on-line medical references through the automated patient medical record system
- handle refill of medications (medications where the number of refills identified on the previous prescription has run out and where the prescription must be re-approved by a physician or nurse practitioner to continue)
- contact an on-call physician to get further medical advice
- contact an on-call pharmacist to get further advice on medications
- call physicians, nurses of physicians, or others in the call center directly or send messages to them (via a messaging system such is described in section 7.7.3)
- make all appointments, including when there is no available time in the physician's schedule, based upon physician or HMO protocols, or contact HMO appointment clerks associated with specialty areas to make the appointments
- for a follow-on appointment that the patient wants canceled and that the automated system marks as requiring special consideration when canceling, take efforts to reschedule or contact a specialist physician or primary care provider to determine if the appointment can be canceled without rescheduling
- make referrals to specialists based upon protocol
- give the member lab test results if allowed by protocol; otherwise, transfer patient to physician or send message to physician to return lab test results
- be aware of experimental programs and alternative medicine, and understand when they are appropriate.

A team of advice nurses could be associated with a facility, whether they are located at the facility or at a centralized call center, and assist caregivers at the facility and their nurses with care of their patients. An advice nurse could, for example, convey important care information personally to a physician or the physician's nurse within the facility, later returning a call to the patient. When located in a call center, the advice nurses could also serve as a resource providing information on the facility caregivers to other advice nurses in the call center.

Through the automated patient medical record system, an advice nurse should be able to document her conversations with a patient and include this in the patient medical record. Calls should be tracked and also recorded in the patient medical record.

With the availability of a complete automated patient medical record for each member calling in, a physician could also serve in the call center, providing consultative support to the advice nurses, providing expert medical advice to a member who does not require an in-person outpatient visit, or providing advice to a member on whether or not the member should come in to the clinic or to the ED.

Other participants in the call center could include pharmacists, who could provide medication advice, refill an existing prescription, issue "grace" refills on most drugs, or discuss drug reactions with the patient. The availability of the patient chart would be useful here also.

For certain sections of the U. S., touch-tone access should be provided for non-English speakers (e.g., in Spanish and Cantonese). For such communities of foreign speakers, there should also be both healthcare services representatives and advice nurses, and possibly appointment clerks, who speak these languages. Additionally, translators during the time of the visit should be even more widely available; when there are few members of a language group, use of a family member to translate may be appropriate. Additionally, AT&T provides telephone translation services that could be used. In all cases, HMO personnel should be trained to be culturally sensitive.

To enable caregiver communication such as between the appointment clerk and advice nurse, the advice nurse and physicians and nurses in the unit, a *caregiver messaging system* such as described in section 7.7.3 should be available. This messaging system would enable messages to be sent from the "initiating caregiver" (e.g., the advice nurse) to the receiver caregiver (e.g., the patient's physician) and for the "receiver caregiver" to respond with the response optionally sent to a "responding caregiver" (e.g., a nurse working with the physician), who calls back the patient. The message could be marked as "closed out". The message could be assigned an "importance level" or priority identifying the maximum length of time before the message should be closed out. The various caregivers could be informed when a new message is received and when a message has not be closed out in the prerequisite time.

CTI enables telephone calls from patients to an HMO to be directed to a category of caregivers (e.g., an advice nurse or appointment clerk); this capability should also be supported for e-mails. For example, a patient might send an e-mail with a health question to an advice nurse, which could be answered by any available advice nurse. A re-fill request could be sent to the patient's personal physician who could approve it and send it to a pharmacy. Such e-mails are most easily handled through the Internet, which would tack on the correct category or recipients, rather than having a patient do this himself or herself.

8.2.7 Primary Care Physicians and Nurse Practitioners, and Associated Care Teams

Primary care is a department which would be the first point of contact in the HMO for a given episode of illness. A primary care physician is chosen by the HMO member, with the physician or an associated nurse practitioner providing the bulk of primary care to the patient. Primary care physicians and nurse practitioners may be in internal medicine, pediatrics, family practice, and gynecology/obstetrics. Primary care physicians and nurse practitioners work together with nurses, medical assistants, and others in the department in formal or informal care teams.

The chosen primary care physician would also be a coordinator of the overall care of the member. The chosen primary care physician would keep track of the member when the member comes in for specialty care, comes in to the emergency department, or is admitted to a hospital. With other care team members, the primary care physician would insure that the patient was educated in providing self care and that the patient's family, where appropriate, participated in the patient's care.

With the automated patient medical record, a physician will be able to immediately view any part of a patient's medical record that the physician has the authority to view (see section 13.9.2 for protected health information). In addition to enabling a physician to always have the patient medical record at the time of an appointment, this will enable a physician to look at the patient medical record prior to drop-in visits, quickly respond to communications from advice nurses and case managers, and quickly evaluate prescription refill requests. This makes unscheduled and ad hoc telephone visits or consultations with the patient now feasible, whereas this was previously only possible with appointed visits or telephone contacts appearing on the provider's schedule, where the patient's medical record could be preordered. It makes consultations with specialists easier as both the primary care physician and specialist will concurrently have the patient's medical record. And it makes telemedicine more feasible, with the caregiver seeing the patient having the patient medical record while a remote physician or nurse practitioner would also have the patient medical record. Patient medical records will no longer be fragmented and in many different places; the complete patient medical record will be available to each caregiver.

A primary care physician or nurse practitioner should track the health of patients on his or her panel, communicating with the patient directly to emphasize health advice, convey important diagnoses and communicate significant diagnostic test results. The primary care physician or nurse practitioner or other caregivers in the department could set *alerts* or *reminders* to inform future caregivers at the appropriate time of special needs of the patient (e.g., sight, hearing, speech or mobility impaired), of safety or caution considerations (e.g., possible violent patient), or other matters (e.g., patient should be transferred over to a case manager upon calling in).

The primary care provider serves as the initial evaluator of what health problem ails the patient and as a gatekeeper for specialists. Further, the primary care provider provides long-term treatment for some chronic conditions, and is in charge of most types of preventive care (e.g., blood pressure checks, that might be scheduled for the patient via a letter, through a *life care path*).

The primary care provider could set up a *trend document* (e.g., to graph the patient's blood pressure) that automatically records a reading whenever taken, with the system automatically informing caregivers to take the reading whenever the patient comes in. Additionally, the patient can be trained to call in readings to an appointment clerk or advice nurse, or to input it via the Internet. Whenever, a reading is recorded that is of concern, the primary care provider can be immediately messaged by the system.

Prior to a visit, a caregiver could get a quick overview of the patient's medical history both by looking at the patient's *overall clinical summary* and by scrolling through *synopses* of past encounters, optionally after filtering to pick out the encounters matching the medical concern of interest.

During a visit, a primary care provider uses the automated patient medical record, displaying clinical information and creating documentation for the automated patient medical record either directly through input to the computer or through forms later entered into the computer. The nurse also inputs to the patient's medical record through the automated system, creating documentation for the automated patient medical record (e.g., a vital signs document).

If this is not an "episodic" (i.e., one-time) visit for the patient for a problem, the primary care provider may initiate a *defined outcome case* for continuing care.

Alternatively, the primary care provider could initiate a *referral request* to a specialist. If the specialist starts a defined outcome case, the automated patient medical record system could combine the referral request and encounter with the referring provider in the defined outcome case. The personal care provider could ask the automated patient medical record system to inform him if the referral did not result in an appointment within a specific period of time and to inform him when the referral appointment is scheduled.

When the primary care provider recognizes that the patient has a chronic condition that dictates tracking of patient compliance with medications and other treatments, a *chronic care management case* could be established with the assignment of a case manager with immediate or future assignment of primary care or specialty care physicians, nurses, pharmacists and/or other caregivers in providing care. A *significant health problem* could be recorded for the patient.

Methods for use of computers during the patient interview need to be studied. An approach that allows caregiver access to the patient medical record during the patient interview is to use a pen computer during the interview. The pen computer could either be used to input informal notes and orders during the interview, which could be later read by the caregiver and input to patient chart via a desktop computer, or the pen computer could be used to directly input to the patient chart during the interview.

Through the automated patient medical record system, before and after the encounter, and depending upon the input method, possibly during the encounter, the primary care physician and nurses will have access to medical references, including those on best practice guidelines, on foreign travel disease risk and prevention from the Centers for Disease Control and Prevention (CDC), etc. If the HMO member has recorded biomarkers or a recorded social, family, environmental and genetic history, then these could be used to anticipate future diseases for which the patient may have a propensity to develop. "Expert systems" could be available to assist in diagnosis and preventive measures (see section 17.4.7). Other clinical decision support systems could automatically make recommendations of better practices, such as equally as effective but lower cost drugs (see section 17.4.9).

Most often best practice treatments and procedures should be followed, but the HMO should make a concerted and controlled effort to have primary care physicians also try other treatments and procedures with the consent of the patient, with the physician documenting these treatments and procedures in defined outcome cases or chronic care management cases. This insures that the HMO actively participates in the evaluation and the improvement of best practice guidelines.

Immediately after the visit, the physician instructions and orders could be printed at a nursing station for a nurse, who would in turn give the printout to the patient, *a post visit report.* The nurse would re-explain instructions and orders given to the patient during the physician interview. An alternative approach would be to send the instructions and orders to the patient by mail. The instructions and orders would re-emphasize the physician's care decisions. Where appropriate, family members who assist the patient in taking medications or following physician orders could be included in this review of physician orders and instructions. Ideally, information presented to the patient and the patient's family should be presented in language clearly understandable by the patient and the patient's family.

Nurse practitioners and physician assistants are under the constant supervision of a physician. Having an automated patient medical record allows for "concurrent review" by a supervising physician of the care being given by the nurse practitioner or physician assistant, where "concurrent review" means "the investigation of patient care while it is in progress, with the intention of modifying that care if appropriate". In fact, both the physician and nurse practitioner or physician assistant could be viewing a patient's chart at the same time, despite being in different locations.

The nurse taking vital signs and the physician examining the patient currently use vital sign, history and physical, and progress note document forms on a clipboard. When this process is computerized, the ideal computer would be a lightweight wireless handheld computer that would not get in the way of patient care and that could substitute for the documents and clipboard. Since a keyboard is impractical for a handheld computer, what fits this description is a tablet computer, a pen computer with a document size screen. For such a tablet computer, entrance of information might best be accomplished through selection of templates and selection from drop down lists (see section 6.7.1, Documenting Patient Care) as input of textual information is slower on a pen computer. A nurse could be entering vital signs for a patient at the same time a physician is reviewing the chart and entering information in the chart; therefore, concurrent entrance of information in the automated patient medical record at the same time should be allowed. For nurses just entering vital signs, an even smaller pen computer, a PDA, might be appropriate. In all cases response time should be quick, perhaps within ½ second. When the computer is turned off, data entered must still be there.

Consideration should be given to supporting all the following:

- the physician switching from use of a desktop computer to a tablet computer for the same patient, possibly with the desktop computer in a secure room still on-line
- the nurse entering vital signs at the same time the physician is viewing or entering information for the same patient
- the nurse and physician consecutively sharing the same computer.

Use of computers when examining or interviewing the patient is referred to as *point-of-care computing.* Other computing involving display or updates to the automated patient medical record when there is no direct patient contact happening at the same time is best done on a desk top computer with a typewriter style keyboard and large screen, rather than pen computer. Computers of any kind—other than perhaps a small PDA—may be inappropriate in any situation when the caregiver has to carry a lot of other equipment around (e.g., a respiratory therapist and many nurses).

Orders for the patient could be sent immediately to the pharmacy and ancillary departments through the automated system, recording them in the medical record. When the caregiver enters an order it would be immediately checked for correctness. More appropriate medications, test or procedures could be suggested. *Clinical checking* of a medication order with other prescribed medications could be done to verify that would be no drug/drug interactions.

Medication orders could be sent directly to an HMO pharmacy, say with a pick-up number being returned at the time of the order. When the patient came to the pharmacy, there would be less, or no, waiting time for the medication (note: this may however result in more medications being returned to stock however).

When results of clinical laboratory tests came back, the caregiver could be informed of results by the automated patient medical record system. An *alarm* would come back to the caregiver or his care team when the results were abnormal or corresponded to STAT orders. The automated patient medical record system could also assist the caregiver in informing the patient of results. For example, it could

- automatically send letters to patients to inform them of normal results, perhaps giving the patient a number for an advice nurse to discuss the results
- specifically inform the caregiver, so the caregiver or his nurse can call the patient to report abnormal results and record in the medical record that he or she did so
- allow the caregiver to print results, annotate them and send them to the patient.

Many activities of a primary care physician, nurse practitioner, physician assistant or other primary care caregiver do not involve direct contact with patients, but handling communications from other caregivers, from the call center, from automated re-fill lines, and directly from the patient via telephone calls or e-mail. Such communications with patients and other caregivers, could include results reporting, giving advice, approving refills, opening up schedule time, and consulting with or supervising other caregivers. A messaging system that combines, but also segregates, clinical messages, e-mails, orders, orders with results, and orders pending results, would assist this process. A caregiver could send out a clinical message or e-mail; an order made by the caregiver would be automatically recorded as a message that both the caregiver and his or her care team could view. A caregiver could receive and look at messages for the caregiver, for the caregiver's care team(s), or for an entire nursing unit. The requirements for such a messaging system were discussed previously in section 7.7.3.

For example, the primary care physician or nurse practitioner could receive clinical messages from the call center regarding a patient (for example, a message indicating that the physician's schedule is full but that a patient may need to be seen soon, that a patient wants a medication refill, etc.) The caregiver could respond to the message and close it out, or respond and send it to another caregiver to call back the patient, who would then close out the message. Messages that are not closed out in a the required period of time, say based upon priority, could be redirected to other caregivers; when the primary care physician or nurse practitioner is unavailable, their messages could be redirected to other caregivers.

The primary care provider could identify to the automated system that he or she be informed when a specific patient completes a particular care activity or any patient on the provider's panel starts a particular kind of care activity. For example, the automated patient medical record system might be designed to automatically inform a primary care physician or nurse practitioner when a patient on his/her panel enters the Emergency Department, is admitted to the hospital, or is seen by a specialty care physician or another primary care physician. Also, the provider can request to be informed of curtailment of care by the patient, so that the caregiver could insure that a treatment is continued.

The primary care provider could get a list of a specific type of patient on his/her panel. For example, he should be able to identify all patients with diabetes or all patients over 70, so he could, for example, send out preventative health letters. The automated patient medical record system could send out these preventative health letters for sigmoids, blood pressure checks, pap smears, or other preventative health reason, with scheduling of the care activities including the scheduling of preventative health appointments via critical pathway documents based upon patient characteristics. The appointment scheduling system could sent out the preventative health letters so they are coordinated with the availability of appointments in the provider's schedules.

A *paradigm* is an original pattern or model of which all things of the same type are representations or copies. This section and the next assume the current paradigm for outpatient care described in section 8.4.1 and figure 8.2. Other proposed future paradigms for outpatient care are also presented in section 8.4.2.

In the future, an individual's genetic information could be recorded within the automated patient medical record; this could provide *biomarkers* for genetically determined diseases. The increased use of an automated patient medical record could provide research information to identify other biomarkers and associated diseases. Together, these biomarkers could be increasingly used to predict and diagnosis disease. Non-altering biomarkers for an individual could be recorded permanently in an individual's patient record, while changeable biomarkers could be periodically recorded via trend documents.

8.2.8 Specialty Care Physicians and Nurse Practitioners, and Associated Care Teams

Referrals are made to specialty departments by primary care physicians, and sometimes by nurse practitioners in limited cases, who determine that the patient needs specialty care. In addition to making referrals to specialty physicians, primary care physician can directly *consult* with specialty care physicians, often via direct physician to physician contacts via telephone. With an automated patient medical record, the primary care physician and the specialty care physician can simultaneously access the patient medical record during the conversation, as opposed to the paper medical record where only one of the two can possess the medical record.

Upon determining that there is a problem that can be solved quickly, the specialty provider seeing the patient could initiate a *defined outcome case* that starts with the referral. For a potentially long term problem, a *chronic care management case* can be initiated. To begin with, the case would identify the initial treatment plan, expected final outcomes for the patient for a defined outcome case, and the case managers and the care team. Optionally, a clinical pathway could be associated with the case and/or a *trend document* to track associated *biomarkers* associated with the disease.

A formal or informal care team for the specialty area could include specialty area physicians, nurse practitioners, nurses, and others in the specialty department. Physicians in the specialty area could have sub-specialties (e.g., a retinal expert in the ophthalmology department).

An agent could be set up by the specialty department that could be initiated automatically when any patient appointment is made with a specialist in the department, with the agent collecting patient chart information for all previous encounters associated specifically with the specialty area and organizing the information in a form useful for the specialist; this could supplement other information in the patient's medical record. Prior to the visit, the caregiver could get a summary of the patient's medical history by looking at the patient's *overall clinical summary* and scanning through *synopses* of encounters pertinent to the appointment.

Upon seeing a patient, the specialist *documents* care either through a computer using the automated patient medical record system or on a form whose information is later transferred to the automated patient medical record system. Upon seeing a patient as part of a case, the treatment plan could be optionally changed, treatment notes could be added, the clinical pathway could be followed or changed, or information could be added to the trend document. *Care notes* are less formal than case documentation—they can be set up for caregivers or care teams and associated with encounters within the scope of care of the caregiver or care team and speculate on future treatments.

A specialist seeing the patient must identify the completion of a defined outcome case. Later, a quality manager could evaluate *actual outcomes* of the treatment by contacting and interviewing the patient.

Specialists could also be involved in the long-term treatment of a chronic condition using a *chronic care management case*. A chronic care management case is particularly suited for the periodic scheduling of telephone "visits" between the patient and caregiver. Telephone visits becomes more feasible with the automated patient medical record always being immediately available to the caregiver. This may be better for patient and more convenient for the patient, as well as almost always being more cost effective for the HMO than return visits in the clinic.

For conditions of a significant magnitude, a specialty care team could be assigned to the patient through the defined outcome or chronic care management case with a designated case manager who has responsibility for insuring that a patient comes in for care. By there being a defined outcome or chronic care management case identified with a specific medication condition, advice nurses in the call center would know to transfer patient phone calls for the identified medical condition to the specialty department, using a telephone number in the defined outcome or chronic care management case.

A *clinical pathway* document could be set up based upon medical condition of a patient that could send out letters advising members to make appointments for preventive care in specialty departments, for example, for a sigmoidoscopy by a gastroenterologist and controlling subsequent care activities based upon the results.

Specialists could use the same chart input methods as for primary care physicians and nurse practitioners discussed in the previous section, for example, inputting informal interview notes to a pen computer or to forms during the interview and using the informal pen notes or forms for later input to the patient chart via a desktop computer or, alternatively, inputting directly to the patient chart via the pen computer during the interview. Like for a primary care visit, the patient could be given a printout of the visit record and orders immediately after the visit, reemphasizing care decisions made during the visit.

Orders would be sent immediately to the performing area, with the results returning back through the automated system to the caregiver. Orders could be checked, with checking for drug/drug and other interactions for medical orders. The caregiver would be alerted of results for STAT orders coming back or of abnormal results.

Specialty caregivers would also have a messaging system that could combine together or separate out e-mails, clinical messages, and orders and results. Through this system the caregiver could receive, send and display these messages.

The automated patient medical record also enables specialists to follow best practice guidelines and to do concurrent review of nurse practitioners being supervised.

All other capabilities for primary care departments would be available to a specialist department.

8.2.9 Urgent Care and Emergency Department Care Teams

Since ordering of a paper chart ahead of time is often not feasible in the emergency department (ED), one the major benefits of an automated patient medical record is that it would be immediately available to the ED caregiver. The automated patient medical record also is likely to be much more complete, including information from multiple facilities and healthcare organizations. (One of the reasons for going through the clinical data collection effort of an extensive H&P in the ED is to make up for the possible lack of chart information; with existence of the automated patient medical record, this may be a less necessary step in ED care.)

For a universal patient record, as long as the patient has an ID, the patient medical record would be available to the emergency department physician, even if the patient was unconscious or could not speak the language of the physician.

Triage is assessment of patients' medical problems to determine urgency and priority of care in the emergency department to determine which patient is to be seen next. The ED triage process can be speeded up by triage documentation entered through the automated patient medical record that can be used to prioritize patients according to severity of illness. Patients on the triage list could be moved over to the *emergency department census* identifying empty rooms and what patients are in each room.

Additionally, after identification of the problem during the triage process, the system, at the approval of the triage nurse or ED physician, could automatically schedule caregivers and equipment when time is critical, for example, immediately schedule an MRI for a possible stroke. This could be done with a clinical pathway related to the medical problem, identifying and scheduling care activities. When a patient comes into the emergency department often for a defined medical condition—for example, epilepsy—then there should be a capability for a patient's family member to call in to a predefined telephone number to identify that the patient is coming in to the emergency department for care, thus initiating a clinical pathway that starts care activities for the medical condition before the patient comes in, including informing the patient's case manager.

During the visit, the urgent care or ED practitioner may *consult* directly with a specialist by telephone. Again, with an automated patient medical record, the urgent care or ED physician and the specialty care physician can simultaneously access the patient medical record during the conversation, as opposed to the paper medical record where only the urgent care or ED physician is likely to have access.

Care within the ED could be improved by the speed up of *ordering* and the receipt of results and the speed up of housekeeping notification of newly empty ED rooms to be cleaned. Clinical laboratory results could be returned to the ED physician at the instant they became available, instead of results being returned on paper, hand carried back from the laboratory. Medications can be more quickly prepared and transported to the ED. This is important, because unlike for the outpatient visit, the patient in the ED usually remains until the results of a test are received back.

After the patient is stabilized, the ED physician may—through the automated patient medical record system—discharge the patient to home or discharge the patient to the hospital, initiating an *admission* through the ADT clinical system. Upon discharge to home, the caregiver could initiate a follow-up appointment from the automated patient medical record through the appointment system or *refer* the patient to a specialist.

8.2.10 Inpatient Care

Upon a patient's admission to the hospital, the automated patient medical record system will automatically create two documents for the duration of the patient's stay, which summarize information collected from other patient medical record documents, and which will disappear after discharge:

- *Inpatient Clinical Summary:* A document equivalent to the Kardex, which is a summarization document to quickly identify the current status of the inpatient and may include the following among other information:
  - the patient's name, age, sex, marital status and religion
  - medical diagnoses, usually by priority
  - nursing diagnoses, usually by priority
  - current physician orders for medications, treatments, diet, IV's, diagnostic tests, procedures, etc.
  - consultations
  - results of diagnostic tests and procedures
  - permitted activities, functional limitations, assistance needed, and safety precautions
  - care plan.

- *medication administration record (MAR):* Medications the physicians order for patients, including times and routes of administration in a nursing unit. Nurses record the times that the listed medications are administered to the patients.

The Inpatient Clinical Summary and the MAR are not part of the patient medical record but use information from existing documents in the patient medical record, and thus can be automatically generated by the automated patient medical record system. The Inpatient Clinical Summary comes from various documents input by inpatient physicians and nurses, and unit assistants during the stay.

The MAR information comes from medication orders which were input into the automated patient medical record system by a physician or a nurse with the approval of a physician. The medication orders are transmitted to the pharmacy system for fulfillment and displayed on the MAR at the nursing unit of the patient. Nurses record on the MAR when a medication is administered to the patient.

(Note that the Inpatient Clinical Summary only exists during the patient's stay and disappears at discharge—although it could be recreated. The *Overall Clinical Summary*, which collects information from outpatient, inpatient, ED and other documents, exists at all times for a patient and provides a more complete view of the patient's health.)

Always available in an inpatient nursing unit (e.g., a "critical care unit", 'Medicine/Surgery unit") will be a *unit census* listing all patients in the unit and their room locations. When a patient is admitted through the ADT (admission, discharge and transfer) clinical system—which would also input information such as financial data, admitting and attending physician, nursing unit, room number—ADT would pass this information to the automated patient medical record system which would update the corresponding unit census, putting the patient, room, physicians on the unit census. Transfer of a patient to another unit—which could be done by the automated patient medical record system in coordination with ADT—might update the unit censuses in both units, taking the patient off one unit census and putting the patient on the other.

The normal process of admission which would occur through ADT would be (1) a pre-admission through ADT during a prior outpatient visit to enter some admission information with the actual admission through ADT occurring when the patient shows up at a future date for admission to the hospital; or (2) an admission through ADT immediately following a visit to the emergency department.

In addition to this "normal" admission process would be a "quick admission" for situations where the patient ends up in the unit and is not yet admitted. Rather than through ADT, the quick admission will occur when the patient is put directly on the *unit census* by a nurse or unit assistant. The quick admission would be sent to the ADT system and other clinical systems. Users of the ADT system could then collect additional information to complete the admission or the quick admission could be set up to collect this information from the patient in his room.

Notification of admission to the unit, discharge from the hospital, and transfer to another unit is important to the automated patient medical record system and to other clinical systems (the pharmacy system, clinical laboratory system) because it locates the patient, which is necessary for ordering through those systems (e.g., the clinical laboratory system would know a patient's unit, room and bed).

Through use of the unit census, nurse assignment could be automated, allowing assignment of nurses using the unit census. During this assignment process, the nurse supervisor doing the assignment could be presented with information from other clinical systems to assist in the assignment, such as nurse scheduling and patient acuity system—the patient acuity system identifies how sick the patient is so nurses with a larger number of very sick patients could be assigned fewer patients.

Upon a pre-admission, upon admission through the ED or upon a quick admission, the automated patient medical record system (via agents incorporating current HMO business policies) could automatically order patient chart information, including CPR information and source documents from multiple locations, including within the HMO and outside healthcare organizations. Medical documents on paper could also be ordered.

Physicians and nurses caring for patients—including the admitting physician, attending physician, and on-call physicians and nurses—and their unit assistants would have immediate controlled access to the patient's medical record and could play an active role in the patient's care no matter where he or she was physically located. With an automated patient medical record, a physician caring for patients could *consult* directly with a specialty care physicians, with them both having simultaneous access to the complete automated patient medical record, and again, with both being located virtually anywhere.

Access to the automated patient medical record would include the ability, if authorized for the caregiver, to *order* medications, clinical laboratory tests, procedures, etc. Again, the ordering of a medication would automatically add the medication to the medication administration record (MAR).

With the automated patient medical record and case information, treatment of a patient could formally be viewed in a multi-disciplinary context, with care being provided across outpatient visits and inpatient stays and tracked via a *defined outcome case* or *chronic care management case* that allows collection of information across different types of encounters, both outpatient visits (in the ED, follow-up visits) and inpatient stays.

Care of an inpatient includes (1) care directly seeing the patient and (2) care not directly seeing the patient. Using computers, and an automated patient medical record system, at the same time the patient is being seen is referred to "point-of-care" computing. These situations where the patient is being seen include the following: (1) admission of the patient, especially when admitting occurs within the patient's room or the ED, (2) during the physician's examination and the nurse's assessment of the patient, and (3) during the time that the nurse is recording interventions, especially when flow sheets are being used. Pen or portable computers might be appropriate for "point of care" computing.

For other situations, during the inpatient stay, the patient is not being seen. These situations include the following: physician review of the patient chart without the patient, nurse creation of care plans using the computer, nurse or unit assistant completion of chart information, ancillary department review of patient charts within the inpatient unit, and automated system notification of the patient's discharge. In such situations, a desktop computer with a large screen and typewriter type keyboard might be a better choice.

Any nurse, physician, unit assistant or ancillary personnel input to the system, will be automatically summarized by the automated patient medical record system on the Inpatient Clinical Summary for the inpatient stay, similar to what currently occurs on a Kardex.

Upon nurse or physician notification to the automated patient medical record system of the patient's discharge from the hospital, the automated patient medical record system could automatically inform caregivers of discharge activities to perform and/or automatically schedule discharge activities bases upon diagnoses and protocols. Examples of these activities could include system ordering of medications for use at home and scheduling of follow-up appointments.

8.2.11 Measuring and Insuring Quality Patient Care

The HMO wants to measure the quality and effectiveness of patient care. The HMO physicians feel that the best patient care (1) uses the most appropriate care plans for a medical condition, including best diagnostic tests, treatments, and procedures based upon best medical evidence (*evidence-based medicine*), (2) has the patient and family involved in the patient's care, which could include patient education and self care, and (3) provides continuity of care, with an assigned personal physician coordinating overall care for the member, the patient coming in most often with the same caregiver or care team for the same medical condition, with caregivers following a consistent plan of care for the patient. (Lawrence 2003)

Often, patient care and treatments are carried out by *care teams*, with care teams consisting of physicians, nurses and others, either in specialty or primary care departments. Some treatments could involve outpatient care and inpatient care and thus the care team may be a multi-disciplinary team of caregivers. Care must thus be evaluated for care teams as well as single clinicians.

In order to evaluate care—care given by both individual clinicians and formal and informal care teams—an HMO quality manager or medical research department could use statistical methods to select and evaluate treatment plans as carried out by the various clinicians and care teams, comparing treatment plans for similar treatments and taking into account the patient condition and other relevant factors in the evaluation of the treatment plan. Looking at *defined outcome cases* (and associated treatment notes, clinical pathway documents, trend documents and references to clinical practice guidelines followed) the quality manager or medical research department would compare different treatments for the same disease. Each patient's medical record would also provide the quality manager or researcher with information to evaluate the physical condition of the patient at the start of the treatment and other factors, so these could be taken account in the evaluation of the treatment plan.

A treatment plan for a patient is evaluated by the actual outcomes of the treatment. Some groups consider outcomes to be related to the patient's perception of his or her health after the care is finished. A good outcome occurs for a disease (e.g., knee replacement, BPH) if the patient's perception of his quality of life is good. One method of evaluating these outcomes is a questionnaire given to a patient. SF-36 and HSQ-12 (Health Status Questionnaire 2.0) are examples of questionnaires measuring outcomes of treatments (Yeomans 1999).

Sometimes outcomes can be directly measured. For example, the outcome of a treatment to lower a patient's blood pressure is directly measurable. Indeed, in such a case and others, the patient may not perceive that his health has changed or improved. The outcomes of some treatments can be evaluated by statistically measurable quantities such as mortality rates (death rates), morbidity rates (those who are sick versus those who are well), returns to the hospital after treatment, and infection rates after surgery.

One HMO, Oxford Health Plans, has stated that they intend to compare care teams as to success of treatments and treatment plans so that future patients requiring the same type of treatment could make selections of the best care team. Evaluations of treatments by different care teams could also give the HMO information on how to improve care for various treatments, assuming the care team having the best outcomes would also have the best treatment plans, with resultant determination of "best practice guidelines".

Together with physicians in the HMO who want to evaluate new treatments, medical researchers in the HMO can develop new treatment plans. After completion of the new treatment, medical researchers can compare the new treatment with existing treatments for the same health problem with consideration of the cost of the treatment.

Automation of the patient medical record also facilitates calculation of actual costs associated with various treatments.

Outcomes of long-term treatments for chronic conditions can be done with quality managers using the chronic care maintenance case in place of the defined outcome case. Outcomes of chronic care maintenance cases could involve comparing costs, quality and patient satisfaction for patients being tracked by chronic care management cases with patients with similar chronic conditions who are not being tracked; for example, patient satisfaction, patient quality of life, number and costs of hospital stays and outpatient visits, primary versus specialty care given, readmission rates, duplicated service, mortality and costs of medications could be compared.

With a universal patient record supplying patient medical information without the identity of the patient, researchers throughout the world could identify biomarkers for different diseases. This information could be used for diagnosis and prediction of diseases.

Other duties of quality managers and personnel in associated departments could be hiring of outside organizations to evaluate individual clinicians especially after they are first hired, (1) to do credentialing and re-credentialing of physicians, nurse practitioners, and other clinicians, verifying that clinicians have the valid licenses to practice and (2) to do quality checks of healthcare organization clinicians and the care they give, *auditing* of medical records to evaluate the quality of a clinician's care, also called *peer review* because it involves the review of medical professionals by other medical professionals. Auditing can either be done afterward the patient care is given, or while the patient care is being given—the latter is called "concurrent review". An automated patient medical record would support auditing, supporting quick access by auditors to a patient's medical record and supporting concurrent review, viewing a medical record at the same time care is being given to a patient.

Quality managers and related personnel also do evaluations of the overall care and cost-effectiveness of care given in a healthcare organization to identify differences with other healthcare organizations so that improvements in care can be made if necessary to match the care given in the other healthcare organizations. This is called a *utilization review*, reviewing the necessity, quality, effectiveness, or efficiency of medical services, procedures, and facilities provided within a healthcare organization as compared to other healthcare organizations. A utilization review could again be done by comparing "defined outcome cases" and "chronic care management cases" in the various healthcare organizations and the recorded outcomes and variances from expected outcomes of these cases as related to the physical condition of the patient at the start of treatment.

The automated patient medical record would also be of benefit to JCAHO and other healthcare regulatory agencies that do periodic quality checks of all affiliated hospitals. Besides visiting the healthcare organization, JCAHO auditors could view medical records via the automated patient medical record system, with the possibility of concurrent review of care. The automated system could also do automated checking for compliance with recommendations from JCAHO or other professional organizations.

An automated patient medical record would also assist in the review of rare occurrences referred to as sentinel events (Moore 1998). The healthcare industry equivalent of the airline industry airplane crash is a "sentinel event". JCAHO defines a *sentinel event* as "an unexpected occurrence involving death or serious physical or psychological injury, or the risk thereof" occurring within a hospital or clinical setting. Examples of sentinel events are medication errors causing death, suicide of a patient, or deaths related to delay of treatment. JCAHO wants to review each sentinel event to determine what went wrong, so new regulations could be established and so healthcare organizations could learn how to prevent these sentinel events.

Sometimes medications or other medical products can be identified as suspected causes of a serious adverse medical event or of a product problem (MedWatch 2004). The United States government FDA runs a safety information and adverse event reporting program termed

MedWatch that enables reporting on these suspected associations to the product company and to the FDA. In turn, such suspected associations may be reported back to healthcare organizations. The automated patient medical record system could assist in MedWatch reporting to product companies and the FDA and could warn caregivers who order or use a product of FDA warnings about reported products.

The automated patient medical record system can also be designed so it automates reports for accreditation organizations and disease registries, for example for the *NCQA (National Committee for Quality Assurance) database*, a national database for evaluating HMOs, and include information for generation of the *HEDIS (Health Plan Employer Data and Information Set)* report, an HMO "report card".

8.2.12 Case Managers

A case manager may be assigned to a "high risk" and "high cost" patient, such as an elderly and frail patient or a worker's compensation patient, for overall care through a *patient case*. Along with physicians or nurses, a case manager may be assigned to a patient with a chronic conditions through a *chronic care management case* or assigned to a patient with a high cost, high risk, treatment through a *defined outcome case* to insure that the care is being given using a consistent treatment plan and to insure that the care is being followed by the patient.

The case manager may be involved in care activities in a *clinical pathway* document, which may or may not be part of a case document. The clinical pathway might identify care maintenance activities by the case manager or by other caregivers, and also identify what should be done by the case manager, or others, when problems occur.

The case manager might closely follow a patient's health progress. The case manager might serve as a "go between" between the patient and caregivers and thus communicate with caregivers. When necessary, the case manager could initiate care activities, such as making *appointments* for the patient.

After a "high risk" or "high cost" patient is discharged from the hospital, the HMO could assign a case manager or a clinical social worker to oversee the patient's follow-up care. That person could be in charge of insuring that post-hospital care activities, such as discharge to a SNF or a treatment plan that extends beyond the inpatient stay, are properly implemented or followed. Such follow-up activities could be part of a clinical pathway, possibly one extending across the hospital stay to the outpatient follow-up activities.

The identity of the case manager for a patient will appear in the automated patient medical record, specifically the *overall clinical summary*. This identification of the patient's case manager to a caregiver looking at the automated patient medical record, would allow the caregiver to inform the case manager of care decisions and, if necessary, to participate in these care decisions, so the case manager could provide guidance to the patient and the caregiver on the most cost-effective care choices.

When a patient has an overall case manager, an appointment phone could automatically transfer incoming appointment calls to the patient's case manager if the patient had one—if not answered, the call could then be transferred to an appointment clerk. This approach would insure that the case manager participated in the patient's outpatient care decisions.

8.2.13 Home Health and Hospice

Case managers are often assigned to home health and hospice patients. Such patients often switch between home, hospice, the hospital, outpatient clinics, nursing homes, and SNFs (skilled nursing facilities). Often the person providing home nursing care for the patient is also the patient's case manager.

Having one complete chart of all visits, home stays and inpatient stays would be beneficial medically and would be beneficial also for case management, especially to track the patient for purposes of reimbursement, especially through Medicare and Medicaid. Documentation of home visits would be greatly facilitated by the use of a mobile computer—perhaps a pen computer—to access the automated patient medical record system through a wireless network, which would allow the caregiver to quickly input and verify information and would enable the caregiver to quickly consult with a physician about care decisions.

A possible future use of computers mentioned previously is to provide the patient with a means for self-care through a Guardian Angel system. See section 5.3.2.2.

Telemedicine, with the home health nurse at the patient's home and a consulting physician or nurse located remotely, is possible given an automated patient medical record system that allows nurses and physicians to concurrently access the patient's medical record.

8.2.14 Compliance Management

Patient compliance with a caregiver's clinical prescription does not always occur. This is especially true for life style changes: Making life style changes, such as stopping smoking or changing eating habits, is especially difficult for a patient, but can make a crucial difference in the patient's health. *Patient compliance* is "The extent to which the patient's behavior, in terms of taking medications, following diets, or executing life style changes, coincides with the clinical prescription"(Haynes, Taylor, and Sackett 1979) (Sackett et al. 1991).

In order to assist a member in complying with a physician's treatments and instructions, the physician can refer the member to a *compliance manager* who (1) can advise the patient on community and health organization resources such as classes for making life style changes or (2) can periodically contact the member to monitor, advise, and encourage the member in complying with treatments and changes. Using a compliance manager in this role is more cost-effective than a physician and provides communication with the member over a more continuous period of time, encouraging the member to develop good habits. Despite the word, compliance needs to be done with the consent and commitment of the patient to be effective.

8.3 PATIENTS

The patient medical record is centered around the patient and patient care should be centered around the patient.

8.3.1 Patient Care in Perspective

We are all patients, some of us all of the time.

Arthritis, pain, diabetes; menstrual, menopause or prostate problems; paraplegia, heart disease, the aftereffects of a stroke—these are all everyday conditions of some people, not just when they seek care.

Newborns, infants, children, and everyone, are injured some days, or are sick or just feel bad on others. Women are pregnant. People forget to take their medications or don't remember whether they did or not. Patients—people who live life—must learn what to do when these problems and situations occur. Should they seek care or not? Can they afford to seek care?—Can they afford not to?

What can a person do today to avoid health complications later in life? What can a caregiver do? What can society do?

Patient care is as much an educational process of people in how to live their lives, than it is in alleviating or fixing acute or chronic problems. Patient care occurs all the time—Sometimes patients come in to be seen by caregivers.

For a caregiver, patient care is giving the patient exactly what the patient needs to stay healthy and to participate in life. And patient care is best if the patient is not dependent upon the caregiver, as each person needs to be in control of his or her own life.

It should always be up to the patient to determine when care is not to be given. This should include the patient's right to get only the right pain medication without any other treatment. When the patient is unconscious or not lucid, advance directives or a durable power of attorney for healthcare should apply.

Caregiving is both common and uncommon—Everybody depends upon everyone else to survive in the world, but "We are all angels to the people who need us the most!"

Patient care is for everybody. Caregiving is for everybody to do, but angelic caregiving is for the privileged few in each of our lives.

And we are all patients, and all caregivers.

8.3.2 Post Visit Report

Physicians, nurse practitioners and other caregivers seeing patients often are very busy, pre-occupied or forgetful. As a result, they often do not put forth all necessary information to the patient pertaining to the patient's problems.

On the other side, patients may not be knowledgeable about their medical conditions or may be emotionally distraught or sickly. As a result, patients often do not hear or understand the information given to them by their caregivers.

It is therefore my proposal that all medical problems (and associated diagnoses) be given a code number (such as the ICD-9 code) and all procedures be given a code number (such as the CPT-4 code). After an outpatient visit, a physician could identify the medical problems and procedures to the automated patient medical record system via these code numbers.

Through the automated patient medical record system, the diagnosis and procedure codes could be expanded to produce a **usually one page** *post visit report* that the patient can take home and carry with him or her. For patients who do not comprehend English, where appropriate and feasible, this report should be in the written language of the patient (e.g., Spanish, Chinese).

First there would be the **overall doctor s comments**.

For each **medical problem**, the following could be displayed on the report:

- diagnosis
- possible causations
- external and internal symptoms
- preventions
- treatments (which may include medications, purposes and dosages)

- doctor's comments on medical problem
- follow-up care (e.g., a referral, a phone number to talk to an advice nurse to schedule follow-up care, etc.)

For each **procedure**, the following could be displayed on the report:

- description of procedure
- why it was done
- results
- doctor's comments on procedure
- follow-up care.

Special precautions should be listed (e.g., "Since you are allergic to Septra, an antibiotic, and other Sulfa drugs, inform any doctor of this who might prescribe any antibiotics or other medications for you.").

Probabilities of future conditions based upon preceding conditions and risk factors, and preventives should be listed (e.g., Since you smoke, you have an XX% chance of developing heart disease compared to an X% chance for someone who does not smoke; if you stopped smoking now you could decrease the risk to X%. For every 100 people with hepatitis C, 20 recover on their own, while 80 develop chronic infection; of the 80 people who develop chronic infection, 60 remain clinically well despite chronic infection, while 20 develop cirrhosis (Harvard Medical School 2000). This information could come from medical research based upon information from other patient medical records.

Also, *immunizations* and *allergies* for the patient should be listed, with the patient verifying that they are complete and correct. If any are incorrect, then these would be corrected through the nurse, with this information updated within the patient medical record.

The above report involves translation of medical problems into a patient medical language, a language for medical problems and procedures that all patients can understand.

The system could verify that each prescribed medication is appropriate for one of the identified medical conditions. Prescriptions could be printed out avoiding wrong medications accidentally being given to the patient due to a pharmacist not being able to read the physician's handwriting.

The resulting post visit report—and any prescriptions that the physician chooses not to print out when the patient is being seen by the physician—could be printed at the nursing station. The report and prescriptions could be given to the patient by a nurse immediately after the visit. The nurse could explain the report, including medications and precautions, to the patient and, if appropriate, to accompanying family members who care for the patient.

Finally, the post visit report could include as e-mail address for the physician or nurse practitioner and a phone number for a nurse in order to enable the patient to get answers to later health questions.

8.3.3 Patient Discharge Summary

Currently, when a patient is discharged from the hospital, the patient receives a *discharge summary* that identifies prescribed outpatient medications for the patient or family to pick up, proscribed activities, and follow-up appointments to schedule.

However, like for a post visit report for an outpatient visit, the patient should be given a replacement discharge summary—a *patient discharge summary*—that contains the same information as the discharge summary but is in a language easily understood by the patient. The patient discharge summary should be reviewed with the patient by the discharging physician or a nurse prior to discharge.

8.3.4 Patient Medication Schedule

Now, one of the hardest things for **any** patient to do after a visit, especially where a new medication is prescribed, is to schedule or reschedule times to take his or her medications. Proposed here is the creation of a personalized *patient medication schedule*.

A *patient medication schedule* is a schedule for patients on when to take medications. A medication scheduler is a person who assists in creating such medication schedules.

A patient's lack of ability to take his medications at the correct time is one reason that many people are not independent and are in nursing homes. A patient's lack of ability to take his medications at the correct time is one reason that many people suffer detrimental side effects from medications (e.g., they forget to take a medication or take a medication more often than prescribed)!

Proposed is that this personalized medication schedule would be created by a computer used by the medication scheduler and created as follows:

1. The patient would look at a list of his medications from the automated patient medical record system. The patient would identify medications he currently takes and add those he currently takes that are not on the list.
2. Medications could be checked against the patient's medical problems. If there were any discrepancies, then a physician would be informed.
3. Expired and incompatible medications and interactions between medications could be identified by the computer program. A physician or pharmacist could be informed if this is the case.
4. The patient would verify medication dosages. Any discrepancies would be corrected. The patient may be informed of proper dosages.
5. The patient would be tested to insure that he could identify each medication and the he could otherwise deal with the medication schedule. Otherwise, he might be trained, or less ideally, a caregiver would have to be involved in administration of the medications.
6. The patient would inform the medication scheduler of the ideal times to take medications in order of preference of times.
7. A ***medication scheduler computer program*** would produce a patient medication schedule that tries to match the patient's ideal times with the medications and dosage frequencies, **minimizing the number of times medications would need to be taken**. In order to do this, the program may have to make compromises on the dosages (e.g., taking some medications earlier or later than identified, adjusting for medication interactions, etc.)
8. The printout could identify what to do if medications were accidentally skipped.

The final result might be a complete medication schedule, say for a week, which could be put onto a usually one-page paper, which might be put into the patient's wallet!

8.3.5 Patient Education Classes, Patient Mentors and Medical Research

An HMO member will be able to take patient education classes to learn about a disease or medical condition and parent education classes to learn about how to take care of children when they are injured or sick. For example, through a class, a new parent could learn when self care for a baby, infant or child is appropriate, and when the child should be brought in to be seen. Through a class, a member with diabetes or severe asthma could learn how to take care of himself or herself, and when it is critical for the patient to come in to be seen.

An HMO member, (1) who may require a future surgery (e.g., a knee replacement, a hip replacement), (2) who has developed a medical condition (e.g., cancer), or (3) who may undergo a significant treatment for a disease (e.g., chemotherapy), will have the opportunity to talk to other members (*patient mentors*) who have had the surgery, disease, medical condition or treatment. The HMO member should be able to talk to both patients who were happy with their surgeries or treatments and those who were not. Patients can volunteer to be patient mentors. To put things in perspective, the patient will also given probabilities of future conditions based upon the surgery or treatment (e.g., if the patient has the knee replacement at age XX, then there is a YY% probability that the knee replacement will need to be re-done in Z years).

HMO members will also have the opportunity to learn of organizations who do research on medical conditions (e.g., a psoriasis society) and to talk to the HMO research department to learn about potential new treatments and surgeries, or about current and future clinical trials they might be able to participate in.

Patients education through the Internet might also be possible with the URL of an individualized patient education course being sent to the patient via e-mail. An e-mail or instant messaging address could be included to allow the member to ask follow-up questions.

8.3.6 Simple, Cheap Transportation

Transportation by ambulance for an emergency situation is sometimes important, but transportation for pre-emergent situations may be an even bigger saver of lives.

These various forms of non-ambulance transportation can be given simple and very "understandable" names. For example, an HMO, such as one which uses the automated patient medical record system, could provide a service which it calls "pre-ambulance transportation" for patients who are unsure whether they need ED care or not.

For anyone who suspects they have a problem, they get an advice nurse. **The advice nurse assumes that the patient needs to be seen in some way**, and only **changes her assumption** if **the patient does not want to be seen** and it is very clear that the patient **should not** come in. Simple, cheap or free, and appropriate transportation if not otherwise available would be sent to pick up the patient and take the patient to a clinic to be immediately seen!

Why is this useful and important? The reasons are many.

It may be unclear to the patient whether he or she needs to be seen immediately. The patient may be alone and not be able to get transportation of any kind and may be reluctant to use an ambulance due to its great expense. Or the patient may be a driver but the only person in the family who drives, and is not in a condition to drive safely. The patient may be too embarrassed or too proud to come in for medical care, such as often is the case for elderly people. Or, the patient may be too macho to come in for care, such as is often the case for men.

For children, a special phone number (similar to '911') just for them might be more appropriate. The advice nurse would first contact the parent or guardian before continuing or contact the appropriate authorities.

8.4 NEW OUTPATIENT CARE PARADIGMS

A *paradigm* is a pattern or model of which all things of the same type are representations or copies. This section presents paradigms for outpatient care.

Figure 8.2 presents a paradigm for outpatient care as it traditionally occurs. Figure 8.3 presents a paradigm that produces a post visit report to be given to a patient after the appointment. Figure 8.4 presents a paradigm that includes a pre-visit gathering of information from the patient.

8.4.1 Traditional Outpatient Care Paradigm

Figure 8.2 shows outpatient care as it traditionally occurs. The patient comes into the medical center and waits in the waiting room. The patient is called into the clinic where the patient's temperature and blood pressure is taken by a nurse. The patient is then escorted to a room where he meets with the physician or nurse practitioner. The physician or nurse practitioner interviews and examines the patient and then gives advice and determines treatments, procedures or medications, giving advice to the patient. The patient thereafter leaves the medical center.

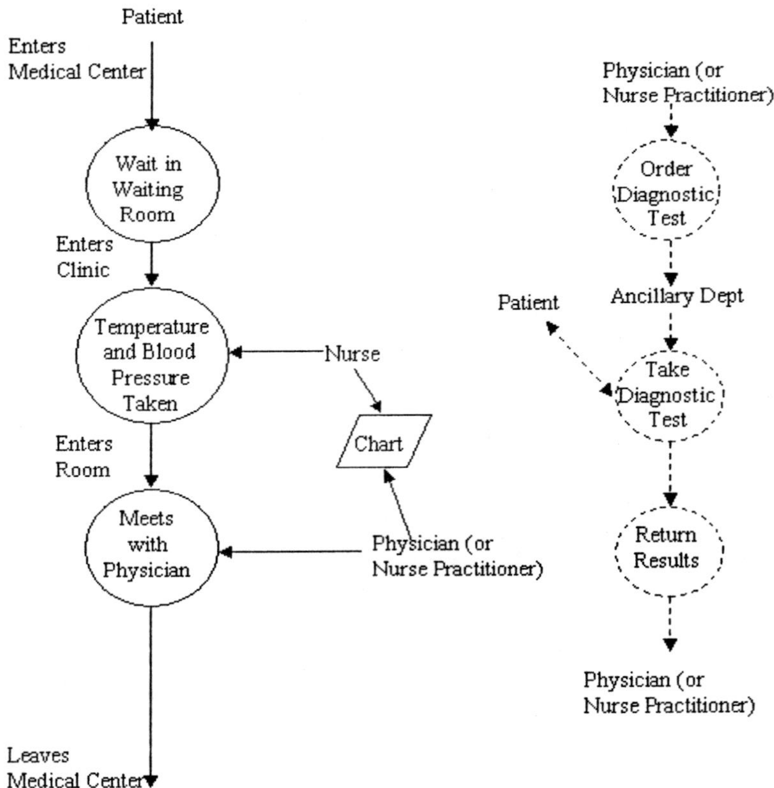

Figure 8.2 Traditional Outpatient Care Paradigm

As part of care, the physician or nurse practitioner could order a diagnostic test for the patient either before or during the visit. The patient would come into an ancillary department for the test—a clinical laboratory test, an x-ray, etc.—before or after the outpatient visit. With results being returned to the caregiver either during or after the visit.

For example, at the time a member makes an appointment for a suspected urinary tract infection, the member could be told to come in to the clinical laboratory for a routine urinalysis. The member could asked to go first to a nursing station to pick up the physician's or nurse practitioner's order.

8.4.2 Outpatient Care Paradigm Modified to Include Post Visit Report

Figure 8.3 shows the traditional outpatient care paradigm—without the diagnostic test—modified to include a post visit report: a report in the language of the patient. A *post visit report* would be generated from physician or nurse practitioner identification of diagnoses, procedures, treatments and medications, and from practitioner comment. The post visit report would be available to the patient if the patient wanted it.

Either the nurse would review the post visit report with the patient and/or his or her family members immediately after the visit, or the post visit report could later be sent to the patient.

The advantage of the post visit report is that it would improve patient compliance with following treatments and taking medications, and encourage patients to play an active role in taking care of his or her medical problems.

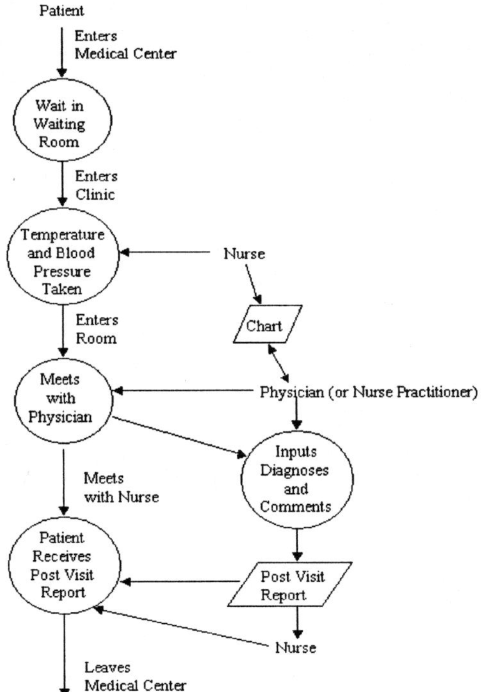

Figure 8.3 Changed Paradigm with Post Visit Report

A possible structure for a post visit report is presented in section 8.3.2. This should be a clear report understandable by a non-medical person, preferably of one page in length, which the patient would use every day.

8.4.3 Adding Value to Outpatient Care

In an HMO, payment is via a periodic capitation fee rather than payment per visit. As a result, it is financially advantageous for an HMO that care be accomplished as efficiently as possible and in as few visits as possible. It is also advantageous for the HMO member in that the member can spend more time living life or working instead of coming into the HMO for care.

Making outpatient care more efficient can be done by not only providing care at the time of the visit, but also before and after the visit.

8.4.3.1 Care Before a Visit

Providing care before the member visits the HMO could result in a visit being unnecessary or in care being provided quickly in the emergency department before the condition becomes more severe.

See figure 8.4. Outpatient care before a visit starts off with an advice nurse located in a call center or a facility. The advice nurse answers calls from members seeking medical advice. Based upon a protocol related to the member's chief complaint identifying questions to ask the member, the advice nurse either

- diagnosis
- schedules the member for an outpatient appointment,
- or advises the member to come directly to the emergency department.

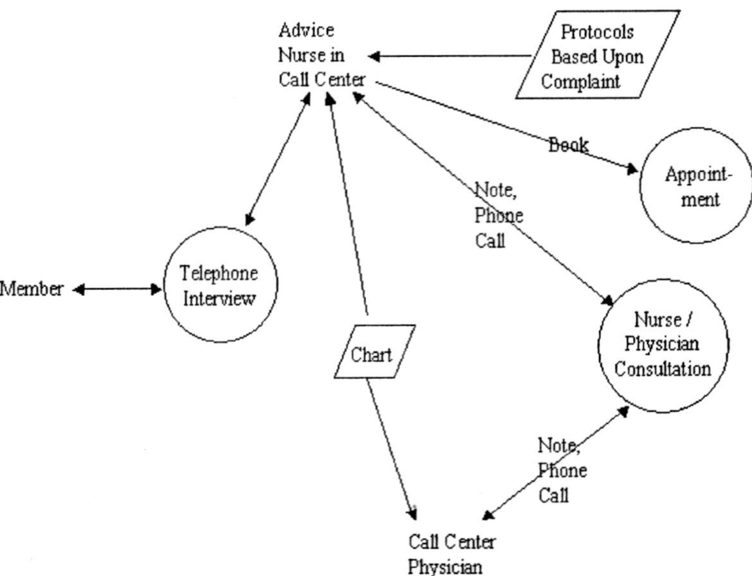

Figure 8.4 Care Before a Visit

The advice nurse could also consult with a call center physician. The member's automated patient medical record would be available to both the advice nurse and physician during this consultation.

8.4.3.2 Care After a Visit

After an outpatient visit, the patient could have questions that he forgot to ask during the visit or have questions about the Post Visit Report. Answering the patient's questions might obviate additional visits or may result in a greater likelihood that the patient would follow the provider's care decisions.

See figure 8.5. In order to enable the patient to ask a question about the visit, a telephone number and e-mail address could be included on the Post Visit Report. Upon calling the telephone number, the patient would enter his medical record number. If the patient had more than one recent visit, the patient would select the visit from a list. The patient would then be connected to a nurse who could view the patient's medical record and the Post Visit Report. The nurse could either answer the patient's question or the nurse could telephone or send a note to the visit physician to get an answer to the question. The patient could also e-mail the visit physician directly. In all cases, the nurse and physician would have concurrent access to the patient's automated medical record.

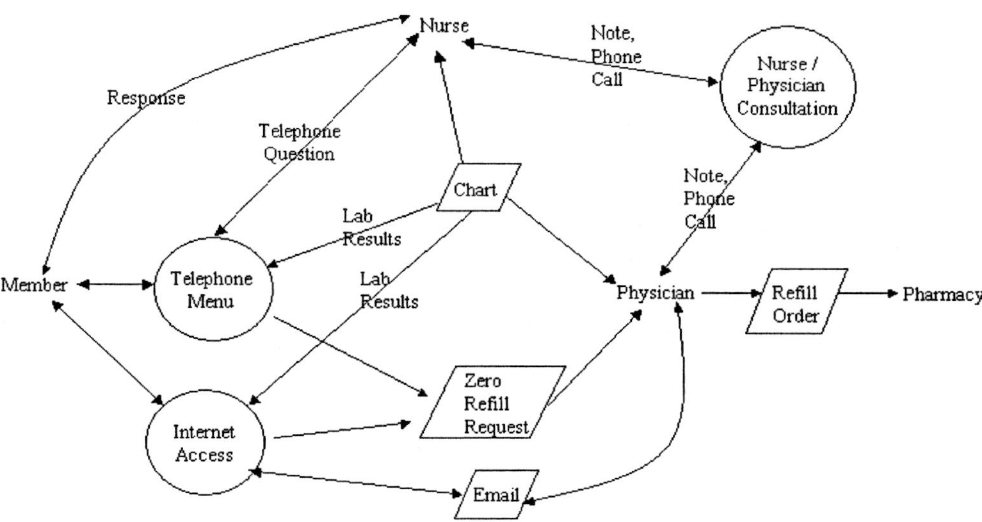

Figure 8.5 Care After a Visit

Other capabilities that could be provided over the telephone or over the Internet along with the e-mail capability could be

- the ability to see lab results for a specific visit if the results have come back from an ancillary system
- the ability to refill a medication.

8.4.4 Care Beyond a Single Encounter

The previous sections describe paradigms for outpatient care with care all occurring during a single encounter. But, as noted earlier, outpatient care often extends beyond the single encounter for a number of reasons:

1. There may be a single encounter resulting in a first, preliminary, diagnosis that is revised after the results of a clinical test that come back after the visit. As a result, care—informing the patient of the results and providing a treatment—occurs after the encounter. Additionally, tests could occur before the encounter and care could start before the encounter.
2. Acute care could occur across two or more encounters (where encounters could include inpatient care as well as outpatient care).
3. Care could be for a chronic condition, in which case there may not be a final outcome.

This book advocates the use of defined outcome cases and chronic care management cases to combine these encounters and events (tests and test results) so that a comprehensive view of the treatment for a condition can be easily identified and so that continuing care can be provided.

Within some HMOs, continuing care is facilitated by setting up care teams, a set of physicians, nurse practitioners, and others who work closely together and have an understanding of how the team members treat patients for a particular medical condition. This facilitates consistent care, continuing the same treatment plan when a physician might be away, having the patient see another physician on the same team or having the patient see a nurse practitioner who works closely with the missing physician.

Use of defined outcome cases and chronic care management cases potentially allows for more flexibility than restricting the patient to being seen by a care team or a single physician at a particular facility. As long as caregivers are willing to understand and abide by the treatment plan of the key caregiver and the key caregiver continues to take an active role in the case, then a treatment plan in a defined outcome case or chronic care management case allows care to continue anywhere—inside or outside the HMO—using the same treatment plan. This requires a change in the way physicians currently function in their work: physicians must be willing to follow the treatment plans of other physicians

How the outpatient paradigms in figure 8.2, 8.3, 8.4, and 8.5 relate to care beyond a single encounter is unclear. Is there a Post Visit Report after the treatment is finished or only after an encounter?

8.4.5 Intermediate Care

In most HMOs, outpatient services provided to patients fall into three categories: standard medical care, patient education classes, and recently, alternative medicine (also referred to as "complementary medicine"). I think that this view of outpatient care is way too narrow. This book views patient care as being a means (1) to help a patient live his or her normal life, and (2) to not set up a dependency situation where the patient loses his or her independence.

People often encounter life situations that affect their health. This is a normal part of living. Some of these life situations lead to stress, insomnia, depression, raced thoughts and moderate to severe anxiety.

Further, during such situations, little things are magnified, and the body's resistance or tolerance breaks down. Situationss that one used to be able to cope with, now, are unbearable.

One of medicine's cures for these life situations are medications, whether this is standard or alternative medicine. A patient's remedy for some of these situations may be drugs or alcohol. In either case, what may result is the patient's dependence on the drug, medication or alcohol, rather than coping with the problem.

Another of medicine's cures for these life situations is psychiatric care. This treats these life situations as abnormal, instead of a normal part of living and may stigmatize the patient, at least in the patient's mind.

A better model for handling such life situations, instead of drugs, is to use the equivalent of the inpatient nursing care model for handling such life situations when they occur in the hospital setting: Treat the life situation as a "nursing diagnosis" and set up "interventions" to mitigate or alter the life situation. Where drugs are needed, the patient could be encouraged to take the least amount of the drugs that can handle the problem, so a dependency on the drugs is not set up. Because a little problem may be magnified (for example, the patient may be effected by a minor allergy), the full cure may not be needed (perhaps a lesser amount of an inhalant than the prescribed dose would be better).

Instead of looking at medical care as either standard medicine or complementary medicine, an HMO should instead put an emphasize on what I call *intermediate care*: off-chart, and strictly confidential, counseling by a psychologist or a clinical social worker (CSW) to either (1) provider the patient with a means to cope with the life situation, (2) refer the patient to appropriate medical care if this is necessary, or (3) suggest patient education classes to take. This solution better serves the patient than traditional or alternative medical care in that (1) it is a better way than medical care and medication to allow a patient to live his or her normal life, and (2) it probably will not set up a dependency situation such as the medication solution might.

"Intermediate care" is thus a preventive for more complex problems such as drug or alcohol dependence or more severe anxiety, and, thus a preventive for more costly standard medical care. In some cases, "intermediate care" is a preventive for suicide or for a patient lashing out against others.

Situations where "intermediate care" is most appropriate include the following:

- Work or personal stress
- Marital or relationship problems
- Parenting problems
- Loneliness or depression
- Alcohol or drug use
- Getting along with co-workers
- Health-related issues
- Caregiving for someone
- Loss and grief
- Domestic violence or abuse
- Family matters
- Stress from financial or legal pressures
- Anxiety
- Aging or aging relatives
- Eating problems.

Medicine involving the brain has special considerations. See section 17.8.

8.5 AUTOMATED HELP IN DIAGNOSING AND TREATING DISEASE

According to a physician I talked to, disease diagnosis is first based upon **risk** and **time**. If the condition has a risk of getting worse or is time sensitive, then such a situation must be recognized and the patient must be given priority for immediate treatment.

Advice nurses often access risk and time criticality through a protocol based upon the patient's chief complaint, asking a series of questions of the patient to determine cases where the patient should get immediate care or where a doctor should be contacted. Automating such a system could insure that care is consistent and that is based upon best practice guidelines. Similar protocols are used in the emergency department to triage patients and determine which patients should be seen first.

The physician told me that 90% of medical conditions are routine and are not difficult for any physician to diagnosis or are conditions that get better by themselves whether care is given or not. For the other 10%, exact diagnosis is often not important as many diseases that fall into the same general category all respond to the same treatments. Where exact diagnosis is important, a specialist in the area should be consulted who would know the difference between the diseases.

Diagnosis is both a science and an art. Some people exaggerate symptoms while others minimize them—the physician must be astute enough to determine the difference. A person's facial expression could identify the true severity of a problem. And if a patient comes in for one condition, say a cold, the physician should also look for other more significant conditions, for example, a melanoma.

One inpatient registered nurse told me that nurses are often in a better position to recognize medical conditions than inpatient physicians, as nurses provide the bulk of primary care for patients while they are hospitalized, while inpatient physicians often spent very little time with the patient. One physician suggested that an automated system could allow the inpatient nurse to flag significant events recorded during the inpatient stay, which could help the physician in making diagnoses and treating the patient. (Note that the inpatient physician is responsible for reviewing the total of the data entered by the nurse not just single events, so the recording of these significant events by nurses are best if they are only transitory and not preserved in the permanent record.)

An automated system could provide diagnosis and treatment assistance in the following ways: expert systems to identify diseases based upon answers to a series of questions; protocols to identify the next step in care (advice, the patient coming in to be seen, a physician being contacted); alert systems to warn a caregiver of care situations that require special notice; or medical references.

An automated system could alert caregivers of inconsistencies in the care being given (for example, when a patient with already low blood pressure is prescribed a medication that lowers blood pressure), could alert the physician of test results that are out of range, or could alert the physician of a patient who is at high risk of developing a particular disease or medical condition, thus identifying a patient who should receive preventive care. A possible disadvantage of alert systems is that they could get in the way of care because they could provide obvious, already known, or irrelevant information to the caregiver.

An automated system could provide expert systems assisting the physician in making diagnoses. In the past, expert systems to identify diseases have not gained large acceptance. One of the reasons is the large amount information they require and the time to enter the information. Another reason is that expert systems may cause the physician to overlook the artistic, experiential, intuitive, face-to-face, and touching sides of diagnosis.

Another basic problem with expert systems is the issue of responsibility. The physician cannot just say that this diagnosis was chosen because this computer program told me it was the correct one. The physician must fully understand the reasons the diagnosis was chosen and take responsibility for one choice over another.

A proposal to limit the amount of information and physician time required to use expert systems is to have the expert system accept a tentative diagnosis from the physician and return conditions that must be satisfied for the diagnosis to be correct (Dankel and Russo 1988). Such a system would help a physician in picking between potential diagnoses.

Capabilities mentioned in this section—expert systems, protocol systems, and alert systems—fall under the category of *decision-support systems*. Professor Shortliffe, the principal developer of the MYCIN expert system, has a discussion of such systems in the book in reference (Shortliffe 1990). (MYCIN was one of the earliest expert systems—It was used to diagnose and recommend treatment for certain blood infections (Alison 1994).)

The diagnosis of disease may be more of a problem in developing nations than developed nations for many reasons: including the unavailability of clinical laboratories and medical devices to do diagnostic testing and the unavailability of specialists to diagnosis hard-to-diagnose diseases. However, even more of a problem than the proper diagnosis of disease in developing countries could be the unavailability of medical supplies to treat properly diagnosed medical conditions and the unavailability of specialists to treat conditions that require specialty care. Perhaps, the automated patient medical record system could be used to help dispense medical supplies and specialty care in a developing nation based upon criticality of need, thus providing assistance in allocating these scarce resources. (However, there may be other problems with medical supplies and specialists it cannot solve: costs and transportation logistics; storage and delays in receipt of medical materials; politics; and the unavailability of infrastructure.)

Caregivers in developing countries or anywhere who want to improve their practice could ask for physicians anywhere, perhaps even volunteer physicians who have retired, to randomly or selectively review their automated medical records and provide *mentoring*, each asking questions about the medical record and discussing alternative medical practices.

Another problem in proper medical care, whether in developing or developed countries, is having the patient remember and follow the prescribed treatment. As mentioned in section 8.3.2, to insure that the patient has properly understood what the physician has told him, a written set of instructions produced by the automated system could be printed after a visit, with the physician's instructions gone over by a nurse. (According to reference (Sackett et al. 1991) non-adherence to treatments can run from 22% to 72%, with the largest percentage occurring for adherence to life-style changes.)

Of course, there are many other factors influencing the quality of treatment and diagnosis, and more generally the quality of medical care: the educational background, culture and experience of the caregiver. Some caregivers have mentors and reviewers to tell them when they are or were wrong; others do not have that luxury.

And in any case there is no certain way of identifying whether a diagnosis or treatment was correct. The most conclusive way of determining if a diagnosis was correct is doing an autopsy, but that obviously can only be done after the patient dies. And autopsies are seldom done.

For those in remote areas where there are few colleagues to be mentors or provide review, in particular review by specialists, the automated patient medical system could be used to discuss disease diagnoses and treatments with other caregivers located remotely.

In the future according to IBM™ who is using computers to do gene research: DNA information for an individual, " . . . will probably become a key component of medical diagnostics and even individualized medical treatments, which tune a medical treatment or drug protocol to the genetic makeup of an individual and his or her medical condition (Swope 2001)." A universal patient record may be an appropriate place to store an individual's DNA information when this becomes feasible—because it is so costly to analyze a person's DNA, a mechanism is needed to record the analysis for use throughout the individual's lifetime. In the future, diagnoses and treatments could be partially based upon an individual's DNA.

8.6 DISEASE PREDICTION

This book views *disease prediction* as any approach to predicting that a patient will get a disease, or to predicting when a patient will get a disease, when a disease will worsen, or when a treatment decision for a disease will need to be made, most often expressed in terms of the probability of that event happening compared to the probability of that event happening for the general population or for an applicable population group.

Analytic disease prediction is predicting disease based upon the patient having known risk factors for a disease (e.g., the person has an increased probability of getting lung cancer later in life because he or she smokes) and having known protective factors against the disease. A caregiver recognizing and recording such risk factors is a normal part of current medical care. The automated patient medical record could assist in this process by insuring these factors are recorded and are communicated to later caregivers. If a patient has risk factors, the automated patient medical record system could inform the caregiver of this information and report to the patient on the Post Visit report something like the following: "Because you have risk factors or _______, ______, and ______, you have a probability of X% of developing the disease ______ instead of the Y% for the normal population of _______. Risk factors that can be controlled are the following: ______, ______, and ______. We recommend that __________."

Disease progression analysis is determining the probable progression of a disease or progression to a disease by measuring medical values over time that are predictive of that disease and identifying risk factors and protective factors. Examples of such medical values are blood pressure as a measure of potential future heart disease, bone density as a measure of future osteoporosis, and x-rays of a knee as a measure of the degeneration of cartilage in a knee.

This book views disease progression analysis as consisting of the following steps:

1. recording a medical value or medical values over time for a patient as a measure of a potential disease, say using trend documents—biomarkers
2. recording risk factors and protective factors
3. identifying controllable risk factors
4. prediction of the future changes in the medical values
5. countermeasures against the disease including removal of controllable risk factors
6. prediction of the probable time of when a treatment decision would need to be made, or of the probable time of unset of a disease or of a debilitating condition—a *treatment decision point* is a point in a disease before which therapy is either more effective or easier to apply than afterward
7. prediction after countermeasures
8. identification of treatments or potential future treatments that could be applied at a treatment decision point.

Through the automated patient medical record and trend documents, disease progression analysis can track medical values and risk factors measuring the potential for a disease for a patient over a long period of time (e.g., a patient's blood pressure, bone density through bone density tests, x-rays of a degenerative knee). By using trend documents of many different patients, changes in these medical values state can be predicted for a patient, and predictions can be made of when treatment decisions would need to be made, when a disease might occur, or when a condition might become debilitating.

For the disease, a physician can propose countermeasures (e.g., blood pressure lowering, LDL lowering, and HDL raising medications for heart disease or exercise for low bone density). By using trend documents for many different patients who used the same countermeasures, a new prediction can be made of the unset of the disease or debilitating condition (e.g., the onset of heart disease). Through this approach, the physician could determine the long-term effects of the countermeasures and whether or not they would be effective.

Although there may or may not be any countermeasures for a disease, predictions of the onset of the disease, of the onset of a debilitating effect, or of an appropriate time to make a treatment decision could still be useful for a patient: The patient could plan for the future. The patient could be informed of current and potential future treatments (those currently in clinical trials) that applied at a treatment decision point.

Treatment decision points will vary according to the patient and to the disease. Reference (Sackett et al. 1991) views critical points in the natural history of disease as (1) biological onset, (2) early diagnosis possible, (3) usual clinical diagnosis and (4) outcome (recovery, disability, death). It also views another critical point, a "treatment decision point": a point in the disease before which therapy is either more effective or easier to apply than afterward. There are a number of factors to be considered in the use of such treatment decision points, including time of earliest detection of the disease, invasiveness of detection or treatment, false positives and false negatives in detection, risk of not treating, and individual characteristics of the patient.

Treatment decision points could potentially occur anywhere in the life cycle of a disease, for example, before its biological onset as a preventative measure, or much later after its onset (e.g., a hip replacement). Predicting potential treatment decision points may be as critical as predicting a disease.

For example, for a man with BPH (benign prostatic hyperplagia, enlargement of the prostate) over a number of years there may be progressive blockage of urine flow. As a result, the man's bladder may, over time, become distended and less elastic, and, consequently, any measures to unblock the obstruction may, as a result, not recover the normal flow of urine. However, since prostate surgery to remove the blockage could affect the man's ability to have children or affect sexual performance, there may be good reasons to delay surgery. Disease progression analysis could be used to determine how long such a man could delay prostate surgery before these detrimental effects of inelasticity of the bladder would occur.

The incorporation of disease progression analysis into medical care may require that physicians change their view of medical care from being almost exclusively re-active, to also being very proactive. In the past, preventive care has not been tailored for individuals but for groups of people (e.g., all women over 50 should have yearly mammograms); disease progression analysis enables preventive care for a medical condition to be tailored to the environment history or genetics of the patient.

In doing trend analysis, care must be given to not over-test. Performing clinical lab tests, taking x-rays, etc. more often than is needed to do the disease progression analysis may increase the cost of medical care as well as potentially harm the patient. Identifying disease early and taking the correct countermeasures early should instead decrease the cost of medical care.

Descriptive disease prediction is identifying common patterns in the automated patient medical record for patients who all develop a particular disease, and then looking for these same patterns for other patients. In this way, these patterns might be used to predict these diseases for these other patients.

All these disease prediction approaches become more feasible with an automated patient medical record.

There is increasing study of biomarkers for disease where a biomarker is "cellular, biochemical, molecular, or genetic characteristics or alterations by which a normal, abnormal, or simply biologic process can be recognized, or monitored (NIH 2004)." There already are many biomarkers to predict diseases; for example, high PSA levels could predict prostate cancer and measuring blood glucose levels could detect diabetes. There could be more complete sets of biomarkers for diagnosing and predicting diseases. In the future, some of these biomarkers could come from an individual's fixed genetic material, the individual's genome, while other biomarkers could be measured over time and be recorded through trend documents. The automated patient medical record could be a storage place for such biomarkers, and biomarkers could be combined with other risk factors for disease in disease prediction; further, the automated patient medical record could be used to identify new biomarkers via descriptive disease prediction.

Whether disease prediction measures are appropriate for a patient is partially dependent upon the patient's values. Would the patient want to know about a future disease if it could be predicted? Would it depend upon the specific type of disease? These questions could be asked of the HMO member as part of the healthcare questionnaire described earlier in this chapter.

8.7 IMPLEMENTATION OF BUSINESS POLICIES

It takes many people in a healthcare organization to implement organizational business policies, in particular business policies dealing with patient care. And as stated in sections 2.5.4.3 and 7.6, some business policies could be implemented via agents: a combination of code and tables, interfaces between systems, databases, user interfaces (possibly all spread across a number of different software systems), and administrative and operational procedures followed by employees implementing the business policy. Agents are a way to make this set of items implementing a business policy distinct from other parts of the automated patient medical record system so that the business policy can be changed by people who are responsible for the business policy rather than only by technical people.

Before automation, business policies were probably all assigned to business employees to administer. With automation, some of these business policies are embedded in code and must be administered by technical people, who may not really understand the business policy. This book proposes returning this administration back to business employees.

This book proposes that agents, in a number of ways, be treated like employees. An agent should be assigned a business manager who is responsible for the agent and knows everything about the business policy the agent implements. Periodically, the agent should be evaluated by the manager and the manager's managers to determine if the business policy should be changed. An agent can be "fired", removing the business policy, or "replaced", changing the business policy.

8.8 ADDITIONAL BUSINESS REQUIREMENTS FROM THIS CHAPTER

Additional business requirements were identified as part of this analysis of future systems and the future environment. Table 8.1 lists these additional business requirements.

Table 8.1 Additional Business Requirements Determined From Projected Future Environment and Systems

Number	*Organizational Objective*	*Project Objective*	*Project Objective Addressed in this Chapter?*	*Business Requirement*
1	Provide quality medical care	Re-evaluate the entire clinical workflow of the HMO to completely eliminate unnecessary steps and restructure non-productive steps while incorporating the automated patient medical record system.	No	
		Create a complete and always available patient medical record.	Yes	The automated patient record will be available for view by any number of authorized caregivers at the same time. See section 8.2.1.4.
		Allow simultaneous viewing and update of the patient medical record.	No	A research area. See the chapter 17.
		Enable a caregiver to quickly find relevant information in the patient medical record by methods such as providing summarization information, organization, information retrieval and tailoring of information related to the type of caregiver.	Yes	A clinical summary for the member and a list of current medications will be identified at the time of an initial interview visit for new members and at the time of an introduction appointment of the member with the member's chosen primary care physician. See sections 8.2.2 and 8.2.3.
		Provide methods to track a treatment for a particular condition across multiple encounters, possibly with multiple different caregivers, potentially in different departments and in different geographic locations.	Yes	Use defined outcome cases and chronic care management cases to track care across encounters. For members with high risk or high cost conditions, assign case managers. See sections 8.2.2, 8.2.8, 8.2.10, 8.2.11, 8.2.12 and 8.4.4.

Automate caregiver ordering and results reporting to make ordering easier, quicker and more accurate and integrate it with the automated patient medical record system.	No	
Do automated clinical checking of medications, such as drug/drug interactions and patient allergy checking. Reduce errors including reordered tests, adverse drug reactions, billing errors, etc.	Yes	See section 8.3.4 for a proposal to create a patient medication schedule that also clinical checks medications.
Provide information to caregivers on best practice guidelines using NGC and/or local guidelines; provide medical reference information.	No	
Collect clinical outcomes information to further evidence-based medicine (identifying best treatments and practices for diseases which produce the best outcomes as determined by the best scientific evidence).	No	
Where possible, automate the identification of trends in the patient's health, especially in cases where there is an emerging health problem (e.g., an increase in the patient's blood pressure).	Yes	Initiate trend documents as needed to measure a health problem over time, often at the first visit with the member's primary care physician. See section 8.2.1.
Generate letters to patients to come in for preventative health exams (e.g., colonoscopies) based upon age, sex, family history and other factors.	Yes	Use 'life care paths' to schedule preventative health letters based upon age, sex, medical characteristics, etc. See section 8.2.1.

		Provide the ability to record a detailed social, family, environmental and genetic history of HMO members who agree to provide this information. Identify family members of these HMO members and their relationships to the HMO member, especially family members who are themselves HMO members.	Yes	Collect a detailed medical history for new members. See sections 8.2.1.1 and 8.2.1.2.
		Explore predicting diseases from information in the automated patient medical record, including from risk factors and biomarkers.	Yes	See section 8.6.
		For medical research purposes, enable useful access to clinical information without providing the identities of patients.	No	
		For medical research purposes, enable controlled access to clinical information to identify patients who are appropriate for specific clinical trials and other medical studies.	Yes	Collect a detailed medical history for new members. See sections 8.2.1.1 and 8.2.1.2.
2	Promote HMO Member Satisfaction	Reengineer the care process to eliminate roadblocks that inhibit the patient from receiving prompt care.	Yes	See section 8.2.11.
		Pre-schedule activities, both generically and for specific individual patients, and, where possible, pre-fill paperwork or fill in paperwork when care is given, such as insurance forms.	Yes	For members with severe medical conditions requiring frequent care, there should be a capability to call in to a predefined telephone number to identify that the patient is coming in to the emergency department for care, thus initiating care activities before the patient comes in. See section 8.2.9.

After an outpatient visit, provide the patient and the patient's family information on clinician orders and other encounter information to promote compliance with physician instructions and orders. After clinical laboratory results are returned, enable physicians to print and annotate results, sending them to the patient.	Yes	See section 8.3.2 for a proposed post visit report. See section 8.3.3 proposes a more patient-friendly discharge summary. See section 8.4.2 for a proposal for using the post visit report.
Where appropriate, provide the patient with automated scheduling of medications and determination of alternative medicines or dosage choices.	Yes	See section 8.3.4 for a proposal to create a patient medication schedule.
Have each HMO member chose a primary care physician. Have the automated system identify a patient's primary care physician(s) and associated caregivers.	Yes	See section 8.2.3.
Store genetic and other information to enable individualized treatments and medications in the future.	Yes	In the future consider storing the member's genome and other biomarkers. See section 8.2.1.
Personalize care for the patient through personal profiles.	Yes	A discussion of patient-centered care is presented in section 8.2.1.5.
Get patients and their families more involved in the patient care process.	Yes	See section 8.2.1.5 for patient-centered care. See section 8.3.2 for a proposed post visit report for the patient and family to follow after a visit. See section 8.3.4 for a proposal to create a patient medication schedule to help members in administration of their own medications .
Record advance directives in the automated system.	No	

		Evaluate the feasibility of the automated patient medical record system receiving input from monitoring systems, including "Guardian Angel" systems.	No	
		Incorporate patient education information in the automated system for the patient.	Yes	See section 8.3.5.
3	Support healthcare workers and improve their efficiency	To reengineer the care process based upon input from employees so that employees' work activities match the most productive and least stressful methods of providing care.	Yes	Employees would have an input into identifying how the automated patient medical record would be used.
		Check for or insure consistent terminology in the medical record.	No	
		Automate the process of identifying situations where patients are not complying with orders that seriously affect the patient's health.	Yes	The provider can request to be informed of curtailment of care by the patient, so that the caregiver could insure that a treatment is continued. See section 8.2.7.
		Provide other automated assistance to the caregiver in providing care, including the following: alerts, trends, assistance in diagnosis, conformance to best practice guidelines, identifying inconsistencies.	Yes	See section 8.2.7 for alerts, alarms, and trends. See section 8.5 for automated help in diagnosing and treating diseases. See section 8.6 for disease prediction.
		Provide on-line medical references for the caregiver to use when providing care.	Yes	Provide medical references for physicians, nurse practitioners, and advice nurses.
		Eliminate redundant entrance of information in clinical systems, eliminating possible contradictory information.	No	

Enable printing of test results so the patient could understand them and so the physician can add his or her comments and send the results to the patient.	Yes	See section 8.2.7.
Use techniques to simplify documentation listed in section 5.3.3.3.	Yes	See sections 8.2.7 and 8.2.8.
Support automated care documentation, including computerized generation of nursing care plans.	Yes	See sections 8.2.10 and 4.4.1.3 for using the computer to create nursing care plans.
Automate coding of diagnoses, procedures, and supplies (such as ICD, CDT, DRG codes). and unit census.	No	
Automate non-chart documentation done manually, such as the Inpatient Clinical Summary, MAR, emergency room census.	Yes	See 8.2.10.
Where possible, validate as correct all information input by the caregiver.	Yes	See section 8.2.7 for checking by the automated patient medical record system. The Post Visit Report can be verified by the nurse with the patient; see section 8.3.2. At time of creation of a Patient Medication Schedule, clinical checking of medications can be done; see section 8.3.4.
Alert attending physician when discharge is pending so discharge procedures can be quickly accomplished.	Yes	See section 8.2.10.
Evaluate the feasibility of using digitized diagnostic images with the automated patient medical record system. Enable quick transmission of images to medical professionals who can interpret them.	No	

4	Making and Saving Money	Re-evaluate the entire clinical workflow of the HMO to eliminate or revise costly processes while incorporating the automated patient medical record system.	Yes	See the total chapter.
		Support demand management in all its forms.	Yes	Section 4.6.2 describes demand management. Compare this to activities described in sections 8.2.8, 8.2.9 and 8.2.10.
		Reduce errors including reordered tests, adverse drug reactions, billing errors, etc.	Yes	Reordered tests are reduced by visibility of information within an automated patient medical record. Adverse drug reactions are caught by clinical checking. Automation reduces billing errors.
		Identify and report on potential patient abuse such as "drug jumping", going from facility to facility for narcotics orders.	No	
		Identify suspicious charges for medications and services when payments are to be made to outside healthcare organizations.	No	
		Support automated collection of payments for medical services from the government and insurance companies via EDI. Support automated payment for medical services. Support automated collection of Medicare payments using HIPAA standards.	No	

Support electronic commerce, in particular DME ordering such as over the Internet.	No	
Provide automated advice on least cost best practices, including lower cost medications that provide equal or better benefits, including advice to use generic medications rather than brand name ones.	No	
Record services, tests and procedures given to patients, supplies and medications, provider time caring for patients, hospitalizations and visits, and trends in membership growth and patient utilization for prediction of HMO costs in the future.	Yes	See section 8.2.11.
Where possible, standardize hardware, system software and clinical systems within the organization.	No	
Standardize clinical system interfaces using industry standards (such as HL7).	No	
Design the automated patient medical record system to eliminate documentation errors identified in table 5.1 to protect against costly lawsuits.	No	
If the healthcare organization considers outsourcing or consolidation of medical services (where the patient is not seen) to be useful, then implement this.	No	
Evaluate the possibility, feasibility and cost-effectiveness of off-site storage of automated patient medical record information.	No	

5	Fulfill the Requirements of Government and Public Health Agencies, Accreditation Organizations, Laws, and Industry Standards	Automatically collect registry information based upon patient diagnoses and alert a caregiver when registry information should be collected.	No	
		Provide automated recognition of infection outbreaks.	No	
		Automate quality control checks that insure that clinical information complies with accreditation agency (e.g., JCAHO) and government standards and which generates proof of compliance.	Yes	See section 8.2.11.
		Provide support in reviewing sentinel events.	Yes	See section 8.2.11.
		For reporting based upon medical-related information (e.g., HEDIS), set up automatic generation of these reports and transmission to outside agencies (e.g., the NCQA).	Yes	See section 8.2.11.

Key Terms

admission
advice nurse
alarm
allergies
analytic disease prediction
appointment
appointment clerk
auditing
automated call distribution (ACD)
decision-support system
defined outcome case
descriptive disease prediction
disease prediction
disease progression analysis
document
emergency department census
MedWatch
mentoring
overall clinical summary
paradigm
patient-centered care
patient discharge summary
patient medication schedule
patient mentoring

automated speech recognition (ASR)
biomarker
call center
caregiver messaging system
chronic care management case
clinical checking
clinical pathway
clinical summary
computer telephony integration (CTI)
genome
high-risk patient
immunizations
Inpatient Clinical Summary
intermediate care
life care path
low utilizer
Medication Administration Record (MAR)
medication scheduler computer program
peer review
personal profile
post visit report
predictive modeling
preventive care
primary care physician
referral request
sentinel event
significant health problem
synopses
team care
treatment decision point

Study Questions

1. Name some purposes for anticipating the future organization once the project is complete.
2. Explain the different effects of high-risk patients and low-utilizers in managed care verses "fee-for-service" organizations.
3. What part of what document is the overall clinical summary most like? What kind of biomarker that does not change does this book propose being recorded in the future?
4. For what categories of patients is case management appropriate? For what categories of patients is a life care path appropriate? What is predictive modelling?
5. Why are encounter synopses problematic?
6. How can a paper chart become unavailable? How can an automated patient medical record become unavailable?
7. This book proposes four items that do not currently exist: a post visit report, a personal profile, a patient discharge summary, and a patient medication schedule. What is a post visit report and its purpose? What does a personal profile allow an advice nurse to do? What does this book suggest be given to a discharged patient instead of or in addition to the discharge summary? Why? What is a patient medication schedule?
8. The information in an overall clinical summary is most like information on what kind of document?
9. A patient having only one personal physician in medicine or pediatrics provides what primary potential benefit for the patient?
10. What is a call center? What are the two primary types of agents in the call center? What types of agents would have access to an automated patient medical record?
11. What is point-of-care computing? How do nurse practitioners and physician assistants differ from physicians in providing care? Name some ways that an automated patient medical record system could assist a physician in providing care to the patient?
12. What is a referral? What are some documents that can be used in tracking care of a patient over many visits with a particular problem or disease.
13. What is triage in the Emergency Department?
14. What paper document does the inpatient clinical summary replace? How long does an inpatient clinical summary exist and how long does an overall clinical summary exist? Who creates these documents?
15. Who creates the automated MAR? How long does the MAR exist for a patient?
16. Name some organizations that receive quality of care information from an HMO (and could potentially automatically receive this information through the automated patient medical record system)? What are sentinel events? What is MedWatch? What is HEDIS?
17. What is a paradigm? According to this book, how would a post visit report change patient care? How would an advice nurse change patient care?
18. In this book what does "intermediate care" mean?
19. Discuss diagnosis being related to "risk" and "time". Identify ways that computers could be used in improving medical care. Why have expert systems not caught on in medical care? What is it that this book calls "mentoring"?
20. What are "treatment decision points"? Discuss "disease prediction".
21. Discuss the idea that many healthcare organizations put too much trust in technical people to implement business policies in software.

CHAPTER 9

Determining Whether to Go Ahead With the Project

CHAPTER OUTLINE

9.1 PROJECT CONTEXT: THE DECISION TO CONTINUE, TERMINATE OR CHANGE A PROJECT AFTER THE INITIAL BUSINESS ANALYSIS

Our business analysis step in the initial overall design of the automated patient medical record project has looked at project objectives and business requirements only dealing with the beneficial aspects of the project. In the next chapter, we will deal with the obstacles to the project, i.e., the costs and complications of introducing an automated patient medical record system. Both benefits and obstacles will be used in the evaluation step.

After initial identification of both benefits and obstacles, an initial evaluation of the project should be done by upper management. This evaluation is very important so the project can be terminated or changed if necessary before the project consumes too much money. The evaluation step is also very complex.

The evaluation step is shown in figure 9.1, which is the same as figure 2.5. This evaluation step asks the question: "Given the benefits and obstacles identified to developing and implementing the project (an automated patient medical record system), is it worthwhile for the organization (an HMO) to do so?" The answer to this question lies in the answers to some other questions:

1. Is there at least one solution that is feasible and which benefits the organization?.
2. Will the project (the automated patient medical record system) support the mission, objectives, business strategies and goals of the (healthcare) organization?

3. Will the projected return on investment of the project (the automated medical record system) support its costs? Or if not, is there another justification in going ahead anyway?—for example, regulatory requirements.
4. What are the obstacles to the success of the project? Can these be managed?
5. Are there more important projects that need to be done instead, that are lower cost or can better fulfill the mission, objectives, business strategies and goals of the company?

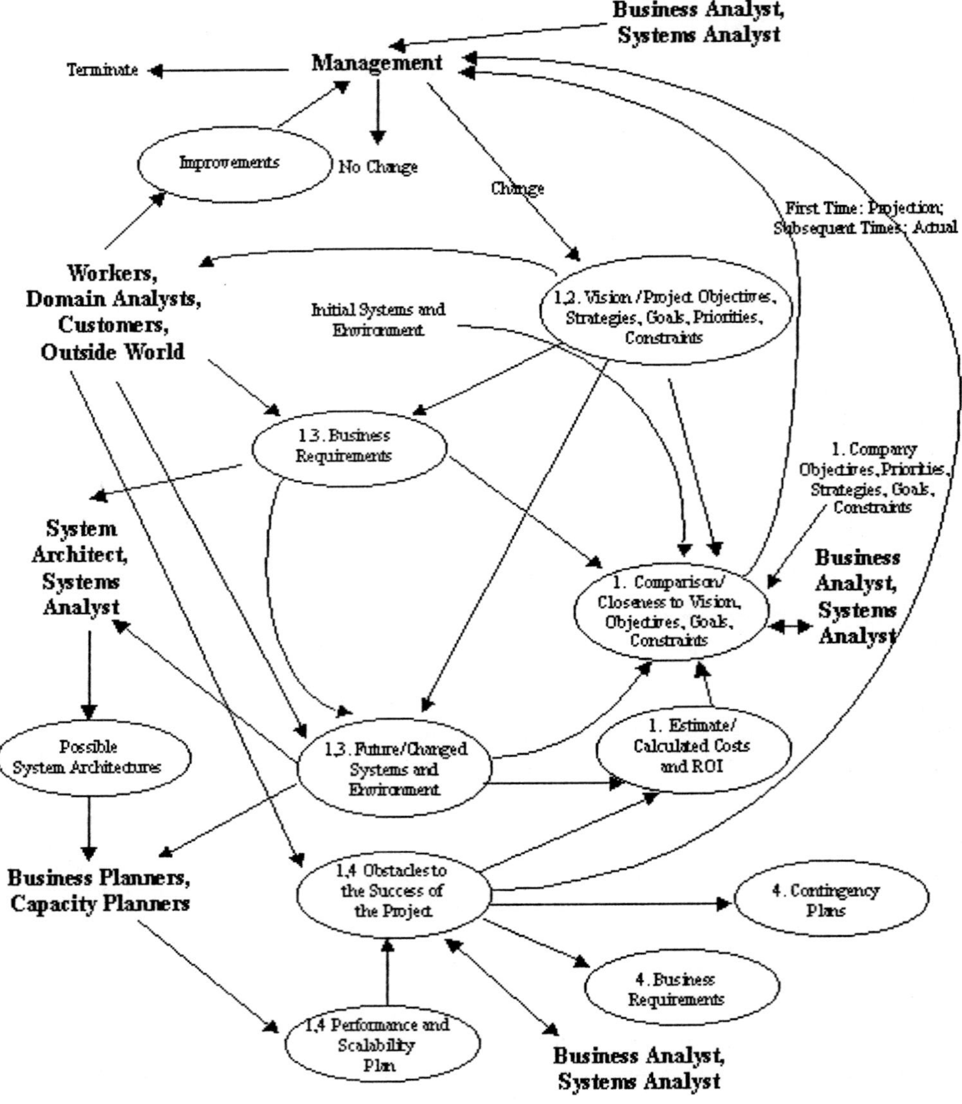

Figure 9.1 Evaluation step.

The initial evaluation falls into the category of a *feasibility study* (Sommerville 2000), evaluating projected—instead of actual—costs and obstacles versus benefits. This initial evaluation step is done by business analysts and is presented to upper management.

At this point, upper management must decide whether or not to continue with the project. Note that return on investment values are likely to be very gross ones at this point and will be more accurate after the project is completely scoped out in the project plan step, where the project will be broken up into phases. Upper management should take this into consideration. And they may decide to continue the project for re-evaluation after the project plan step, when more accurate return on investment values are likely to be available.

If management decides to continue the project, they should make one or more of the following decisions:

1. to continue the project until the step to break up the project into phases and determine then whether to continue with the project, as more information on the project will be known at that time, including more accurate return on investment estimates
2. to determine that the project is going largely the wrong direction, and change objectives, strategies or constraints as a result, possibly requiring that the business analysis step be re-done
3. to defer the project until later
4. to determine that the project is going the right direction, but to change, delete or add objectives, objective priorities, strategies, constraints or business requirements
5. to identify now how the project should later be broken up into phases
6. to identify how the project could be improved
7. to pare down the project
8. to give an absolute go-ahead for continuing the project to the next evaluation point without changes.

There is a potential danger in paring down a project: losing the context of the project. If the intent is to later do the larger project, then the business analysis work done so far should not be lost, so that the pared down project could be developed so it could later be extended to produce the larger project. This may, for example, require building the pared down project with additional information in databases or building the application as if the larger system was there, but leaving out the actual code or interfaces.

See figure 9.1 again. A business analyst involved in the analysis reports to upper management on how the project objectives achieve the organizational objectives. The business analyst reports on the future systems and environment and how they change the existing systems and environment. And the business analyst identifies obstacles to doing the project and makes an analysis of whether they are manageable or not, including whether the obstacles are so significant that management should consider not doing the project at all. The technical group presents technical obstacles, such as potential system performance and scalability problems.

Upper management uses this information to compare the project against other possible projects, and give directions on how to proceed. As a result of this process, upper management may choose to change strategies, goals or constraints, reprioritize objectives or to make the project more compatible with organizational objectives. The business analysis step might, as a result, be redone, with changes to business requirements and the future, changed, system as a result of changes to project objectives, strategies, goals or constraints. Additionally, the business analysis step may have to be re-done, adding or changing business requirements as a result of the identified obstacles to the project.

In the evaluation step, upper management has a chance to review and update the description of the future environment and systems. This is important because this description presents a clear description to the organization of how the project results will be used in the future.

The next chapter looks at the part of the evaluation step that deals with obstacles to the success of the project.

An evaluation step should not only be done in the overall design or overall redesign but also should be done at various points in the project. For the overall (or re-)design, the evaluation step should be done early on. Evaluation steps within phases of the projects, called "gates", are done at any time during the project as warranted by the project, particularly when significant risks have been identified. See section 14.2.1.

Key Terms

evaluation

feasibility study

gate

Study Questions

1. When is an evaluation step done in a project? What is another name for the evaluation step when it occurs later in a project?
2. What is a feasilbility study? Why is a feasibility study not done in later evaluation steps?
3. What does this book suggest to do if the project is pared down?

CHAPTER 10

Obstacles to Success

CHAPTER OUTLINE

10.1 PROJECT CONTEXT: OBSTACLES TO THE SUCCESS OF A PROJECT

Obstacles to the success of the project influence business decisions to continue or change the project and often provide additional business requirements for the project. Obstacles to the project might be so overwhelming that management might determine that the project is not possible or is too costly to continue. Some obstacles may have to be taken care of immediately, while other obstacles with no certainty of occurring might require a contingency plan to take specific actions if the obstacle does occur during the project.

Obstacles often result in additional business requirements or changes to previously determined business requirements. Technical obstacles, such as computer system capacity and performance constraints, are determined by specialized technical staff rather than business people; these technical obstacles should be included in a performance and scalability plan document.

Development, or even installation, of an automated patient chart system in a healthcare organization is a project of major proportions. There are many obstacles to doing so. This chapter explores these obstacles and how to overcome them. Contingency plans and additional business requirements that might result from the obstacles are listed in the last section of this chapter. Goals that could be used to measure the business requirements are also listed. A *contingency plan* is a plan of action to minimize or negate the adverse effects of a risk should it occur.

10.2 PHYSICIAN ACCEPTANCE OF THE AUTOMATED PATIENT MEDICAL RECORD SYSTEM

Automation of the patient medical record will not be successful unless physicians and other caregivers use the system. Physician usage is particularly important. Physician decisions in the care of their patients account for more than three-quarters of all health care costs (Anderson 1997). Therefore, it is extremely important to accurately and thoroughly record and later retrieve for analysis these decisions by physicians. This can only be done if physicians, or less ideally, caregivers working for the physicians, use the automated patient medical record system.

Studies have shown that physicians, even more so than other caregivers, are reluctant to use clinical information systems (Anderson 1997). A major effort must be made by HMO management to convince physicians, and other caregivers, to use the automated patient medical record system.

The experience of one facility of an HMO in the Northwest in this regard was that approximately half the physicians refused to use their facility's automated patient medical record system and simply left the organization. These physicians were replaced with computer-literate physicians who did use the system. Physicians left even though the HMO facility chose the least automated input method: keeping point of care documentation on paper within the exam room while providing a computer system in the physician's office. Did the facility make mistakes in implementation of their system, or will it always be the case that a large number of physicians will not want to use an automated patient medical record system?

For a caregiver to use the automated patient medical record system, the system must fit into a workflow that the caregiver is comfortable with. This is why workflow analysis before implementation of an automated patient medical record system is so very important (see chapter 11).

Of particular importance is to have quick log-on and sign-off of the system(s) the caregiver uses; otherwise, the caregiver is spending significant time logging on and off the computer. A goal should be that, with the automated system, care processes should not take longer than without the system.

Some people also contend that a caregiver will only use the automated patient medical record system if he also benefits from the system. For example, it must supply the caregiver with more useful information than without the system.

A caregiver must not only use the system, but must use the system well, so there is complete, accurate and organized information in the patient medical record. The accurate recording of chart information could be a particular problem if the caregiver does not directly input chart information himself during the patient interview, and either relies on others to input the information or inputs the information much later himself.

But most significantly, if any healthcare provider does not use or does not output information to a patient's automated patient medical record or delays in doing so, then that patient's automated patient medical record will either become permanently incomplete or be incomplete for a period of time. The same is true of the universal patient record. Caregivers may then mistrust the information in the automated patient medical record (or universal patient record).

10.3 MANY PAPER CHARTS IN MANY LOCATIONS

Another obstacle to automation of the patient medical record in an HMO is the situation that there may currently be many paper charts in many different facilities in the HMO for a patient, as well as in many different locations outside the HMO.

Consider figure 10.1 also presented in an earlier chapter. This diagram shows a possible set of charts that could exist for a patient in an HMO. For each facility in the HMO where the patient was seen as an outpatient, there could be a different outpatient chart. For each facility in the HMO where the patient had a hospital stay, the patient could have an inpatient chart. Psychiatry and genetic departments keep their own charts in the HMO. With alliances with hospitals and clinics outside the HMO, further charts could exist in these alliance organizations. With "point of service" agreements, allowing patients to also be seen outside the HMO, still other charts could exist. Charts before the patient joined the HMO could also exist.

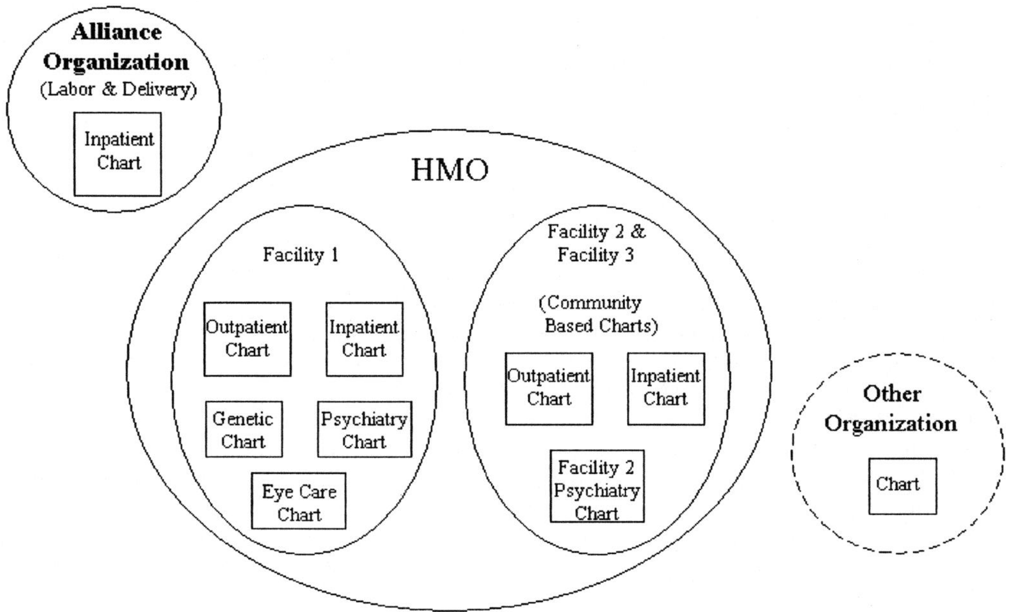

Figure 10.1 An example of the existing charts for an HMO patient.

Thus, for a single patient, there is likely to be many charts in many locations. Even after automation of the chart, this is likely to remain true, as the HMO is unlikely to have control over charts outside the HMO; this complicates the process of automating the chart, especially if the intent of automation is to produce a single complete patient medical record for a patient (sometimes referred to as a *lifetime* or *longitudinal patient record*).

There will be many different types of documents in a chart, each with a different format. Even if the documents from different organizations are of the same type, they are also likely to use different formats and have different formats for the same field (e.g., names, dates, etc.). The identifier for the patient is likely to be different in different organizations (Garling 1996), and other types of identifiers are also likely to be different (e.g., perhaps one location would use a numeric identifier for a physician, while the other might use an alphabetic mnemonic). Terminology used in each chart is also likely to differ, by organization, location or even caregiver (AHCPR 1994).

Retrieving chart information pre-existent to the automated patient medical record is a challenge. Building an automated patient medical record system that combines patient medical record information in charts is a challenge.

Especially challenging is identifying that dispersed medical record information belongs to the same patient. One problem is that there is no common patient identifier used by all healthcare organizations. And even if there were, there is no guarantee that there would not be multiple such identifiers for the same patient. Merging of medical record information for a patient, or alternatively, splitting medical record information between two or more patients due to inadvertent merging, could be required.

One way to include HMO patient medical records previous to automation with the automated patient medical record is to scan them in. Doing so is usually not cost-effective.

10.4 LACK OF AGREED UPON STANDARDS OR INADEQUACY OF STANDARDS

Another obstacle to automation of the patient medical record is sometimes the lack of standards for the patient medical record and clinical information, and sometimes, the multiplicity of different, competing, standards. See the appendix.

Presumably, one of the reasons an HMO would want to implement an automated patient medical record system is to get a competitive advantage over its competitors. However, for the automated patient medical record system to evolve into the longitudinal patient record and to thus work in the long run, there must be agreement on standards for the automated patient medical record information between the HMO and its alliance hospitals and also eventually among other healthcare organizations. At first glance, agreement with other healthcare organizations on standards seems contradictory to the HMO trying to get a competitive advantage. However, assume, that the HMO goes it alone and develops its own proprietary system for storage of the patient chart, which the HMO demands that alliance hospitals also follow. If eventually, other outside organizations agree upon non-proprietary standards, then the HMO is suddenly at a competitive disadvantage. The HMO is thus best off if it works with other healthcare organizations in developing standards for the patient medical record information prior to implementing the system, even though this approach may appear to cause the HMO to lose its competitive advantage in the short run.

Further, a large HMO that first develops an automated patient medical record system using standards can have a large influence on the direction of standards and thus can insure that the standards entirely fit the needs of the HMO. This could provide a significant competitive advantage to the HMO.

The standards that are required are those for storing the detailed patient medical record information and the indexing necessary to retrieve this information; also, there must be some standard for recording patient encounters and uniquely identifying patients. With such standards, the HMO could also have a competitive advantage based upon additional summary information, compatible with the standard clinical information, that the HMO could keep in its own computers and upon the methods it uses to tie together the different parts of the patient chart.

Agreeing upon standards on storage of patient medical record information and indexing to retrieve it has the additional advantage that the principal information in the patient chart could be stored in a remote location instead of the HMO's chart rooms and would be readily available to other health care organizations, including alliance hospitals given agreed upon security standards.

My prediction of the future, as discussed in chapters 6, is that there will be a computer-based patient record (CPR) that will be stored in a repository outside the healthcare organization. The CPR will be a standardized longitudinal (i.e., lifetime) patient record from many healthcare organizations that summarizes clinical information from each of the organizations' patient records. See figure 10.2.

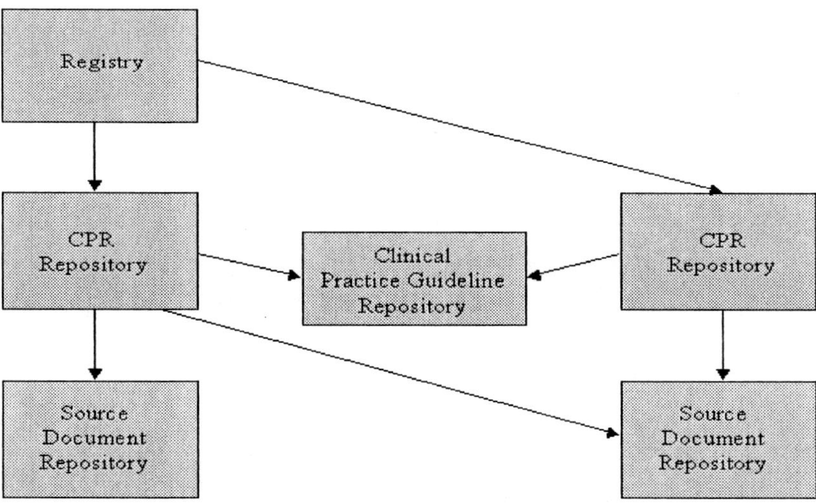

Figure 10.2 Predicted Repositories and Registry

Each healthcare organization may have its own patient information in its own format in terms of "source documents" (e.g., progress notes, incident reports). A healthcare organization may opt to save its source documents off site, replacing its chart rooms. These source document depositories may be in the healthcare organization or perhaps in telecommunication or computer companies—Pacific Bell, now SBC, at one time proposed the development of a source document depository for diagnostic images (Kohli 1996).

Ideally, the CPR repository would identify the locations of all medical documents for each healthcare encounter, whether these documents are on paper in the healthcare organization or electronically stored in source document repositories. In order to locate the CPR repository for any patient, a patient registry might also be set up. The CPR might also reference clinical practice guidelines; repositories for these clinical practice guidelines might exist within healthcare organizations or nationally (e.g., the *National Guideline Clearinghouse* database (NGC 1998-2004)).

When transmitting information over a network from one computer to another, sets of header and trailer data are tacked on to the data transmitted; this is called a layer of information. These layers are used by hardware or software to route, interpret or verify the transmitted information. After the layer is used by the hardware or software, it is stripped off. An existing network protocol standard at the applications level for healthcare is Health Level 7, HL7 (Health Level Seven 1997-2003); this is the innermost layer used by healthcare software to interpret healthcare information. Using this protocol within the HMO is highly beneficial to the HMO, as almost all commercial clinical systems use this protocol for interfacing between their system and others. One standards organization, the ASTM (the American Society for Testing and Materials) has defined a standard for the CPR that also uses HL7 to communicate CPR information to a CPR repository (ASTM 2002)—this standard, the ASTM E1384 standard for a CPR, is referred to throughout this book.

"Clinical Document Architecture" (CDA) is a standard for storage of source documents, although it is not intended to be used to define standard formats for source documents. Section 6.6.5 proposes a way where to define standard formats for different types of source documents where an healthcare organization can add or delete data elements as necessary.

The HMO must join standards organizations and have an influence over these standards.

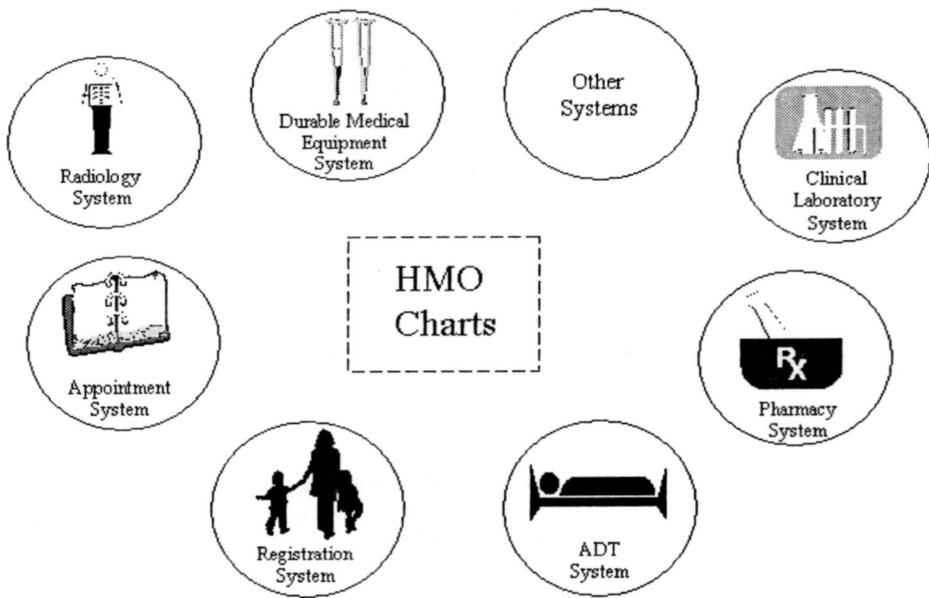

Figure 10.3 Other HMO Clinical Software Systems.

10.5 EXISTING CLINICAL SYSTEMS

Another obstacle to automation of the patient medical record is that the HMO automated patient medical record system must be integrated with existing HMO clinical systems.

In a highly automated HMO, there is likely to be a large number of existing clinical systems prior to creation of an automated patient medical record system. See figure 10.3. The creation of the automated patient medical record system would require an interface with these clinical systems to insure the consistency of clinical information.

In order to develop a completely automated patient medical record, the HMO must move from relatively independent automated clinical systems, possibly using proprietary interfaces between them, to a fully integrated automated patient charting system as illustrated in figure 10.4, most likely using the HL7 standard for healthcare networking.

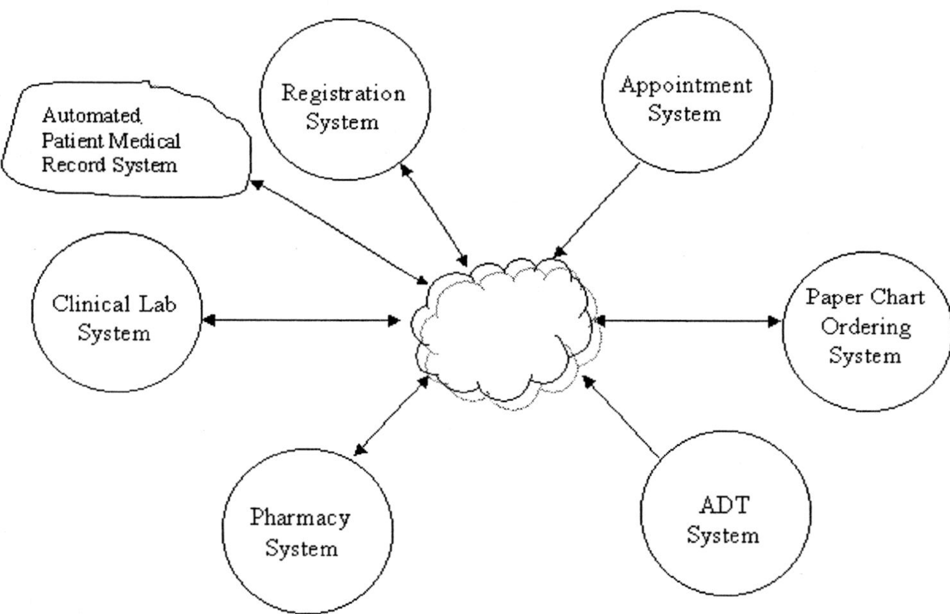

Figure 10.4 Proposed Interfaces Between Clinical Systems.

The information in the existing clinical systems is likely to be redundant and possibly contradictory, with the likelihood that the same information was being re-entered in multiple systems. It is also very likely that the information in these systems is not organized to support an automated patient medical record. Thus the creation of the automated patient medical record system might involve (1) interfacing with these other systems, making sure information is no longer redundantly entered, (2) changing or replacing these other systems so they supply information organized according to the requirements of the automated patient medical record system, or (3) conversion in format of information or restructuring of databases to match the needs of the automated patient medical record system.

During the development of an automated patient medical record system, the paper chart will be phased out and existing clinic systems will be changed or phased out. There thus will be many intermediate steps in development of the automated patient medical record as the automated patient medical record system evolves. I think that the proper development process should be to first attempt to design the complete final future data base for the automated patient medical record system, and then develop an approach that evolves toward use of this final data base, incorporating changing requirements as they occur (e.g., changing standards for storage of the patient chart).

As stated in the previous section, a standard for interfacing clinical systems is *HL7 application level network protocol.* Assume a clinical system uses this protocol. An upgraded version of the clinical system also using HL7 protocol could then replace the existing one, with minimal change to the previous interface.

Although redundancy and inconsistency in data and lack of communication between clinical systems is a potential obstacle in implementing the automated patient medical record system, correcting such problems could provide a significant benefit to the healthcare organization above and beyond the benefits gained from the automated patient medical record system. Creating a common, although perhaps distributed, data base that would result from synchronizing clinical data and getting rid of redundancies would result in a database with much greater integrity of data—data that is more likely to be correct. In this process, synchronization of data could go beyond clinical databases, into financial, personnel and other databases.

As we will see later, besides removing the possibility of redundant information, interfacing these systems with the automated patient medical record is also necessary to enable ordering through the clinical systems (e.g., the pharmacy and clinical laboratory systems) and for the automated patient medical record system to know about encounters (outpatient visits from the appointment and registration systems, inpatient stays from the ADT system, etc.) which could be used to organize the patient medical record.

10.6 REQUIRED REENGINEERING OF THE ORGANIZATION

In order for the automated patient medical record system to be successful, the entire HMO care process **must** be reengineered, as such a system will change the way caregivers work, but, at the same time, the system must fit into the operations of the HMO, be comfortable for caregivers to use and provide more productivity in the care process.

This *reengineering* must be planned along with planning the development of the system. Because the automated system will evolve over time, incorporating more and more of the paper patient medical record into the automated one, needed reengineering will also evolve over time as the system evolves over time. See chapter 11 for a discussion of *reengineering*.

10.7 CONTINUED MAINTENANCE OF THE PAPER CHART OR OF SCANNED DOCUMENTS

Another obstacle to automation of the patient medical record is that paper chart documents will continue to be needed. Such documents could include consent forms and other documents requiring patient signatures, incoming letters such as referral letters, clinical results where ordering is not yet automated such as EKGs, sketches, and documentation from healthcare organizations that have paper charts. Such documents could also include chart documentation previous to automation.

Such documents could be scanned and included as part of the automated record, indexing the documents so they could be found, with index information either entered by a human after scanning, input from a bar code on the document, or read from the document via OCR. (A *bar code* is an array of rectangular marks and spaces in a predetermined pattern, usually used for automatic product identification or for input of encounter or other information on a scanned document.*OCR* (optical character recognition) is process wherein a printed page is scanned and the resulting image of the page, line, or part of a page is interpreted and translated into a sequence of characters.)

Scanned documents, like other parts of the automated record, can be viewed concurrently by multiple users, and including scanned documents enables the automated patient medical record to become completely automated, with there no longer being a need to have paper documentation. However, a disadvantage of scanned documents over automated documentation is that, other than text that is part of the index, text in scanned documents is usually not available for searching.

When the automated system is down, care would probably be done through paper documentation. This paper documentation could later entered through the automated system or, alternatively, be scanned and included in the automated record.

10.8 EMERGING TECHNOLOGY

Another obstacle in the automation of the patient medical record is that it likely requires new technology that has not yet matured, or perhaps does not even yet exist. An automated patient medical record system may require distributed technology and perhaps Internet type technology, i.e., distributed but independently controlled systems. In order to make this feasible, very high-speed networks will be required.

Multiple caregivers may be viewing or updating the patient chart at the same time. This requires *group communication* capabilities (UsabilityFirst 2002) that enable control over view of the patient chart information by multiple caregivers at the same time with possible updating at the same time.

Use of a computer during examining and interviewing the patient, could potentially detract from patient care. Use of a pen computer during the examination of the patient, where the pen computer has the appearance of the paper chart, can create greater personalization of care. Pen computers fall into two categories: a *handheld* computer (a pen computer that can be held in one hand) and a *tablet* (sometimes also called a *slate*) computer (a pen computer about the width and length of a standard, 8 ½" x 11", sheet of paper); the one appropriate for direct medical care is the tablet computer (Jones 2002). Pen computers have various methods of conveying information between the pen computer and the automated patient chart system; wireless communication, if it had no complications, would provide for the most personalization of care. Research is required to determine if the wireless communication considered, whether infrared or spread-spectrum, will have complications; some reports of conflicts of cellular phones with defibrillators have been reported, which indicate that there may be problems with spread-spectrum, but, on the other hand, infrared has its limitations also—infrared is point of light communication and thus cannot go through walls or turn corners.

Both where the patient medical record will be stored and the standards to be used for the format of the stored patient medical record need to be determined. Storage and quick retrieval of the large volume of information in the patient medical records for an HMO may require super high speed networks and archival storage media capable of storing huge amounts of information cost effectively, perhaps tape cartridges or optical disk, and SANs (Storage Area Networks).

Automation of the patient medical record involves distributed n-tier technology, where computers of different types and manufacturers, and having differing operating systems, can be connected, whether through an Intranet or other connections.

Much of the above is, at the very least, emerging technology. Research dealing with such technology is discussed more in sections 17.2 and 17.3.

10.9 TECHNICAL OBSOLESCENCE AND OBSOLESCENCE DUE TO CHANGING STANDARDS

Because technology needed for automation of the patient medical record is changing so rapidly and because standards for a national or international patient health record have not be agreed upon as of yet, any system to automate the patient medical record has the potential of becoming quickly obsolete with upcoming technical changes and changes in standards. This is another potential obstacle to the automation of the patient medical record.

Also, because personal computers, networks, distributed systems and operating system software are changing so rapidly, any hardware or operating system that is bought now will become virtually obsolete in about two or three years. However, this is simply a fact of life about current personal computer and distributed system technology. Early large-scale investments in a hardware or distributed system infrastructure may thus not be cost effective; one approach might be to delay implementation at a location until just before the hardware is needed at the location so as to maximum the life of the hardware.

10.10 SECURITY AND CONFIDENTIALITY

Another obstacle to the automation of the patient medical record is that patient medical record information would potentially become available to more people, and thus there is greater potential of problems with the security and confidentiality of patient medical information.

Laws and **standards** must be set for patient medical record information electronically transmitted outside the HMO. Where HMOs have direct alliances and "point of service" agreements **direct agreements** between the HMO and the outside organizations might also apply. Where HMOs are dealing with patient medical record information in non-affiliated healthcare organizations, laws and standards only must suffice. Healthcare organizations should also have **confidentiality agreements** with its employees.

Together, these laws, standards, direct agreements, and confidentialty agreements would determine

- who is allowed to view the patient medical record information
- who is able to update it
- at what points the patient medical record for a particular encounter can no longer be changed
- the legality of electronic signatures
- who may do ordering
- who may order narcotics
- etc.

Laws and organizational standards may exist for certain categories of information in the chart, including HIV and genetic test results, psychiatric care, abortions, etc. There may also be standards across healthcare organizations.

Patients are entitled to confidentiality of their own health care information. Claims for invasion of privacy might be made against a health organization that allows release of patient medical record information to an unauthorized person. For example, the patient must be protected against the fear of being discriminated against because he is tested HIV positive, the fear of being harassed due to having an abortion, or the fear that an insurance company might drop her due to having a gene that predisposes her to breast cancer or colon cancer (e.g., women with the mutated BRCA 1 gene have up to an 85% chance of developing breast cancer and up to a 60 percent chance of developing ovarian cancer sometime in their lives).

In some healthcare organizations there may be department specific security rules that were developed and agreed upon at a facility or healthcare organization level, but getting an agreement to extend such security rules beyond the single healthcare organization level may be very difficult or impossible. For example, at one healthcare organization, the genetics department wanted its charts viewable only by personnel in the genetics departments; on the other hand, oncologists would want to know if a woman had the BRCA 1 gene. The psychiatry department wanted its charts viewable only by personnel in the psychiatry departments; on the other hand, ED physicians wanted the whole patient's medical record available to them. This agreement in one healthcare organization might be difficult to extend beyond the healthcare organization.

Laws on security and confidentiality of patient charts may differ from state to state and thus complicate creating a national, or international, patient record.

Access to patient medical record information without identification of the patient might be provided to research institutions. This allows for large-scale studies of a drug, procedure or treatment plan and allows for picking of ideal target patient populations for clinical research (although the researcher might have to be restricted from knowing the identities of the patients).

Methods of legally identifying caregivers, e.g., by user logons and passwords, and methods of auditing chart information access (keeping an *audit trail*), must be established. There must be methods of controlling what information a user is allowed to access or change, of insuring that information is not sabotaged or accidentally destroyed, of insuring that information is not made inconsistent with other information, and of insuring that medical information that is signed off and part of the patient's permanent record will be preserved, yet can be corrected.

A report on electronic medical records systems privacy was done by a committee of the National Research Council in 1997 and commissioned by the National Library of Medicine, an agency within the U.S. Public Health Service's National Institute of Health (CSTB 1997). The committee's recommendations on improving electronic medical record security included the following (Morrissey 1997):

- Every employee with a legitimate need to know about information in a record should have a unique identifier or password, and anyone who shares a password or leaves records unattended at computers should be punished.
- Organizations should use additional access controls to restrict employees from getting information not necessary for their jobs. Electronic audits should be conducted routinely to track all access to clinical data.
- Points in a system that are vulnerable or set up for remote access should be strongly protected through special software, encrypted passwords or "dedicated" modem lines that carry no other electronic traffic.

- Organizations should encrypt all patient-identifiable information before transmitting it over public networks such as the Internet. That includes e-mail and messages between caregivers.
- HHS and the U.S. Office of Computer Affairs should develop a visible, central point of contact about privacy issues—a privacy ombudsman. The government ombudsman could field complaints from patients about privacy breaches.

These and other security ideas were considered for the final version HIPAA, a law governing security of electronic transactions to Medicare for government payment of medical services and all medical communications between healthcare organizations and groups or people outside the healthcare organization. HIPAA is the Health Insurance Portability and Accountability Act (HIPAA) of 1996 for Medicare and Medicaid programs (CMS 2004). HIPAA includes standards for security and electronic signatures (as well as standards for provider identifiers and taxonomy, electronic transfers, and employer identifiers). Section 13.9.1 and the appendix have more information on HIPAA.

An approach for caregiver security developed in Europe for the European Commission is to provide personal smart cards (computer chips imbedded in credit cards) to caregivers to gain access to healthcare systems, using RSA encryption algorithms (TrustHealth 1997). The project's name is Trustworthy Health Telematics (TrustHealth).

Encryption is the transformation of confidential plain text into a cipher text in order to protect it from being read by a third party. Encryption may have its own problems, including slowing performance, making it more difficult to detect computer viruses, and making it harder to detect when someone outside your system is maliciously accessing your patient or other information.

Perhaps smart cards could also be used for patient access to their own records through the automated system. A patient could also carry the equivalent of the CPR with him/her on a smart card. This is an approach fraught with large potential security problems such as unauthorized use and possible legal problems due to the data not being up-to-date. However, accurate information would be extremely beneficial, especially in emergency care situations. In 1987, Mark Landis started a company, Health Information Technologies, to store a patient's medical history and to store patient insurance information, supplying healthcare organizations with card readers. The liability of inaccurate information and patient unwillingness to pay for such cards limited the success of this endeavor (Kaplan 1996).

10.11 UNAVAILABILITY OF THE SYSTEM

The automated patient medical record system may become unavailable at any time, requiring caregivers to go back to a paper system or some lesser-automated system. This might even occur in the middle of a visit.

With the system down, automated clinical practice guidelines and physician and nurse protocols would also be unavailable. They would now have to be on paper.

Unavailability of the automated patient medical record in the outpatient clinic and Emergency Department (ED) is no different than situations that commonly occur now: the chart can be found, the chart has not arrived, the patient has not been seen before.

Unavailability of patient information in the inpatient setting could be a much bigger problem than unavailability in the outpatient setting. If the automated patient medical record system came down in the hospital, then suddenly all the patient information that the clinical staff was using, and relied upon for communication between them and for patient care, might suddenly disappear.

One possible solution to this is to periodically print the automated patient medical record information at the unit. Such printed information, though not necessarily up-to-date, would most likely provide enough information to smoothly continue taking care of the patients in the unit.

Another possible solution is to save the current inpatient chart information at the unit for all patients in the unit on storage media that could later be available to the local computers. When other parts of the automated patient medical record system went down, the local computer could use this stored information. This works as long as the local computers do not go down also.

Thus, in summary, if the automated patient medical record system came down, then two ways of continuing are the following: (1) Run from local computers from previous patient information stored locally. (2) Continue care from paper, possible using patient information printed periodically, and either input the patient information later into the automated system or scan the paper documents to include them in the automated system.

Once the failed component(s) come back up, patient medical record information recorded when the system was down must be sent to the automated patient medical record system. If the information was recorded in a local computer, it must be uploaded. If the information was recorded on paper, it must first be entered into the system; this could be done either by entering information into the automated system directly or by scanning the paper documents to include them in with the automated patient medical record in image form together with textual indexes.

It is absolutely essential that patient medical record information not be permanently lost because of a disk failure. A number of ways exist to protect against such disk failures, referred to as "fault tolerance". Methods of fault tolerance include disk mirroring, writing the same information on two different disks with two different controllers, and striping using three or more disks and controllers and keeping the data on one disk and parity data on another disk; if data is lost, it can be reconstructed from data on the other disks. A method of using standard, lower cost, disks to do this is called RAID technology with RAID-1 being disk mirroring and RAID-5 involving striping (Patterson, Gibson, and Katz 1987).

Other forms of fault tolerance handle abnormal termination of programs due to software errors via *checkpoint/rollback*, rolling back database updates occurring during the program so the database(s) are not inconsistent or otherwise corrupted.

Methods of assuring the parts of the automated system do not go down for very long after a power failure are to provide emergency power in servers via generators and UPSs (uninterruptible power supplies) for workstations.

Excluding these short unplanned outages every now and then (and recovery procedures), the automated patient medical record system must be available 24 hours a day, seven days a week, every day of the year.

10.12 RELIABILITY, PERFORMANCE AND SCALABILITY REQUIREMENTS

Reliability is the measure of how well a software system provides the services expected of it by its users, including up time, accuracy of information, and speed in operation. (Up time was discussed somewhat in the last section, specifically, what to do when the system is not up.)

Reliability is an intertwined web. Unless caregivers use the automated patient medical record system for input of virtually all patient clinical information, then this information will not be easily accessible, as much of the information will still be stored on paper in chart rooms—which would defeat the whole purpose of an automated patient medical record system—scanning the paper documents can be an alternative, although a costly one. If the system is down quite often, slow in operation, or does not provide significant benefits to the users, the users will not use the system unless perhaps coerced. Coercion, in turn, makes for a high turnover of users, which also decreases the reliability of the system.

Part of reliability is accuracy of patient clinical information. If a caregiver questions the data, then it is much less useful, as any time-savings that would be accrued from immediacy of information through an automated system, would be eaten up by the caregiver having to extensively re-verify significant portions of the patient clinical information. An important aspect of accuracy of information is real-time communication between clinical systems, as data that must be entered many different times in many different systems without immediate synchronization, has a high probability of being inconsistent.

When a computer system is not powerful enough to handle all the users, then the users may have to wait an unduly long period of time to receive back responses to what they have entered; such lack of system *performance* could cause a user to lose his or her train of thought. Performance monitoring, measuring the performance of an automated system while it is in operation, to monitor response time as well as other performance characteristics is important in a system as large and complicated as the automated patient medical record system with its many computers, networks and users. Highly loaded parts of the system, and bottlenecks in the system, should be identified as soon as possible so that these parts of the system could be enhanced ahead of time. In computer terms, a *bottleneck* is a system component that limits the performance of the system (Cline 1999).

Performance testing is a carefully designed, repeatable experiment used to evaluate the performance characteristics of an automated system, hardware or application (Cline 1999). Performance testing should first be done immediately before the automated system is implemented in the implementation step. Performance monitoring could be based upon scripts mimicking user input developed in the business reengineering step; see section 11.7.

Capacity is the ability of an automated system, including computer, hardware, software and network systems, to handle an anticipated number of users and customers and is related to performance. Automated systems must not only handle the anticipated initial number of users and customers but additional ones later in the future. *Scalability* is the ability of an automated system to handle the future number of users and customers and is related to future performance.

Business planners and capacity planners should be significantly involved in the evaluation step, advising the organization about the feasibility of planned hardware, including networks, and planned system software to handle the current capacity and performance required and advising the organization about the future scalability of the system to take care of anticipated increases in capacity. Capacity and scalability evaluations are difficult at this stage because (1) during the project, the system is likely to be used at more and more locations with increases in capacity required; (2) the requirements for the system are likely to change over the lifetime of the system with resultant increase in the demands of the system; but (3) technology to handle the capacity is likely to change, allowing for increased capacity.

The business planner would anticipate future changes in business requirements for the system over time. The capacity planner would determine if there were indeed capacity and performance concerns.

In the evaluation step, a performance and scalability plan document should be started to record anticipated capacity requirements for automated systems, anticipated needs for upgrading the system, and to identify how and when capacity and performance measurements should be done to evaluate the system.

10.13 OVERWHELMING SIZE OF PROJECT

A major obstacle to automation of the patient medical record is the huge size and cost of such a project.

The amount of work in completely automating the patient chart is overwhelming. Because it is so large, the project must be an iterative, evolutionary, one. But to make this iterative development possible, the entire project must be extensively pre-planned.

For example, an HMO may be composed of a number of regions (e.g., the East, the Midwest, the West and the South) with many facilities in each region. Each region may have alliances with other health care organizations where their patients may also be seen. Because an automated patient medical record system works well when implemented for a single facility or region does not necessarily mean that it can be upgraded to work well for multiple facilities or regions. If the system is not pre-planned to be designed for multiple facilities, regions and organizations, then it is very unlikely that the system would be able to smoothly evolve into a system that could be expanded to completely automate the patient medical record, creating a longitudinal patient record.

As part of implementation of any part of the automated system, criteria for the success of that part of the system should be established with criteria that can be measured. This criteria for success may be improved service for patients, timesaving, improved accuracy of information, or greater monetary reimbursements. Measurements should compensate for a temporary overhead of having both a non-automated and partially automated patient medical record.

Redesign might be required where the success criteria are not realized, with a reconsideration of the effects of the redesign on the entire system. The success criteria of certain parts of the system might simply be that these parts of the system have been completed, as they might not provide any measurable benefit other than being absolutely required to eventually create a useful automated patient medical record system (e.g., establishment of a network, hardware and system software infrastructure, and of other infrastructure items).

10.14 COSTS

A major obstacle to automation of the patient medical record is the huge size and cost of such a project. The costs of an automated patient medical record system could be enormous. Costs are of at least four types:

1. **infrastructure costs:** the costs of virtually everything that is hidden that is connected with the automated patient medical record system. This includes the costs of user, technical and other meetings to design the system, the "blueprints" for the system, the costs of planning for, and making changes, to buildings, including new wiring for the system, logical database design, etc. (These costs are usually substantial and all occur without any visible payoff.)
2. **development and implementation costs:** the costs of developing, installing, and implementing the automated patient medical record software system. This includes the physical database design and the programming, and this includes putting the computers in the pre-planned places in the medical centers.
3. **training and personnel costs:** the costs of training; of lost personnel time due to learning and training, and not doing their normal jobs; and the costs of resistance to the system.

4. **maintenance costs:** the costs of preserving the system so it is not deteriorated and so necessary changes are made to it. The costs include the substantial costs for maintenance staff to service installed hardware and software, support the controlled documentation and identify, prioritize and quickly make maintenance fixes to any parts of the system that may be used by users, with the feedback of these fixes to development staff. (This is a huge cost mainly due to the long time frame that the system undergoes maintenance.)

This section will discuss the minimization of these costs based upon the following ideas:

1. Build the automated patient medical record system correctly
2. Standardize to control scope
3. Build the organizational infrastructure first
4. Measure feasibility before implementing
5. Build iteratively, if possible, identifying and initiating subprojects with early payback
6. For infrastructure outside the organization, use someone else's infrastructure.
7. Encourage component adaptability in the healthcare industry for systems that interface with the automated patient medical record system (e.g., clinical laboratory systems, ADT systems, etc.)

10.14.1 Build the System Correctly

According to reference (Fayad and Cline 1996), costs of any computer system can be minimized via the following means:

- **Design the system right to begin with:** develop requirements for the automated patient medical record system that fit the needs of both the HMO and the general health care community
- **Develop the system right:** make sure that these requirements are built into the system when the system is being developed
- **Build for the next:** build for expandability for the future and anticipated future changes in requirements.

I would also add the following to the list because an automated patient medical record system is such a large project and thus must be developed incrementally:

- **Build for the current and previous:** because the automated patient medical record system must be done gradually, enable current systems, for example, the paper chart system, to function also. (Building the automated patient medical record system is sort of like building a superhighway in the right of way of an old highway: you want old highway to be useable while you build the new one, and thus have to do additional engineering work to do so.)

An additional reason for building for the current and previous is that it is desirable to also include patient clinical information for HMO patients from outside health care organizations that the HMO may have little control over (e.g., hospitals who have alliances with the HMO).

To design the system right to begin with and to do it economically, I think you have to treat such a system, which is largely untried, like other such projects that were new and untried: NASA and the space program, or the building of the Panama Canal. Put together a nucleus of people that have a strong academic interest in the area and are willing to reason out the best ways of doing things, based upon their intellectual interests in the area. Consider the project to be consisting of a number of research areas to be studied (e.g., a CPR repository, searching through the automated patient medical record, distributed systems and network technology, etc.) See Chapter 17 for a discussion of many of these research areas.

Developing the system right is a matter of creating good design requirements, hiring good people, and executing a lot of discipline in following the requirements. Further, the overall design must be validated first before deploying it in possibly many thousands of computers.

For the concept of "build for the next", I will use the term "flexible". For the concept of "build for the current and previous" as well as build for the initial version of the automated patient medical record system, I will use the term "broad". Costs for development and infrastructure can be minimized by creating a system that is *broad* and *flexible*. "Broad" means that it can handle current non-sophisticated solutions for the patient chart (e.g., paper patient charts and e-mail) as well as initial automation of the patient medical record. "Flexible" means that the automated system can be upgraded in capabilities without having to be extensively changed (e.g., the initial automation of the patient medical record can be extended to include a national Patient Health Record with clinical information from other healthcare organizations; business policies can be changed without large changes to the automated patient medical record system).

Examples of "broadness" are the following:

- The automated system can order paper charts, for later manual transport, as well as gather automated patient medical record information transferring the information over computer networks
- Small facilities can send e-mails/messages summarizing patient encounters to the automated system and repositories, while large facilities could send complete patient clinical information
- Besides providing direct input of clinical information through specially formatted GUI (graphical user interface) screens, or through pen input, while interviewing the patient, the system gives the user the option of inputting documents through automated forms that duplicate the paper form so information from paper forms can still be used.

Examples of "flexibility" are the following:

- Interfacing clinical systems are set up to communicate with the automated patient medical record system via established standards (principally via HL7 (Health Level Seven 1997-2003)—see section 12.11.6) so they can be more easily replaced when other improved clinical systems become available
- The automated patient medical record system supports the ability to integrate products from multiple vendors (such as by use of Cooperative Business Objects—see section 11.2.2). (The system must follow "open standards".)
- Future technology, such as gigabit WAN networks and gigabit Ethernet LAN's for transferring diagnostic images and multi-media information or voice technology transcription, can be implemented as needed without large changes to the system. (The future technology must be compatible with open standards.)
- If necessary, systems are developed or purchased that are "portable", i.e., a system is able to run on the different computer system architectures that will be used
- An important part of flexibility is "scalability", those characteristics of system structure that allow it to grow gracefully: the number of users or distributed computers or the data volume can be increased and the system still works and still works efficiently

- Changed health organization business policies can be implemented quickly without significant changes to the system (see section 7.6).

"Broadness" and "flexibility" decrease costs in that the system does not have to be implemented all at once, but can be implemented incrementally. New health care institutions can be quickly made part of the system, even when they currently use unsophisticated technology. The infrastructure required for the automated system (e.g., high-speed networks) can be incorporated as it is needed, not before it is needed.

10.14.2 Standardize to Control Scope

Some CIO's of large corporations (Hewlett-Packard and 3M Corporation) have stated in computer conferences that the way to minimize costs of a new large system is to use only standard, already matured, systems. This means that where more expensive technology is needed in the automated system (e.g., PACS systems), systems should have been around a number of years rather than being state of the art, and, in all other cases, well established standard, preferably identical, computer, server and workstation systems should be implemented throughout the healthcare organization. Only organizationally approved software is allowed. There are a number of reasons this philosophy could minimize overall costs:

1. Standardizing on systems greatly decreases maintenance costs, as there can then be company-wide standard procedures for fixing systems and for providing help to users.
2. Standardization of systems opens up the possibility of remote distribution of new software; otherwise, personnel would have to load the new software individually on each machine.
3. Implementing systems that follow open standards offers greater future flexibility in replacing and matching up systems that make up the automated patient medical record system.
4. Systems would be able to communicate with each other when necessary (e.g., one PACS system could transfer diagnostic images: x-rays, CT scans, etc.) to another system, whereas incompatible systems may not be able to do so).
5. Unique new non-established technology is likely to become obsolete very quickly, as the technology industry either tries to sell a better product or more of an established product in quantity.
6. Problems with incompatible software that does not work together could be avoided.
7. The cost of brand new technology decreases in price as it matures; delaying its implementation usually greatly decreases costs.

10.14.3 Build the Organizational Infrastructure (Correctly) First

The *infrastructure* is virtually everything that is hidden that is connected with the automated patient medical record system. This includes the costs of user, technical and other meetings to design the system, the "blueprints" for the system, the costs of planning for, and making changes, to buildings, including new wiring for the system, logical database design, etc.

The infrastructure of a computer system is analygous to the foundation, structural components, plumbing, electrical works, etc. of a house. If the infrastructure of the house is not done right then something is going go seriously wrong with the house later on, even to the extend that the occupant might get killed by house falling down.

Likewise, many, many future costs of the automated patient medical record system could be saved by doing its infrastructure first and doing it correctly.

10.14.4 Measure Feasibility Before Implementing

Despite any standardization approaches chosen, the automated patient medical record system involves new technology and ideas. Any implementation may involve thousands of workstations and many other computers. Any implementation involves implementing many ideas over and over again. In order to minimize the risks of accidentally implementing a very costly idea, the following should first be done:

- create a *test bed* system where new ideas can be tested and validated
- implement and evaluate the system in a pilot site first
- build the system iteratively, continually evaluating the system, especially early on before too much money is spent.
- do a complete overall design of the system first so every part you build will fit together.

10.14.5 Build Iteratively, Identifying Stand-alone Subprojects with Early Payback

Development and implementation of the automated patient medical record system is of such large scope that it should be broken down into subprojects if possible. Rather than being termed a "project", the automated patient medical record system should probably be termed a "program" consisting of a number of "projects" in order to build it.

Because implementation of the total automated patient medical record system program is of such large scope and will in total have quite a long payback period before it makes money for the HMO, it would be monetarily and psychologically beneficial to search for a phase within the project that could both stand-alone and have a much shorter payback period. Section 5.4.2.8 mentions one such potential subproject: standardize HMO clinical systems with standardized interfaces so they can later be easily integrated with the automated patient medical record system. Such a subproject might have a quick payback in that it would allow the HMO to standardize on "best of breed" clinical systems and thus decrease future costs for system maintenance.

10.14.6 For Infrastructure Outside the Organization, Use Someone Else s Infrastructure

The automated patient medical record system could use the Internet or an equivalent multi-organizational TCP/IP network to get information from CPR's, patient registries and source document repositories. Ideally, the project to automate the patient medical record should piggyback upon the development of the national initiative to create a high-speed gigabit/sec information network often referred to as the National Information Infrastructure (Chatterjee 1997). As reference (Chatterjee 1997) notes, a reason that such a network does not yet exist is that there is not as-of-yet a "killer app" that justifies it. Reference (Chatterjee 1997) postulates that there might be such a set of applications that together constitute this killer app and include the Web, HDTV, healthcare, LAN interconnections and telephony.

Reference (Clark 1998) predicts that, in the future, the Internet will be connected via very high bandwidth fiber optic networks using *WDM (wave length division multiplexing),* essentially using different colors of the spectrum. Such a technology would support data/voice/video integration (DVVI). Such a network could potentially be used by many companies to connect up the Patient Health Record network.

The proposed universal Patient Health Record is an example of a "cross enterprise" system, i.e., a system providing information for multiple businesses, in this case healthcare organizations. With the automated patient medical record system, there are many other possibilities for such systems. Outside organizations could store "source documents" electronically in source documents repositories for healthcare organizations; a healthcare organization might eventually no longer need to have its own chart rooms or source document repositories. Interpretations of diagnostic images could also be done by other companies, with the electronic diagnostic images being electronically sent to them and the interpretations returned electronically. The automated patient medical record system could organize worker's compensation related medical information for a patient and send the information directly to insurance company of the patient's employer. There is the potential for many different forms of "cross enterprise" transactions.

There are new techniques for securing information sent through the Internet or similar multi-organizational networks. One approach is the Virtual Private Network (VPN). A VPN provides encryption to the sender and decryption by the receiver so the connection across the Internet is secure. This is done by a technique called "tunneling". Tunneling works by encapsulating a network protocol (e.g., that of the automated patient medical record system) within packets carried by the other network (e.g., the Internet).

10.14.7 Encourage Component Adaptability in the Healthcare Industry

Component adaptability is the use of various strategies to procure, develop or structure a system or component of a system so that the system or component can more easily be replaced in the future by another equivalent system or component. As a result of component adaptability, parts of the automated patient medical record system could be replaced to scale or improve the system rather than having to replace the entire system—this could save significant money for the healthcare organization.

For example, healthcare organizations can insist that clinical laboratory systems have standard interfaces that allow one clinical laboratory system to be replaced by any other. Section 13.12 later explains component adaptability in more detail.

Component adaptability is particularly pertinent to the healthcare industry where there are already many existing standards. The appendix describes many of these standards.

With even more stringent healthcare standards such as the development of strict standards for interfaces for the various types of clinical systems (e.g., admission, discharge and transfer hospital systems, clinical laboratory systems) and standards for a computer-based patient record, component adaptability would become even more of a reality. Healthcare organizations with an interest in implementing an automated patient medical record system should encourage the healthcare industry to work toward such component adaptability standards.

10.15 ADDITIONAL BUSINESS REQUIREMENTS AND CONTINGENCY PLANS DUE TO OBSTACLES

These obstacles to creation of an automated patient medical record—more formally termed risks—can be resolved in a number of ways (1) creating new business requirements that *mitigate* the risk, (2) developing a *contingency plan* to follow if a risk, which is not guaranteed to occur indeed occurs, (3) waiting for future advancements (e.g., new standards), (4) doing research on the risk. Table 10.1 identifies obstacles (risks) and how they could be resolved.

Besides goals being set for project objectives, goals can also be set for business requirements. For each business requirement, obstacle or research product, table 10.1 also identifies a goal that might be used to measure progress toward and final achievement of the business requirement, resolution of the obstacle, or success of the product developed by the research.

Table 10.1 Obstacles and Business Requirements, Contingency Plans or Required Research

Number	*Obstacle*	*Previous or New Requirement / Contingency Plan / Research*	*Requirements / Contingency Plans*	*Metrics for Goals Measuring the Business Requirement or the Success of the Contingency Plan*
1	Physician Acceptance of System	Previous Requirement	Reengineer the care process based upon input from employees so that employees' work activities match the most productive and least stressful methods of providing care.	Survey employees to determine if they feel they are providing quality care, are productive or are under stress.
		New Requirement	Provide quick log-on and sign-off of the system, so the caregiver spends very little time logging on and off the computer.	Is there a way to quickly log on and off and then back on the system? Do the large majority of caregivers agree with the approach?
		Previous Requirements	Provide demonstrative benefits to all caregivers who use the system. Various requirements do this.	Survey caregivers to determine if the automated patient medical record provides overwhelming benefits to caregivers.
2	Existing paper charts	Previous Requirement	Include the recording of the location of paper charts within the automated medical record system.	Determine the percentage of encounters in the automated patient medical record system for which there are paper charts and whose locations can be immediately identified.

3	Lack of agreed upon standards	Previous Requirements	Use existing standard HL7 for communication with other healthcare organization clinical systems. Study creating common clinical systems within the organization.	What are the numbers and percentages of clinical systems using HL7? Of common clinical systems compared to the total of clinical systems?
		New Requirement / Research	Create a Master Patient Index to translate patient identifiers or equivalent approach to translate local information to national formats. This requires further analysis.	For each set of clinical systems, determine if the identity of a patient can be recognized in one clinical system that was entered in another clinical system.
		Contingency Plan	Working with applicable standard organizations to get standards compatible with what the HMO needs.	Can a chosen standard handle the requirements of the HMO?
4	Existing clinical systems and redundant information	Previous Requirement	The automated patient medical system and other clinical systems when gathering information on patients, providers, encounters, orders and results will communicate this information to the other clinical systems via network interfaces or databases.	If a clinical system is the first to learn about an encounter, order or result, is the automated patient medical record system immediately informed about it? If the automated patient medical record system is the first to learn about it, are all clinical systems that make use of the information immediately informed of the information?
		New Requirement	Use common databases and interfaces between the automated patient medical record system and other clinical systems to insure all clinical information needs to be entered only once.	Count the cases of redundant information in clinical systems.

5	Required Reengineering	Previous Requirements	Do reengineering along with development of the automated medical record system.	Count unnecessary and high cost steps in caregiver workflow.
6	System, because of its size, is an evolving one	New Requirement	Completely design the system first so you can build in the "hooks" for future parts of the system and include necessary information.	Identify future additions to the system and determine the percentage of these where the "hooks" for future interfaces and the projected necessary data is built into the system.
7	Maintenance of the paper chart must be continued	Previous Requirement	Include the recording of paper charts within the automated medical record system.	Take a representative set of patients and determine what percentage of the time the system knows the location of all paper chart information for a patient.
		New Requirement	Plan on keeping, but phasing down chart rooms, for paper charts.	Count the number of chart rooms and number of chart room personnel. Count the number of medical records still on paper.
		New Requirement	Study scanning of current paper charts or archiving on media such as optical disk.	Count the number of scanned and archived medical record documents.
8	Emerging technology	Research	Do research on use of the Internet for display of the automated patient chart.	Compare provider satisfaction with use of the Internet for display of the automated patient medical record versus other methods, and identify any security considerations.
		Research	Do research on system software necessary to incorporate group communication capabilities, i.e., multiple caregiver access to the automated chart.	Query caregivers to determine the usefulness of creating, updating and view of the automated patient medical record by multiple caregivers. Is data corrupted? Does locking unnecessarily restrict caregivers?

		Research	Do analysis on best input techniques, including possible use of pen computers.	Survey caregivers to determine if they are happy with the input methods provided and that they care receive adequate information on the patient? Survey patients to determine if input methods provided get in the way of care.
		Research	Study requirements for high volume, high speed, storage for the automated patient medical record and available hardware.	Based upon stress testing software running the automated chart system, verify that the system can handle the peak load expected in X months. Based upon vendor hardware specifications and contractual guarantees, insure that system software and hardware is scalable for Y years.
9	Technical obsolescence	New Requirement	Plan for the future to not be technically obsolete.	(Non-measurable goal)
10	Security and confidentiality laws	Contingency Plan	Lobby for laws that allow sharing and security of chart information in different states, especially those where the HMO is located.	Count the number of favorable and unfavorable laws past. How significant is the favorable or unfavorable law that was passed?
		Contingency Plan	Work for standards or lobby for laws on privacy of special category patient information such as psychiatric information, genetic information.	Count the number of favorable and unfavorable special category laws past and standards agreed upon. How significant is the favorable or unfavorable law or standard?
		New Requirement	Use HCFA standards for electronic signatures.	Are HCFA standards for electronic signatures followed?
		New Requirement	Keep an audit trail of those who access the chart.	Is there an audit trail of every user, including external users, who access the patient medical record?

		Previous Requirement	Provide medical research databases (data warehouses) to allow access to clinical information without determination of the identify of the patient.	Is access to patient identity disallowed for categories of users who do not have the need to know? Survey medical researchers to determine if they are satisfied with the information they can retrieve from this medical research data warehouse.
		Previous Requirement	Provide a controlled ability to get names of patients for clinical trials based upon identified clinical criteria (patient is post menopausal and has migraine headaches).	Is access to patient identity allowed for categories of users who do have the need to know? Survey medical researchers to determine if they are satisfied with the information they can retrieve which identifies the patient.
		New Requirement	Provide authentication (identification of the user) and authorization (identification of what the user can access).	For a representative sets of users, does the system appropriately exclude or allow user access to the system? Does it appropriately exclude or allow user access to resources?
		Research	Do research on smart cards, biometrics, time out and other techniques for user access security.	Select a representative of users and sophisticated non-users and verify access is allowed or disallowed for each. Measure the speed of access. Survey users for satisfaction with access.
		Research	Do research on encryption for securing access across networks.	Tap network line before and after encryption verifying information is encrypted.
11	Unavailability of the system	New Requirement	Allow entrance of information through a local computer when a server or host computers are down.	Disconnect connection to servers. Observe care both before and after disconnection and evaluate negative effects, if any. Survey users for problems giving care, if any, when servers are disconnected and recovery procedures are followed.

		New Requirement	Build in fault tolerance into the system such as RAID disk drives, checkpoint/rollback, etc.	Create checkpoint/rollback situations and verify that interrupted tasks are rolled back correctly and system otherwise functions.
		New Requirement	Provide methods to keep the system up 24 hours, 7 days of the week, such as mirrored systems.	Record and total all downtimes. By hardware manufacturer specifications, bring down one set of mirrored drives to verify system still functions correctly.
		New Requirement	Enable use of documentation on paper forms that may be input into the computer later.	Have caregiver input by supported paper forms with input later within the automated system or scanning of the paper documents. Survey users or personnel entering the information about their satisfaction with the process.
12	Reliability requirements	New Requirement	Insure data is accurate by keeping it synchronized with other automated systems.	Identify where data is not synchronized by testing multiple systems to identify where data used by one system is not passed from another system where the data is entered.
		New Requirement	Use performance monitoring to identify bottlenecks in the system. Take actions to correct the bottlenecks before they hurt the system.	Count bottlenecks. Keep mean time to identify and fix each bottleneck.
13	Size of project	New Requirement	Pre-plan as much of the system as possible, using open architecture, so the system is can grow (i.e., is scalable).	Are there plans for scalability "x" months into the future? Were the plans for scalability "x" months ago adequate to handle the true scalability?

		New Requirement	Define mechanisms to evaluate the success of the system, such as improved service for patients, time savings, improved accuracy of information, return on investment.	Measure wait times for patients and caregivers, cost per patient encounter relative to condition, patient satisfaction, etc.
14	Costs	New Requirement	Build the system for flexibility and broadness as defined in this chapter.	Survey business, system and technical analysts to determine if they think flexibility and broadness has been built into the system according to specifications s or the actual system.
		New Requirement	Standardize on hardware and software.	What percentage of the clinical systems, including the automated medical record system, software and hardware in the system is standardized?
		New Requirement	Create a test bed for testing new ideas before implementation on a wider scale.	Is there a test bed? Have technical personnel verify that it is useful in predicting the future system.
		New Requirement	Design as much up front as possible. Build the system iteratively.	Count the number of instances of redesign. What percentage of time is the redesign not anticipated?
		New Requirement	Standardize on "best of breed" clinical systems using agreed-upon healthcare computer system standards such as HL7.	Push for component adaptability in the industry for clinical systems. What percentage of clinical systems are standardized? Of the existing clinical systems, what percentage use HL7 to communicate with other clinical systems and use other identified healthcare computer system standards?

		Contingency Plan	Encourage development of a national, shared cost, very high speed, secure network for healthcare.	Is there a national, shared cost, very high speed, secure network for healthcare? If not, push this effort, developing a network that could evolve into such a network.
15	Current and future capacity, performance and scalability	Contingency Plan	Determine if the anticipated systems, with current technology, could handle projected capacity and performance requirements, including number of users, database requests and network traffic. Inform the organization if the system is not currently feasible. If feasible, identify the maximum number of users and database requests, and maximum volume of network traffic that can be handled.	Is there a contingency plan to handle growth beyond maximum limits?

Key Terms

audit trial
bottleneck
broad
capacity
checkpoint/rollback
component adaptability
confidentiality agreement
contingency plan
direct agreement
flexible
group communication
handheld computer
HL7 application network protocol
infrastructure
laws
obstacle
performance
performance testing
reengineering
reliability
scalability
slate computer
standardization
standard
tablet computer
test bed
WDM (wave length division multiplexing

Study Questions

1. Obstacles are studied for what two principal purposes? What is a contingency plan?
2. Why is physician acceptance of the automated patient medical record system important?
3. What are two ways of integrating paper medical records into the universal patient record?
4. What information does the automated patient medical record system need from other clinical systems?
5. Why is reengineering of the healthcare organization needed when the automated patient medical record system is implemented?
6. What U.S. law has resulted in definition of major security and confidentiality standards for the medical record?
7. If the automated patient medical record system went down, what are two potential ways that documentation could be recorded?
8. What is reliability? Performance? Capacity? Scalability?
9. What are ways of making an automated patient medical record system or universal patient record less costly?

CHAPTER 11

Reengineering the HMO for the Automated Patient Medical Record

CHAPTER OUTLINE

11.1 PROJECT CONTEXT: BUSINESS REENGINEERING OF AN ORGANIZATION FOR A PROJECT

Business reengineering is rethinking and redesigning business processes to achieve quantum improvements in the performance of the business, which may be improvements in cost, quality, service or speed. In the business reengineering step of a project, employee workflows, user interfaces, and business policies would be determined that would accomplish these improvements. These changes would be determined from

1. talks with employees
2. future organizational business policies of the organization
3. the anticipated new way the organization would function (in our case, as identified in chapter 8, describing the future environment and system).

For our automated patient medical record system project in an HMO, the future users include inpatient and outpatient physicians, inpatient and outpatient nurses, and others. Future workflows are determined for each category of user.

Figure 11.1, previously shown in figure 2.2, shows the business reengineering step within the overall design: the first part of a project is to plan the complete project.

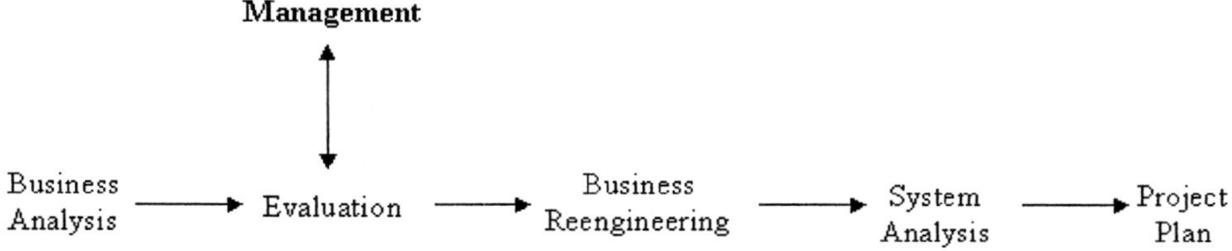

Figure 11.1 Steps Within the Overall Design.

Figure 11.2, previously shown in figure 2.6, shows the details of the business reengineering step. The business reengineering step consists of the following activities:

1. Define the workflows of various categories of caregivers
2. Define the business policies of the organization
3. For automated systems, define the business objects to be used in user interfaces, define the user interfaces for each category of user, and keep user interfaces in synchronization with databases and interface information from other systems.

11.1.1 Define the Workflows of Various Categories of Workers

A *workflow* is sequence of activities of a business. Different categories of workers have different workflows.

Different categories of workers impacted by the project are identified, such as listed in section 4.2. For each category of worker, a changed workflow as it would be after the project or phase was complete is developed.

11.1.2 Define the Business Policies of the Organization

A *business policy* is a policy to be applied throughout an organization. Business policies may be implemented in number of ways:

- by changed employee procedures, workflows and user interfaces—see section 11.4
- by storage of data on databases, by code, or by interfaces between systems—this will be discussed in later chapters.

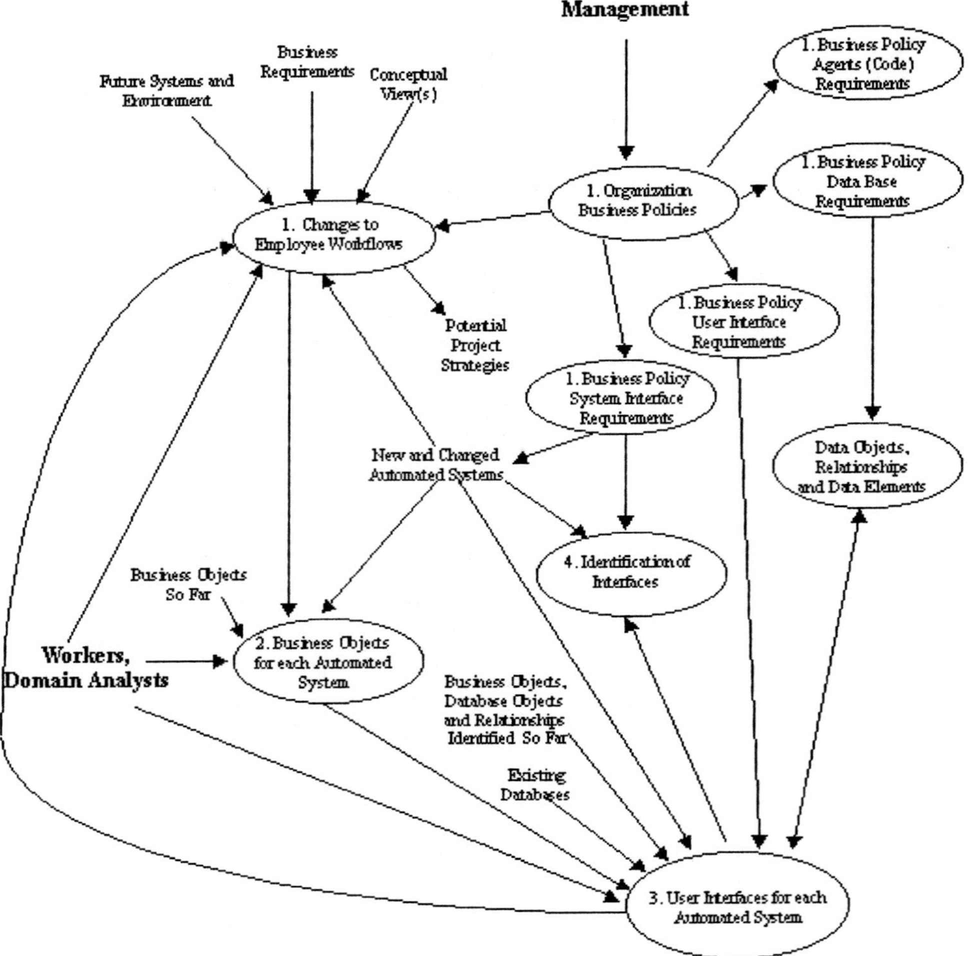

Figure 11.2 business reengineering step: workflows and user interfaces.

11.1.3 Define the Business Objects to be Used in the User Interfaces

In order to make user interfaces easier, it is useful to first define *business objects* that are objects that the users use in real life in the business, e.g., patients, the patient chart, etc. User interfaces may be defined in terms of these business objects. See section 11.5.3, Model User Objects. These business objects are used both within any new user interfaces and within databases.

11.1.4 Define the User Interfaces

A *user interface* is the part of a computer program that displays on the screen for the user to see and the user interactions it allows. A *graphical user interface (GUI)* is a user interface that makes use of every addressable pixel on the screen and thus makes it possible to create detailed visual symbols for user navigation, characters, pictures, and lines; a GUI consists of dialog boxes. A *dialog box* is a window that a GUI program displays to prompt a reply from a user.

The user interfaces may be defined in terms of dialog boxes and user interactions, written requirements for these user interfaces, or both. For vendor systems, only written requirements are likely to result. For a new system developed in house, a complete description of the user interfaces for the entire system would result; for a changed system developed in house, a description of changed user interfaces would result. When user interfaces are defined in terms of screens without any underlying functioning code or databases, this is referred to as *prototyping*.

A monitor with a screen and a keyboard or other input devices is a *terminal.* A typewriter-type *keyboard* comes with terminals for all types of computer except for a few pen computers. A pen computer enables *pen* input by the user printing or writing and selecting on a screen via a stylus.

A *cursor* is a flashing line, square, rectangle or other symbol on the computer screen that moves when you move the mouse or other pointing device and can also be moved around via characters or character combinations entered through the keyboard. For some terminals connected with mainframes (very large computers) only keyboard input is supported. For PCs, pointer devices are included.

A *pointer device* allows a user to move the cursor and make a selection at the cursor point. Examples of pointer devices are the *mouse* (a device when moved across a flat surface, a ball on the bottom causes the cursor to be moved on the screen), the *touch pad* (A pointer device that works by sensing the user's finger movement and downward pressure) and the *trackball* (a pointer device that is essentially an upside-down mouse that rotates in place within a socket.).

11.1.5 Keep User Interfaces in Synchronization With Databases and Data from Other Systems

Most all of the data displayed or input through user interfaces comes from or will be stored on databases. Thus user interfaces and databases must be kept in synchronization. Additional data for user interfaces may come from direct interfaces with other systems; this data must also be identified. Other information comes from data entered by the user that is transitory.

11.2 PROTOTYPING

When a new computer software system is being introduced as part of the project, there is a way to evaluate the system's effects upon the organization prior to completion of the system. This approach is called prototyping.

Prototyping is the process of developing and interacting with a partial version of a system in order to gain user feedback and to evaluate feasibility. A prototype appears to provide all the functionality of the final system, but parts of the system are left out (e.g., there are likely no databases, no interfaces to other systems, and the actual functioning of the system is missing).

Prototyping is vastly misunderstood. To explain prototyping better, we use an analogy of building a house.

In designing a house, potential buyers, the architects, civil engineers, plumbers, electricians, city building code people and others get together. Blueprints are created to capture the agreed-upon design of the house, including floor plans, foundations, roofs, structural components, electrical fixtures, etc.

A scale model of the house may be created for potential buyers to look at. Potential buyers may look at the model to see if this is the kind house they would want to buy.

Then the contractors, carpenters, plumbers, electricians and others get together to actually build the house. Building the house is based upon the blueprints.

Now, by the time the scale model was created, lots and lots of hard work has already been done. This work includes all the thought-work in designing the house along with buyers, electricians, plumbers, civil engineers, etc., and in doing the blueprints. The building of the house may in fact be a much easier process than the design part, with the building part only being hard because of the time consumed to do it. Of course, you could have created a quick scale model without the design process, but there is no guarantee that such a house would be structurally sound, fit the appropriate lot, or pass building inspections.

What is the purpose of the scale model of the house? To have *potential* buyers look at the proposed house. These potential buyers would determine if they liked the house or not. If enough potential buyers liked the house, then the contractor probably would go ahead with building one or more houses.

On the other hand, if no potential buyers liked the scale model of the house, then the contractor would probably either (1) scrape everything! or (2) start all over again with the design process (and probably create a completely new scale model)!

What has this to do with the automated patient medical record system? Well, the design part up to creating blueprints for the house is equivalent to getting users, database people, technical people, caregivers, patients, and others together to design the automated system, and the business analysts and software engineers to write all the specifications for the system. The scale model of the house is equivalent to creating a prototype of the automated patient medical record system, usually including screens. And the actual building of the house is equivalent to actually building the automated patient medical record system, i.e., programming it.

For the house, potential buyers look at the scale model to see if this house is acceptable to them. Likewise, for the automated patient medical record system, potential users look at the prototype to see if the system is appropriate for them—the results of this process are similar that for the house: (1) the users either accept the system, only making cosmetic changes that do not structurally change the design, (3) the design is started over again, or (2) everything is scraped.

What have we learned here about prototyping? A lot of design work precedes prototyping, and if the users do not like the prototype, then what is likely to happen is that the previous design will be scraped and the design process must be started all over again!

What are the advantages of doing a scale model or a prototype? If we started the building of the house instead of doing the scale model for the potential buyers, then many houses may have been built that no buyers would have bought! Likewise, if we started building the automated patient medical record system instead of doing the prototype for the potential users, then a system may have been created that few users would want to use!

A prototype is not to be confused with a conceptual view. A user interface can be presented as a conceptual view, but it must be treated as such: the conceptual view is presented to generate or demonstrate ideas that provide input in the design process. A "conceptual view" is like a "rough sketch". A "prototype" is a potential product that must fit together in all respects.

11.3 DEFINING CHANGED WORKFLOWS

Changing workflows as a result of a project involves

1. identifying the future users of the project and its software systems,
2. determining their current workflows, and
3. changing workflows to anticipate needed workflows once the project or phase is complete.

For our automated patient medical record system project in an HMO, the future users include inpatient and outpatient physicians, inpatient and outpatient nurses, medical assistants, and others. Future workflows are determined for each category of user.

For the current workflows,

- identify current processes within the workflow
- identify processes with a high potential for improvement
- identify processes of high value to patients, caregivers or the organization that should be kept
- identify the roles and responsibilities of individuals in the organization involved in the workflows
- understand the goals of the overall organization
- understand how departments work together and how the organization works with outside organizations.

For the future workflows,

- provide a mechanism for extensive employee input into workflow changes, as changing workflows is a social, as well as a technical and business process
- develop new, more efficient, processes within each workflow identifying processes that should be kept, added, changed and eliminated while preserving the relationships between the processes
- align individual roles and responsibilities with those of the business, modifying processes if required
- optimize interdepartmental communications and communications with other organizations, often with medical assistants. (A *medical assistant* is a healthcare professional who performs a variety of clinical, clerical and administrative duties within a healthcare setting)
- formulate complete blueprints for revised workflows
- design the automated system to support the workflows and overall goals of the organization
- allow enough room for employee initiative, expertise and creativity, and control over their own destinies
- provide fallback modes of operation when things go wrong (such as computer failures, power failures, etc.) or unusual circumstances (such as emergency situations)

- set future ways to measure and monitor success of the organization with respect to the workflows and automated systems.

A diagrammatic method for modeling current workflows and new workflows in detail are *Data Flow Diagrams (DFDs).* For example, see figure 11.3 for a DFD showing a simplified workflow for a nurse practitioner (NP). In the DFD, a named curved line identifies communication of information. A bubble, called a process, portrays transformation of information. A straight line points to a data store, a place to store information (a data base, paper document or other medium of recording information).

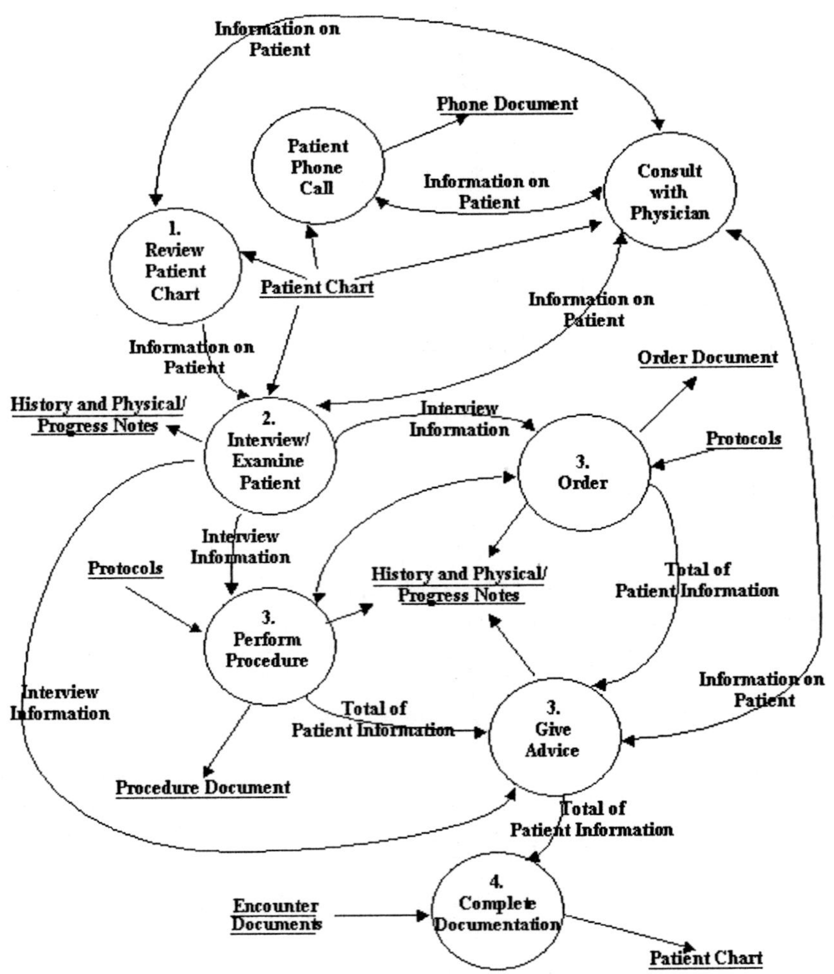

Figure 11.3 Simplified Nurse Practitioner Workflow.

The DFD shows the following: A nurse practitioner sees patients or makes phone calls to patients. In all her major activities, the nurse practitioner consults with a lead physician or follows protocols. Before a patient comes in, she reviews the chart. When the patient comes in she examines and interviews the patient, usually creating a History and Physical or Progress Note document to be put in the chart. Nurse practitioners can make orders or perform procedures according to protocol; she documents these activities, which may require a physician to co-sign a **document. In the last part of the patient encounter, she gives advice to the patient, documenting this information. After the patient leaves, she may complete all her documentation on the patient, and she puts the documentation in the chart.**

Reengineering workflows has been referred to as Business Process Reengineering (BPR). Although popularized by Michael Hammer and James Champy in the 1993 book, *Reengineering the Corporation: A Manifesto for Business Revolution* (Champy and Hammer 1993), BPR is quite old. In fact, the process of workflow analysis has been automated, using more sophisticated models than DFDs.

There are at least two types of software systems to model workflow: *workflow systems*, where a business is described by processes, discrete activities that make up the business practices of an organization or of a part of a business, and where these processes are analyzed, and *discrete event simulation* (Law et al. 1999), where, in addition to defining the business processes, the time of each process takes is statistically evaluated and the total expected time of a workflow can be evaluated. A standard for the former, workflow systems, has been established by consortium of companies by the Workflow Management Coalition (Pyke 2004).

Within the workflows for each category of user, the use of existing and new automated systems is then identified. For each new automated system, an analysis must then be done for each class of users to define appropriate user interfaces, with commonality between interfaces also identified so these parts of the user interfaces for the new automated system can be combined; section 11.5 describes a process for defining user interfaces. For each existing system, changes to user interfaces are identified.

11.4 IMPLEMENTING BUSINESS POLICIES

Organizational *business policies* are sets of rules and procedures for running an organization. Through workflows, user interfaces, databases, code or interfaces between systems, organizations implement important business policies. For example, one HMO business policy might be the rules for assignment of an HMO member with a primary care physician.

In order for an organization to keep control over the implementation of business policies, documents describing organizational and project business policies should be developed and kept up to date. Such documents should also describe how the policies will be manifested by databases, program code or tables, by user interfaces, by interfaces between systems, and the manual operations of employees in the organization.

To not have such documents would require that implementation of the business policy be under the control of computer programmers. The project business policies document should be used to test the project-automated systems to verify that all business policies have been implemented correctly.

A business policy consists of the business rules for implementation of the policy in total in the organization, including the implementation of the policy within organization automated systems and databases. Thus documentation of a business policy combines business information and information technology information.

Consider again the business policy defining the rules for assignment of an HMO member with a primary care physician. This might be implemented operationally, telling employees how to talk to a patient to encourage that patient to select a primary care physician; implemented by adding information to databases, such as including information on databases to record the patient assignment with a primary care physician; implemented through user interfaces, by providing fields on the screen to allow input of the assignment; and implemented through code, which incorporates the rules for assigning the patient to a primary care provider in code.

11.5 DEFINING USER INTERFACES

This section assumes that graphical user interfaces are used for all user interfaces. A *graphical user interface (GUI)* is a user interface that makes use of every addressable pixel on the screen and thus makes it possible to create detailed visual symbols for user navigation, characters, pictures, and lines. The next chapter discusses other possibilities besides GUIs and why this assumption of use of GUIs was made.

Reference (Redmond-Pyle, Moore, and Pyle 1995) describes a method for designing, evaluating and refining the design of GUI based software systems, which is presented in summary form in this section. This model, referred to as *GUIDE* for "Graphical User Interface Design and Evaluation", is diagrammed in figure 11.4 (Redmond-Pyle, Moore, and Pyle 1995). Boxes represent processes and lines represent how products are produced by one process and input to another. The steps of this process of defining a GUI user interface is presented here for the automated patient medical record system.

11.5.1 Define Users and Usability Requirements

The principal users of the automated system are identified and described. For the automated patient medical record system, users will be put into the following classes:

- outpatient physician
- hospitalist/inpatient physician
- outpatient nurse
- medical assistant
- ED triage nurse
- nurse practitioner
- physician assistant
- inpatient nurse
- unit assistant
- ED physician
- ED nurse
- advice nurse
- appointment clerk
- case manager
- clinical social worker
- allied health professional
- health care service representative/ombudsman

- quality manager
- medical researcher
- ancillary department personnel
- medical transcriptionist.

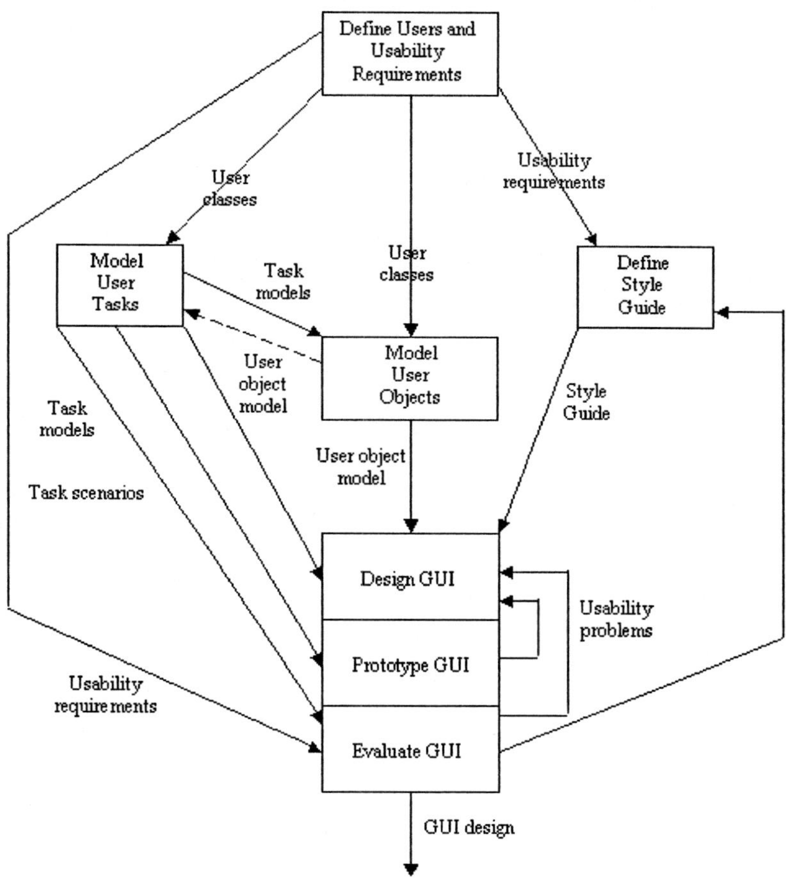

Figure 11.4 Overview of the GUIDE Process (Redmond-Pyle, Moore, and Pyle 1995).

For each class of user there should be an evaluation of the following so the system can be designed to best accommodate each class of users:

- type of users (direct user of the system, indirect user in that other people use the system for the person, remote user who works at a different location than the system, support user who helps other users)
- mandatory or discretionary user
- probable computer experience and skills

- motivation for using the system.

For example, direct users and mandatory users must become computer-literate. For indirect users an efficient communication mechanism must be set up to communicate information from the caregiver to the input specialist. Remote users require set up of remote connections. The system must be developed to provide payback to each user class, whether a direct or indirect user, so they are motivated to use the system.

For each class of user, usability requirements should be established. *Usability* is the extent to which a computer system is easy to learn and effective to use for the given business tasks and users. According to Jakob Nielsen (Nielsen 1998) usability consists of five characteristics:

- **Ease of learning:** How easy it is for a new user to learn the system.
- **Efficiency of use:** How fast an experienced user can accomplish his or her tasks.
- **Memorability:** If the user used the system at an earlier time, how quickly she can pick it up at a later time.
- **Error frequency and severity:** How often the user makes errors and how severe these errors are.
- **Subjective satisfaction:** How much the user likes using the system.

After implementation of the automated system, these characteristics could be used as a quantitative measure of how effectively each category of user uses the system and could then be used to evaluate the GUI design. The most effect standards and input styles could be evaluated for the sets of users, resulting in the production of a style guide that can be used for the system.

Identification of the user classes would enable work tasks for each class of users to be developed and user objects for each class of users to be identified.

11.5.2 Model User Work Tasks

The purpose of a computer system is to help each class of user perform their work tasks (i.e., their jobs, their workflow) more effectively and efficiently while allowing the users to concentrate on their jobs. This step uses the workflows described in section 11.3 to identify how a class of worker performs his job. Parts of the workflow dealing with the automated system are identified and the user interface is viewed in the context of these work processes.

11.5.3 Model Business Objects

The intent here is to create real world, independent *business objects* that correspond to the objects the user uses in doing his or her job. These will be objects within the user interface, thus enabling the user to think in the same terms as he or she currently does. Section 12.2.2 in the next chapter explains this idea in more detail.

For the automated patient medical record system, these objects might be as follows:

- patient demographics information
- patient lists
- patient clinical summaries
- encounter synopses
- chart display

- cases
- orders
- chart documentation input
- appointments
- e-mails/messages
- medical references.

These business objects would be used in the GUI interface.

11.5.4 Match User Interfaces with Databases and Interfaces

A *database* is a collection of permanently stored data used by one or more applications. What is displayed through user interfaces is

- data from one or more databases,
- data input by the users,
- transitory data determined during display of the information (e.g., by calculation), and
- data from other applications coming via interfaces (such as via a network or magnetic tape).

However, databases should not be developed based upon user interfaces in the business reengineering step but rather upon business objects and the relationships between these business objects determined in the business analysis step.

These business objects that define databases and the relationships between these business objects are often described by entity-relationship (E-R) diagrams. See section 13.8.

Some of the databases used by the user interface may already exist in the organization—*corporate databases*—and some may be new and created just for the application—*application databases*. Sometimes additional data is added or removed from existing databases. Thus an important part of the process of defining user interfaces is defining data within these databases and creating additional user interfaces or changing user interfaces so the correct data for the databases is collected at the right time.

There are corporate databases that may be used across many applications and application databases used by only the new application. Further, an application database may migrate to become a corporate database if it is determined that it could be used by other applications. When databases are split amongst different computers, whether they are application or corporate databases, we refer to them as *distributed databases*, often connected via a network to the computer running the application.

Databases are often optimized to support on-line operations (i.e., to support quick user access to information to display through the user interfaces).

For more information on databases, see sections 13.8 and 13.13.

Matching of user interfaces with databases also involves implementation of business policies and business rules for the data: In order to have good data, business rules for the data must be established at the time the user interface for entrance of the data is created. If the user interface allows data values that the business rules do not allow, then there almost certainly will be bad values on the database.

11.5.5 Define Style Guide

One basic principal of quality software design is to have a consistent and useable set of screen display and input standards as this decreases the complexity of the system and makes the system more intuitive for the user and more useable. Developing a *style guide* based upon business objects does this. In addition, it gives the users an impression of a uniform 'look and feel' for the system. And it makes program maintenance for programmers much easier, as code controlling the user interface can simply be replicated and used over and over again. The style guidelines chosen must enhance usability requirements determined previously.

Thus a *style guide* is a guide to be used in the development of a particular user interface that defines screen display and input standards based upon business objects. Some important points about screen and input standards are the following:

- **The system should help the caregiver do his or her job and never get in the way:** Make the system transparent so a user can forget the system, use it intuitively, and concentrate on his job.
- **Ordinary users and technical users of software systems are different:** Ordinary users like simplicity while technical users may or may not be comfortable with complexity.
- **Make the most used parts of the system conspicuous and very simple to use, while hiding the most complex parts:** Make the fundamental functions obvious and easy to find and use. It is also okay to have powerful complex functions, but they should be hidden from users who do not need them and they should be extremely useful for those who do use it.
- **Consistency:** Have absolute consistency of everything, so users know exactly what to expect of the system at all times (e.g., have scroll bars, list selections, etc., all work the same, as identified in the style guide).

  Consistency includes consistency of error messages. Wherever the same named field appears on any window or screen, it should give exactly the same initial result (e.g., a date is a date, an address is an address, a city is a city, and a zipcode is a zipcode no matter where it appears in the system). This consistency is accomplished by first doing *single field edits*, using the same computer program code for any like field, and only then doing *relational edits*, edits which combine two or more fields. Relational edits could be ordered too, with edits within the same line done first and then edits between lines, edits between sections of data on the screen, etc. An important first step though is doing the single field edits first, so the user, for example, doesn't enter a zip code correctly in one place on the screen and makes exactly the same error in another place, he gets exactly the same error message. Additionally, edits (e.g., all single field edits) should be done in the order the fields appear on the screen top to bottom, left to right, so, when the user corrects one error, it goes to the next one, if any.
- **Initially, on each window or screen put the cursor or focus on the location where a reader would normally start reading on the page of a book for English, this is on the upper left part of each window or screen:** A window or screen is potentially very large, containing a large amount of information. The user often does not see the whole area. Simplify the window or screen and hide the complexity on the by putting the absolutely essential stuff in the upper left part so, most of the time, the user only has to look at that. If she needs more information some of the time, she can then find it on other parts of the window or screen.

11.5.6 Define the Graphical User Interface (GUI)

The GUI design is developed from the four main products mentioned so earlier:

1. The user object model
2. The user work task model
3. Available data (from databases and interfaces)
4. The application style guide.

The objects making up the GUI design comes from the user object model. Windows would be in the style determined by the style guide. What the entire system must support are the workflows in the user work task model for the various classes of users. Data displayed comes either from databases, interfaces with other systems, or user input.

11.5.7 Prototype and Evaluate the GUI

Prototyping is the process of developing and interacting with a partial version of a system whose interface functions the same as the final system in order to gain user feedback to evaluate usability. A prototype appears to provide all the functionality of the final system, but other parts of the system are left out (e.g., updates to databases, interfaces, etc.)

The reasons for using a prototype rather than the real system are the following:

1. the prototype system can be developed long before the real system
2. the prototype system can be changed much more easily than the real system

Developing a prototype system enables users to test out and critique the system. It enables business process analysts to determine when usability requirements are not met. When problems are found, the design must be changed, and the prototype changed and re-tested.

The purposes of prototyping are to do the following:

- validate the style guide
- reach agreement on how the GUI is to support each task in the workflows
- explore the appearance and behavior of each screen
- satisfy usability requirements.

11.5.8 Other Considerations

In developing user interfaces from workflows there are many considerations, including the following:

- **Different locations of the organization may want different workflows:** You either have to have user interfaces that accommodate these many different workflows or you must change the workflows of one or more locations.
- **The organization may want to standardize workflows:** An organization may want to standardize on a particular user interface to force everyone in an organization to use the most efficient workflow or to enforce a required process (e.g., collect information required by a regulatory organization).
- **What may seem like the best workflow may later not be:** An anticipated workflow may have to later be changed, possibly making the associated user interface obsolete.

- **User interfaces can be general, accommodating many different workflows or can be tailored to a specific workflow:** More general workflows are more likely to succeed.
- **A system that is extremely flexible may be more costly to develop and may be more difficult to train, use, and maintain.**
- **Systems with user interfaces that do not accommodate a workflow will not be stable:** Either the workflow will change or the user interface will not be used as expected
- **Accommodating workflows is just a starting point:** Many things, including workflows, change in an organization over time.
- **To insure that a user interface is used, you must have user buy-in to the user interface by a large number of users:** The best approach is to have significant involvement of a large number of users in the development of the user interface, with consensus agreement that they can "live with it". Beyond that, you need good facilitators to work with the users, as well as user interface designers who recognize good designs and are very flexible in absorbing, and accepting, other people's ideas.

11.6 WORKFLOWS AND THE DISADVANTAGES OF A SUPER COMPETENT EMPLOYEE

It is important to recognize all workflow activities, especially those that are hidden. For example, a workflow may consist of activities A, B, C, D and E, but a super competent employee may automatically take care of B, C and D for the department, so the needs for B, C and D may be hidden to a naive manager.

For example, a Spanish-speaking physician may cover for the need of a department to serve Spanish-speaking patients. But what the healthcare organization really needs instead is to have Spanish-speaking interpreters who can cover many different departments, not just one.

By being willing to take all the Spanish-speaking patients, the physician may be assigned predominantly to patients who speak Spanish, and may thus be penalized for her special capabilities by seeing many more patients than the average physician and at times be overworked. Further, Spanish-speaking patients may all be directed to her department (e.g. internal medicine) instead of the more appropriate one (e.g., cardiology). But the need of having interpreters for all departments does not go away.

If the physician leaves, if the physician is unavailable or is replaced by an average competence employee, then all the missing processes (and needs) resurface.

Therefore, it is important for managers to recognize real needs and processes, which again, can be covered up by having super competent employees. Sometimes it is better to fail than to patch things up through super competent employees. Sometimes it is better to have average competence employees so missing processes can be identified.

Super competent employees need to be treasured. They need to be recognized for the special contribution they make, and they should never be penalized.

11.7 USABILITY, RESPONSE TIME, AND SYSTEM PERFORMANCE

Usability is a quality of a system to assist a user in doing his job, to be easy to use, and to be intuitive for the user. *Response time* is the time for an automated system to respond back to the user upon entrance of input; bad response time may disrupt the user in doing his job. Good *system performance* is the ability for the system to handle all its users and perform all its activities in a timely manner.

Caregiver scenarios are useful for the analysis of all three items: usability, response time, and system performance. A scenario is a common workflow of a user during which the user uses the automated system—an example is the workflow for an outpatient physician seeing a patient for an urgent care visit while using the automated system, or the workflow of an inpatient nurse in caring for a patient in the hospital while using the automated system.

Taking the set of common scenarios and analyzing the automated patient medical record system with respect to each of these scenarios enables the system to be created to maximize usability of the system. Potential system architectures for the automated patient medical record system can be selected based upon which ones can best handle the scenarios together with all the other supporting activities of the system (given the relative frequencies of occurrence of each of the scenarios).

Once potential system architectures are selected, these architectures can be simulated in a *test bed*, a smaller scale hardware and software system that mimics the automated system. Response times and other system performance characteristics can then be estimated through testing within these test beds with subsequent determination of which of these architectures will work the best.

Once the system architecture is selected and after the automated patient medical record system is created later in the development step, the scenarios can then be used in scripts to drive performance testing. A *script* mimics the input of a caregiver in using the system; using a number of scripts together can mimic a large number of users using the system, without there being actual users. During performance testing using the scripts, network throughput, disk drive efficiency and other elements of the system can be measured, thus identifying bottlenecks in the system. Through correction of these bottlenecks, system performance can be enhanced, including lowering of response time.

Key Terms

application database
business object
business policy
business reengineering
corporate database
cursor
Data Flow Diagram (DFD)
database
dialog box
discrete event simulation
distributed database
graphical user interface (GUI)
GUIDE (Graphical User Interface Design and Evaluation)
keyboard
mainframe
mouse
pen
performance
pointer device
prototyping
reengineering
relational edits
response time
script
single field edits
style guide
terminal
touch pad
trackball
usability
user interface
workflow
workflow systems

Study Questions

1. What does an organization hope to achieve by business process reengineering?
2. Business process reengineering may involve the following: workflows, business policies, and user interfaces. What are these? How do business objects, databases and interfaces business objects relate to user interfaces?
3. When a new computer software system is being introduced as part of the project, there is a way to evaluate the system's effects upon the organization prior to completion of the system. What is this?
4. In defining new workflows, what kind of activities within current workflows should be considered for removal or changing, and what kind of activities should be kept? Why is it important to involve current employees in redefining workflows? What are DFDs?
5. What is an organizational business policy? How is a business policy implemented?
6. What is a user interface? What kind of user interface does this book recommend? What is GUIDE? What hardware devices exist to enable a user to interact with what is displayed on the screen?
7. When defining user interfaces, why is it important to identify categories of systems users? What is "usability" and how can usability be increased?
8. What are business objects? What might the business objects be for a cafe? How do business objects relate to user interfaces?
9. How are databases related to user interfaces? What are corporate databases? What are application databases?
10. How does a style guide improve a user interface?
11. When there are automated systems being developed, the last part of the business reengineering step is creating a prototype of the user interfaces. What are the purposes of such a prototype?

CHAPTER 12

Example User Interface for the Automated Patient Medical Record

CHAPTER OUTLINE

12.1 PROJECT CONTEXT: USER INTERFACE

This chapter presents an example user interface for the automated patient medical record system. The user interface was developed to handle the composite of workflows of the caregivers within our HMO.

Caregivers who provide patient care in the HMO are listed in section 4.2. The organization wants to preserve all current workflows, as described in section 4.3 but removing unneeded paperwork and duplicated entrance of information. New capabilities described in chapters 7 and 8 need to be supported.

The previous chapter describes a process that could have been used to identify this composite user interface. This user interface was chosen because it can handle all the workflows for all caregivers in the HMO; the user interface would be tailorable by type of caregiver as well as by each individual caregiver.

As a basis for the description of the composite user interface and the workflows, we start with the conceptual view of the system previously presented in section 7.9 and figure 7.15 and now shown here in figure 12.1.

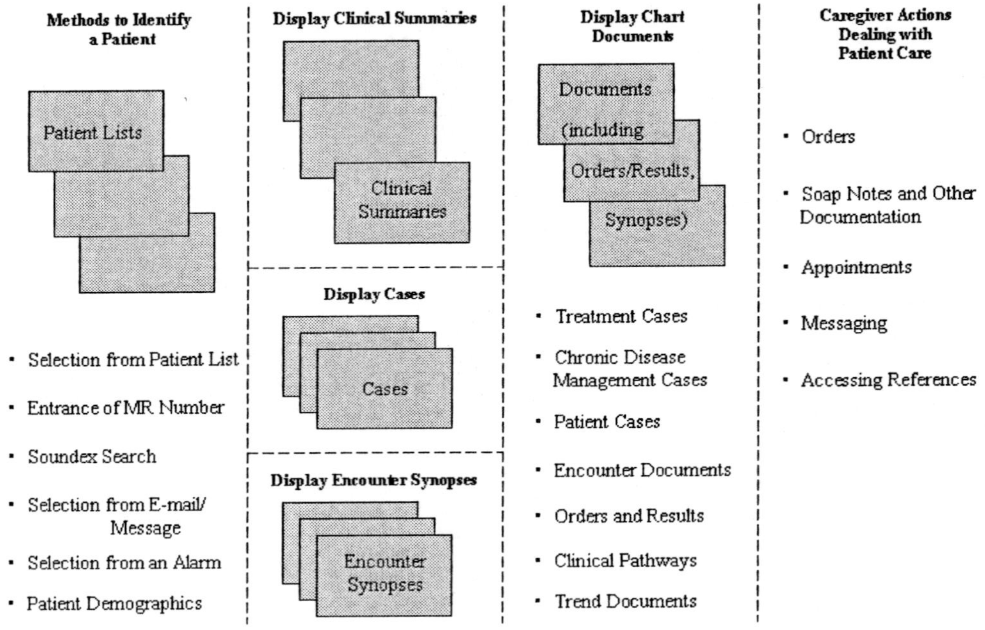

Figure 12.1 Basic Elements of an Automated Patient Medical Record.

This conceptual view includes the following parts:

- **methods to identify patients of interest to a caregiver:** methods tailored to the specific caregiver to select a patient and verify that the correct selection has been made
- **a quick overview of clinical information for a patient:** a summary of patient clinical information tailored to the caregiver (e.g., current medications, past encounters, immunizations, etc.)
- **defined outcome cases, chronic care management cases, and patient cases for a patient:** a list of defined outcome and chronic care management cases (identifying treatment plans and related information) and patient cases (identifying case notes for a case manager)

- **synopses of past encounters for a patient:** a list of caregiver or automated system generated summaries of each encounter; synopses could also exist for a case and a clinical pathway
- **documents making up a patient s chart:** the set of documents making up the chart, with documents organized by encounter, defined outcome case, chronic care management case, patient case, or clinical pathway. These are the "source documents"
- **the ability to perform and record actions dealing with the patient s care:** this covers all activities to schedule or perform services and record care, including the following: (1) ordering clinical lab test, medications, diagnostic images, etc., and receiving back results, including alarms of abnormal results; (2) documenting patient care, producing documents in the chart; (3) messaging between caregivers; (4) making patient appointments; (5) viewing medical and HMO reference information, including HMO guidelines and drug formulary.

The proposed automated patient medical record system would be tailorable by job category or individual caregiver. For example, the type of patient lists immediately available to a caregiver (inpatient census versus outpatient schedule) might be dependent upon type of caregiver (inpatient physician versus outpatient physician). Patient medical record information might be organized differently for an ophthalmologist versus an internal medicine physician. The following sections describe how the user interface might look to different types of caregivers and describes additional aspects of user interface design.

What is presented here are screens of the automated patient medical record system, equivalent to a *prototype* of the system. A prototype is a realistic model of a system, usually described in terms of the user interface of the system, which looks like the real system. Although it looks like the real system, it does not function like the real system in one or more ways (e.g., it probably has no databases or underlying code or its screen navigation is likely to be in some ways unlike the real system).

Why prototype? Prototyping is for experimenting—showing a system to users for their evaluation without going through the hard, time-consuming work of actually building the system.

12.2 USER INTERFACE MODELS FOR A WORKSTATION

A *workstation* is a micro- or minicomputer system with a network attachment that is used for providing information, computation, and/or network services directly to an end user.There are two categories of workstations: *desktop computers* (microcomputers using the traditional full-size case, monitor, and keyboard that is designed to be used in a stationary "desk-centered" environment), and *portable computers* (microcomputers that are easily moved from place to place and that normally use battery power for use on the go). Two categories of portable computers are *laptop computers* (briefcase-sized computers with capabilities similar to the desktop computer) and *pen computers* (computers that mainly use a pen stylus for input).

There are several choices for user interfaces for the automated patient medical record system workstation: character-based, Graphical User Interface (GUI), pen computer interface, or Internet-like with hypertext.

Character-based user interfaces still exist largely because of the success of the *IBM Corporations Customer Information Control Systems (CICS),* one of IBM's most popular *mainframe* (very large) *computer* software systems, which supports creation of applications on character-based terminals (Janossy and Samuels 1995). In the next section, 12.2.1, we will explore the limitations of character-based interfaces. (CICS is discussed further in section 17.3.1.)

A *Graphical User Interface (GUI)* is the proper interface for many parts of the automated patient medical record. GUI is a user interface that makes use of every addressable dot (called a *pixel*) on the screen and thus makes it possible to create detailed visual symbols for user navigation, characters, pictures, and lines.

A *pen computer* enables input via a stylus pen, by the individual's own writing or printing and, more commonly by stylized printed input where each printed character must follow a specific format. However, with a pen computer, the easiest input approach is selection by radio button or check mark. Pen computers allow for much lighter weight computers than those with a keyboard, and thus pen computers are appropriate for use when the caregiver is interviewing the patient or when the caregiver is on-the-go.

Internet/Intranet/Extranet hypertext documents must be formatted in HTML or XML together with HTML. Many medical references are available through documents in such a form on the Internet. Whether it is feasible to also present documents making up the patient chart in the form of such hypertext documents is explored in section 12.4. An *Intranet* is a part of the Internet reserved for use within an organization. An *Extranet* is a part of the Internet reserved for use within multiple organizations.

12.2.1 Character-Based User Interfaces

Let us compare *character-based systems* such as IBM's CICS versus GUI PC systems. First consider a CICS character-based approach for an automated patient medical record system. The initial character-based screen might be a menu as pictured in figure 12.2.

```
CHRTMNU                                   Patient Chart Menu

Select one of the following:

_  1.Patient Information
   2.Patient Lists
   3.Patient Clinical Summary
   4.Encounter Synopses
   5.Chart Display
   6.Case Display
   7.Ordering
   8.Documentation
   9.Appointment
   a.E-mail/Messaging
   b.Medical References







F1=Help  F3=Exit  F12=Cancel
```

Figure 12.2 Character-Based Menu Screen.

The list of menu selections in figure 12.2 are as follows:

- **PATIENT INFORMATION:** Identify a patient by entrance of a patient identifier and display associated patient demographics information
- **PATIENT LISTS:** Select a Patient List for display, such as a particular provider's outpatient schedule
- **PATIENT CLINICAL SUMMARY:** Select a Clinical Summary of the patient's clinic information (e.g., medications, previous encounters, etc.) for display
- **ENCOUNTER SYNOPSES:** Display summaries of previous encounters
- **CHART DISPLAY:** Display documents in the chart
- **CASE DISPLAY**: Display defined outcome cases, chronic care management cases, and patient cases
- **ORDERING:** Enable various types of orders to be executed, including clinical laboratory tests, prescriptions, charts, etc.
- **DOCUMENTATION:** Enable selection of a type of chart document and allow entrance of information into the document
- **APPOINTMENT:** Make an appointment
- **EMAIL/MESSAGING:** Allow e-mail, messages to be sent to other people
- **MEDICAL REFERENCE:** Allow display of a medical reference such as MEDLINE.

Selection of PATIENT INFORMATION from the menu might bring up a screen to display and collect patient demographics information. See figure 12.3.

```
PATINFO                          Patient Information

Type Information.   Then Enter.                                Page 1 of 2
                                                             More:       +
Patient Id ..... :  6347730211
Patient Name.... :  Cindy S Brady
  First.........    Cindy___________________
  Middle........    S_______________________
  Last..........    Brady___________________
  Suffix........    ___
  Birth Date/Age    01 / 01 / 1991   :    7:02
  Sex...........    F                 : Female
  Day Phone.....    ( 415 ) 333 - 3333 EXT 1000
  Eve Phone.....    ( 808 ) 359 - 6817 EXT ____
  Mail Address..    2222 Miami Ave__________
  City..........    Palm Springs____________
  State.........    CA   Zip  97956 - 0120

Contact Name....    Sarah Rogers____________
  Relationship..    Mother__________
  Day Phone.....    ( 415 ) 333 - 3333 Ext ____
  Eve Phone.....    ( 808 ) 359 - 6817 Ext ____

Enter  F1=Help  F3=Exit  F7=Bkwd  F8=Fwd  F12=Cancel
```

Figure 12.3 Character-Based Information Screen.

Selection of PATIENT LISTS from the menu might bring up a list of patient lists available to **the user for display. The user can select the type of patient list to display and enter a date if required to identify the patient list to display. See figure 12.4.**

As shown by this example, some characteristics of a character-based user interface are the following:

- **The user can do only one thing at a time**: The user selects what to do from a menu. In order to start a function, any other function being executed must first be completed. Two or more functions cannot be handled concurrently.
- **The character-based structure enforces business rules but guides and restricts** the user through all processes.
- **The character-based structure does not easily handle indefinite and large lists (i.e., menus) of different types of selections** such as might occur within the PATIENT LISTS function (with possible display many different types of patient lists), the CHART DISPLAY function (with possible display of many different parts of a chart), the CASE DISPLAY function (with possible display of many defined outcome cases, chronic care management cases and patient cases) or the DOCUMENTATION section (with a possible capability to enable entrance of a large number of different types of chart documents).
- **The screen structure is inflexible:** the screen is of fixed size, a fixed number of characters wide by a fixed number of characters in height. Images, line drawings, waveforms, etc. cannot be displayed.

The first two characteristics, one thing at a time and enforcing business rules, limit the way the user can work; however, guiding the user through the processes may assist new users. The last two characteristics, difficulty in handling indefinite lists of selections and variable information, and information limited to the size of the screen, we shall find, greatly limit character-based approaches for use with the automated patient medical record.

Other problems with character-based user interfaces are as follows:

- Character-based user interfaces do not support standard word processing capabilities for text, such as word wrap (forcing a word which is at the end of a line to the next), insertion of text, or deletion of text.
- Without mouse support, it is difficult to go from field to field. Cursor movement is generally restricted to be from field to next field, left to right and top to bottom. Not so obvious key combinations allow cursor positioning to the first field, the last field, the next field, the previous field and the next line.
- Character-based user interfaces do not provide the equivalent of the GUI message box. *Message boxes* can pop up and inform the user of an important event or warn the user of a potential problem. For example, the GUI message box in figure 12.5 shows an alarm being presented to the caregiver showing a clinical laboratory test result that is out of range.

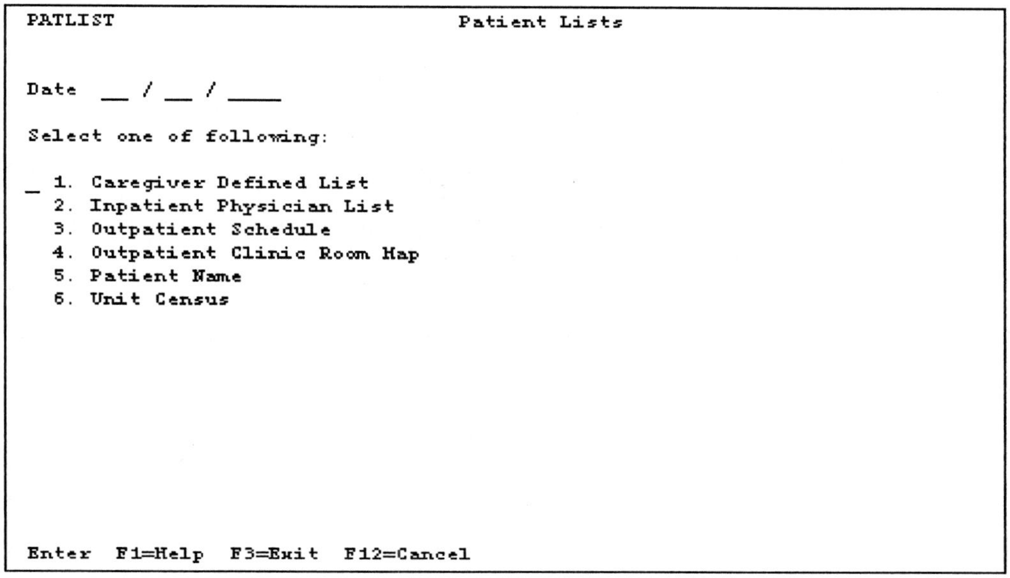

```
PATLIST                                  Patient Lists

Date  __ / __ / ____

Select one of following:

_ 1. Caregiver Defined List
  2. Inpatient Physician List
  3. Outpatient Schedule
  4. Outpatient Clinic Room Map
  5. Patient Name
  6. Unit Census

Enter  F1=Help  F3=Exit  F12=Cancel
```

Figure 12.4 Character-Based List Screen.

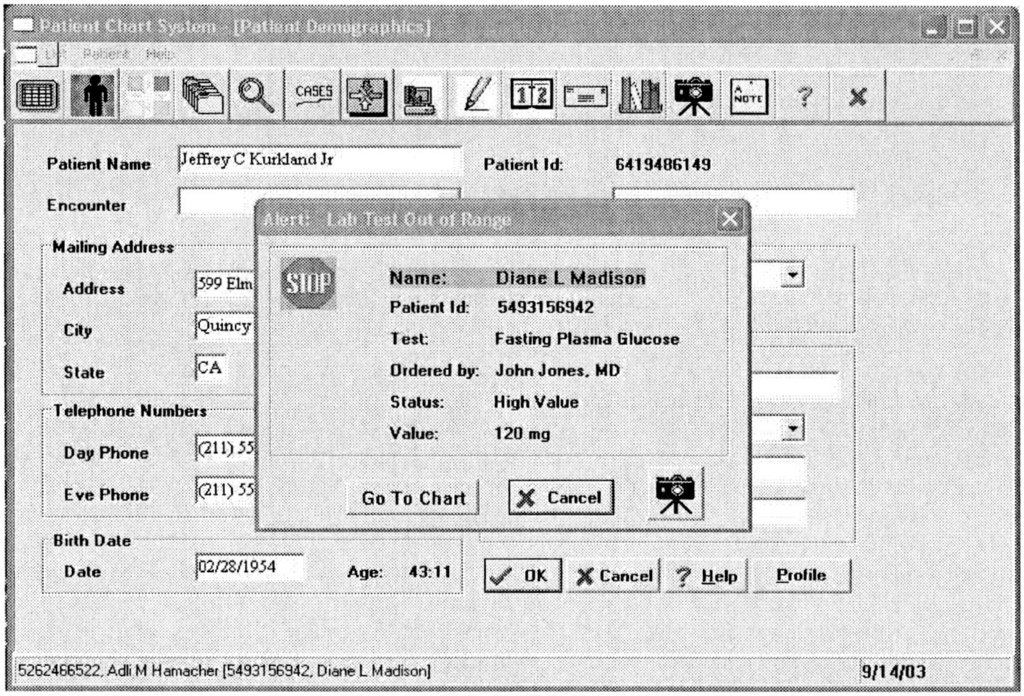

Patient Chart System - [Patient Demographics]

Patient Name Jeffrey C Kurkland Jr Patient Id: 6419486149

Encounter

Mailing Address

Address 599 Elm

City Quincy

State CA

Telephone Numbers

Day Phone (211) 55

Eve Phone (211) 55

Birth Date

Date 02/28/1954 Age: 43:11

OK Cancel Help Profile

Alert: Lab Test Out of Range

STOP

Name: Diane L Madison

Patient Id: 5493156942

Test: Fasting Plasma Glucose

Ordered by: John Jones, MD

Status: High Value

Value: 120 mg

Go To Chart Cancel

5262466522, Adli M Hamacher [5493156942, Diane L Madison] 9/14/03

Figure 12.5 Message Box.

12.2.2 Graphical User Interfaces (GUIs)

With a *Graphical User Interface (GUI),* the user has many graphic elements available, including windows; bitmaps and drawings; drop-down menus; message and dialog boxes, and *controls* of various types, including group boxes, static text boxes, scroll bars, input fields, single-selection lists, radio buttons, check boxes, tabbed structures, and controls specific to pen input. Reference (Johnson 2000) describes these controls and the screens and windows starting at figure 12.5 in this chapter collectively show many of these controls. *Windows* are a rectangular part of a computer screen that contains a display different from the rest of the screen.

Input in a GUI system is by keyboard, pointer devices (mice, trackballs, glide points, etc.) or pen. Various processes can be selected via pointer device selection of buttons with icons; icons can appear as part of tool bars (see figure 12.6).

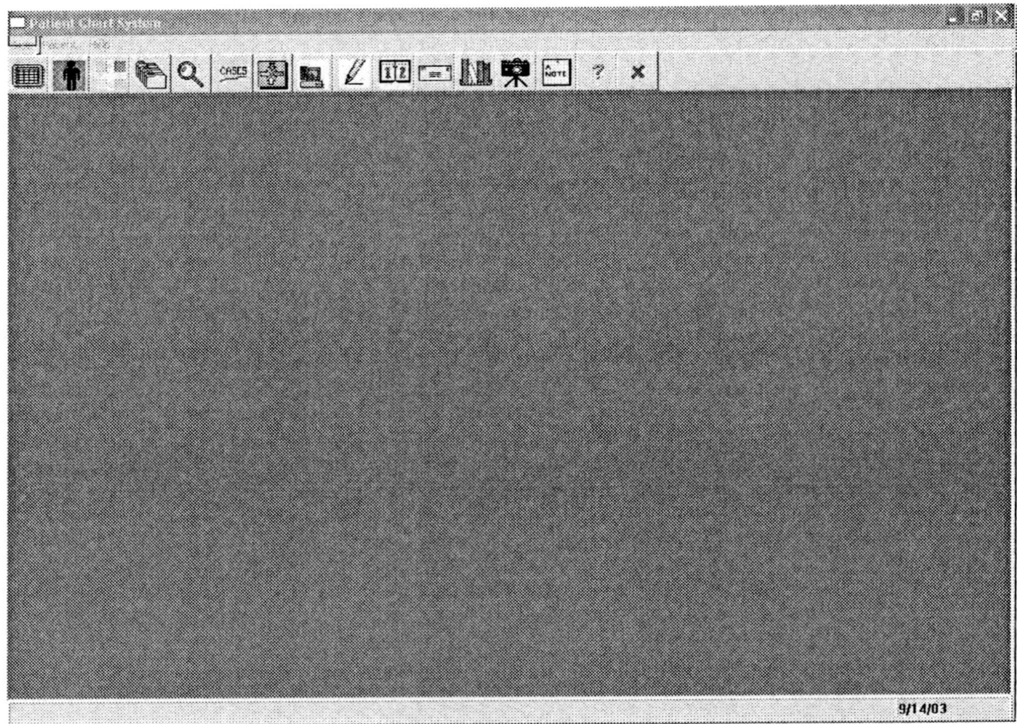

Figure 12.6 Business Objects in Terms of Icons.

Reference (Sims 1994) recommends to think of systems and GUIs in terms of real world independent "business objects" that the user of the system uses in real life to do his or her job where these business objects can cooperate with each other allowing the transfer of information between business objects. The term used is *Cooperative Business Objects (CBOs)*. For example, for the automated patient medical record system, CBOs might include the following: patient, chart, documentation form, order form, appointment form.

Like real world objects, a number of these objects could be in use at the same time (e.g., an H&P document can be created concurrently with display of the patient chart). A number of instances of the same object could be in use (e.g., two patient lists, a physician's outpatient schedule and the inpatient census could be in use).

CBOs are "cooperative" in that they would be built to allow communication between them. CBOs could be developed by different parts of the healthcare organization, completely different healthcare organizations or by outside vendors. This cooperativeness might be as simple as allowing cutting and pasting of text from one CBO to another via a clipboard; this cooperativeness might involve transfer of data in one field in one CBO automatically to the same format field in another CBO; or this cooperativeness might be transferring of objects and all associated processing from one CBO to another (a spreadsheet with all its functionality). Another method of cooperativeness is *drag-and-drop*, such as dragging a patient's name from a patient list or Emergency Department triage document to a room shown on a room map, indicating that the patient has been assigned to that room.

One principal advantage of a CBO is that, since CBOs are relatively independent from each other, one CBO can generally be replaced by another similarly functioning CBO when the new CBO is an improvement over the earlier one, with minimal changes, if any, to the other CBOs. This is again an example of "component adaptability", implementing a component so it can be more easily replaced later by an improved component.

The following are example CBOs making up the automated patient medical record system. Each CBO is represented by a selection button shown in the tool bar on the screen in figure 12.6:

- Patient List (identified by a "table" icon)
- Patient (identified by a "person" icon)
- Clinical Summary (identified by an abstract icon)
- Patient Chart (identified by a "chart with tabs" icon)
- Search (identified by a "magnifying glass" icon)
- Patient Cases (identified by a "cases" icon)
- Encounter Synopses (identified by an abstract icon)
- Order Form (identified by an "Rx order" icon)
- Documentation Form (identified by a "pencil writing" icon)
- Appointment Form (identified by a "calendar" icon)
- E-mail/Message. (identified by an "envelope" icon)
- Medical References (identified by a "set of books" icon)
- Snapshot (identified by a "camera" icon)
- Note (identified by a "note" icon)
- Help (identified by a "question mark" icon)
- Exit (identified by an "X" icon).

Another term for a GUI interface using CBOs is an *Object Oriented User Interface (OOUI).*

Consider an example scenario for a physician who works both as an inpatient and outpatient physician and say, works in an outpatient clinic in the morning and in an inpatient unit in the evening. She or he might select the Patient Lists icon and create an instance of his Inpatient Physician List and an instance of his Outpatient Schedule for today, selecting each of these patient lists from a scrollable list. Thus two patient lists could be open at the same time, and the automated patient medical record and another application could be open at the same time. See figures 12.7 and 12.8.

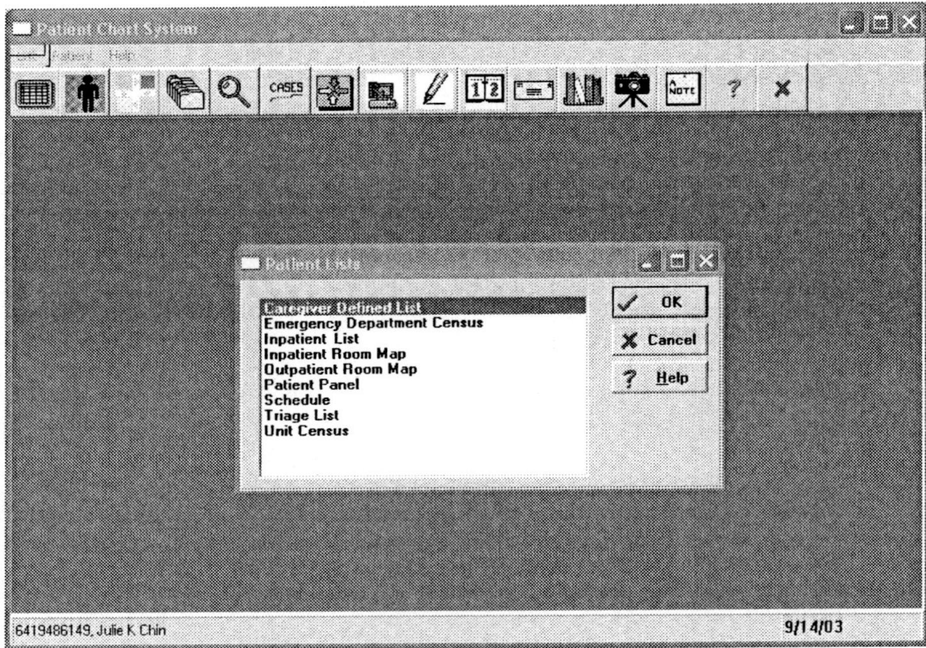

Figure 12.7 Patient Lists.

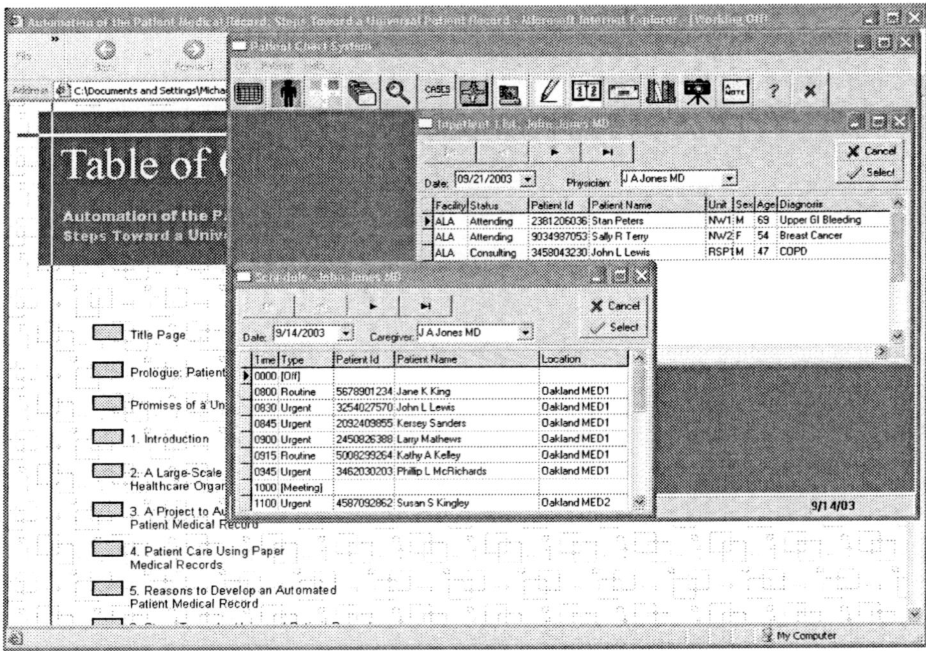

Figure 12.8 Multiple Open Patient Lists and Applications.

Operating systems often provide a number of different ways to switch between these dialogs, for example between Patient Lists and between other applications. When selected, a Patient List or application can be closed by selecting the "Cancel" button or 'X' button in the right-hand corner. Applications and dialogs can be generally be resized to be larger or smaller (when smaller often displaying scroll bars to scroll to the now out-of-view areas).

From a patient list, a patient can be selected (Kathy Kelley from the outpatient schedule in figure 12.9). Alternatively, the Patient icon could be selected, allowing entrance of a patient identifier fo rthe patient (see figure 12.10).

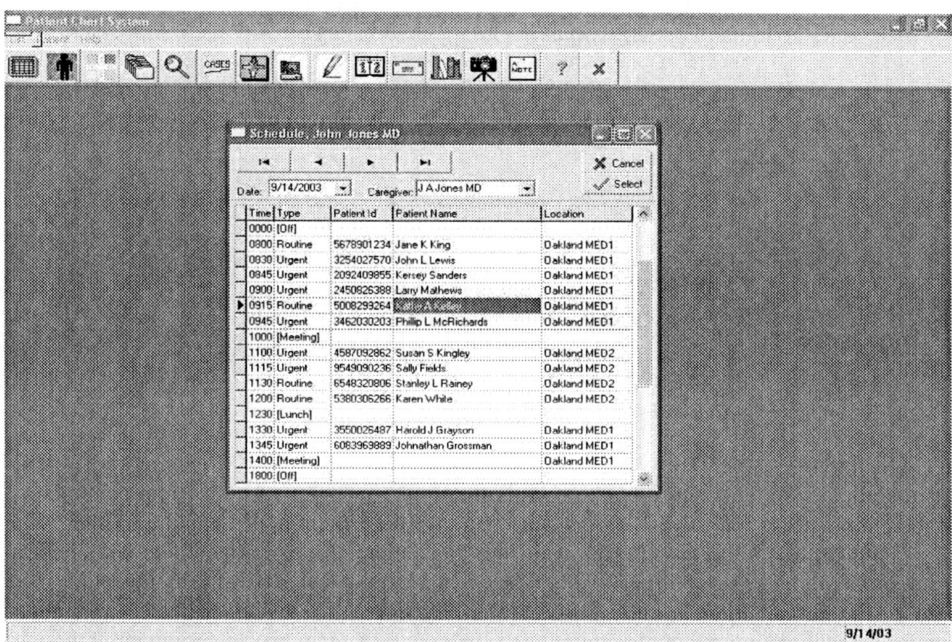

Figure 12.9 Schedule with a Selected Patient.

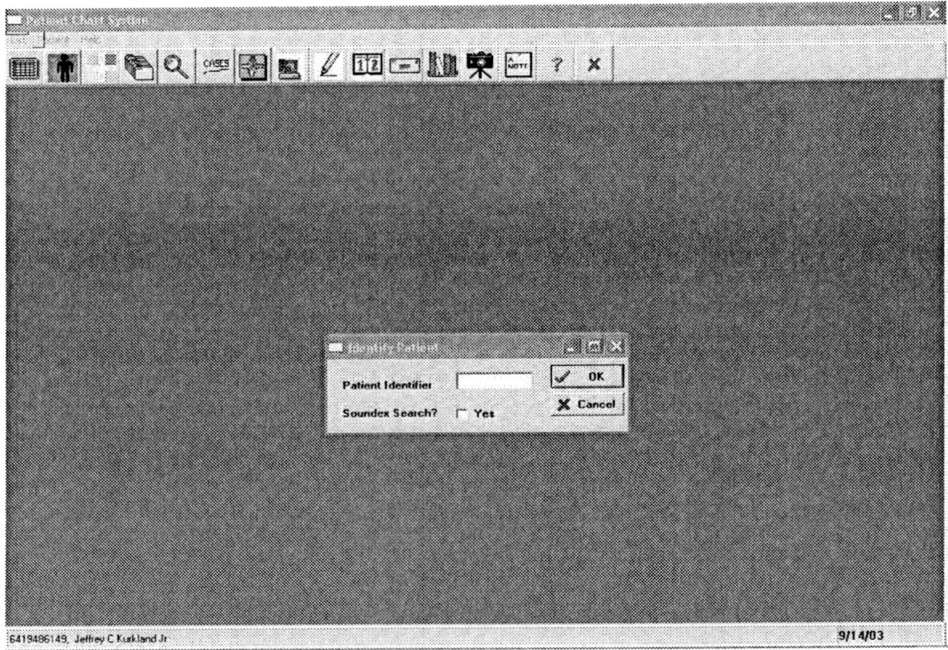

Figure 12.10 Selection of the Patient After Selecting the Patient Icon.

After selection of a patient either from a patient list or by entrance of the patient's identifier, patient demographics might be displayed to allow the user to verify that the correct patient was selected (see figure 12.11). *Patient demographics* displays the patient's name, address, telephone number, sex and other information that identifies the patient. From patient demographics, a *personal profile* of the patient might available describing personalized information about the patient, to assist the caregiver in taking care of the patient and the patient's needs (see figure 12.12). For example, from a personal profile for the patient, transfer to the personal profile for the patient's wife, husband or children might be possible (see figure 12.13) and transfer of a phone call to a specialist or the patient's case manager might be possible.

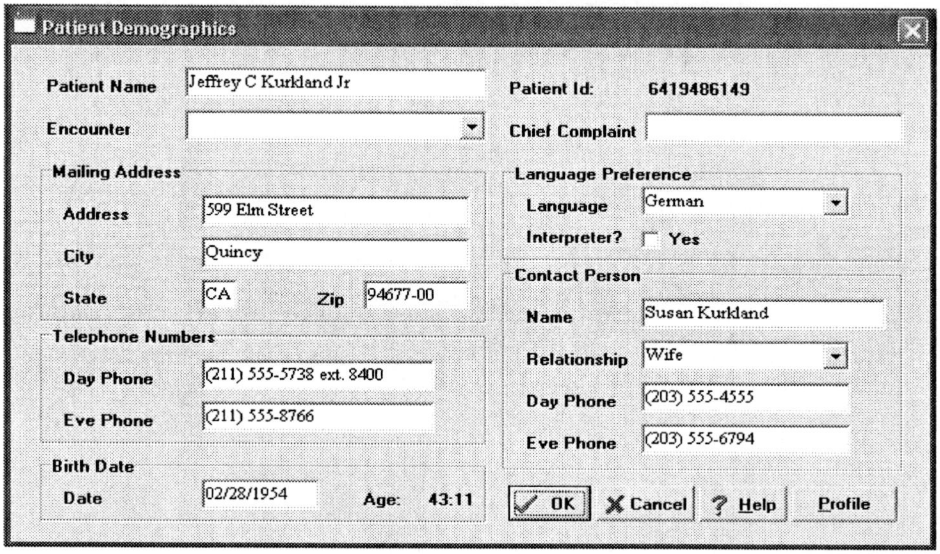

Patient Demographics

Patient Name: Jeffrey C Kurkland Jr
Patient Id: 6419486149
Encounter:
Chief Complaint:

Mailing Address
Address: 599 Elm Street
City: Quincy
State: CA Zip: 94677-00

Telephone Numbers
Day Phone: (211) 555-5738 ext. 8400
Eve Phone: (211) 555-8766

Birth Date
Date: 02/28/1954 Age: 43:11

Language Preference
Language: German
Interpreter? Yes

Contact Person
Name: Susan Kurkland
Relationship: Wife
Day Phone: (203) 555-4555
Eve Phone: (203) 555-6794

OK | Cancel | ? Help | Profile

Figure 12.11 Patient Demographics.

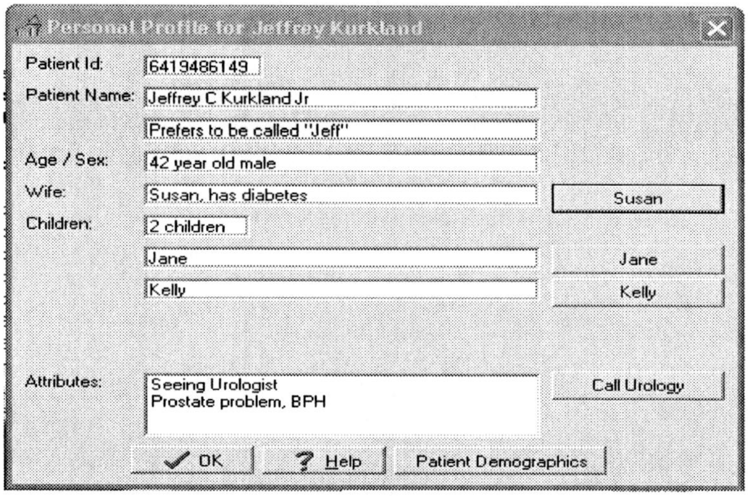

Personal Profile for Jeffrey Kurkland

Patient Id: 6419486149
Patient Name: Jeffrey C Kurkland Jr
Prefers to be called "Jeff"
Age / Sex: 42 year old male
Wife: Susan, has diabetes — Susan
Children: 2 children
Jane — Jane
Kelly — Kelly
Attributes: Seeing Urologist
Prostate problem, BPH — Call Urology

OK | ? Help | Patient Demographics

Figure 12.12 Personal Profile from Patient Demographics.

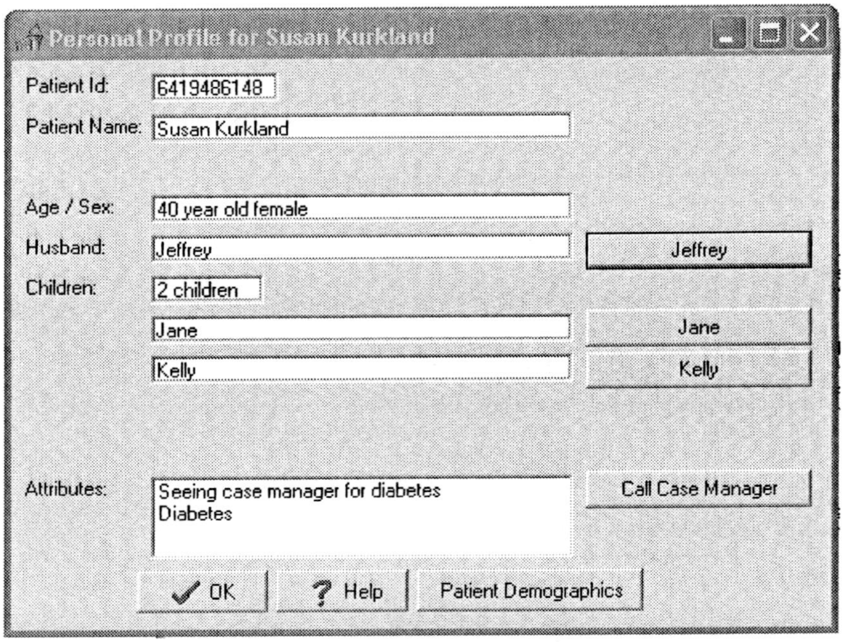

Personal Profile for Susan Kurkland

Patient Id: 6419486148

Patient Name: Susan Kurkland

Age / Sex: 40 year old female

Husband: Jeffrey | Jeffrey

Children: 2 children

Jane | Jane

Kelly | Kelly

Attributes: Seeing case manager for diabetes
Diabetes | Call Case Manager

OK | Help | Patient Demographics

Figure 12.13 Personal Profile of Wife from Husband s Personal Profile.

After selection of the patient, other icons related to the patient could be selected: Clinical Summary, Patient Chart, Search Patient Clinical Information, Patient Cases, Encounter Synopses, Order Form, Documentation Form, and Appointment. For example, by selecting a patient, Julie K Chin and pressing the Summary icon, the list of Clinical Summaries available for the patient might be displayed (see figure 12.14). Julie Andrew's Overall Clinical Summary could then be selected (see figure 12.15). (Other patient icons deal with multiple patients rather than just one: Patient Lists, E-mail/Message, Medical References, Snapshot.)

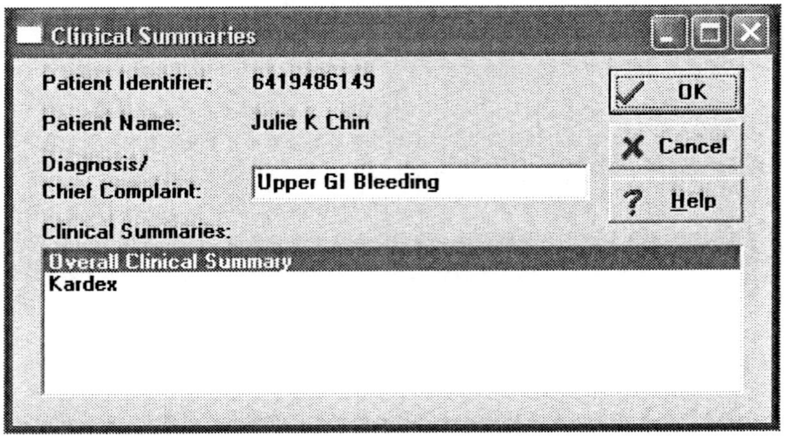

Clinical Summaries

Patient Identifier: 6419486149

Patient Name: Julie K Chin

Diagnosis/
Chief Complaint: Upper GI Bleeding

Clinical Summaries:
Overall Clinical Summary
Kardex

OK | Cancel | Help

Figure 12.14 Clinical Summary List.

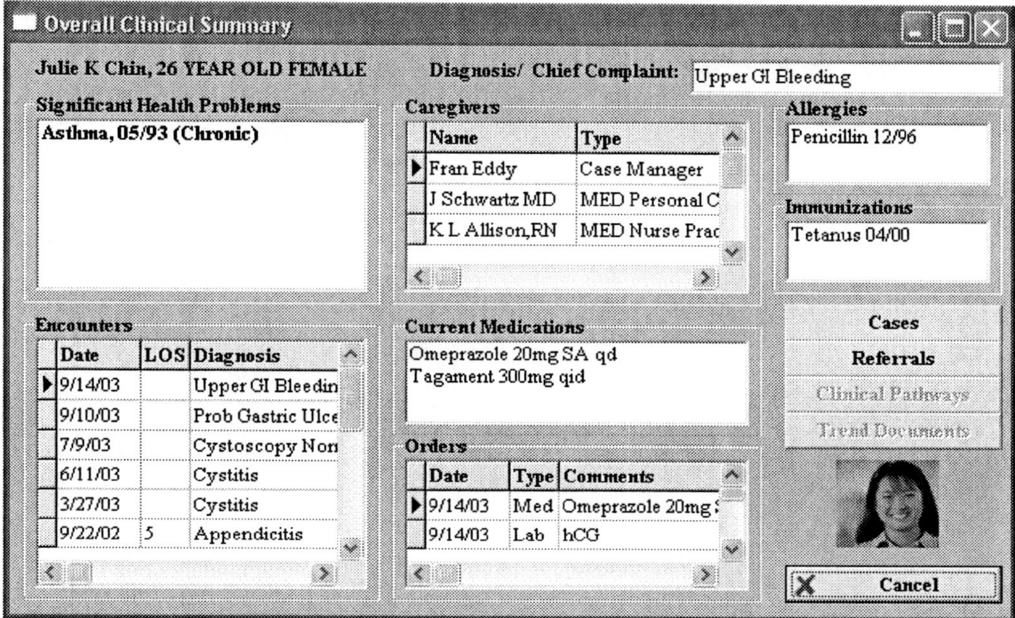

Figure 12.15 Overall Clinical Summary.

The overall clinical summary consists of various scrollable lists summarizing patient information and buttons to display documents. Unavailable button selections might be dimmed; for example, Julie Chin has cases, referrals, but no clinical pathways or trend documents.

Either pressing the "Cases" button on the Overall Clinical Summary or the "Cases" icon on the tool bar would bring up Julie Chin defined outcome, chronic condition management or other cases.

The physician could see the patient's chart by pressing the "Chart" icon on the tool bar, or if the physician had set up a relationship between encounters and the chart, see the chart for a selected encounter(s) by selecting and highlighting the encounter(s) and double-clicking. For example, selection of the 9/10/03 encounter on the overall clinical summary for Julie Chin might bring up the chart so it shows the chart for that encounter (see figure 12.16).

The patient chart would show the main tab and a visit synopsis. Selection of any date would open up encounter information below the document date on a *document list*. The physician could select other tabs either by selecting the tab on the tabbed structure or selecting the section in the document list under an opened encounter date. When the Vital Signs tab is selected for the 9/10/1998 encounter, both the visit synopsis and the vital signs might be displayed. For example see figure 12.17.

At any point after a patient was selected, the caregiver could select the Snapshot icon resulting in the patient identifier and name being made an entry on the menu. Thereafter, the patient could be reselected by selecting the patient off the menu. See figure 12.18. Selecting "Close" on the "Patient" menu selection, would close and remove the current patient. The previous patient could be restored by selecting the "Previous" menu selection.

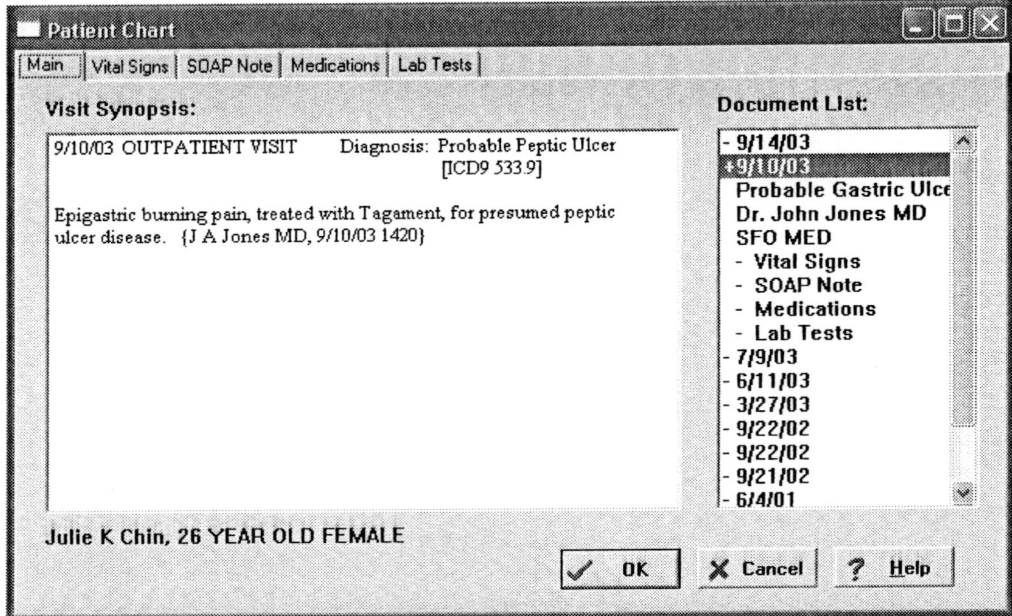

Figure 12.16 Patient Chart / Visit Synopsis.

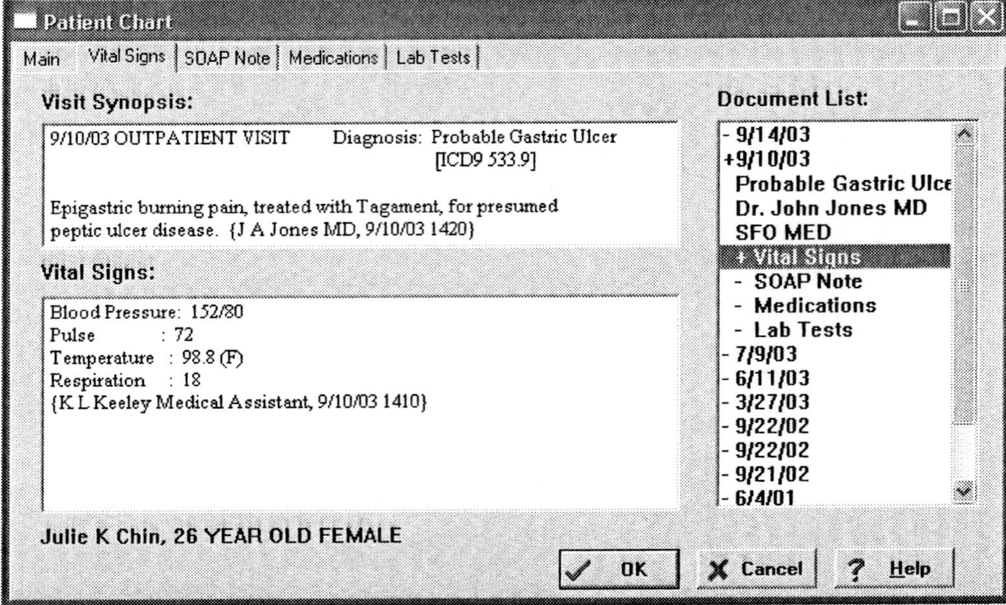

Figure 12.17 Patient Chart/ Vital Signs.

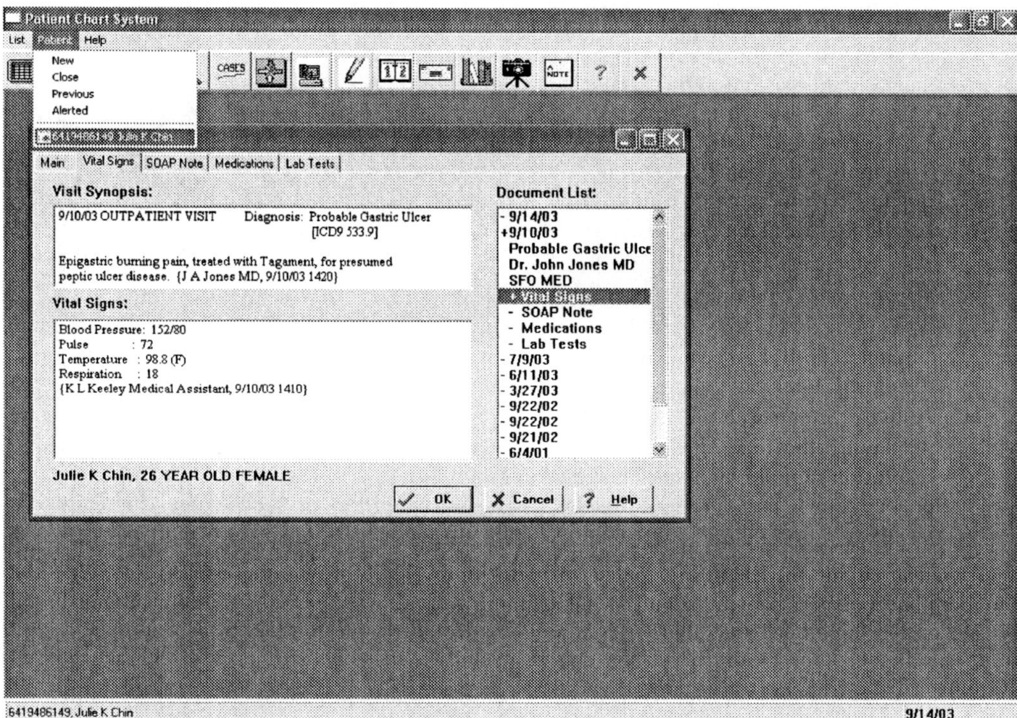

Figure 12.18 Patient Menu Selection Created by Snapshot Icon.

Also, when a caregiver is on a particular section of the chart, the caregiver can select the "Note" icon and mark a place in the chart where he/she can come back to. The caregiver could also optionally set a time she or he is to be alarmed and re-informed about the note.

The following are some observations about GUI interfaces:

- ***Concurrency*:** Two different windows could potentially be displayed at the same time, for example, the patient's Overall Clinical Summary and the patient's chart.
- ***Multiplicity*:** The physician can work on two instances of an object at the same time, say two patient lists (see figure 12.8) or the patient's chart for two different encounters. (Generally, GUI systems enable an application to identify whether or not multiple instances are allowed or not; if not, selection of an icon where there already is an instance will return to the single instance rather than create another one.)
- ***Direct Manipulation:*** Information could be transferred from one window to another, for example, from a medical reference to an H&P. The medical reference could be cut and pasted into the H&P.
- ***Multimedia* Can be Supported:** graphs, voice, video, pictures, drawings, scanned images, diagnostic images (such as x-rays or CT scans), and waveforms.
- **Decision-based *Message Boxes*:** These are windows that inform the caregiver of alternative decisions and choices. When an error occurs, the error can be displayed with buttons displaying choices on how to correct the error. Also, the automated system could make recommendations on better choice care decisions, such as recommendations on less

costly medications, and allow selections of these alternate medications, or selection of the original one, via buttons. And as pictured in figure 12.5, the caregiver can be informed of an alarm during other processing.

Other general attributes of GUI systems are the following:

- The application can be controlled largely by a mouse that can move around anywhere quickly on the screen, from control to control, where controls are buttons, text fields, scroll bars, etc. Text entry by keyboard is also possible.
- Windows can be moved around, brought in and out of focus (i.e., be identified as the selected one), and put side by side.
- A window and areas of windows can potentially be made smaller or larger. When made smaller, scroll bars can be added allowing non-displayed parts of the screen to be displayed. Images can be scaled, though the resolution might change.
- With *scroll bars*, larger than window or screen size images can be displayed while displaying the images with high resolution. This might be useful for display of high resolution digital diagnostic images that require more dots (or "pixels") than is available on the screen is to properly display them—although use of such images for diagnosis usually requires a larger size monitor than a physician uses for direct patient care.

Because of all these attributes that provide more flexibility to the user, I feel that the (cooperative business object-oriented) GUI interface is far superior to the character-based interface. On the other hand, some users are uncomfortable with this flexibility and have a hard time learning GUI or mouse-based systems, especially when being trained on character-based systems.

A basic principal of quality software design, for whatever interface is chosen, is that a consistent and useable set of screen display and input standards be chosen and followed on every screen. This decreases the complexity of the system and makes the system more intuitive for the user. This use of a consistent set of screen display and input standards applies whether the screen metaphor chosen is GUI or character-based.

Where there is an industry standard for the screen metaphor, this industry standard should be followed.

12.2.3 Pen-Based Interfaces

A disadvantage of using a desktop or laptop computer, whether GUI or character-oriented, is that it cannot be easily used during the time the patient is being interviewed, the keyboard and extra weight due to it get in the way. A pen computer simulates the current clipboard with notepad and is thus much more natural for a caregiver to use during direct patient care. A pen computer mainly uses a "pen" for input, "writing" on the screen. Such pen input can control a GUI application and can be based upon GUI "controls" such as buttons, check boxes, etc.

Pen computers are also compatible with the use of detailed clinical pick lists based upon a standardized medical vocabulary to create comprehensive clinical documentation without use of a keyboard. This usually also results in the automatic coding of diagnoses and procedures. For some, this seems like an excellent way to create medical documentation that is very consistent, even with different users, for others, this approach appears much too rigid.

Pen computer input also supports input of either handwriting or printing, usually printing that is stylized. For example, Palm™ PDA computer input uses a stylized printed input called "Graffitti" where some characters are shortened (for example an "A" is input as an upside down

"V") and some characters are standard printed character (for example a "C" is input as a "C"). A new version, "Graffitti 2" allows input of characters closer to normal print and an easier way to identify a capital letter.

Also, via some pen computers, a user can enter "gestures" to edit text. For example, if a user enters via pen an "x" with a circle around it after selecting text, this cuts the selected text for pasting into the text in some other location.

Sometimes notes verbatim without interpretation can be entered into the computer, which could include printed or cursive characters, pictures or doodles, which are recorded exactly as entered. The system could potentially determine whether to interpret the data or leave it as is from the context.

When used during patient care, a pen computer is unlikely to have a keyboard, or if it does, it is likely to have a very small keyboard or screen to compensate for the extra size or weight. A pen computer will therefore not be a complete substitute for a desktop or laptop PC. A desktop or laptop PC is probably still necessary when completing input of patient clinical information when the caregiver is back in his office, when a full size keyboard is essential. Pen computers and desktop/laptop PCs thus could complement each other.

For desktop/laptop and pen computers to practically be used as complements to each other, they should probably not be two entirely different systems; otherwise, the operator would need to be trained on two completely different systems. In order to avoid this, the PC system must be "ported" to the pen computer system and be largely the same, functioning nearly the same. There are some complications to doing this: for example, currently, desktop systems for the automated patient medical record often require super VGA screens while pen computers most often use lower resolution VGA screens (see section 17.2.5).

A relatively new type of pen computer is the *Tablet computer* that is the size of a clipboard and can be held like a clipboard, which may also have handwriting and voice recognition capabilities. Without a keyboard, the computer is relatively lightweight. With a wireless radio connection, it can be made even more lightweight by sending all inputs to a server and not needing a hard drive that adds weight itself and consumes energy and thus requires a heavier battery. Tablet computers are well-suited for computing at the point-of-care, such as physician interviews of patients or nurse care of patients in the hospital. Microsoft has come out with a Tablet computer that runs using a version of the Windows XP operating system. See references (Waegemann and Tessier 2002) and (Nobel 2003).

A type of very small, pen computer is a *PDA* or *personal digital assistant.* These are computers small enough to be carried around in a coat pocket or handbag. These computers may be most useful when a caregiver, such as a nurse, needs to go quickly from room to room where carrying around a larger computer may not be feasible. Ideally, the PDA would automatically transfer information over to the medical record, such as by wireless. See section 12.3 for more about computing at the time that the patient is being seen.

12.2.4 Tailoring by User

The automated system could be *tailored* dependent upon the needs of the user. For example, it could be tailored differently by caregiver. There could be a standard system, with optional tailoring by caregiver type (e.g., inpatient nurse, outpatient physician), by caregiver department (e.g., ICU) or by the individual. This could be done via agents. Agents are also discussed in sections 7.6 and 13.7.2.8 of this book.

Tailoring could include

- the Patient Lists available to the caregiver (see section 7.7.5 and figure 12.7).
- the Patient Clinical Summaries available to the caregiver and the identification and format of clinical items in each of the summaries (see section 7.7.4.1 and figure 12.14)
- the escalation procedure for reporting on STAT, abnormal or other results when the ordering caregiver is unavailable (e.g., an alarm is sent to nurse practitioner Pat Smith if the ordering caregiver, Dr. Sally Jones, does not respond to the alarm in a given period of time) or for reporting on "unresponded-to" messages when the receiver is unavailable (see sections 7.7.2 and 7.7.3.)

12.3 POINT-OF-CARE AND NON-POINT-OF-CARE INPUT METHODS

For purposes of a discussion of input methods, it is useful to distinguish computing where the patient is being seen by a caregiver and computing when the patient is not being seen. The general term for use of computers at the time a patient is receiving care, whether in the inpatient setting with a terminal at the bedside, or in the outpatient setting while interviewing the patient, is *point-of-care computing*. As stated earlier, it is the author's opinion that desktop computers can get in the way of patient care and are not appropriate for point-of-care computing.

Various input methods are listed in table 12.1. These input methods are presented in terms of a point-of-care computing part where interview information is gathered, and a potential later part not a the point of care to complete the process, for example to correct errors occurring during point-of-care.

Table 12.1 Example point-of-care input methods

Point-of-Care Input Method	*Later Additional Input Required*	*Advantages*	*Disadvantages*
None—patient interview recorded on paper	Input at workstation from paper notes	Does not get in the way of patient care. This is the least expensive alternative. It requires learning only one new system. Freehand input possible. No problem of a computer system going down.	The chart is not available during the interview except on paper or by going to a workstation. Two steps are required for input of interview information, rather than one. There is a question of what to do with the informal paper notes. Re-inputting freehand input may be difficult. There is the potential for late, inaccurate, or contradictory input.

Pen computer input directly to the automated patient record	Corrections of non-structured input at a workstation	The entire patient chart is available during the interview. Actionable information is available. Inputting the interview information can be done concurrently with the interview. Freehand input may be possible. The weight of a pen system is likely less than a desk-top computer.	May get in the way of patient care. The caregiver probably still needs to learn two systems, as the pen computer does not work 100% of the time in inputting text and correction might have to be made via a workstation or keyboard connected to the pen computer. Problems if system goes down.
Workstation input directly to the medical record	Corrections of mistyping may be required later at a workstation	The patient interview is input in one step. The entire patient chart is available during the interview. Requires learning only one new system. Actionable information is available.	May get in the way of patient care. May slow down patient care because caregiver might have to interrupt the interview, going to the workstation. Freehand input may not be possible. Problems if system goes down.
Portable input device connected to a workstation input directly to the automated patient record	Corrections at a workstation	Can be smaller and lighter than a pen computer. Dependent upon input device, interview information may still be recorded if system goes down. Inputting the interview information can be done concurrently with the interview. Freehand input is possible.	The chart is not available during the interview, except on paper or by going to a workstation. Most input devices do not work 100% of the time in inputting text, so input corrections are probably required at the workstation. Problems if device or connected system goes down. Unproven technology. Other possible disadvantages depend upon type of input device.

Let us first consider the paper input approach: A caregiver uses paper to jot down notes while interviewing the patient, then the caregiver or a medical transcriptionist later uses a workstation to input the notes to the automated patient medical record. The advantage of this approach over point-of-care computing is that during the patient interview, the caregiver can spend more time caring for the patient as the caregiver is not distracted by inputting to a computer.

The disadvantages of the paper input technique for point-of-care computing are the following:

- The patient's medical record information would not be immediately available on-line to the caregiver during the interview.
- Inputting information to the automated patient medical record would be a two-step, rather than a one-step, process.
- There is the potential of the caregiver, or someone else, inputting the incorrect information into the computer due to the caregiver or someone else not being able to read the handwritten notes.
- The caregiver must remember to perform the second step of inputting information into the chart, especially in situations where this second step may be delayed due to an emergency situation.

Another input approach is for a caregiver to use a pen computer, inputting directly to the automated patient record during the patient interview. Advantages are

- The pen computer is similar to the current paper chart clipboard and thus may not unduly get in the way of care.
- The entire patient medical record is available on the pen computer during the interview.
- There is no additional input step, like there for the approach of first recording the patient interview on paper.

It has the disadvantages in that

- Pen computers cannot guarantee completely accurate computer interpretation of text input with the pen—the text input may later have to be corrected.
- Like for laptop computers, a pen computer may be heavy or alternatively have too small a screen to substitute for a paper chart.
- The pen computer going down could disrupt the care process, potentially losing collected information.

A caregiver inputting information during the patient interview to a desktop workstation has similar advantages and disadvantages to a pen computer; however, its use during the patient interview can severely interfere with the patient interview, as the caregiver would have to move away from face-to-face contact with the patient to use the workstation.

An approach that is similar to recording patient information on paper is using a portable input device that records patient information on a piece of paper for backup purposes and at the same time sends the information directly to a workstation. One such input device is the Anoto digital pen (Anoto 2004) that reads dots on the paper it writes on. The Anoto digital pen requires the use of special paper, referred to as *digital paper*. Such a device has the same advantages and disadvantages as paper input, but turn the two-step process of inputting patient information during the interview into something simpler: instead of having to re-input the patient interview information, the user would only have to make corrections to the small parts of text information that the workstation could not accurately interpret.

A recent digital pen input device requires neither special paper or special ink: Jian Wang in China invented a pen that was perfected through Microsoft Research Asia in Beijing. (Huang 2004)

These new portable input devices require that recorded information be sent to the workstation or a server. Likewise, pen computers can be used as input devices (or "front-ends") for workstations. At least seven interface methods exist for transporting this information from the input device to the workstation or a server. These seven interfacing methods are listed in table 12.2, which also lists the characteristics of each of these interfaces. There are other interfacing methods that have a much greater range, but they are not recommended as their signals would go outside the building cause interference or security problems.

Each point-of-care input approach, and the non-point-of-care approach of recording to paper, has its advantages and disadvantages.

Note that the critique that a workstation may get in the way of patient care does not apply to visits via telephone or to telemedicine where the patient is remotely located from the caregiver. In such cases, a workstation may work as well as a pen computer or digitized pen.

Table 12.2 Interfaces for portable input devices

Interface Type	*Capabilities*
Direct wire connection after recording the input	Two step operation. Not real-time. Slow total process. Fast transmission after the connection is set up. Serial, USB or IrDA connection possible.
Infrared	Fast. Line of sight. Cannot go through walls. Real-time.
Bluetooth	Real-time. Can penetrate objects. Supports communication within 33 feet (10 meters). Selection between Bluetooth discovered devices. Security to provide only authorized access. Requires very little power. 720 Kbps. 2.4GHz devices may disrupt connection. Supports voice as well as data. So far, not very popular. An interface type for the Anoto™ pen.
HomeRF	Real-time. Requires PC card. Requires much more power than Bluetooth. Supports up to 127 nodes. Transmission rate much slower than Wireless LAN. Supports voice as well as data. Supports 50 meter transmission range. Can penetrate objects, such as walls.
80211a Wireless LAN	Real-time. Can penetrate walls. Intended for LAN connection over distances of up to 75 feet. Requires more power than Bluetooth or HomeRF. Speed up to 54Mbps. Not compatible with 802.11b and 802.11g.
80211b Wireless LAN (Wi-Fi)	Real-time. Can penetrate walls. Intended for LAN connection over distances of up to 150 feet. Requires more power than Bluetooth or HomeRF. Speed up to 11 Mbps. 2.4GHz devices may disrupt connection. The most dominant wireless LAN standard used today.
802.11g Wireless MAN	Real-time. Can penetrate walls. Intended for LAN connection over distances of up to 150 feet. Requires more power than Bluetooth or HomeRF. Speed up to 54 Mbps. 2.4GHz devices may disrupt connection. Because of bandwidth, it may be appropriate for departments requiring transmission of high volumes of information, such as radiology.

12.4 USE OF THE INTERNET

The *Internet* is a worldwide network of interconnected computers. The Internet, with the use of the Java language or Microsoft .NET, HTML and XML on Web servers, is becoming more versatile. The Internet can now be used to program very sophisticated GUI-based systems using these products. The user could communicate with the Web server through a large variety of devices, including PCs, PDAs and other types of pen computers, and wireless telephones, with a variety of input methods including keyboard, pen input, and voice. Point-of-care input methods described in the previous section also apply to the Internet.

Many completely in-house systems are being moved to work partially or entirely on the Internet or variants of the Internet. Variants of the Internet are an intranet, a part of the Internet that is internal to an organization, and an extranet, a part of the Internet that is shared by multiple designated organizations. With future changes in Internet technology, including increases in bandwidth (speed because of optical networks), quality of service, and security, moving in-house systems to the current Internet or a future Internet, or to its variants, will likely become even more prevalent.

Should the automated patient medical record system use the current or future Internet or its variants? The author views the automated patient medical record system, as described in chapters 6 and 7, as consisting of many parts. Each part should be evaluated individually to determine its appropriateness for use of the current or future Internet:

- for large healthcare organizations, a full-featured local automated patient medical record system
- for smaller healthcare organizations, an automated patient medical record system through an *ASP (an application service provider* that can provide an automated patient medical record system on a rental, pay-as-you-use, basis)—see chapter 6
- source document repositories for storage of individual patient records
- a computer-based patient record (CPR) consisting of a summarized history of the patients encounters, health problems, medications, allergies, etc
- a patient repository identifying the patient and healthcare and insurance organizations who would receive medical record information on the patient
- medical references available over the Internet
- patient access over the Internet to healthcare organization information of benefit to the patient.

Figure 12.19 shows the interconnections (interfaces) between these parts of the automated patient medical record. Each line in the diagram represents an interface that could potentially occur over the current or future Internet, or an intranet or extranet.

Clearly, the interfaces of medical center personnel with medical references and the patient with healthcare organization information should take place over the Internet. Should the other interfaces occur over the Internet?

Any interface that goes outside a single healthcare organization should have the characteristics of speed, security and reliability and have the ability to reach any healthcare organization in the world. This could involve an extranet, future versions of public networks such as the Internet, or perhaps a combination of both.

The Internet should be viewed as a changing network, with future likely changes including increased bandwidth, increased quality of service and greater security from unauthorized use, with changes agreed upon by a standards organization such as the *World Wide Web Consortium for the Internet (W3C)* (W3C 1994-2004). In the future, the Internet is likely to use more and more optical fiber, making it faster and faster, and likely to handle different type transmissions, voice, video, and data. The next version of the Internet will have more addresses and better security and is being developed by the *Internet Engineering Task Force (IETF)* (IETF 2004). Japan, South Korea and China are collaborating to move from today's IPv4 protocols to the next-generation Internet protocol addresses, Ipv6, that are 128 bits in length to increase the number of addresses, as these countries, as opposed to the US, are quickly running low on Internet addresses. (Lyman 2004)

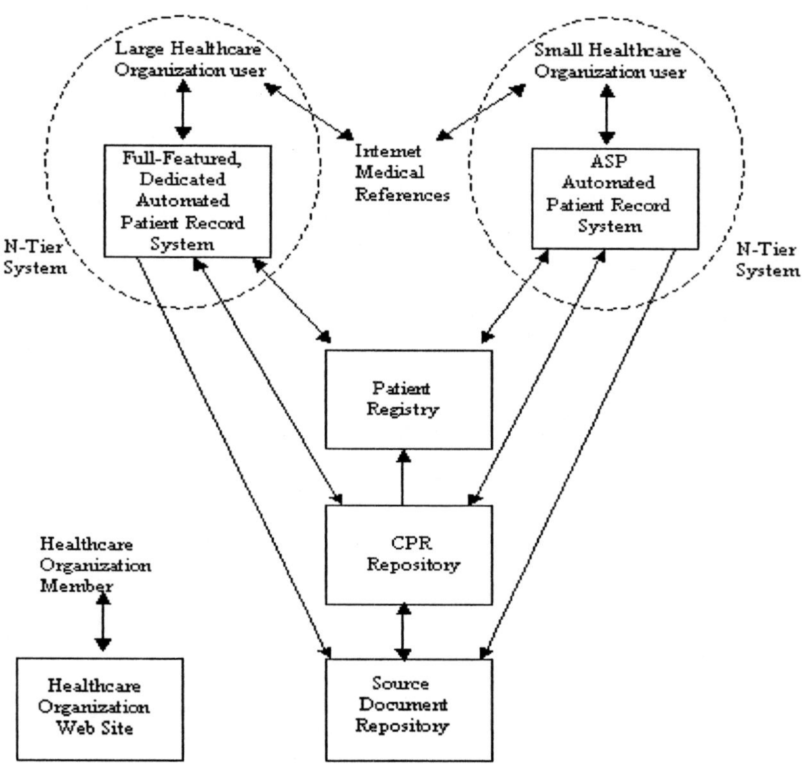

Figure 12.19 Proposed Intranet or Extranet Connections with an Automated Patient Medical Record System.

There are already alternative versions of the Internet available—*vBNS (very high-speed Backbone Network Service)* is one existing alternative version of the Internet, reserved for scientific applications, that can transfer data much faster than the current Internet (vBNS+ 2004). The North Carolina State University's Department of Computer Science has developed a new Internet protocol, BIC-TCP, which stands for Binary Increase Congestion Transmission Control Protocol, and is 6000 times as fast as DSL. (Kroeker 2004) The U.S. Department of Defense and 30 network vendors are testing an IPv6 version of the Internet, termed MoonV6, with the Department of Defense mandating its use within the department by 2008 (Reardon 2004).

The feasibility of use of the current and future Internets for the interfaces in figure 12.19 is dependent on the following:

- ***bandwidth**:* the speed of network traffic needed to handle the transmission—Dedicated network connections between healthcare organizations are the fastest. Is the current Internet fast enough or do we have to wait for a future Internet?
- ***quality of service (QofS)**:* the ability to differentiate between classes of network traffic and users and give the highest priority and error correction to the most critical

messages—The current Internet does not support QofS, but future planned networks will, and QofS within intranets or extranets is currently feasible and practical.

- **security**: keeping intruders out and limiting access of information to the appropriate users. Should all or part of the solution be a network dedicated to healthcare to insure the utmost security, as well as bandwidth; security within the Internet (PKI and other encryption techniques) increases network traffic, requiring greater bandwidth.
- **standards**: following agreed upon standards that can result in common networks that efficiently support healthcare transmissions. Such standards should include use of XML for source documents.
- **legal matters**: legally being able to share patient medical record information with those with a need to know.

The connection between the full-featured automated patient medical record system and medical center personnel, unlike the other connections, involves one healthcare organization. There is less of an advantage to use of the common network connection such as the Internet in such a situation; never the less, organizations are increasingly making use of the Internet within an intranet or extranet through *n-tier systems* for their in-house systems.

An n-tier architecture connected to the universal patient record is as shown in figure 12.20. "n" refers to an integer that might be any value, while *tier* refers to a category of computer. Thus an "n-tier system" consists of "n" different categories of computers.

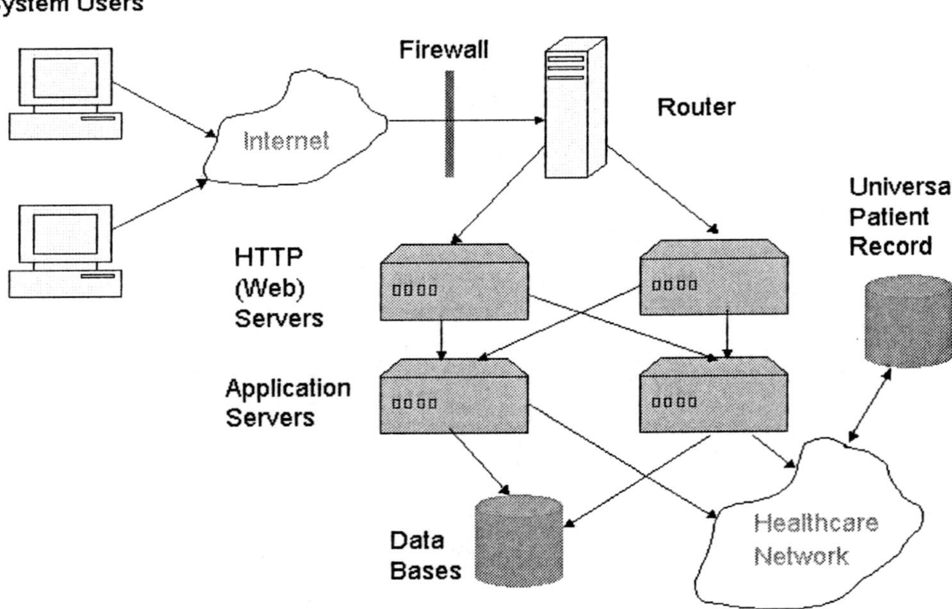

Figure 12.20 An N-Tier System Connected to the Universal Patient Record.

Such an n-tier system might include:

- ***thin clients* using *browsers* (often the Microsoft Internet Explorer or Netscape Navigator):** This provides the interface for the user. Interfaces can occur with PCs, pen computers, PDAs, and other devices.
- **communication over the Internet:** Communication between the user and the "n-tier" system is over the Internet.
- ***firewalls:*** This is a computer that keeps out users outside the intranet or extranet organizations and employees who are not authorized to use the system—The firewall is the part that turns the Internet into an intranet or extranet.
- **duplicated *Web servers* multiply connected so if one goes down, the other can still perform the same functions:** A Web server is a computer that handles the display of information to users through the Internet.
- **duplicated *application servers* multiply connected so if one goes down, the other perform the same functions:** An application server is computer that runs an application, such as the automated patient medical record system.
- **Sometimes *legacy systems:*** Legacy systems are existing healthcare organization systems.

The n-tier structure is also the typical architecture for ASPs—see chapter 6—although ASPs seldom handle legacy systems.

The Internet is currently being used on a limited scale for access to an automated patient record. For example, reference [11] describes the actual usage of the Internet for display of patient chart documentation at the University of Missouri's Health Sciences Center. Additionally, there is much medical reference documentation currently available on the Internet both in the category of public domain and commercial (e.g., Medline).

Also, use of the Internet could provide a valuable method for informing emergency department personnel (no matter where the emergency department is geographically located) of alerts and warnings for a patient (e.g., this patient is allergic to penicillin or has a pre-existing heart condition). Before this is feasible, there must be a certain threshold of patients with patient information on the Internet. Where available, the automated patient medical record could provide this information; with a significant implementation of a national or wider and more comprehensive automated patient medical record system, this approach might be superseded.

Although not really part of an automated patient medical record, many healthcare organizations currently provide access to HMO health care and non-health care information via the Internet to patients [12]. These systems are primarily made for HMO members, although some of these systems are also available for use by caregivers, other HMO employees, and designated personnel in organizations who contract with the HMO to provide medical care for a group of members (e.g., a company contracting with the HMO to provide medical care for its employees). Some information and capabilities that could be provided over the Internet are the following:

- information on the member's benefits*
- information on the member's healthcare services representative, primary care physicians or nurse practitioners, other assigned physicians or nurse practitioners, or case managers*
- ability to make appointments*
- get a list of health care facilities and providers based upon entered zip code
- ability to get information (e.g., biographies) on potential principal primary care and other physicians and nurse practitioners to be assigned with the patient

- ability to select principal primary care and other providers to assign with the patient based upon the most important characteristics (e.g., female, has at least so many years of experience, etc.)*
- directories of caregivers, including name, location and phone number
- information on preventive care recommendations by sex and age
- information on the latest treatments, including alternative medical care provided by the HMO
- on-line medical advice, with the stipulation that the patient should come in to the medical center for emergency medical situations*
- chat rooms with psychiatrists and other medical providers*
- on-line searches
- information on medical center layouts.

If any of the information that has an * is available, then the Internet user must first be required to enter the patient's HMO membership number and a personal identification number (PIN) to verify that he/she is a member of the HMO and to identify the member.

Other connections shown in figure 12.20 could also potentially occur over the Internet. Some connections, such as between the web server, application server, database, and legacy system would likely to be connected by local networks or dedicated connections. Dedicated network connections could also occur between networks of different healthcare organizations outside of the Internet.

There are four different basic types of application system structures: a *mainframe* application, a PC application, a *client-server* application, and an Internet application. The application could be on a large computer, a mainframe system, which runs the application for many users, each at a *dumb terminal*, i.e., a terminal consisting of a keyboard and display screen that cannot run applications itself but can receive and send character data to a mainframe (e.g., a CICS application running on a mainframe); see figure 12.21a for a mainframe application structure. Often, a PC is used in place of a dumb terminal; the PC *emulates* the dumb terminal—it runs a program in a window that mimics the dumb terminal. The application could run on a PC for a single user; see figure 12.21b for a PC application structure. The application could run on a server computer with additional application logic—usually for the GUI part of the application—on each PC client workstation of a user; see figure 12.21c for a client-server application structure. The application could run on a server computer, with a Web server connecting to PCs, with each PC running an Internet browser; see figure 12.21d for an Internet application structure.

An application running through an Internet browser is called a *thin-client*. A thin-client has the advantage over a client in a client-server setup in that it does not require the PC to have application-specific code other than the user interface code; thus, virtually any PC running anywhere can be used as the thin-client, as long as the user can be identified as having access to the application. Because application-specific code runs only on the server, the PC, which can be a portable or pen computer, need not have a hard disk and thus can be more light-weight, and thus more portable.

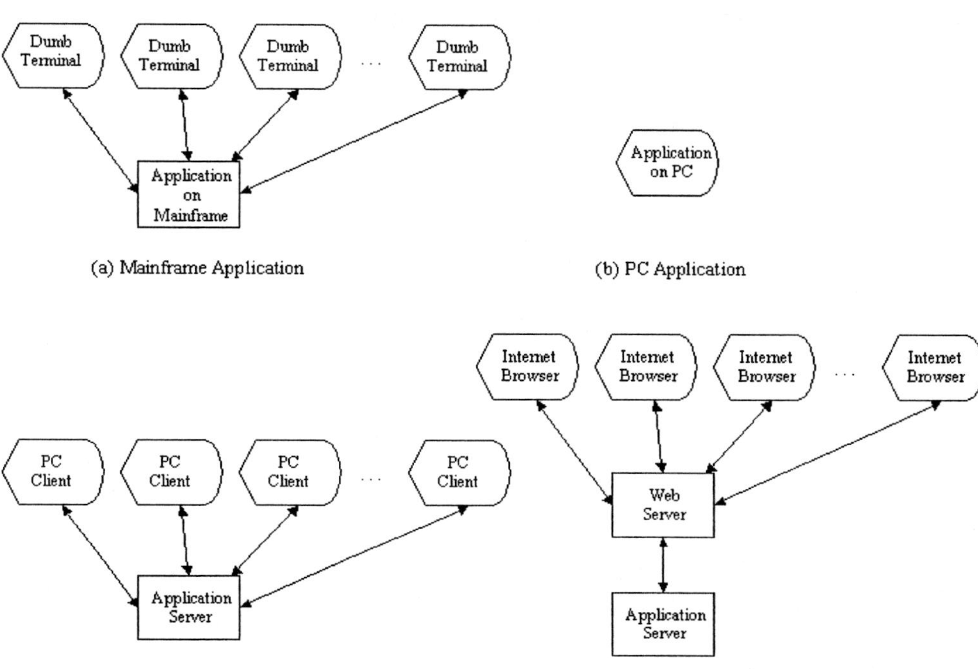

Figure 12.21 Application Structures.

Many applications that have been initially structured as client-server applications that have complex user interfaces, including the automated medical record and clinical systems, can be restructured as Internet systems by a commercial product, the Citrix Metaframe Access Suite™, thus transforming a client-server application to an Internet application, whereby the application's logic executes on the server and only the user interface is transmitted across the network to the client to an Internet browser. This technique of running the application on a server and only the user interface running on the client's browser is referred to as *server-based computing.* Note that computer languages that can be used with the Internet such as Java, enable the user interface code to be transmitted down to the client's browser through the Internet as needed and thus need not be permanently stored on the client computer—see section 13.11.4.

Programs transmitted down to the thin client are called *plug-ins.* Such plug-ins control processing that browser programs cannot efficiently handle. For example, scrolling documents larger than a computer screen (e.g., diagnotic images or large clinical images) might be handled by a plug-in. Such an approach to handling scrolling of medical documents requires that the medical document be shipped down for storage to the thin-client computer—This could result in potential memory and security problems.

12.5 AN OUTPATIENT PHYSICIAN, PHYSICIAN ASSISTANT, AND NURSE PRACTITIONER S VIEW

Outpatient physicians, nurse practitioners and physician assistants, as clinicians, perform similar functions in caring for patients (with the exception that nurse practitioners and physician assistants are under the supervision of physicians). Thus in general, all use the same patient lists and patient chart documents.

Schedule, John Jones MD

Add Patient | Cancel | Select

Date: 9/14/2003 Caregiver: J A Jones MD

Time	Type	Patient Id	Patient Name	Location
0000	[Off]			
0800	Routine	5678901234	Jane K King	Oakland MED1
0830	Urgent	3254027570	John L Lewis	Oakland MED1
0845	Urgent	2092409855	Kersey Sanders	Oakland MED1
0900	Urgent	2450826388	Larry Mathews	Oakland MED1
0915	Routine	5008299264	Kathy A Kelley	Oakland MED1
0945	Urgent	3462030203	Phillip L McRichards	Oakland MED1
1000	[Meeting]			
1100	Urgent	4587092862	Susan S Kingley	Oakland MED2
1115	Urgent	9549090236	Sally Fields	Oakland MED2
1130	Routine	6548320806	Stanley L Rainey	Oakland MED2
1200	Routine	5380306266	Karen White	Oakland MED2
1230	[Lunch]			
1330	Urgent	3550026487	Harold J Grayson	Oakland MED1
1345	Urgent	6083969889	Johnathan Grossman	Oakland MED1
1400	[Meeting]			Oakland MED1
1800	[Off]			

Figure 12.22 Outpatient Schedule.

The principle documents identifying patients for an outpatient clinician, an patient list, is the *outpatient schedule* (see figure 12.22). From a schedule, a clinician can select a patient who is scheduled for an appointment or who was not scheduled but who came in and is registered to be seen.

Also the clinician could press the "Add Patient" button to add a patient to the schedule, bringing up a dialog to enter a patient identifier to identify the patient to be added (for example, as shown in figure 12.10). An alternative design is to not provide this function and have "drop-in" patients only identified by the registration system. In either case, the appointment system should provide a method to book patients anywhere in the schedule.

Another patient list is an *outpatient clinic room map* (see figure 12.23). One possibility is that the patient's name could be "dragged over" from the schedule using the mouse or other pointer device to the room map, perhaps by a receptionist or nurse, which could trigger notification of a nurse and the physician caring for the patient; each nurse and physician could wear an electronic tracker that could identify the room the caregiver is in and thus automatically identify on the room map which caregiver is in which room, and with which patient. When the patient is ready to leave, the patient can be removed from the room on the room map.

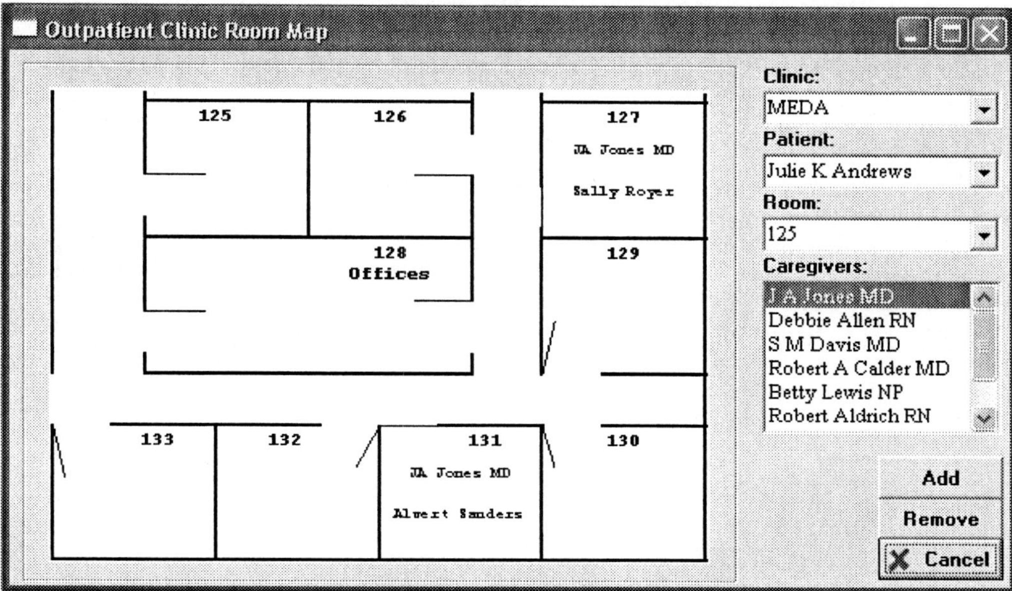

Figure 12.23 Outpatient Clinic Room Map.

After selection of a patient from the schedule or room map, or identification of the patient by entrance of a patient identifier, an overview of clinical information for the patient in the form of a *overall clinical summary* could be displayed, which might include the following (see figure 12.15):

- shortened patient demographics
- a list of significant health problems
- a list of encounters
- a list of primary caregivers (primary care providers, case manager and health service representative), including telephone numbers and ability to select a caregiver on the list to automatically establish a telephone or e-mail connection
- a list of current medications
- a list of clinical orders, results and alarms
- allergies and adverse reactions
- immunizations
- special precautions, made very obvious to the caregiver (e.g., violent patient, court injunction against patient, drug seeking behavior)
- active defined outcome cases/chronic care management cases/patient cases
- referrals
- active clinical pathways (which may include a life care path scheduling preventive care)

- active trend documents.

Buttons for cases, referrals, clinical pathways or trend documents would be highlighted or dimmed dependent upon whether there were or were not such documents. In the example, the list of significant health problems identifies that there is a chronic care management case associated with the significant health problem of "asthma".

Through the overall clinical summary Cases button or through the Cases icon on the tool bar, the outpatient clinician will have access to all defined outcome cases, to all chronic care management cases, and to all patient cases, active and inactive (see figure 12.24). When treatments involve more than one encounter, a *defined outcome case* or a *chronic care management case* may be developed, which may capture the case managers, the treatment plan, notes on the treatment progress, clinical pathways based upon the patient condition, references to clinical practice guidelines, and trend documents (see figures 12.25-12.29); these documents are explained further in section 12.7. Also when it is uncertain that a defined outcome case is needed, a conditional defined outcome case may be developed by a primary care physician, urgent care physician, nurse practitioner, or advice nurse that may be later used to generate a defined outcome case (see section 7.4.1) or be automatically hidden or deleted should it not be used. Case managers, guiding high risk, high cost, patients through the system, may record their actions through case notes in a *patient case*.

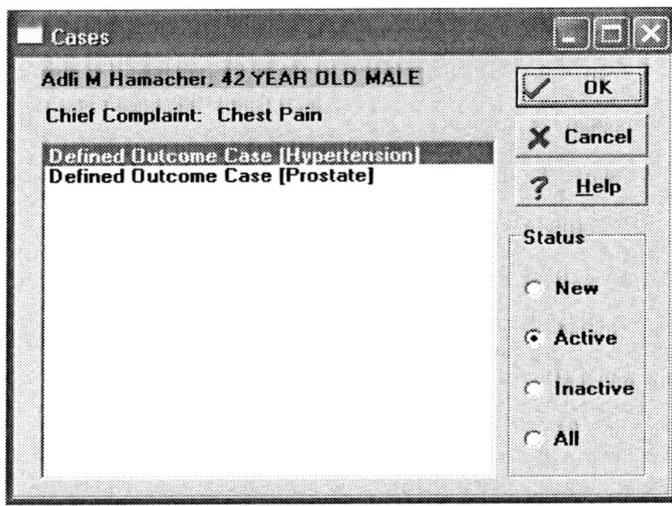

Figure 12.24 List of cases.

On the list of cases for a patient, the caregiver can select active cases, inactive ones that are in the past, or all cases. A new case can be started. Selection of a case goes to a dialog for that case. See figure 12.25. Selecting the "Treatment Notes" button might bring up treatment notes organized by encounter. See figure 12.26.

Defined Outcome Case

Adli M Hamacher, 42 YEAR OLD MALE

Priority: Medium

Case Information

Treatment Id: Drug Therapy for Hypertension

Expectations: Lower Blood Pressure

Appt Phone: (510) 555-2242 Transfer

Documents: Clinical Pathway,Trend Document

Encounters

Date	LOS	Diagnosis
5/20/03		Hypertension
4/15/03		Hypertension
3/20/03		Hypertension
2/28/03		Hypertension

Treatment Plan

Following care path for Drug Therapy for Hypertension, test out medications for hypertension. Patient told to come in or call in periodically for blood pressure check, which will be automatically recorded on trend document.

Case Managers

Name	Type
Fran Eddy	Case Manager
J Schwarz MD	Primary Care Physician

Treatment Notes

Documents

Cancel

Help

Figure 12.25 Defined outcome case for hypertension.

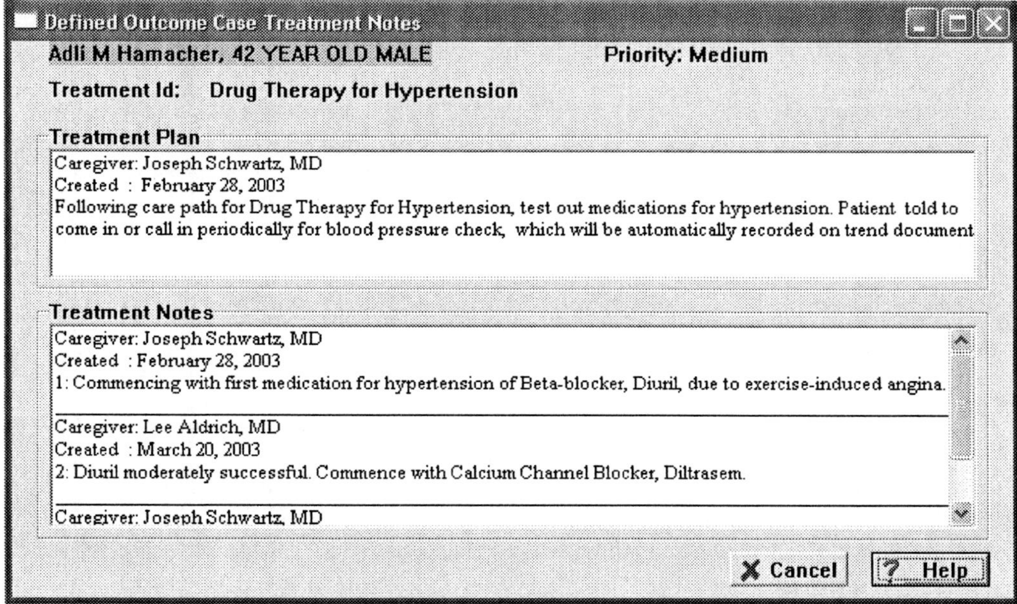

Defined Outcome Case Treatment Notes

Adli M Hamacher, 42 YEAR OLD MALE

Priority: Medium

Treatment Id: Drug Therapy for Hypertension

Treatment Plan

Caregiver: Joseph Schwartz, MD
Created : February 28, 2003
Following care path for Drug Therapy for Hypertension, test out medications for hypertension. Patient told to come in or call in periodically for blood pressure check, which will be automatically recorded on trend document

Treatment Notes

Caregiver: Joseph Schwartz, MD
Created : February 28, 2003
1: Commencing with first medication for hypertension of Beta-blocker, Diuril, due to exercise-induced angina.

Caregiver: Lee Aldrich, MD
Created : March 20, 2003
2: Diuril moderately successful. Commence with Calcium Channel Blocker, Diltrasem.

Caregiver: Joseph Schwartz, MD

Cancel

Help

Figure 12.26 Defined outcome case treatment notes.

Selecting the Document button would display documents created for the defined outcome case. See figure 12.27.

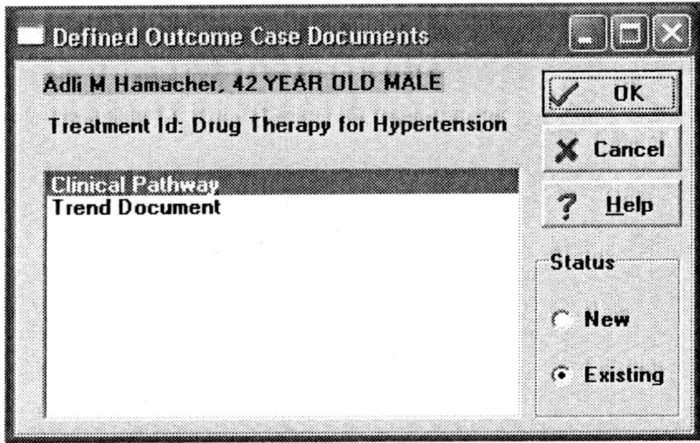

Figure 12.27 List of defined outcome case documents.

Defined outcome case documents could include clinical pathways and trend documents. See figures 12.28 and 12.29.

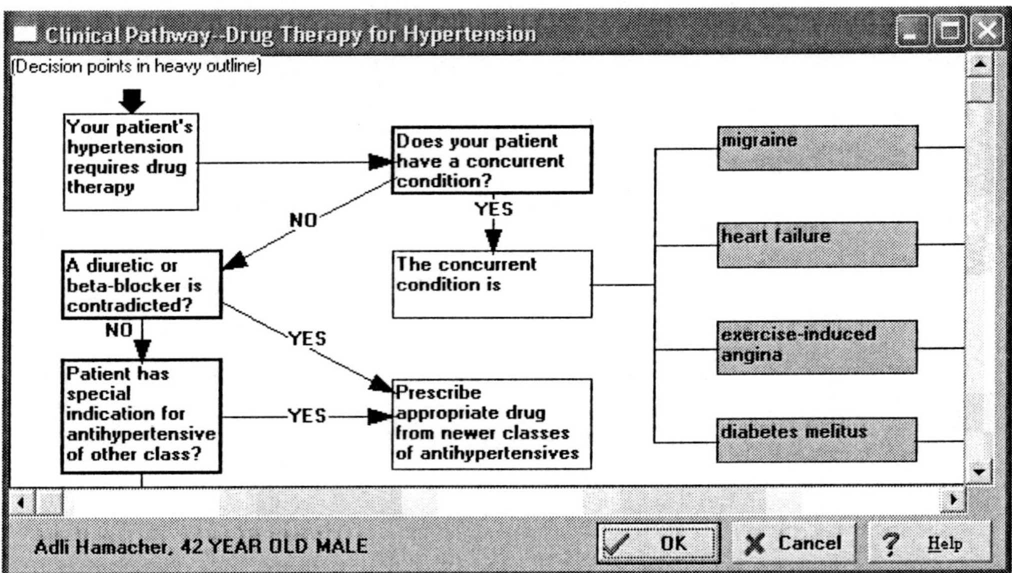

Figure 12.28 Clinical pathway.

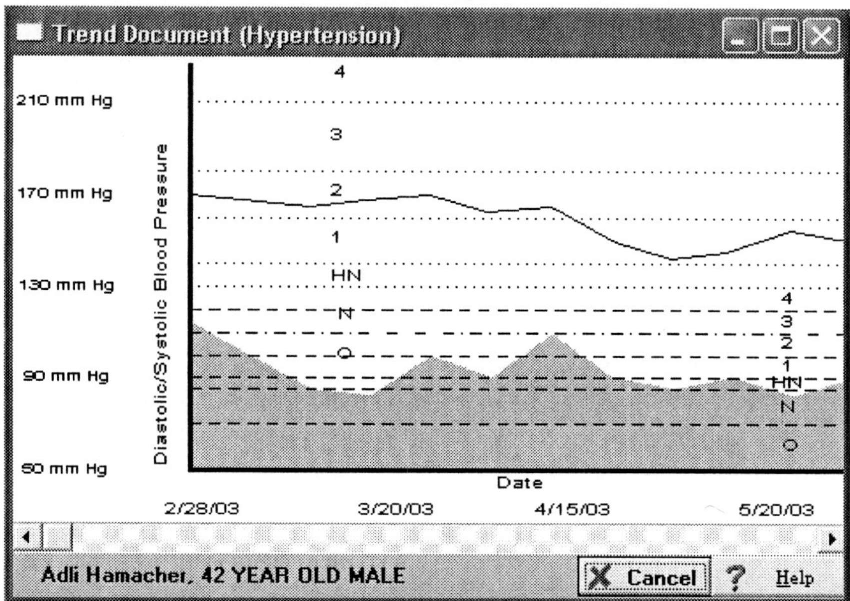

Figure 12.29 Trend Document.

By pressing the Synopses button on the tool bar, the outpatient clinician can indicate to display a list of *synopses of all encounters* (see figure 12.30).

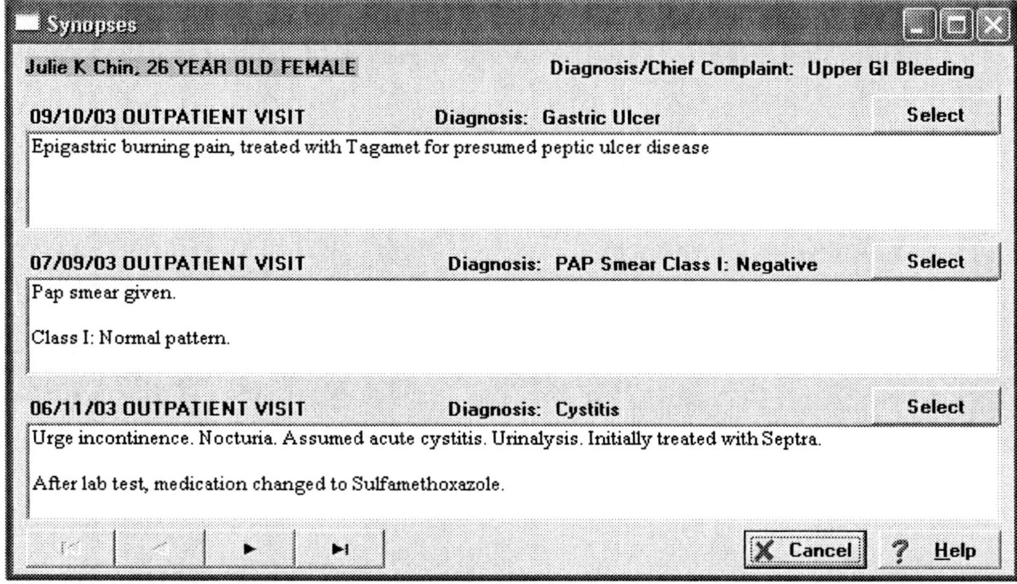

Figure 12.30 Encounter Synopses.

By pressing the Chart icon on the tool bar, a *document list* of all chart documents for the encounter could be displayed along with the patient chart (see figure 12.31). The user could select a particular encounter date in which case the associated encounter (visit) synopsis would be displayed. The user could then select a chart document for display (see figure 12.32).

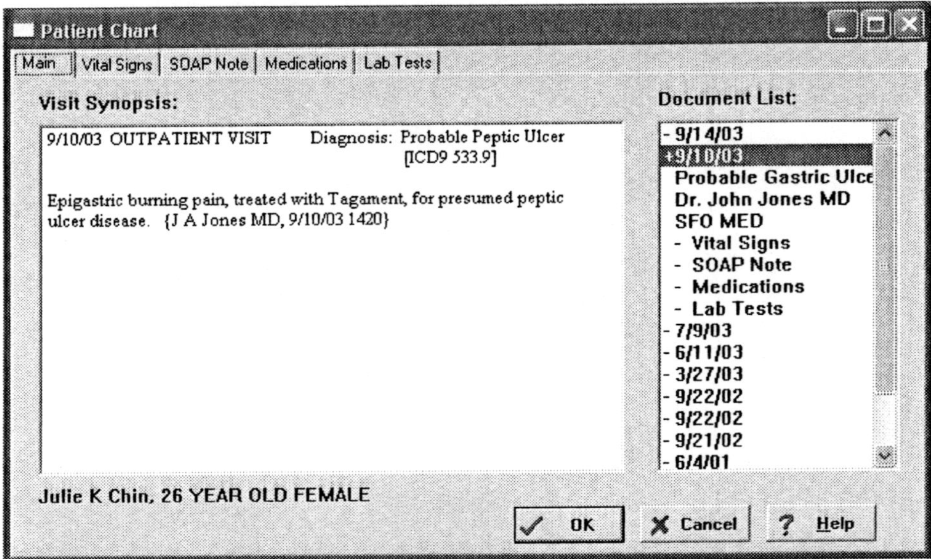

Figure 12.31 The Chart, and an associated Document List.

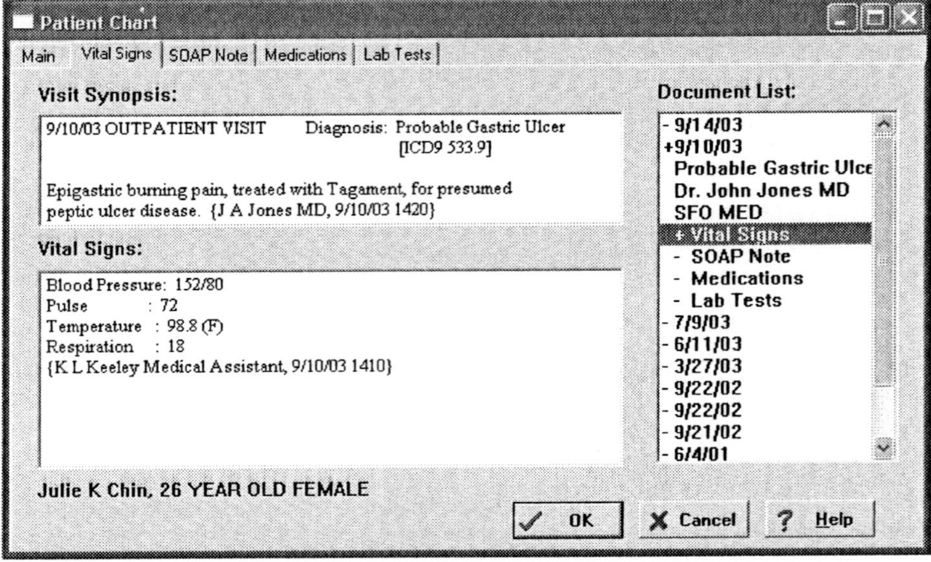

Figure 12.32 Document selected from Document List.

Documents in facilities outside the HMO might display a message box that would allow the clinician to optionally order the document(s) from the remote location (see figure 12.33), or alternatively, agents could automatically order these documents for the clinician when the appointment, registration, admit or pre-admit is made.

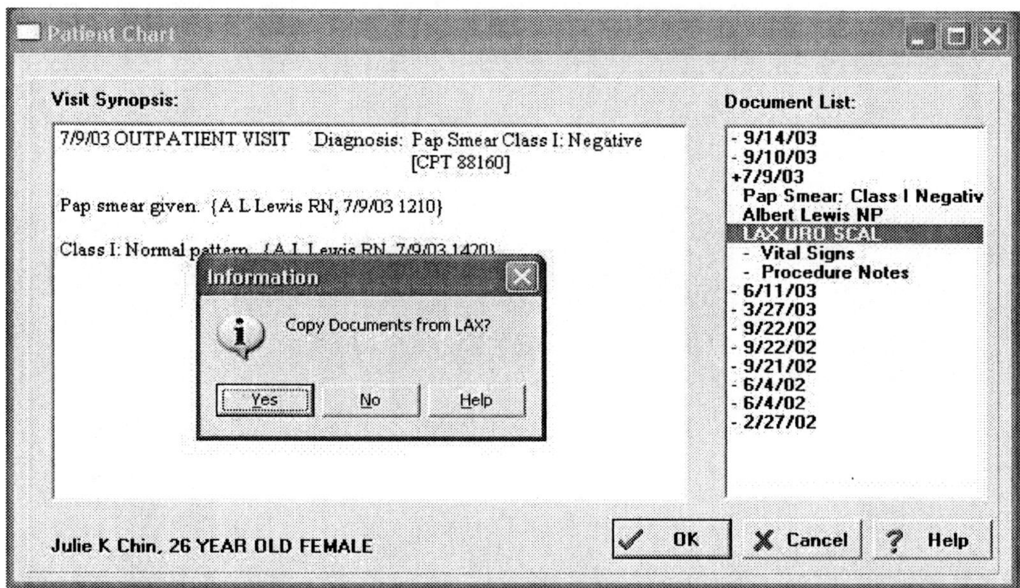

Figure 12.33 Documents located remotely.

By selecting the Search button on the tool bar, the clinician could search through the patient chart for information satisfying particular criteria selecting associated synopses. For example, as in figure 12.34, he can search for encounters dealing with either the "prostate" or "urogenital" body system, resulting in the display of synopses of these selected encounters (see figure 12.35).

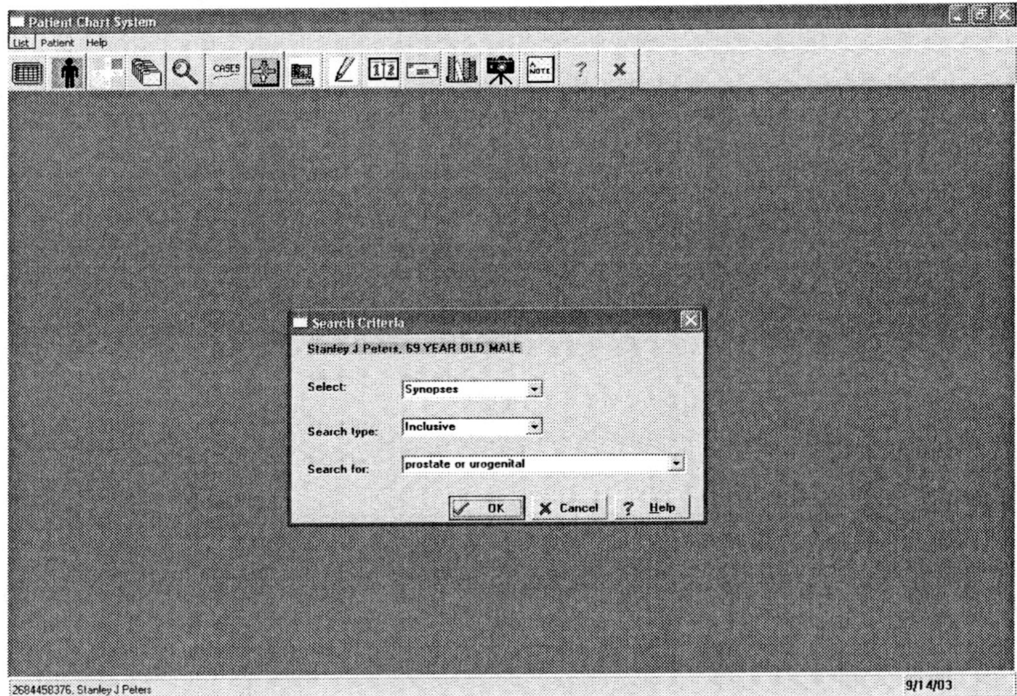

Figure 12.34 Search for encounters meeting criteria.

During the examination of the patient, the outpatient clinician would create documentation, enter orders, make appointments and initiate case documents among other actions. The automated patient medical record system would support the outpatient clinician for the following:

- clinician entered documentation: Selection of the Document button on the tool bar would bring up a list of documents (see figure 12.36). A new or existing document could be selected. For example, a new history and physical (H&P) could be selected. An example of an H&P using templates, abbreviations and pick lists was shown in section 7.7.1 of this book (see figures 7.7, 7.8 and 7.9).

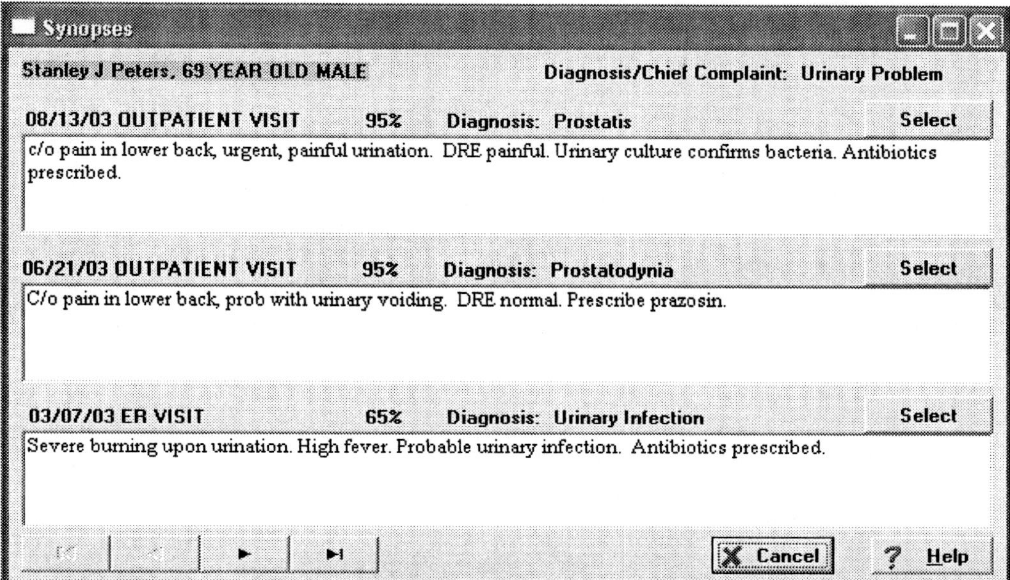

Figure 12.35 Selected encounter synopses.

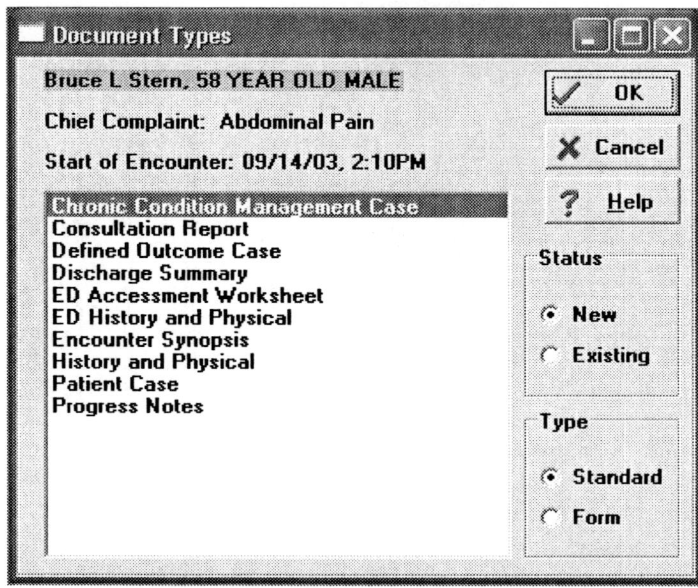

Figure 12.36 List of documents.

- ***orders***: Orders for medications, clinical lab tests, diagnostic imaging, etc. could be made (see figure 12.37).

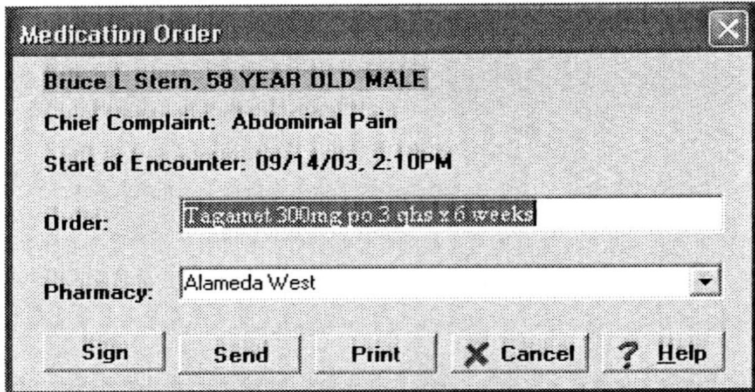

Figure 12.37 Example order.

- ***appointments*:** Future appointments could be made (see figure 12.38), either taking up available time in a caregiver's schedule or being "force booked" and being booked independent of the free time in the caregiver's schedule.

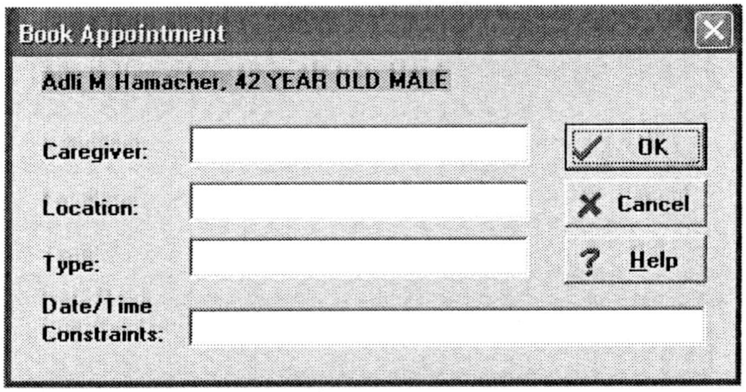

Book Appointment
Adli M Hamacher, 42 YEAR OLD MALE
Caregiver:
Location:
Type:
Date/Time Constraints:
OK
Cancel
? Help

Figure 12.38 Book an appointment.

- **defined outcome case:** Initiate a **defined outcome case** and create **treatment plan and notes** to be included in a defined outcome case to track and monitor a treatment for the patient, most often spanning many encounters. A defined outcome case is proposed to have the information identified later in section 12.7.1 of this paper (see figure 12.25). At the time of the first encounter for a treatment, an initial treatment plan can be created and treatment notes could be successively added after each follow-on encounter (see figure 12.26). The treatment plan can be modified as necessary, with the new treatment plan appended to the previous one.
- **chronic care management case:** For a "high risk" chronic condition initiate a condition management case, similar to a defined outcome case but generally also with the assignment of a case manager
- **trend document:** Initiate or conclude a trend document that automatically records information on the patient over time, also optionally part of a defined outcome case or

chronic care management case, with the system informing a provider if a value is not collected during a visit (see figure 12.29).

- **synopsis of the encounter:** Enable a clinician to enter a synopsis of the encounter after the encounter, say from information in an H&P (see figure 12.39), although such a document could be conceivably generated by the system from other documents.

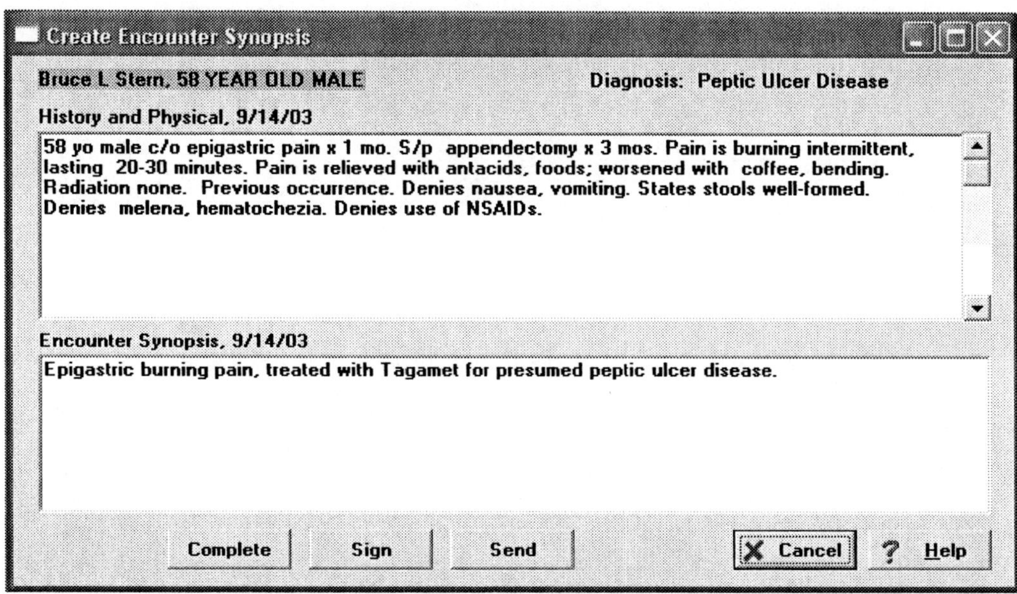

Figure 12.39 Function to create encounter synopsis from H&P.

Other documentation available in the chart might come from automated systems (e.g., clinical laboratory results) or other caregivers (e.g., radiologist or cardiologists results).

The clinician could be interrupted to be informed of new e-mail, new messages or *alarms* as a result of abnormal results coming back from orders, such as for clinical laboratory tests, diagnostic images, or EKGs (see figure 12.40). The clinician could, perhaps, be able to immediately jump over to the results in the patient chart (see figure 12.41), or to the e-mail or message, with the ability to later return to chart for the previous patient. The clinician could also acknowledge the alarm, e-mail or message, and return to it at a later time.

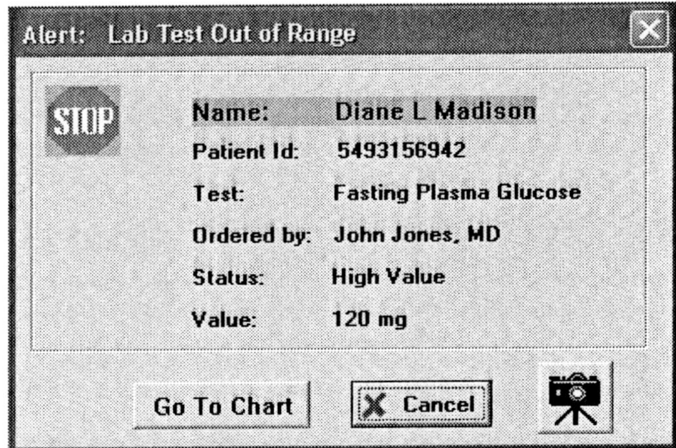

Figure 12.40 Alarm

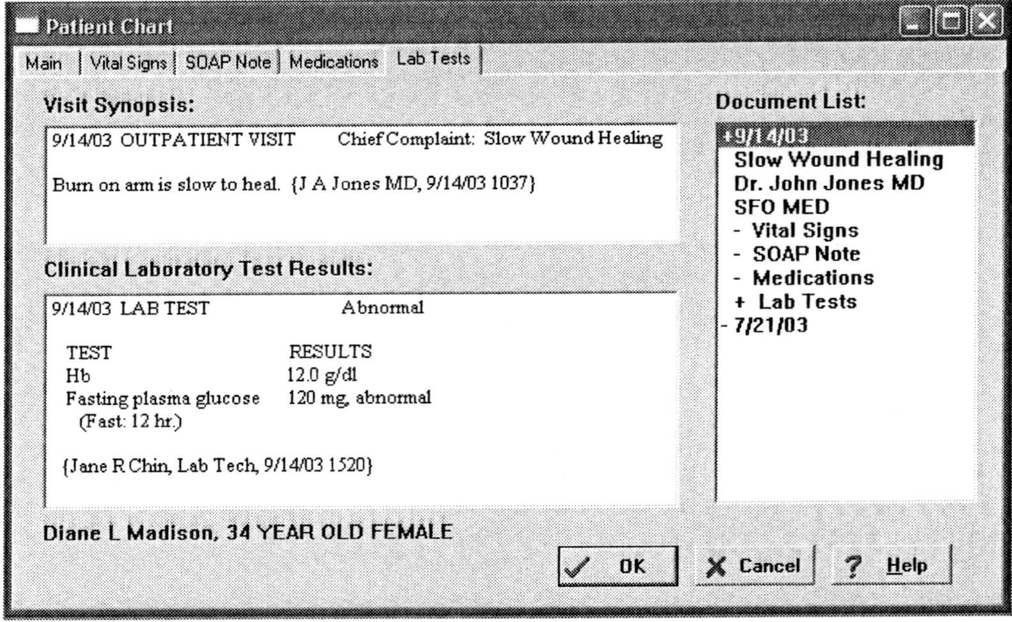

Figure 12.41 Patient chart / laboratory test results.

Pressing the "snapshot" icon on the alarm or while a patient was selected might put the patient on the menu (see figure 12.18), allowing that patient to be selected later; also the last "Selected" patient and last "Alerted" patient could be re-selected. Pressing the "snapshot" icon while a patient list is displayed might put the patient list on the menu (see figure 12.42).

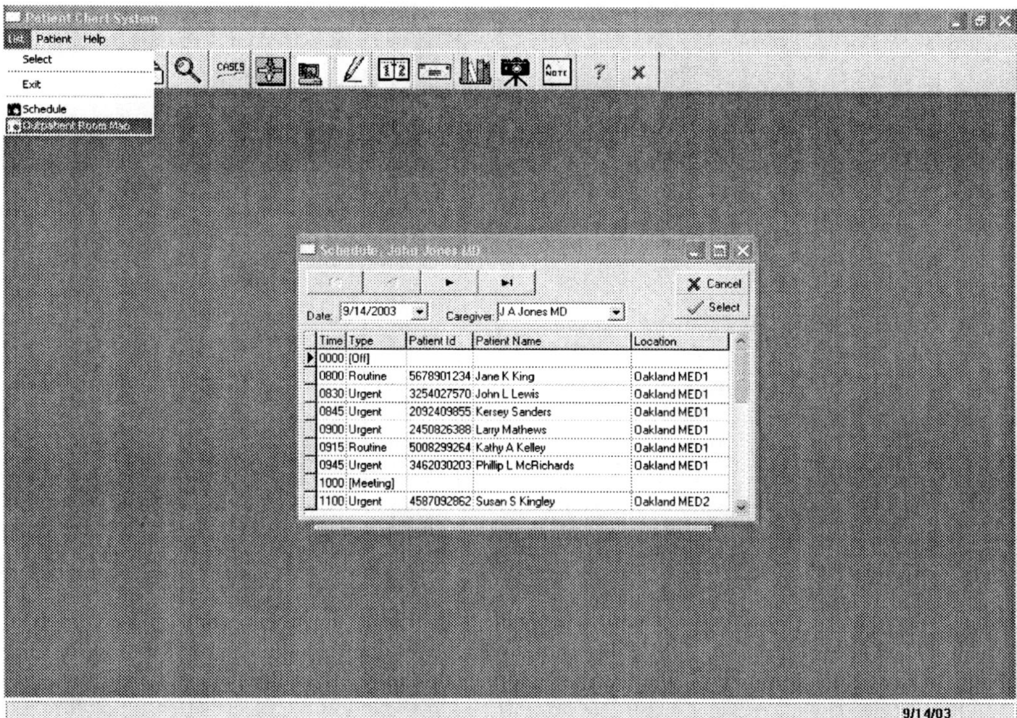

Figure 12.42 Addition of patient lists to menu so they can be quickly selected.

-So far, the automated patient chart, other than patient lists, is centered around a single patient. Another screen not centered around a single patient is an *in-basket,* a collection of a clinician's orders and results, e-mails, and clinical messages (see figure 12.43). Selection of the "messages" icon could allow the caregiver to select to display clinical messages for the caregiver, care team, hospital unit, or patient panel, for all facilities or a particular facility location. (Note that a physician's patient panel is all the patients for which the physician is the primary care physician.) Additionally the caregiver can select to see all his orders and results or all his e-mail.

Selection of the "orders" icons would display the clinician's orders and any returned results; the clinician might then get a screen such is shown in figure 12.43. Selecting an order line, an order/result line for one with returned results, and the "Go to Chart" button might go directly to the order and result in the patient's chart. Selecting the "create" button might allow the caregiver to create a new order, e-mail or clinical message.

Lists could be sorted based upon any displayed field, by selection the column name. This would allow the clinician to find orders of a particular type (medications, diagnostic images, etc.) and/or orders with abnormal, panic or alarmed results and/or for a particular patient and/or within a particular date/time range.

By selecting the Medical References button on the tool bar, the outpatient clinician could see practice guidelines, protocols, standard operating procedure documents and other *medical reference documents*. These might be available through the Internet, an Intranet or Extranet. Also available would be generic medical references such as MEDLINE.

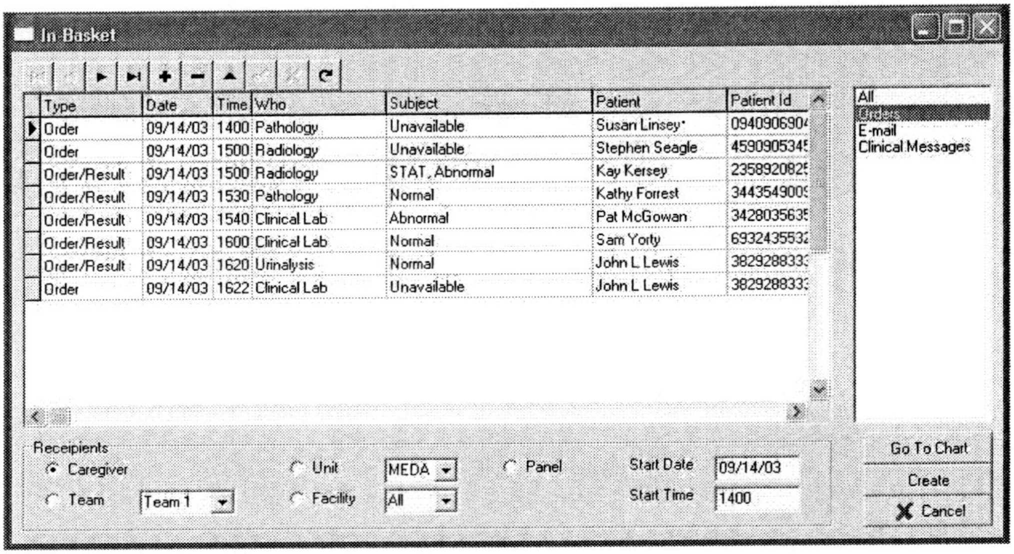

In Basket

Type	Date	Time	Who	Subject	Patient	Patient Id
Order	09/14/03	1400	Pathology	Unavailable	Susan Linsey	0940906904
Order	09/14/03	1500	Radiology	Unavailable	Stephen Seagle	4590905345
Order/Result	09/14/03	1500	Radiology	STAT, Abnormal	Kay Kersey	2358920825
Order/Result	09/14/03	1530	Pathology	Normal	Kathy Forrest	3443549009
Order/Result	09/14/03	1540	Clinical Lab	Abnormal	Pat McGowan	3428035635
Order/Result	09/14/03	1600	Clinical Lab	Normal	Sam Yorty	6932435532
Order/Result	09/14/03	1620	Urinalysis	Normal	John L Lewis	3829288333
Order	09/14/03	1622	Clinical Lab	Unavailable	John L Lewis	3829288333

All
Orders
E-mail
Clinical Messages

Receipients
Caregiver Unit MEDA Panel Start Date 09/14/03
Team Team 1 Facility All Start Time 1400

Go To Chart
Create
Cancel

Figure 12.43 In-basket.

As stated in section 7.7.11, a patient's medical decisions may be partially based upon a patient's HMO coverage. If an HMO does not cover a treatment or requires an extra fee for one treatment or medication or procedure versus another, this may affect the patient's, and thus the caregiver's, decisions on what treatment to follow, medication to prescribe or procedure to perform. Benefits at this level should be available to the clinician.

12.6 SPECIAL SITUATIONS

This section discusses two situations where the availability of a simplified automated system would be useful: (1) the automated patient medical record system is down; (2) a small facility wants its information to be included in the CPR repository but it cannot afford to fully automate the patient medical record.

12.6.1 Use of Forms When the System is Down

In the case of the system being down, a backup approach would be to input documentation on paper forms as is done before automation. Through a "form fill" program showing the exact form on the computer screen, each form could then later be input to the computer or alternatively scanned and stored in the automated patient medical record as images. See figures 12.44 and 12.45. This approach could also be used as a first documentation approach, prior to development of more sophisticated methods of inputting document.

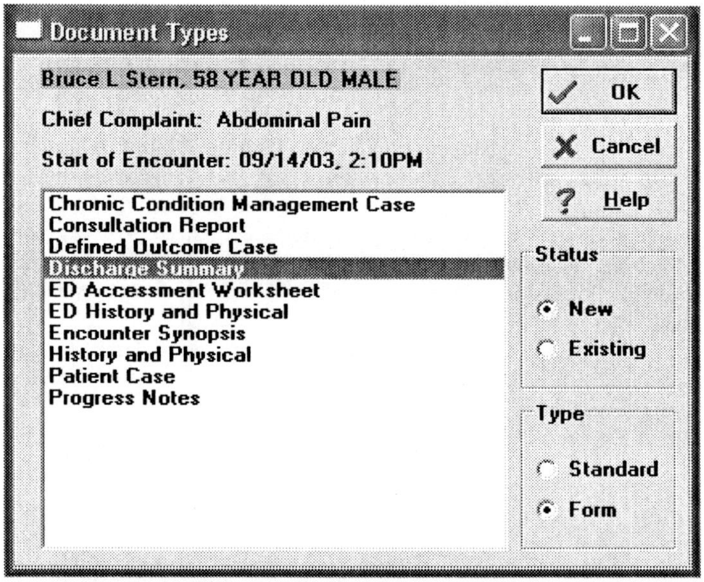

Document Types

Bruce L Stern, 58 YEAR OLD MALE

Chief Complaint: Abdominal Pain

Start of Encounter: 09/14/03, 2:10PM

Chronic Condition Management Case
Consultation Report
Defined Outcome Case
Discharge Summary
ED Accessment Worksheet
ED History and Physical
Encounter Synopsis
History and Physical
Patient Case
Progress Notes

OK
Cancel
Help

Status
New
Existing

Type
Standard
Form

Figure 12.44 List of form documents.

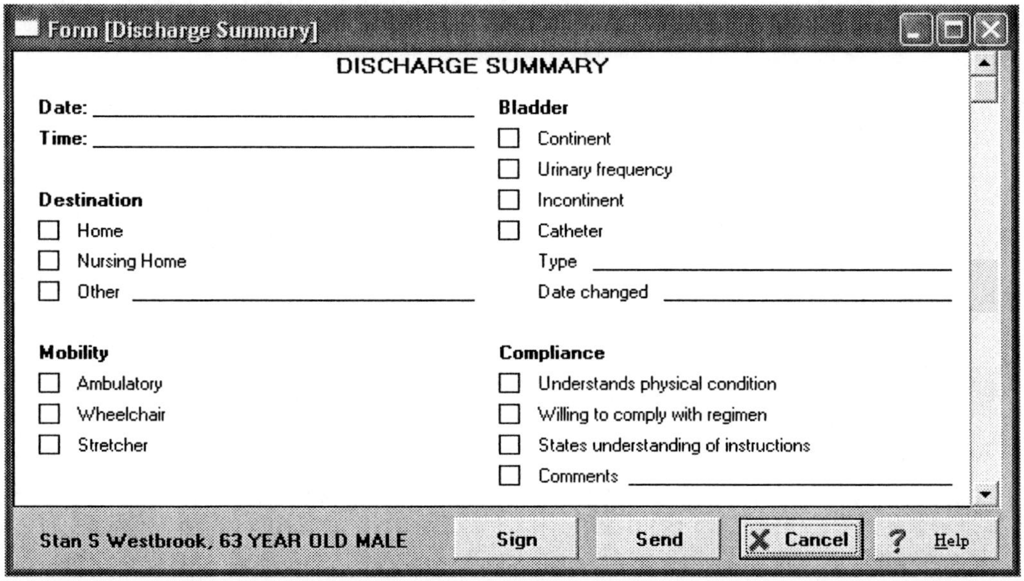

Form [Discharge Summary]

DISCHARGE SUMMARY

Date: ______
Time: ______

Destination
- Home
- Nursing Home
- Other ______

Mobility
- Ambulatory
- Wheelchair
- Stretcher

Bladder
- Continent
- Urinary frequency
- Incontinent
- Catheter

Type ______
Date changed ______

Compliance
- Understands physical condition
- Willing to comply with regimen
- States understanding of instructions
- Comments ______

Stan S Westbrook, 63 YEAR OLD MALE

Sign
Send
Cancel
Help

Figure 12.45 Form document.

12.6.2 Automation for a Small or Medium Size Healthcare Organization

The author feels that, in the long run, small and medium size health care organizations will make use of application service providers (ASPs), outside companies providing automated patient medical record system services (or other software services) on a pay per transaction basis. Through such systems, users could input patient information on source documents, which would be used to create the CPR and source document information for the patient. Because ASPs can be viewed to be similar to utilities such as those that provide electricity to anyone on demand and provide software systems to organizations upon demand, ASPs are said to provide *utility computing* capabilities to organizations (see section 17.3.2).

Prior to the establishment of ASPs, a quick and easy approach to automating the patient medical record for a small or medium size healthcare organization could be to have the provider input an e-mail summarizing a patient encounter, sending the e-mail to the CPR.

12.7 DOCUMENTS AND TOOLS FOR CONTINUITY OF CARE

Continuity of care requires that care be tracked and documented at a level that goes beyond single encounters to insure that the most effective care is provided at the least cost. As discussed in earlier chapters, the treatment process is an iterative one, with a treatment of any complexity extending across multiple encounters. Also, care for elderly, Medicare or high-risk patients should be continually monitored to insure that the least costly and most appropriate alternative care is picked (e.g., care in an SNF or nursing home) This process of tracking a patient across encounters falls into the categories of care management, case management or disease management (see section 7.4.7). This section presents documents that support these various forms of management of patients.

Examples of care situations extending across multiple encounters are the following:

- **extended *treatment plan***: when a treatment plan spans a period of time until it is no longer needed (e.g., when a patient is treated with a number of hypertension medications to find the best one, when a patient has a suspicious pap smear, or when a patient is pregnant)
- ***chronic condition***: when a persistent or long lasting condition is recognized that must be improved or maintained by treatment (e.g., paraplegia and urinary infections, prostate cancer, age-related macular degeneration, degenerative arthritis, juvenile diabetes)
- **high-cost condition**: when the patient has a costly, high risk, disease or condition, such as chronic or end-state renal disease (ESRD), juvenile diabetes or cancer treatment, over a long period of time or over a lifetime, where management of costs and risks must be controlled
- ***worker s compensation***: when the patient has a potential worker's compensation injury or disease where worker's compensation is a state-mandated program requiring certain employers to pay benefits and furnish medical care to employees for on-the-job injuries.
- **the elderly and *Medicare* patients**: when the patient is elderly and must constantly switch between home, hospital, nursing and SNF care, some of which is paid for by Medicare— a federal health insurance program for people over age 65 –some of which is not, where costs must be controlled.

These situations require special documentation that crosses encounters. This documentation was introduced in Chapter 7: defined outcome case documentation for management of treatments across encounters until the condition is improved, maintained or cured, chronic care management case documentation for management of a patient with a chronic condition, and patient case documentation for overall management of a high risk or high cost patient. Chapter 8 identified how these documents could effectively be used within an HMO to improve patient care.

The following sections propose documentation for defined outcome cases, chronic care management cases and patient cases, and describe various other documents that can be used to track the patient across encounters, including *clinical pathways* and *trend documents*.

12.7.1 Defined Outcome Case

As evidenced by the patient care process as described in section 4.4.1.3 and pictured in figures 4.1 and 4.2, the care process is an iterative one: The caregiver selects the most likely diagnosis, treats the patient and observes the results. If the treatment doesn't work, the caregiver considers another diagnosis or another treatment. Further, many of the diagnostic tests, radiological studies, or laboratory tests may not yet be complete before a treatment is started. When the results do come back, there is a likelihood the treatment will be changed. A series of different treatments may thus be tried over a significant period of time.

To emphasize this iterative process, consider a recommended treatment plan for hypertension: "When starting on anti-hypertensive medication, trying one at a time may be the best approach..However, control of blood pressure in some patients may still require a combination of two, or even three, drugs (Margolis and Klag 1996)." Clearly, such a treatment plan requires a lot of communication across outpatient encounters, even if only a single physician is involved; if there are many physicians involved, there is even more of a potential communication problem.

In order to track a treatment over multiple encounters, documentation to track the treatment over multiple encounters should be developed. For a non-chronic condition, this set of documents will be termed a *defined outcome case*. Some parts of a defined outcome case are the following (see figures 12.25 - 12.29 where most of these are shown):

- **priority of treatment** (e.g., minor, medium, major, critical, unknown) so the detriment of curtailment of the treatment can be identified
- **treatment type identifier** (needed to compare treatments).
- **expected outcomes** (caregiver expected outcome and patient's expected outcomes)
- appointment phone number to call for appointments
- **encounters**, including associated caregivers
- **treatment plans**
- ***case managers***
- a ***clinical pathway*** document based upon the patient condition can optionally be attached to the defined outcome case, guiding the treatment—In figure 12.25, a "Documents" button allows access to this and other documents (see figures 12.27 and 12.28)
- a ***trend document*** can be optionally included in the defined management case, which automates collection of particular data values, such a blood pressure over the various encounter, growth charts (height and weight), etc.—In figure 12.25, a "Documents" button also allows access to this document (see figures 12.27 and 12.28)

- **encounter summaries** attached by later caregivers (or the same caregiver) to identify a continuation or change in the treatment—an "Encounter Summaries" button might be added to figure 12.25 to display encounter summaries such as shown in figure 12.30
- references to ***clinical practice guidelines*** followed—not shown.

A defined outcome case will normally be assigned to a particular physician. A defined outcome case involving high risk may also be assigned to a case manager. Because of the importance of a treatment not being interrupted or discontinued, assigned caregivers or the case manager could be informed if a critical event (e.g., a required appointment) fails to take place in a given time. After the defined outcome case is closed, *actual outcomes* could be recorded by independent evaluators.

The defined outcome case could also be available to advice nurses through the overall clinical summary, so if the patient called in to ask a question about the treatment, the advice nurse could more easily answer it. For example, the cases could be available through a "Cases" button on the tool bar or through a "Cases" button on a clinical summary (see figure 12.15) that would bring up a single case or a list of cases to select; see figure 12.24.

In order to facilitate an advice nurse or appointment clerk in transferring a patient over to the appropriate department to make an appointment connected with the defined outcome case, selection of the transfer button next to the appointment phone could result in the patient's call being automatically transferred to that number.

A special situation where a defined outcome case may be useful is for a worker's compensation case. For a possible worker's compensation case, a healthcare institution must follow special procedures. Before care is given, a healthcare worker must first get verification from the employer of the injury, unless the injury is life threatening. The part of the medical record pertaining to the injury is considered to belong to the employer so that the claim can be reviewed by the employer's insurance company. In this context, use of a defined outcome case and assignment of a case manager is a method to tie together all the documentation related to the worker's compensation injury and to assign a person responsible to handle communications with medical personnel, the employer, insurance companies, and the government.

12.7.2 Patient Case

The purpose of a *patient case* is for a case manager to track a high risk or high cost patient independent of the particular condition or disease, usually over a long period of time, so the patient can be guided into receiving the best and most cost effective treatments. A stand-alone patient case is not directly associated with a disease or chronic condition; however, a patient case can report case manager comments on a particular episode of care and be included as part of a defined outcome case or a chronic care management case. Parts of a case may include the following:

- *case managers*
- *case notes* for use by the case manager to track the patient's progress.
- *expected outcomes* (caregiver expected outcome and patient's expected outcomes)
- optional *clinical pathways*
- other case documents.

12.7.3 Chronic Care Management Case

Chronic condition management requires treatments over an extended period of time for a particular chronic condition (e.g., persistent and severe asthma). Additionally, to control costs and provide patient access to necessary services, a case manager may be assigned. Thus, for the *chronic care management case*, the capabilities of the *defined outcome case* to track treatments should be combined with the *patient case* to assist the case manager in tracking the patient.

A chronic care management case, unlike a defined outcome case, usually tracks a condition that never goes away; thus evaluation only of final outcomes is not sufficient. Such chronic condition case management might be periodically evaluated by comparing costs and intermediate outcomes of patients undergoing case management versus those with similar patients who are not. Immediate outcomes could include mortality rates (death rates), morbidity rates (those who are sick versus those who are well), returns to the hospital after treatment, infection rates after surgery, patient feeling of well-being, patient satisfaction with medical care, etc.

12.7.4 A Treatment Plan and Notes Within a Case

See figures 12.24 and 12.25. Within a defined outcome case or chronic care management case, the treatment is described by a dated *treatment plan*. After an encounter, details of what happened during an encounter as related to the treatment would be put in as dated *treatment notes*. A major modification of the treatment might produce another treatment plan. Successive caregivers seeing a patient would add additional treatment notes, and upon change of treatment an additional treatment plan. It is suggested that treatment plans and notes be part of the same document within the case, resembling an e-mail with forwarded messages, with the treatment plan part being distinguished from the treatment notes.

12.7.5 Clinical Pathway

A more structured approach to patient care is a *clinical pathway* (sometimes called a "critical path" or "life care path") document. A clinical pathway encapsulates a care or treatment plan for a specific condition or for patients in a particular category (e.g., preventive care for men over 60).

As stated in section 5.3.1.4, a clinical pathway is a structured way to identify care activities and caregiver workflow needed to care for a patient with a particular condition or disease. Paths through a clinical pathway can be adjusted for the particular needs of an individual patient.

A *standard of care* is the minimum level of performance accepted to ensure high quality of care to patients. Standards of care define the types of therapies typically administered to patients with defined problems or needs.

A *clinical pathway* identifies a *standard of care* for caregivers for a particular *patient problem or condition* with consideration of *risk adjustments*, which may be based upon patient psychological, health and social factors, family/genetic history, patient age, race and sex. Clinical pathways may exist for outpatients, inpatients or patients who will both be an outpatient and inpatient [14]. Clinical pathways may be used for treating illnesses or for managing health and wellness.

A clinical pathway document may be stand-alone or be part of a defined outcome case, chronic care management case, or a patient case. It describes a series of care activities that may be conditionally performed that are either part of a treatment (e.g., for Alzheimer's, kidney stones) or part of a strategy for preventive care (e.g., preventive health activities to be performed on the patient of such a sex and age such as mammography). The latter type of clinical pathway identifying preventive care for a member over a long period of time is termed a *life care path*, as it may exist over the life time of the patient, not just during a specific treatment.

A clinical pathway consists of the following elements:

- *clinical pathway template*: a network structure diagram identifying all recommended alternative paths of care based upon intermediate goals and outcomes. A clinical pathway template consists of a series of *care activities* and *paths* between care activities. For each path, there may be a time between care activities in a path as identified either by a fixed time value or by a *probability density function (pdf)* statistically identifying likely time values for a path (e.g., the time for a fibula to heal). From one care activity there may be one or many paths leading to other care activities. A number of care activities could lead to the same care activity. Network diagram paths eventually may lead to *final outcomes* that identify conclusion of the care path (e.g., discharge from the hospital), or, alternatively, paths may be ongoing. A care activity may consist of text identifying care to be given, a goal, an order to be made or an appointment to be automatically scheduled, a protocol defined elsewhere in the system (e.g., "Implement 'anticoag' protocol"), or another clinical pathway. For example, there may be a clinical pathway template identifying all likely clinical pathways for women over 50 for detection and care of breast cancer, including paths identifying that the patient has been confirmed as having breast cancer and thereafter treating the patient, with a care activity consisting of a different clinical pathway specifically for the treatment of breast cancer. There would be another path identifying that the patient is healthy. One possible final outcome in the breast cancer clinical pathway may be total remission of the cancer. Again, pdf's can be used to estimate time between care activities; figure 12.46, for example, shows a pdf which might

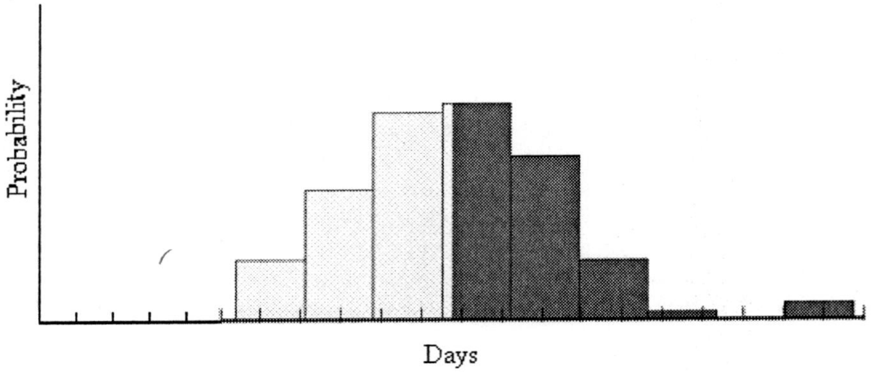

Figure 12.46 Conceptualized probability distribution function (PDF) for bone healing.

identify how many days it takes for a fracture to heal, which might be used to estimate the time between a care activity to put on a cast and later take it off, with the probabilities for the different number of days to heal for the collection of patients adding up to 1.00.

- *selected path*: one of the paths through the clinical pathway template selected by caregiver(s) upon intermediate outcomes or goals, identifying care to be given to the patient as determined by the clinical pathway template. During an encounter between the patient and a caregiver, the caregiver can select the next path to take in the clinical pathway template based upon a goal or an intermediate patient outcome. For example, a clinical pathway may include a care activity that consists of giving the patient a mammogram, with the intermediate outcome that the patient has a normal mammogram, and thus the patient would be scheduled for the next care activity, a mammogram a year later.

- *actual path*: a path identifying actual care activities given to the patient, that tracks the outcome-directed "selected path" except that actual times, if applicable, may be assigned to paths, care activities may be added or skipped, additional intermediate and final outcomes may result. The actual path identifies what actually happened; it may consist of the same path as the outcome-directed path but with actual times between activities or additional care activities within the path.
- *variances*: variance between an actual path and a selected (projected) path, in time, care activities, order of care activities and costs; variance between actual and projected immediate outcomes; and the variance between the actual final outcome and the initially projected final outcome.

During an encounter of a patient with a caregiver, the caregiver can identify the next path to take, adding to the selected path. The next care activity in a selected path may be an encounter and optionally include *automatic scheduling of the encounter* or may put the encounter on a *wait list* to be scheduled. A care activity in a selected path may also optionally *automatically schedule an order*. The caregiver may be informed if a care activity is not performed within the required time (e.g., a patient with a disease condition that must be closely followed does not show up for his appointment and does not reschedule the appointment in the required time). The caregiver can add or skip care activities changing the selected path, and creating an actual path different than the selected path.

After assignment of a clinical pathway to a patient, a clinical pathway can be discontinued, merged with another clinical pathway or identified as completed by a caregiver. Merging of clinical pathways would take into account, *co-morbidity*, i.e., interaction of the care activities in the multiple clinical pathways, where the original clinical pathways were each for different diseases. Care activities in different clinical pathways that are merged might be color-coded by the clinical pathway the care activity came from and highlighted for co-morbidity. As paths are completed, times for actual paths would be included in with the pdf's for the organization in the clinical pathway template.

A clinical pathway structure could also include care activities that a patient himself or herself is advised to follow (e.g., a drug therapy program for the patient). Figure 12.28 shows part of a care path that is a simplified clinical pathway used in our defined outcome case to determine the best drugs to prescribe for a patient with hypertension.

12.7.6 Trend Document

A *trend document* tracks the progress of a health condition over time. A trend document may stand alone or be part of a defined outcome case, chronic care management case or patient case.

A caregiver could be concerned about the patient's blood pressure and start off a "trend document" that records the patients blood pressure over time, perhaps graphing the patient's blood pressure versus high, low and medium blood pressure values for the member's age and sex (see figure 12.29); out of range values for which the physician should be alerted could also be identified. If the patient came in for a visit and the blood pressure was not measured, then the system would inform a caregiver to do so. Additionally, the member could be trained to measure his own blood pressure and call in the result periodically to an appointment clerk or advice nurse—the automated system could verify that the appointment clerk or advice nurse entered the value correctly and alert the appointment clerk, advice nurse or a physician about out of range values. Also, the trend document could be set up so the patient is automatically periodically sent a letter advising the patient to come in for an appointment dealing with the condition, or automatically put on a wait list for such an appointment. The trend document would be available to advice nurses, physicians and other caregivers through the overall clinical summary; see figure 12.15.

Figure 12.29 displays a trend document that shows the member's systolic and diastolic blood pressure values versus general blood pressure classification values. Another approach would be to display the patient's blood pressure values versus mean (systolic and diastolic) values by age and sex; such a trend document might be used in conjunction with a life care path that might identify preventive health care that should be given over a patient's lifetime, based upon patient characteristics. Or it might be used in conjunction with a defined outcome case to control the patient's hypertension as in figures 12.25-12.29.

Other examples of trend documents are the following:

- a growth chart for a child patient who is too short for her age
- mammographies taken over time
- x-rays of a patient's knee over time who has progressive osteoarthritis.

Trend documents could optionally be displayed in terms of graphs or tables or pictures.

12.8 THE CHANGED NATURE OF CONSULTATIONS AND REFERRALS

With the automation of the patient medical record and concurrent availability of the patient's medical record to multiple caregivers, consultations could significantly change. One caregiver could be consulting with one or more caregivers at the same or different locations while all are viewing the patient's medical record, and viewing the patient either in person or via television. All caregivers could potentially input information for the same patient encounter. Multidisciplinary care would be supported, with specialists from many different disciplines consulting with each other regarding a patient's condition.

Primary care physician requests for specialty care (a referral) or for specialty advice at a later time would also change in character. With the automated patient medical record system, a short communication, say a *consultation* or *referral request*, could be sent to a specialist or specialty area. Upon receiving or being assigned the request, a specialist would have immediate access to the patient's automated patient medical record. Upon the specialist giving advice to the primary care physician or after the patient has been scheduled, a *response* could then be sent back to the primary care physician. The primary care encounter notes, request, and response, and later any specialist encounter notes, could be automatically combined in a defined outcome case or chronic care management case, which would be available within the automated patient record.

12.9 A HOSPITALIST S/INPATIENT PHYSICIAN S VIEW

Inpatient physicians take care of patients in the hospital. An inpatient physician who exclusively see inpatients and serves as a substitute for the primary care physician when patients are in the hospital is referred to as a *hospitalist.*

The hospitalist and inpatient physician use the same documents as the outpatient physician except that the principal patient lists are the *inpatient physician list* for a physician and the *inpatient clinical summary* rather than the *overall clinical summary*, although that is used also. The *inpatient physician list* for a physician lists all admissions for which a physician is either the admitting physician, attending physician, consultant, attending resident, primary care physician or hospitalist (see figure 12.47).

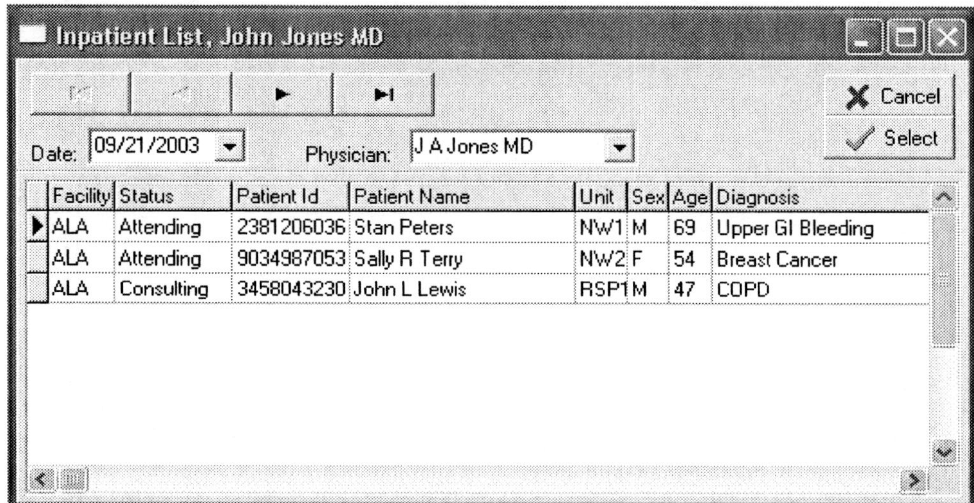

Figure 12.47 Inpatient List for a Physician.

The *inpatient clinical summary* is similar to an overall clinical summary except that it exists only during the time of the inpatient stay and summarizes information during the stay. See figure 12.48. The inpatient clinical summary could be composed of the following information:

- the patient's name, age, sex, marital status and religion
- medical diagnoses, usually by priority
- nursing diagnoses, usually by priority
- permitted activities, functional limitations, assistance needed, and safety precautions
- current physician orders for medications, treatments, diet, IV's, diagnostic tests, procedures, etc.
- results of diagnostic tests and procedures
- consultations
- the inpatient care plan
- access to the Medicine Administration Record (MAR)
- active defined outcome cases/chronic care management cases/patient cases

- active clinical pathway documents
- active trend documents
- important nurse notes.

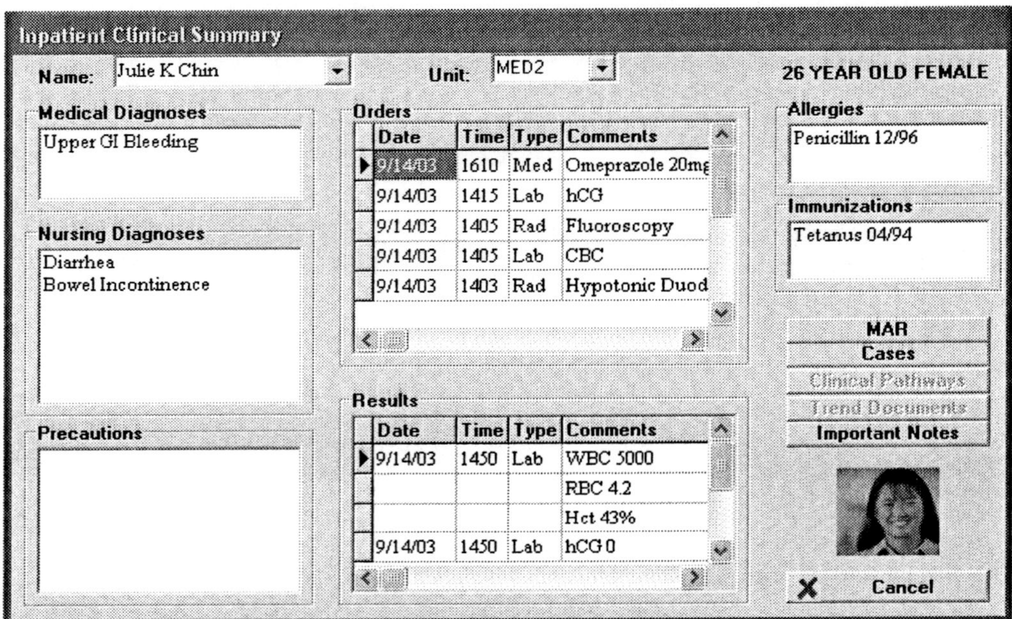

Figure 12.48 Inpatient Clinical Summary.

An active defined outcome case, chronic care management case or clinical pathway document that applies to the inpatient stay would be accessible from the inpatient clinical summary. The caregiver would be able to update treatment plans and add treatment notes in defined outcome cases and chronic care management cases, and the caregiver would be able to update clinical pathway documents. Applicable information for trend documents (e.g., blood pressure, height, weight) would be automatically included in the trend document after it is measured unless the caregiver requested that it not be (e.g., blood pressure is abnormally high due to an illness).

The inpatient physician/hospitalist would be able to view the patient chart (see figure 12.17) and view and add various documents related to the current inpatient stay including the initial *medical history and physical (H&P) examination document*, which might have created in the emergency department (see figure 12.53). When inpatient physicians or nurses enter progress notes, they can highlight the most important notes identifying them as "important notes"; these could be alerted to other caregivers and be available on the inpatient clinical summary, thus assisting communication between physicians and nurses in the care of the patient (see figure 12.48).

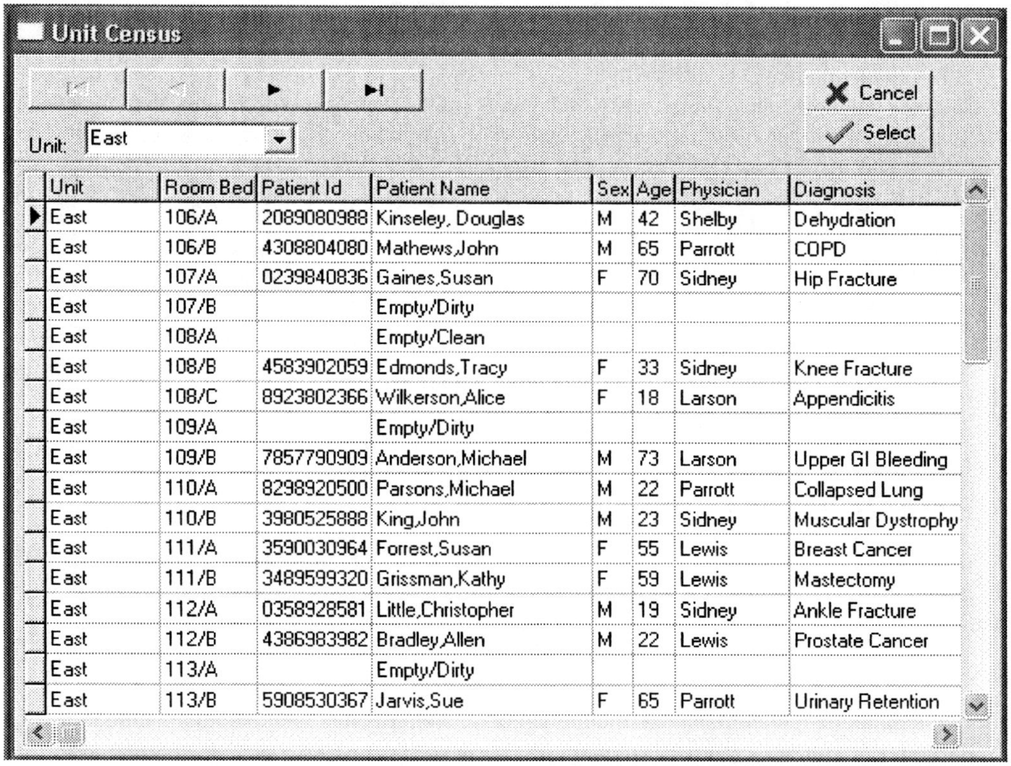

Unit Census

Cancel Select

Unit: East

Unit	Room Bed	Patient Id	Patient Name	Sex	Age	Physician	Diagnosis
East	106/A	2089080988	Kinseley, Douglas	M	42	Shelby	Dehydration
East	106/B	4308804080	Mathews,John	M	65	Parrott	COPD
East	107/A	0239840836	Gaines,Susan	F	70	Sidney	Hip Fracture
East	107/B		Empty/Dirty				
East	108/A		Empty/Clean				
East	108/B	4583902059	Edmonds,Tracy	F	33	Sidney	Knee Fracture
East	108/C	8923802366	Wilkerson,Alice	F	18	Larson	Appendicitis
East	109/A		Empty/Dirty				
East	109/B	7857790909	Anderson,Michael	M	73	Larson	Upper GI Bleeding
East	110/A	8298920500	Parsons,Michael	M	22	Parrott	Collapsed Lung
East	110/B	3980525888	King,John	M	23	Sidney	Muscular Dystrophy
East	111/A	3590030964	Forrest,Susan	F	55	Lewis	Breast Cancer
East	111/B	3489599320	Grissman,Kathy	F	59	Lewis	Mastectomy
East	112/A	0358928581	Little,Christopher	M	19	Sidney	Ankle Fracture
East	112/B	4386983982	Bradley,Allen	M	22	Lewis	Prostate Cancer
East	113/A		Empty/Dirty				
East	113/B	5908530367	Jarvis,Sue	F	65	Parrott	Urinary Retention

Figure 12.49 Unit Census.

Documents locating patients within the unit are the *unit census* (see figure 12.49) and a *inpatient unit room map* (similar to figure 12.23). These could be built from information sent to the automated patient medical record system from ADT (the hospital system—the admission, discharge and transfer system). As a result of a nurse and physician wearing a tracker badge, the inpatient unit room map could also identify the physicians and nurses seeing the patient and the date and time of each. Other documents available to the inpatient physician would be identical to those available to the outpatient physician.

Like for the outpatient physician, standards of practice would be available to the inpatient physician through practice guidelines, protocols, and standard operating procedure documents. Also available would be generic medical references such as MEDLINE.

12.10 AN OUTPATIENT NURSE S VIEW

The *outpatient schedule* (see figure 12.22) besides being important to a physician is important to tbe outpatient nurse. Another document used by the outpatient nurse, a patient list, is an *outpatient clinic room map* (see figure 12.23) showing a map of the outpatient clinic with all its rooms. After a patient comes in, a receptionist or nurse could perhaps drag the patient's name from the outpatient schedule to the room within the outpatient clinic room map. As a result, a nurse could be informed of the patient being in the room. Upon leaving, the patient's name could be removed from the room on the room map.

The outpatient nurse also deals with documentation such as a *vital signs document* (see figure 12.32 showing how the vitals signs document might appear within the patient chart). Additionally, the outpatient nurse records medication taken and injections given in the clinic on other documents.

At the end of the appointment, the outpatient nurse or receptionist may make a future *appointment* (see figure 12.38) for the patient through an interface to the appointment system. Later, the nurse could review the physician's notes and *synopsis of the encounter* (see figure 12.39) created by the physician, possibly using the *overall clinical summary* (see figure 12.15) and documents in the *chart* (see figures 12.31, 12.32 and 12.33) such as the *H&P* (see figure 7.9).

Standards of practice for the outpatient nurse would be available through practice guidelines, protocols, and standard operating procedure documents. Also available would be generic medical references such as MEDLINE.

12.11 AN ED TRIAGE NURSE S VIEW

The triage nurse evaluates and prioritizes patients coming in to the Emergency Department (ED), determining which patients should be seen first. The triage nurse creates a *triage document* (see figure 12.50), which records the patient's problem and condition, including vital signs. The ED room assignment could later be entered through the triage document—one approach is to have the triage document also serve as the history and physical document.

Information on the triage document might be automatically transferred over to a *triage list* (figure 12.51), listing all the patients interviewed by the triage nurse, including the time that the triage nurse was seen (arrival time) and triage nurse determined priority of care.

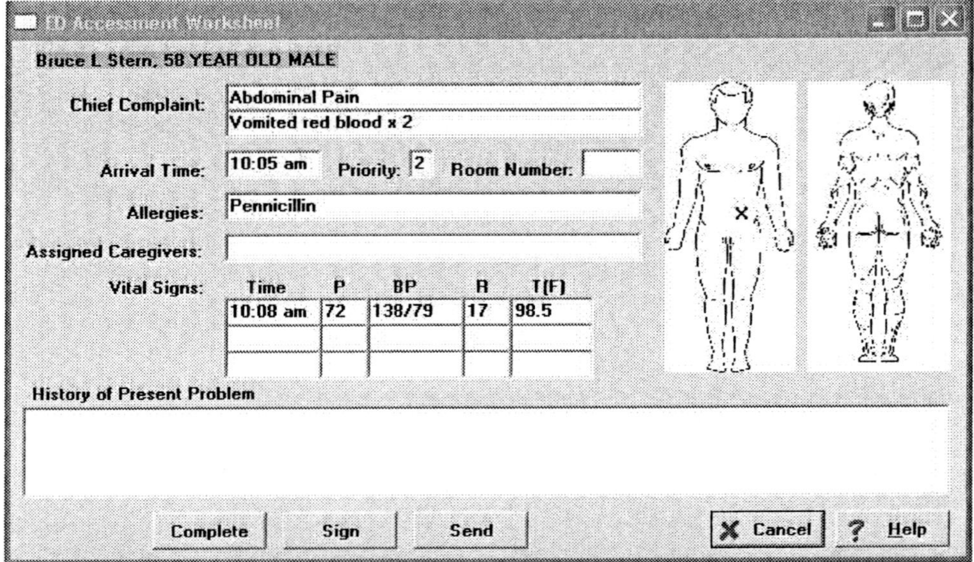

Figure 12.50 Triage document, also used as the H&P.

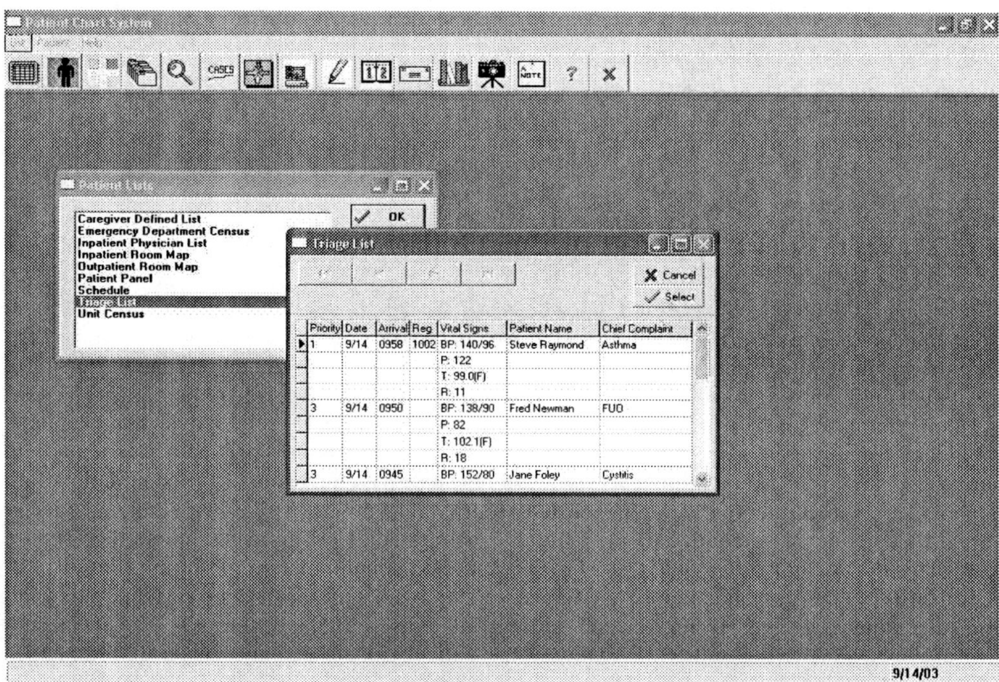

Figure 12.51 Triage list.

Emergency Department Census

Cancel
Select

Room	Patient Name	Sex	Age	Chief Complaint	Assigned	Treatment/Disposition
01	Lesley L Lang	F	42	FUO	Smith	Home
02	Joe S Bugle	M	65	Strep	Cauley	Lab
03	Susan Carlson	F	30	Intestinal Obstruction	Madison	
04A	Jon J Westlake	M	14	Leg Fracture	Johnson	X-ray
04B	Steve Raymond	M	71	Skull Fracture	Alpleby	Admitted
05	Empty/Dirty					
06	Kathy A Kelley	F	33	Subdural Hematoma	Cauley/Young	Home
07A	Steve J Stevenson	M	15	Laceration	Young	Tetanus shot
07B	Empty/Dirty					
08	Jeffrey M George	M	34	Snake Bite	Todd/Sidney	
09	John L Wisner	M	32	Laryngospasm	Cauley	
10	Michael Grishem	M	63	COPD	Ferris/Langley	Admitted
11	Alice N Stodderg	F	27	URI	Alpleby	
12A	Kelley C Kingsley	F	17	Human Bites	Johnson	Lab
12B	Cathy M Forrester	F	61		Johnson	

Figure 12.52 Emergency Department Census.

The triage nurse could use an *emergency department census* (figure 12.52) and a *emergency department room map* (similar to figure 12.23) to determine when rooms become free and locate empty rooms in the ED, so new patients can be assigned rooms in order of priority. The triage nurse could drag the patient's name from the triage list to the emergency department room map, which would also update the emergency department census.

12.12 AN ED PHYSICIAN S AND NURSE S VIEW

The emergency department physician and nurse use the *emergency department census* (figure 12.52) and *emergency department room map* (similar to figure 12.23) to locate patients in the ED. By the triage nurse placing the patient in a room, the system could inform a physician or nurse, so the patient could be seen.

Upon entrance into the room, the ED nurse together with the ED physician or nurse practitioner usually creates a *medical history and physical examination (H&P) document* (see figure 7.7, 7.8 and 7.9) for the patient, recording the patient's initial medical examination and evaluation data; as an alternative approach the H&P could be part of the *triage document* (see figure 12.53), which is a continuation of the document started by the triage nurse (see figure 12.50). This document may include the following: chief complaint, history of present illness, past medical history, family history and social history, marital history, review of systems, physical exam, assessment, diagnosis, impression, rule out, plan and prognosis. The ED physician and nurse provide patient care and try to stabilize the patient, so the patient can be discharged to home, a hospital or to another healthcare institution (e.g., a SNF). Information on the patient's *overall clinical summary* could be transferred over to the H&P document, including medications, allergies, etc.

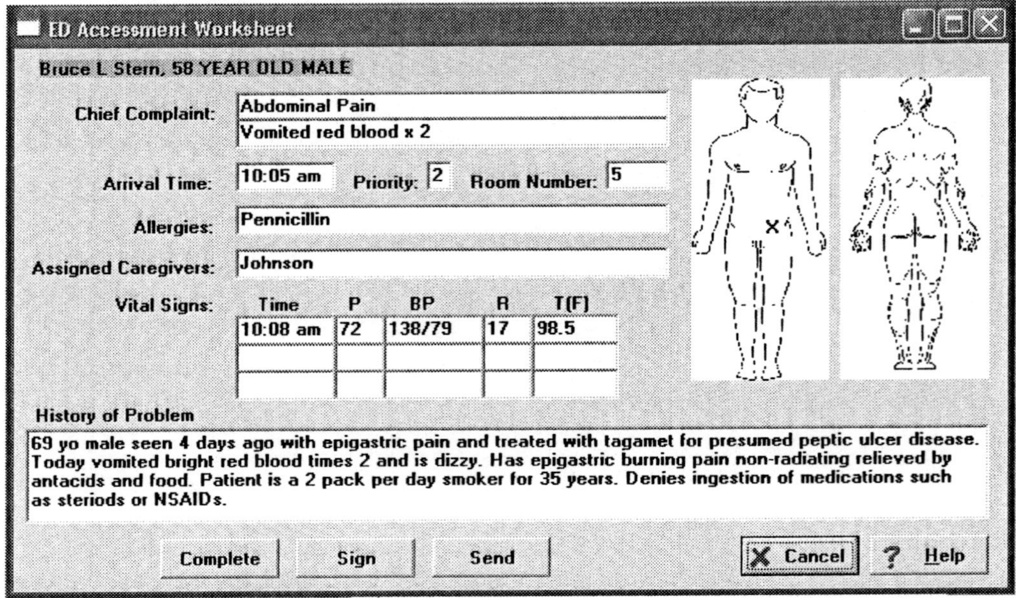

Figure 12.53 H&P from triage document.

Various other ED documents could be created, including discharge instructions, especially for patients returning home. The patient is told what to do upon continuing problems, what follow-up appointments to schedule, etc. This is recorded on a *discharge instruction sheet.*

12.13 AN INPATIENT NURSE S VIEW

The inpatient nurse is the primary caregiver for inpatients providing the majority of direct patient care. The inpatient nurse uses documents locating patients within the unit, the *unit census* (see figure 12.49) and uses the *inpatient unit room map* mapping out the rooms and identifying which patients are in them (similar to figure 12.23). These documents are built automatically by the automated patient medical record system from information sent from ADT (the hospital system—admission, discharge and transfer system).

Before each shift, patients need to be assigned with nurses. Input from other clinical systems could be available for this assignment (e.g., patient acuity systems, such as GRASP, to identify how much nursing care is needed for a particular patient). This assignment could be recorded on the unit census.

Each patient admitted or transferred needs to be assigned with a nurse. An *initial nursing assessment* of the patient is done by the nurse, a *nursing diagnosis (or problem) list* is created listing nurses diagnoses, and a *nursing plan of care* is created. See section 4.4.1.3.

A patient list that an inpatient nurse will use extensively, which summarizes an inpatient's stay from medical record documentation entered so far, is the *inpatient clinical summary* (see figure 12.48). The inpatient clinical summary and other documents give information on diagnoses; on physicians' dietary and other orders; etc. The nurse can find details on the patient in the chart through documents stored there, including nurses' and doctors' SOAP notes (e.g., figure 7.9). In general, input of information into the inpatient clinical summary would not be necessary, as information would be automatically collected from documentation containing the same information in the patient chart.

There is currently an overwhelming amount of inpatient nurse documentation. These documents include H&P's, progress notes, care plans, flow sheets, documents and reports for regulatory organizations, and many, many other types of documentation. These documents would be available on-line as needed (see figure 12.36).

Various techniques exist for simplifying such nursing documentation and reducing the large amount information that an inpatient nurse had to previously enter. These techniques are detailed in section 7.7.1, and include the following:

- non-redundant entrance of information: once information is entered, it need not be entered again (e.g., patient age)
- nursing diagnoses and nursing care plans can be automated using *NANDA* and *NIC* categories; see section 5.3.3.3
- *entrance* of information *by exception,* such as in flow sheets where values are recorded every hour (e.g., skin color), and non-entrance of a value re-enters the previous value (e.g., the value of the previous hour)
- entrance of information via *pick lists,* thus enabling quicker entrance of information
- creation and maintenance of *nursing care plans* and *critical path documents* based upon nursing diagnoses and selection from a predefined list of interventions and outcomes
- automatic system generation of reports to JCAHO and other regulatory organizations.

The inpatient nurse administers medicines according to the *medication administration record (MAR)* (figure 12.54) which is automatically created by the automated patient medical record system from inpatient physician's medication orders; the MAR also serves as a method to record the administration of a medication and return that information to the automated patient medical record system, through the pharmacy system which could send a medication status back to the automated patient medical record system, identifying that the drug has been administered. Other administration records could be built from other completed orders (e.g., injections).

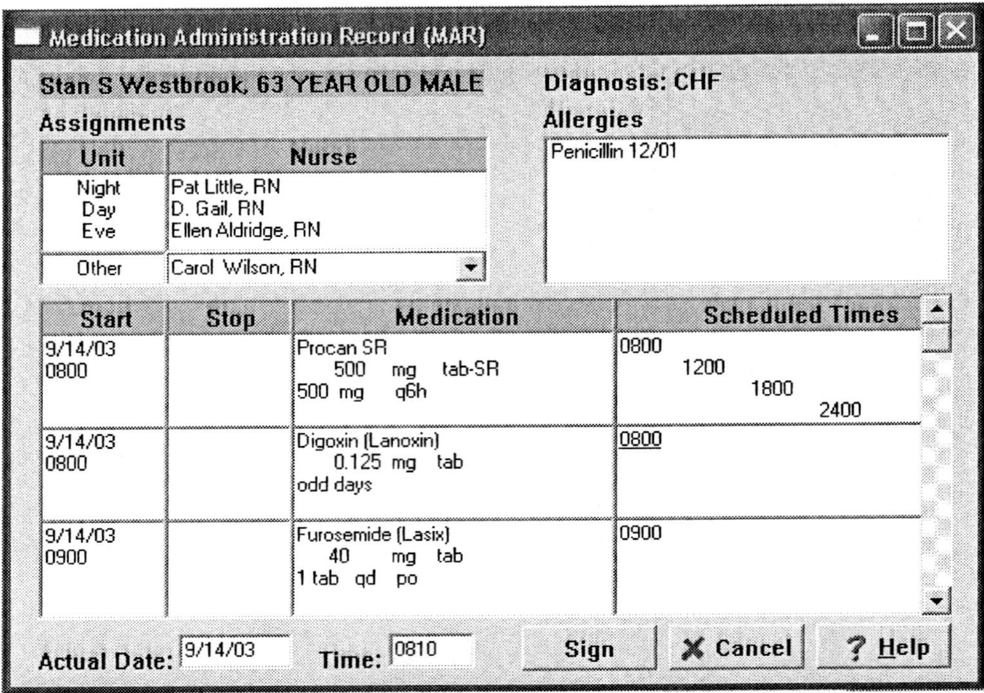

Figure 12.54 Medication administration record (MAR).

Upon a new shift, an inpatient nurse could be responsible for taking an inventory of narcotics. The automated system could assist in this process by generating an inventory list based upon initial stock and dispensed medicine, which the nurse could compare against existing stock.

Information on standards of care for the inpatient nurse, like for other caregivers, would be available through practice guidelines, protocols, standard operating procedure, clinical pathways documents and other *medical references.* Also available would be generic medical references such as MEDLINE.

12.14 CARE TEAMS

Patient care today increasingly involves more than one caregiver working together in a *care team* to jointly care for patients. In the outpatient setting, a care team may include physicians, nurse practitioners and physician assistants working together, receptionists and medical assistants, and sometimes may even include ancillary care specialists and health educators. A typical care team in the inpatient setting may include physicians, nurses and unit assistants who jointly provide direct care to patient or support those providing direct care. A care team in the ED may include physicians and nurses, including the triage nurse.

Care teams may either be very static or change day to day or dissolve once the schedule day is over. A caregiver may have a different care team for every location where he works, for example, a caregiver may have a different care team for each outpatient, inpatient, or ED unit he works in. See section 13.7.2.2 for more detailed information on care teams.

Other caregiver relationships are also important:

- to identify the physician who supervises nurse practitioners, physicians assistants and other caregivers in the care of patients
- to identify to whom else to send STAT or abnormal diagnostic test results if the ordering caregiver is unavailable and to whom to send important clinical messages or e-mail associated with a patient if the recipient remains unavailable
- to identify other physicians who will take over a physician's patients when that physician is unavailable.

12.15 AN ADVICE NURSE S VIEW

An *advice nurse* is either in the call center or within a particular outpatient department. The advice nurse takes telephone calls from HMO members and gives healthcare advice, usually based upon the member's chief complaint and an associated HMO-developed *protocol* or upon communication with a physician. She may make an appointment for the member or insure that the member gets to an emergency department. Some HMOs give the advice nurse the ability to refer a patient for specialty care—in the past, this was a capability that HMOs only gave to primary care physicians. The advice nurse protocols guiding advice nurse actions, especially within the call center, may be on-line.

The advice nurse identifies a member calling in from the member's medical record number or through his name that provides a cross-reference with the medical record number. The advice nurse could then bring up patient demographics for the patient (see figure 12.11) to verify the patient name, address and phone numbers.

From patient demographics, a member's personal profile could be brought up (see figure 12.12). The personal profile may contain some information of use to the advice nurse such as what the patient considers his or her most significant health problems, what specialty departments he or she is being seen in, the case manager if any of the patient, the patient's spouse and children (see figure 12.13). Through buttons on the personal profile, the advice nurse might be able to transfer the call over to the specialty department where the patient is being seen, to transfer the patient over to his case manager, or transfer over to patient demographics for a child or spouse, to make an appointment.

After identifying the patient, the advice nurse could make an appointment. The advice nurse could make an appointment through the appointment system or through the automated medical record system in communication with the appointment system. See figure 12.38.

With an automated patient medical record system, the primary document used by the advice nurse to identify health considerations related to the member other than the protocol would be the *overall clinical summary*. See figure 12.15. She could use this to determine the patient's current health problems, caregivers, and dates and reasons for past encounters. Through the overall clinical summary she could also identify *active defined outcome cases* and *chronic care management cases* and the caregivers involved; see figure 12.24.

If an appointment is needed to continue an active defined outcome case or chronic care management case, the advice nurse could perhaps push a transfer button associated with an appointment phone within the case (see figure 12.25), automatically transferring the patient call to the correct department to make the follow-on appointment.

The advice nurse may communicate with a physician about the patient's problem. In the call center, this could be via a *caregiver messaging system* (see section 7.7.3) to the patient's primary care provider. In a department this could be via message, phone call, or directly talking to a physician in the department who has given care to the patient previously (usually a specialty care physician). Selection of a caregiver on the *overall clinical summary* and the *e-mail/messaging* icon could setup a message template for that caregiver, which the advice nurse could complete and send.

12.16 AN APPOINTMENT CLERK S VIEW

An *appointment clerk* answers calls from HMO members and makes appointments for the member. Also, the appointment clerk must make decisions about whether or not the member should talk to an advice nurse.

The appointment clerk probably would not have the automated patient medical record system available to her, as she would not be making medical decisions, but might have automated protocols on-line upon which she would base her actions. These actions might include sending messages, most often to advice nurses, but also sometimes to case managers, and healthcare services representatives; the messaging system described in section 7.7.3 could be used. The appointment clerk could also transfer the patient phone call to another caregiver.

After the appointment clerk enters the medical record identifier of the member, patient demographics might be brought up (see figure 12.11). After the HMO member is identified, an appointment could be made for the member (see figure 12.38).

From patient demographics, the member's personal profile could be selected (see figures 12.12). This could provide a quick means to make an appointment for the member's child, husband or wife, or transfer the member over to his case manager (see figure 12.13).

12.17 A CASE MANAGER S VIEW

It is efficient to assign *case managers* to high-risk patients. A case manager's job is to move the patient efficiently between segments of the health care system, determining the best, most cost effective ways to do so, with assistance from caregivers in insuring that the best quality care is provided.

The case manager would generally have some medical background and thus should be able to access the *overall clinical summary* for a summary, and the *patient medical record* for details of clinical information on the member.

The case manager may be assigned to elderly patients who have need of nursing home, SNF and periodic in-hospital care and may be assigned to patients suffering injuries related to worker's compensation. In the first case, the case manager may have to be knowledgeable about Medicare rules and the elderly member's Medicare benefits. In the latter case, the case manager may have to be knowledgeable about federal or state regulations involving workers' compensation. Such patients could be tracked through a *patient case* document.

The case manager may be assigned to high-risk patients with chronic diseases. Together with physicians, nurses, pharmacists and other caregivers, the case manager will insure that the patient complies to treatments and medication therapies, and has cost effective access to medical services and quality medical care. Such patients could be tracked through a *chronic care management case* document.

Less commonly, a case manager will be assigned to a treatment for a non-chronic condition or disease (e.g., a pregnancy). Such patients could be tracked through a *defined outcome case* document.

A useful document for case managers is a *clinical pathway* document that could be for care over a long period of time for a particular condition (e.g., diabetes) or for a treatment plan for a shorter period of time.

As patients are assigned to the case manager, the case manager would develop a *patient panel* (as would an assigned primary care provider for a patient), a patient list identifying the case manager's assigned patients.

12.18 HEALTH CARE SERVICES REPRESENTATIVE/OMBUDSMAN

It is suggested that each new member to an HMO be assigned a specific *health care services representatives* (HCS reps) associated with the most likely facility that the patient will visit. The HCS rep will serve as an ombudsman for the patient, being a person who knows the patient, his or her physicians, the medical center and the patient's benefits package. The HCS rep can answer questions, resolve issues and coordinate care where appropriate. HCS reps should be collectively available 24 hours a day, 7 days a week.

Although the HCS rep would not necessarily have a medical background, she or he should have available to him or her the patient's *overall clinical summary*, identifying the patient's *primary care* and other *providers*, *case managers* and current *defined outcome cases*, *chronic care management cases* and *patient cases*. The HCS rep should be able to transfer the patient's telephone call to an advice nurse, call center physician or physician's nurse; send an e-mail to a physician or other caregiver that the patient was requested to contact to answer questions that do not require immediate response; identify primary care physicians with open panels; and add a patient to a primary care physician's panel.

As discussed in section 7.7.10, a patient's medical decisions may be partially based upon a patient's HMO coverage. The HCS rep should be a primary provider of information to patients on their benefits. For example, some patients may have full psychiatric benefits while others do not. Although information on benefits might not be viewed as part of an automated medical record system, a patient's *benefits* should be immediately available to the HCS rep through the system.

12.19 QUALITY MANAGER AND MEDICAL RESEARCHERS

A *quality manager* will evaluate defined outcome cases and the outcomes associated with these defined outcome cases in order to evaluate physicians, nurse practitioners, and associated care teams performing care.

Documents with the automated patient medical record that could be particularly useful for the **quality manager are the following:**

- clinical summaries
- detailed medical record documents
- all case documents
- clinical pathway and trend documents
- clinical practice guidelines.

Also, quality managers may be involved in the evaluation of chronic care management cases, to insure that case management for a particular chronic condition is indeed saving money for the HMO, improving quality of care and/or increasing patient satisfaction.

See section 8.2.11 for more detail on the activities of quality managers.

The medical research department evaluates and conducts epidemiological studies and compares results with current HMO care practices, providing information to improve medical care. Together with HMO physicians they help identify *best practice guidelines* for the HMO.

Patients with life-altering and other significant problems requiring pending or possible future surgery or procedures can meet with the medical research department in coordination with the patient's specialty physician to discuss current care options and to compare them with possible future ones.

12.20 ANCILLARY SERVICES PERSONNEL

An *ancillary department* provides *ancillary services*: support services other than room, board, medical or nursing services to patients, including the following: clinical laboratory, x-ray, physical therapy, injection clinic, pharmacy, optical sales and hearing center.

Automation of the patient medical record could have significant impact on how ancillary department personnel function, including radiologists doing interpretation of diagnostic images, respiratory physicians analyzing pulmonary function tests, and lab workers doing clinical laboratory tests. The ancillary department orders could be put on a *work list* after being directly sent over a network from the clinician through the automated patient medical record system.

After an order for a test requiring interpretation is completed, resulting diagnostic images and pulmonary function test results or other test results to be interpreted could be sent via network to a radiologist or respiratory physician or other clinician doing the interpretation. Final diagnostic findings, once completed, could be immediately sent back via the network to the clinician doing the ordering, or alternatively to the clinician's care team, through the automated patient medical record system. This network communication, in each case, likely replaces much slower hand delivery via couriers. After a test not requiring interpretation is complete such as a lab test, results could be sent immediately back via computer network to the clinician.

Ancillary personnel doing the analysis and interpretation of results could potentially be located anywhere, even out of state or country. The whole patient medical record would be immediately available to them for this analysis and still be available for caregivers outside the ancillary department. When needed, communication between the ordering clinician and ancillary personnel could occur by telephone or e-mail.

Diagnostic findings interpreting the test results could either be typed in or dictated by the analyst. Supporting multi-media, the automated patient medical record system could record voice as part of the diagnostic findings in the chart, although typed input or typed input interpreted by a voice recognition system would be needed to support later information retrieval.

Computer typed results from user dictation (*voice recognition systems*) are quickly becoming a practical input method in place of dictation or typing. Medical dictation is one vertical market strongly supported by voice recognition systems. See section 17.3.6.

Key Terms

802.11
advice nurse
alarm
ancillary department
ancillary services
application server
appointment clerk
appointments
ASP (application service provider)
benefits
Bluetooth
browser
care activity
care path
care team
caregiver messaging system
case manager
character-based user interface
chart
chronic condition
chronic management case
client-server
clinical pathway
clinical practice guideline
clinical summary
co-morbidity
concurrency
consultation
Cooperative Business Objects (CBOs)
cursor
defined outcome case
desktop computer
diagnostic findings
digital paper
direct manipulation
discharge instruction sheet
document list
drag-and-drop
dumb terminal
Emergency Room Census
emulation
encounter synopsis
entrance by exception
Extranet
firewall
glidepoint
Graphical User Interface (GUI)
health care services representative
high-cost condition
history and physical (H&P)
hospitalist
IBM Corporation's Customer Information Control Systems (CICS)
in-basket
inpatient clinical summary
inpatient physician list
inpatient unit room map
Internet
Internet Engineering Task Force (IETF)
Intranet
laptop computer
legacy system
life care path
mainframe computer
medical reference
Medicare
medication administration record (MAR)
message box
mouse
multimedia
multiplicity
NANDA
NIC
n-tier
nursing assessment
nursing care plan
nursing diagnosis list
outpatient clinic room map
outpatient schedule
overall clinical summary
patient case
patient demographics
patient list
pen computer
personal digital assistant (PDA)
personal profile
pick list
pointer device
point-of-care computing
portable computer
probability density function (pdf)
prototype
quality manager
Object Oriented User Interface (OOUI)
referral
response
scroll bars
server-based computing
tablet computer
tailor
thin client
tier
touch pad
trackball
treatment plan
trend document
triage document
unit census
variance
vBNS (very high-speed Backbone Network Service)
voice recognition system
Web server
window
worker's compensation
workstation
World Wide Web

Consortium (W3C)

Study Questions

1. What is a conceptual view? Name ways to identify a patient—Why is this important? What is the importance of a clinical summary? Name documents for tracking a patient's care across encounters. What activities of a caregiver should an automated patient medical record system support and what types of documents are produced?
2. What is a character-based user interface? What is a GUI? What are other types of interfaces? What user interface does this book suggest for desk-top computers?—Why? What is point-of-care computing?—What user interface does this book recommend for point-of-care and why? What are the advantages of GUI user interface over a character-based user interface? Why are character-based user interfaces still used? What are "controls"? What is the difference between a window and a screen?
3. What are Cooperative Business Objects? Why use them in user interfaces?
4. What can be done through pen input that cannot be done easily without pen input? What is the easiest thing to do using a pen? Why can pen-based computers be more lightweight than others?
5. What is the most used wireless interface for computers? How can a wireless capability allow a computer to be more lightweight?
6. How can desktop computers be used together with portable computers in providing patient care with the automated patient medical record system.
7. What is the Internet? An Intranet? An Extranet? This book recommends application service providers (ASPs) for smaller healthcare organizations that want to use the automated patient medical record system—What is an ASP? What is an n-tier system and typical serve types within an n-tier system? Is a typical ASP an n-tier system?
8. Name the four basic types of application structures? What structure most corresponds to the Internet? What most corresponds to a mainframe system? What corresponds to a stand-along PC? What is the difference between a stand-along PC and a client-server set up.
9. What is server-based computing and what are its advantages? The standard Internet and server-based computing have the same application structure—What does a server-based computing application have that a standard Internet connection may not have?
10. What is the basic document of an outpatient physician or nurse practitioner in identifying his patients for the day? What document identifies patients in the ED? In a unit? What is the quickest way for a caregiver to see a patient's medical record in the automated patient medical record system? What if the patient is a drop-in patient, what is done?
11. What documents summarize a patient's health history? Which of these are permanent documents and which of these only exists during the encounter? Where does information for these documents come from?
12. What documents does this book recommend using if care involves multiple encounters? Name different kinds of such documents and when they would be used.
13. How do encounter synopses and searches relate? Why might an encounter synopsis be problematic?
14. In what care situations can patient room maps be used? Why might a patient room map be costly to implement.
15. What is a document list? Name some of the documents that may be in a document list. Who creates these documents? Where could the documents be located?
16. What is an ancillary service? Give examples. By what means does a physician or nurse practitioner use to communicate with an ancillary department performing an ancillary service? Is this two-way or one-way communication?
17. What is an alert? alarm? reminder? STAT? What GUI item is useful for displaying messages associated with these?
18. What is a clinical pathway? What is a life care path? What is a trend document?—How does the automated patient medical record system help the caregiver in getting the information for trend documents?
19. What is a hospitalist? What is a care team? What is triage? What is an advice nurse? What is an appointment clerk? What is a case manager? What are medical references? In what care situations do each of these apply?
20. Name some ways in which the automated patient medical record system could help the inpatient nurse with care documentation. What is the MAR?—Where does information for it come from?

CHAPTER 13

System Analysis: Software and Hardware Design

CHAPTER OUTLINE

13.1 PROJECT CONTEXT: SYSTEM ANALYSIS AND DESIGN

One part of *System analysis* is assessing whether a particular task is suitable for computerization. Another part of *System analysis* is developing the internal design of an automated system—its *system architecture*—necessary to support its previously determined external design including its user interface and to provide the previously determined business requirements intended for the system. Another part of *system analysis* is developing any part of the collective internal design of the automated systems functioning together within an organization—called the *enterprise architecture*—consisting of the combination of all system architectures of all the systems in the organization and their connections.

The automated systems in a healthcare organization together with the employee use of the automated systems and the non-automated processes of employees must support the total business requirements of the healthcare organization.

A system architecture, or an enterprise architecture, the parts of a system or collective systems that a system analyst designs, consists of the following internal structures:

- the various computer systems
- application program design
- databases
- hardware, including networks
- system software such as operating systems
- internal data
- interfaces with other systems
- implementation of business policies.

In the system analysis step—see figure 13.1—the internal design of each automated system is planned, and how organizational automated systems will function together as a whole is planned. System requirements for each automated system are developed identifying an overall design of each system and the design of its component parts: the system's hardware, software, databases, infrastructure, and interfaces with other systems.

In the system analysis step, integration of automated systems is planned so the systems will function together: (1) The overall system architecture of the automated systems functioning together is identified. (2) Requirements for the performance of the systems and their future growth (scalability) are incorporated into the system designs so they fulfill the requirements of the *performance and scalability plan* developed previously by technical personnel in the evaluation step. (3) Requirements for interfaces between systems are identified, adding to those defined during the business reengineering step and identified during the design of other automated systems; the description of the newly identified interfaces are added to an organizational Interface Plan so changes can also be made in systems outside the project. (4) Business policies of the organization are implemented as previously planned, which could potentially be implemented across many automated systems.

A business policy (for example, rules for the assignment of a primary care physician to an HMO member) could be implemented through a combination of employee procedures in handling the business policy, software (ideally kept distinct from other software and referred to as an "agent"), user interfaces, and information on databases. For a particular business policy, the software, user interfaces and database information could be distributed across many different automated systems. Creating a document that describes an overall business policy and its implementation enables non-computer personnel to work together with technical personnel in the implementation of, and any future change to, the business policy.

Potential system designs can be discussed and evaluated by creating models—in this book called "conceptual views"—of the system.

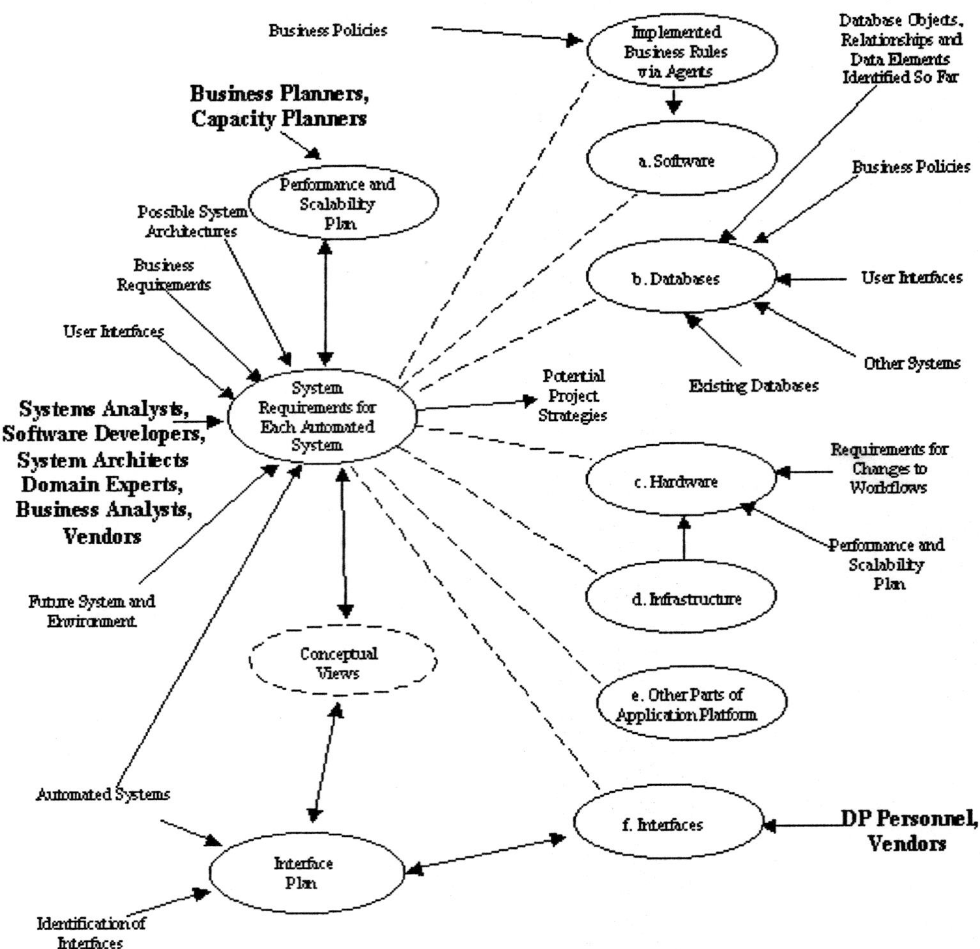

Figure 13.1 system analysis step.

13.2 THE BASICS OF COMPUTER SOFTWARE SYSTEM DESIGN (AND ALSO OF THE DESIGN OF WATCHES)

Designing a computer software system is analogous to designing a watch. Assume that a watch company was designing a new watch as pictured in figure 13.2. There would be designers of the outside of the watch and its external *functions*. There would be engineers to design the internals of the watch.

The external functions of the watch might be the following:

- to tell time in terms of minutes and hours
- to tell seconds via a second hand
- to allow winding of the watch.

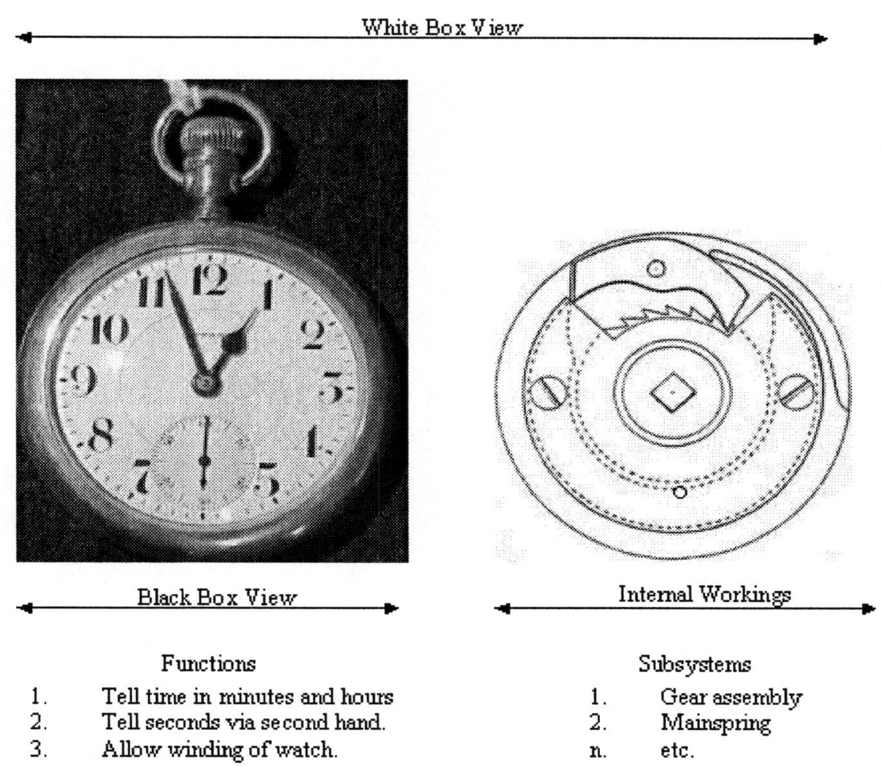

Figure 13.2 Black box and white box views.

The designers of the externals of the watch would have a *black box view* of the watch. It is not required that they look inside the watch to know how the watch functions.

The engineers of the watch would need to have a *white box view* of the watch: they would need to understand the watch's external *functions* and also would need to be able to picture what the inside of the watch would look like. In this way, they could create the *internal workings* of the watch—the gear assembly, the mainspring, etc.—that would support the external functions of the watch.

Design of a computer software system is completely analogous to the design of a watch. There is an external view of the system with its various external functionality: this is the system user's view of the system. The business group and analysts design the external system seen by the users and do not need to know how the internal system works. They would only need a *black box view* of the system.

The system analysts and technical group design the internal system. The internals of the system—the software, hardware, databases and interfaces—are created to support the external design of the system. The system analysts and technical group build the internal system, creating internal subsystems, so it supports the external system and its functions. Thus the system analysts and technical group need to both understand how the system functions externally and how it would work internally. They would need to have a *white box view* of the system.

This chapter identifies the basic tools—the system software, hardware, databases and network interfaces—needed to implement the internals of the automated patient medical record system. And this chapter delves into the implementation of the system using these tools. The application software implementing the automated system—the *internal workings*—would be broken up into *subsystems* (e.g., alert system, display subsystem), portions of code that together implement the external *functions* of the system.

13.3 A SYSTEM ARCHITECTURE CONCEPTUAL VIEW

We start with another conceptual view of the system, a conceptual view looking at the automated patient medical record system from a system architectural point of view. See figure 13.3.

The automated patient medical record system uses information from many other clinical systems in the HMO. The automated patient medical record (APMR) system receives encounters from HMO encounter systems enabling the patient medical record to be organized by encounter. The automated patient medical record system sends orders to other HMO clinical systems and receives results back.

The automated patient medical record system stores information in the distributed universal patient record, consisting of CPR repositories storing summaries of chart information and source document repositories or in chart rooms storing source documents.

The HMO automated patient medical record system will be assumed to be composed of a central HMO system, and local HMO systems, each each local HMO system handling a set of facilities (hospitals and outpatient clinics). This proposed break up of the automated patient medical record system is explained in the next section.

The HMO automated patient medical record systems provide the following capabilities and interfaces:

- **documentation:** A caregiver can create documentation on the patient, which stores patient clinical information within the local HMO database,
- **ordering:** The caregiver can do ordering, sending the order to another clinical system (e.g., the Clinical Laboratory System for a lab order, the Pharmacy System for a medication order, the Radiology System for a diagnostic imaging order, the Appointment System for an appointment or wait list request, the Medical Records System for ordering the paper chart).
- **results and order statuses:** The caregiver can view results and order statuses received back from a clinical system (e.g., the Clinical Laboratory System for lab results, the Pharmacy System for administration of medication, especially within a hospital, say from an automated MAR, the Radiology System for diagnostic images and transcribed interpretations, the Medical Records System for the status of the ordered paper chart).

- **encounters:** Both the automated patient medical record system and the universal patient record (i.e., the CPR repositories and the source document repositories) require that patient clinical documents be tied to encounters. Clinical systems would inform the automated patient medical record system of new encounters and changes in encounter status (e.g., the ADT System would inform the automated patient medical record system of admissions, discharges and transfers; the Appointment/Registration System would inform the automated patient medical record system of new appointments, canceled appointments, the patient showing up, the patient not showing up; the Membership System would inform the automated patient medical record system of new patients to the HMO).
- **receipt of remote documents:** The system can receive remotely located patient clinical documentation from other local HMO systems, other HMOs, CPR repositories and source document repositories.
- **monitoring systems:** The system can receive and filter information from systems monitoring the patient, such as patients in the cardiac or respiratory ICU and from at home Guardian Angel systems (see section 5.3.2.2).

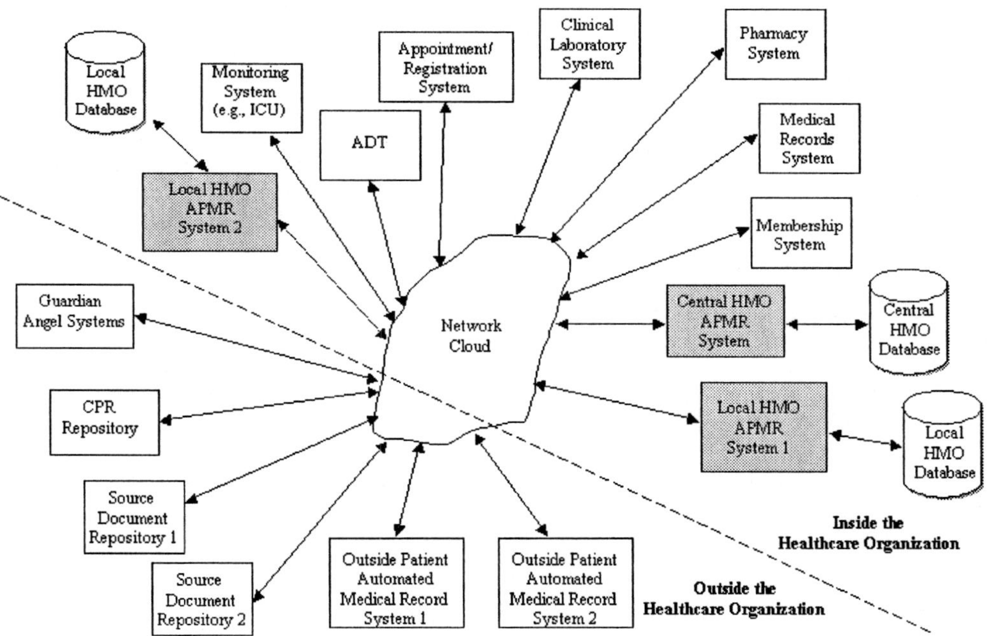

Figure 13.3 Possible system architecture.

- **remote storage of documents:** Periodically, the automated patient medical record system would send source document information to a Source Document Repository and summarized patient clinical information to the CPR Repository, two parts of the universal patient record. Upon sending clinical information to the universal patient record, the automated patient medical record system would also send the associated encounter.

13.4 THE AUTOMATED PATIENT MEDICAL RECORD SYSTEM

There are many possible hardware/software designs for the automated patient medical record system for a large healthcare organization such as our large HMO. This section chooses one possible design and proposes details of the design, justifying choices made. Many other logical choices could have been made for the hardware and software design for our automated patient medical record system.

The following are some possibilities: (1) one central automated patient medical record system, e.g., a mainframe computer, (2) multiple local, facility-based, systems (and no central system) and (3) a central system and one or more local, facility-based, systems. (However, a small healthcare organization might suffice with a single facility-based system.)

Choice 1 simplifies databases by centralizing them and is the least risky because it uses technology that has been around many years (e.g., CICS—see section 17.3.1). It simplifies security, as security can be controlled centrally. Its disadvantages are that it is difficult to make full use of GUI interfaces, it requires a very expensive computer and networks, and a very expensive support staff, and it has potential to have bad user response time due to the processing power being concentrated to one, or a few, computers.

Choice 2 makes it difficult to have any sort of centralized control, which I view as necessary in certain circumstances.

Choice 3 is proposed here. See figure 13.4. The automated patient medical record system would be a *distributed* one, with a central HMO system and local HMO systems, with each local system handling caregivers within a set of facilities within the HMO. A local system would perhaps be composed of a server, a local database and workstations. Each local system is responsible for storing the source documents created in the facilities it supports. Such a set of facilities supported by a particular local system will be referred to here as a "distributed facility group". All the source documents generated at the set of facilities (the distributed facility group) that have not yet been downloaded to a source document repository would be stored in a local HMO system database. In the local system there would be complete summaries of patient clinical information for **all patients currently being seen within the distributed facility group,** together with a list and locations of all medical documents for these patients.

The central system would also keep summaries of patient clinical information, such as in the CPR repository, and a list and location of all medical documents for **all HMO members**. It would not store the medical (i.e., source) documents.

Some reasons to choose the above automated patient medical record system architecture are the following:

- Each local system for a distributed facility group would be responsible for the chart (source document) information it created and not responsible for chart information created by other facilities; this would make the system scaleable if systems in outside healthcare facilities or other regions of the HMO were added.
- The central system could serve as a controller to insure that the local system for a facility where an encounter was to occur had an up-to-date copy of a patient clinical summary and a list and location of medical documents at the time of a patient admission or outpatient visit; this would allow a complete set of this information to be stored centrally when no encounter was occurring and not require complex communication between distributed systems.
- The central system could serve as a focal point to record a patient's clinical activity outside the HMO in the CPR repository and to send out source documents to the source

document repository and the location of medical documents to the CPR repository; this would simplify communication between the healthcare organization and the outside world.

- The central system could serve as a focal point to pick up clinical information from outside the HMO for patients not previously seen by the HMO, such as new HMO members; since this process may not be related to encounters, it is appropriately done by the central system, rather than the distributed systems.

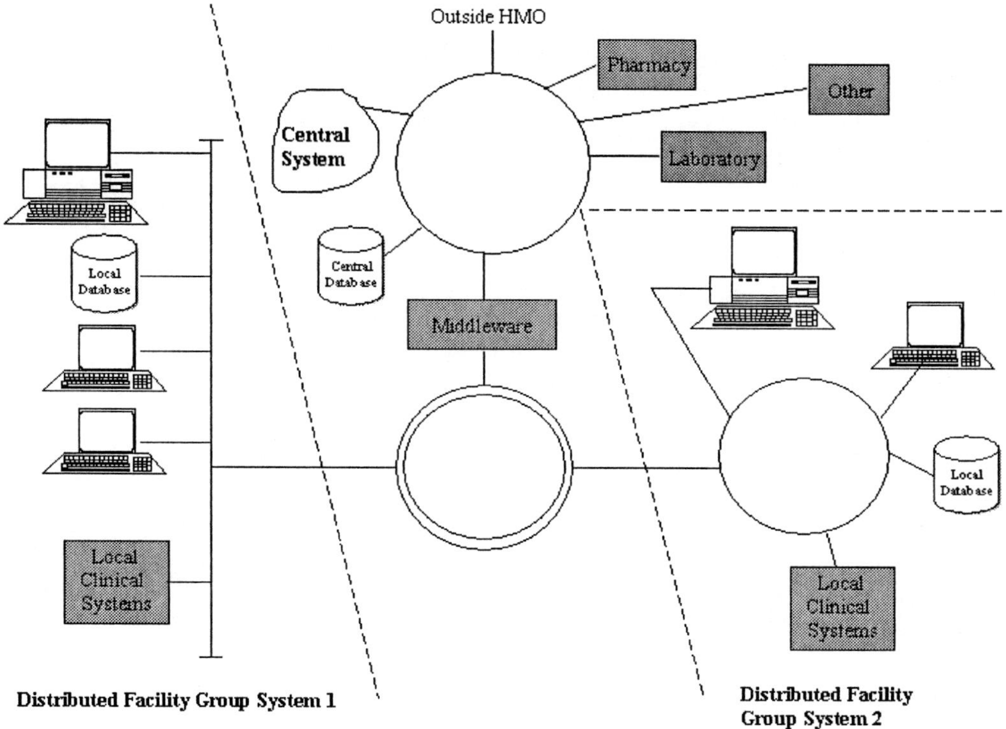

Figure 13.4 Choice 3: A distributed system.

Besides identification of the hardware and software architecture for the automated patient medical record system, in the system analysis step, the actual hardware, operating system(s) and database management systems making up the automated patient medical record system are identified.

13.4.1 Central System

The central system as envisioned here would be a computer system that is a portion of the distributed automated patient medical record system for the HMO. The central system would be responsible for storing patient clinical summary information for all patients in the HMO, responsible for handling communication with the outside world, such as with the CPR and source document repositories, and responsible for processing orders and encounters received through interfaces with other HMO clinical systems.

The central System would store patient clinical summary information such as might appear in an overall clinical summary, preferably in the same format as the CPR repository, perhaps in ASTM E1384 format. This would include patient demographics information, encounters, medications, health problems, etc.

When a patient was identified as scheduled to be admitted, scheduled for a surgery, or scheduled to come in for an outpatient visit (by the appointment system), or when an admission, surgery, outpatient visit or ED visit actually occurred as identified by the ADT, surgery scheduling, or registration system, the central system would inform the appropriate local system of the admission, surgery, pending admission, or visit. Clinical summary information would be sent down to the local system for the facility of the admission, surgery, or visit. The local system might already have much of this information and thus transfer of the total information may not be necessary.

When the membership system identified a new patient to the HMO, the central system would go to the CPR repository to try to pick up clinical summary information for the patient, identifying encounters and clinical summary information from other medical institutions. The HMO could also signal the CPR repository that future outside HMO patient clinical summary information is to be passed down to the HMO.

A local system where the patient was just seen would pass patient clinical summary information for the encounter to the central system so it could be included in the overall clinical summary for the patient. When the location of source documents changed, say from a local system to a source document repository, the central system would be informed so locations of source documents kept in the central system and the CPR repository could be updated.

13.4.2 Local Systems

A local system is a computer system that is a portion of a distributed automated patient medical record system for the HMO. A local system records patient clinical information for a set of HMO facilities and performs all the functions of the automated patient medical record system for caregivers at these facilities.

A local system would control the user interface and associated functions described in Chapter 12 for caregivers working with a set of HMO facilities, with this set of facilities referred to as a distributed facility group. The local system would be responsible for recording caregiver activities within these facilities. These activities would be recorded on documents, such a H&P's and Progress Notes. Orders sent to other clinical systems through the central system would be recorded. Results coming back from other clinical systems through the central system would be recorded. Alarms of abnormal or panic results would be immediately sent to the ordering caregiver. E-mail/messages sent by caregivers within the distributed facility group would be recorded; e-mail/messages coming in to caregivers in the distributed facility group would be recorded; such e-mail/messages may optionally be included in the patient's chart

When the central system informs the local system of an admission or visit or pending admission or visit, the local system would record this on its databases so that future documentation and orders for the encounter could be categorized under this encounter. The central system would insure that the local system would have a complete overall clinical summary for the patient. The local system could have agents related to admissions, surgeries, outpatient visits, or ED visits, which might pick up source documents for previous encounters from other local systems or from outside the HMO; alternatively, these source documents would only be ordered upon caregiver request.

During or at the end of an admission, surgery, or visit, the local system would send information summarizing the encounter and information on the existence and location of associated medical documents to the central system, which would in turn send the changed locations to the CPR repository.

Periodically, the local system could off-load source documents to a source document repository, informing the central system and CPR repository of the new locations of these source documents. Space for the source documents on the local system could then be reused.

Also, determined by agents, space for patient clinical summaries in the local system could be reused, perhaps on a least-recently-used basis, when an encounter had not occurred for a long time. In such a case, the next time an encounter occurred for the patient would result in significant clinical summary information be transferred down to the local system from the central system.

13.4.3 Remote (Outside HMO) and Virtual Systems

A remote system is any part of the automated patient medical record system outside the HMO. In order to minimize network traffic with remote systems for patients being seen or HMO patients seen outside the HMO, CPR repository and source document repository information could be retrieved from remote systems, perhaps at off-hours, and stored on a computer system referred to as a *virtual system*. Thereafter, the virtual system would function like another local system except that it would handle remote, rather than local information.

A virtual system could also potentially be used as a back up system when another local system is down.

13.4.4 Other Clinical Systems

The automated patient medical record system would use data from *clinical systems* for encounters and ordering and would send data to these clinical systems. See the next section.

For generality, our design would be able to handle both clinical systems for the entire HMO (connected to the central system) and clinical systems for particular facilities of the HMO (connected to the local systems for these facilities). For example, there might be an ADT hospital system for the entire HMO connected to the central system and various clinical laboratory systems throughout the facilities connected to local systems.

Clinical systems could be connected to the automated patient medical record system via an interface engine, which, for example, might accept HL7 inputs and convert them to a form where the central or a local database can be updated. See section 13.11.5 for a discussion of interface engines.

13.5 SYSTEM COMMUNICATION WITH OTHER CLINICAL SYSTEMS

As mentioned in section 13.4, the automated patient medical record system needs to receive information from various other HMO clinical systems. The systems fall into the following two categories:

- *encounter systems*
- *ancillary*, or ordering, *systems*.

An encounter system identifies encounters, which would be used by the automated patient medical record system to organize patient medical information by encounter. The encounter system would identify an appointment, outpatient visit, admission, discharge, transfer, or other event that starts a patient encounter or changes the status of such an encounter.

An ordering system would receive orders from caregivers and return results or order statuses through the automated patient medical record system. The automated patient medical record system would send an order to the ordering system for execution. In turn, the ordering system would return changed statuses for the order and eventually any results of the order (e.g., clinical lab order test results).

The following types of encounter systems are assumed:

- a hospital system (identified as an *ADT system* for admission, discharge and transfer)
- outpatient systems, including an *appointment system* and a *registration system*
- a surgery scheduling system.

(When a patient comes in for outpatient care in either an outpatient clinic or the Emergency Department, then the visit is recorded by the registration system, with any fees being paid through this system.)

The following types of ancillary systems to which orders can be sent to a performing area for execution are assumed:

- a *clinical laboratory* system
- an *anatomic pathology* system (examination of body tissue or other items removed from the body)
- a *pharmacy* system
- a *radiology* system (handling x-rays, MRIs, etc.)
- a *durable medical equipment (DME)* system (through which wheelchairs, walkers, etc. can be ordered for a patient from outside the organization).

Also, consultation requests can be sent to individual physicians and to performing areas, which also function similar to orders.

Encounter systems send encounter events (in the form of admissions, pre-admits, registrations, appointments, surgeries, etc.) to the automated patient medical record system, as all patient clinical activities and associated documents are grouped by encounter.

Ordering systems accept orders from the automated patient medical record system, send back order statuses and/or return results and inform the ordering caregiver of alarm conditions (e.g., abnormal or panic results). Orders can most often also be grouped by encounter.

In order for clinical systems to function, there are databases available to these systems which contain the translation information necessary to interpret encounters, orders and results, and other documents created within their systems; these are sometimes referred to as *master files*. This master file information must be transferred down from these other clinical systems to the automated patient medical record system, either upon initial system load of the automated patient medical record system or whenever the information changes within these other clinical systems; or alternatively, this information could be passed down only when needed by the automated patient medical record system or reside on shared databases. This master file information allows the automated patient medical record system to validate caregiver-entered orders, interpret results, organize encounter information and interpret document information.

Included in the master file information passed down to the automated patient medical record system might be the following:

- a *drug compendium* which validates drug orders, includes both HMO formulary and non-formulary drugs, enables clinical checking (drug interaction checking) and enables drug costing
- a *clinical laboratory test directory* to validate clinical laboratory orders, which includes test names, test measurement units and reference ranges
- a *DME formulary*, which lists and describes all durable medical equipment (DME) offered to patients.

Other "master files" existing in other clinical systems include the various information included in section 13.8.2: locations, resources, including caregivers, rooms and equipment, and patients.

The standard for communication between clinical systems, including master files, is HL7 (Health Level Seven 1997-2003), an applications level network communication protocol for health care systems.

Clinical information is shared between systems and is usually stored on a database called the *clinical data repository (CDR)*. This information constitutes a large part of the information needed by the automated patient medical record.

Orders can either come through clinical systems connected with the central system or clinical systems connected with the local systems. Master files might then also exist on the local systems to speed verification of orders and other documents entered by the user.

13.6 A UNIVERSAL PATIENT RECORD

The structure of a universal patient record must be agreed upon by a lot of people and healthcare organizations, insurance companies and government organizations. My conceptions of such a universal patient record have been presented previously in Chapter 6 and section 7.5.1 and are described further in this section.

The universal patient record consists of patient-centered clinical information that may be distributed throughout multiple databases and multiple healthcare or commercial organizations:

- **computer-based patient record (CPR) repository:** Summarization of clinical information for each patient encounter, together with documents that may cross encounters, including defined outcome cases, chronic care management cases, clinical pathway documents and trend documents. The locations of medical documents for each encounter will also be stored. A nationally, or internationally, agreed upon standard format for information in this repository must be developed; an example is the ASTM E1384 standard for patient health records.
- **source document repository:** A place for electronic storage of documents, including orders and results, created during the care of the patient. These documents are ordered by encounter. The format of source documents stored would be that of the healthcare organization where the document was created, in order to preserve the appearance of the document when it was created. The CPR repository could identify where the medical documents are located, whether in a chart room on paper, or in a source document repository in automated form.

- **patient registry:** A mechanism to record the patients that are of interest to each healthcare organization, insurance company or other organization. Whenever a CPR repository detects an addition to the CPR for a patient or a new medical document being created, the CPR repository would inform the patient repository and the appropriate healthcare organization, insurance company or other organization would be informed about it, so the new information can then optionally be picked up by that organization.
- **paper medical document chart room:** A location for storage of paper charts. The CPR repository could identify that paper medical documents for an encounter are located in such a chart room.
- **clinical practice guideline repository:** A place for electronic storage of clinical practice guidelines that may be referenced by source documents or the CPR.
- **patient identifier assigning authority:** An organization to generate patient identification information used to uniquely identify a patient. The location will return either an existing patient identifier for the patient or a new patient identifier. This identifier can be used to uniquely identify the patient for the universal patient record.

13.6.1 A Universal Patient Record Network and Patient Registry

All the elements making up the proposed universal patient record are connected via a network (see figure 13.5). The purposes of the universal patient record are

- to inform a healthcare or other organization of a patient encounter occurring outside the organization for a patient of interest so the organization can pick up the patient encounter information from the CPR repository and from the medical document locations
- to enable a healthcare organization to determine the locations of all previous encounter information for a new member to the healthcare organization, or for a non-member visiting the healthcare organization, so the healthcare organization can pick patient encounter information in CPR repositories and medical document locations.

Figure 13.5 shows what happens, step by step, when a patient encounter occurs for an HMO patient at a healthcare organization other than the HMO.

- **Step 1**: The patient is being cared for during an encounter in a healthcare organization outside the HMO where the patient is a member. Through an automated patient medical record system, documents are created and orders initiated and results received. During this process, source documents and CPR repository information are created. Because a universal patient identifier is used within the CPR repository, if none is yet assigned, an inquiry of an outside assigning authority needs to be done to get the patient identifier for the patient. Documents created could optionally reference a national clinical guideline; in such a case, a clinical guideline repository could be assessed to bring up the latest clinical guideline for a disease or condition for the caregiver.
- **Step 2**: Once the encounter is complete, patient medical record summary information is sent to the CPR repository and medical documents are either saved in paper form in the chart room or sent electronically to a source document repository. Also sent to the CPR repository are the locations of medical documents, whether in a chart room or in a source document repository.
- **Step 3**: The CPR repository then informs the patient registry of the new CPR repository information, and the patient registry informs all healthcare organizations or insurance

companies who have an interest in the patient's encounters. One of these is the HMO where the patient is a member.

- **Step 4**: The HMO requests and receives patient encounter information from the identified CPR repository and from any source document repository. The HMO could also order paper charts from the healthcare organization of the encounter.

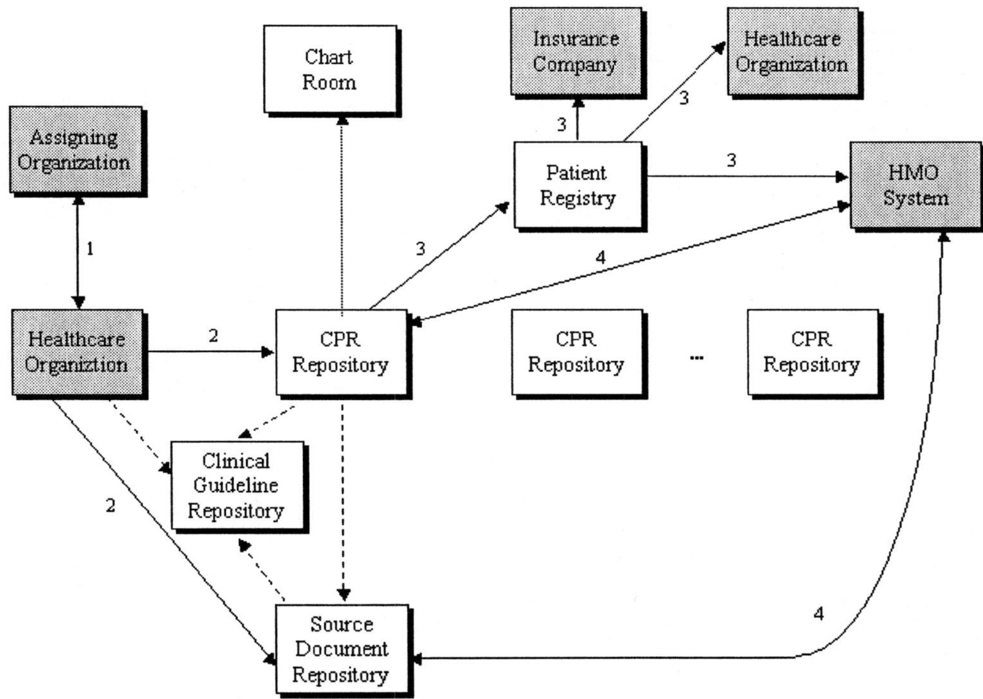

Figure 13.5 Communication within a Universal Patient Record network for an outside HMO encounter.

Figure 13.6 shows what happens, step by step, when an HMO has a new member or a non-member visit.

- **Step 1**: The HMO membership system informs the HMO automated patient medical record system of a new member or the appointment or registration system informs the automated patient medical record system of a non-member visit to the HMO. The automated patient medical record system makes a request of the patient registry to identify all CPR repositories where the new member has clinical information.
- **Step 2**: The HMO picks up patient encounter information from CPR repositories which includes medical document locations.
- **Step 3**: The HMO may request source documents from the source document repositories or request copies of paper patient charts from chart rooms in other healthcare organizations.

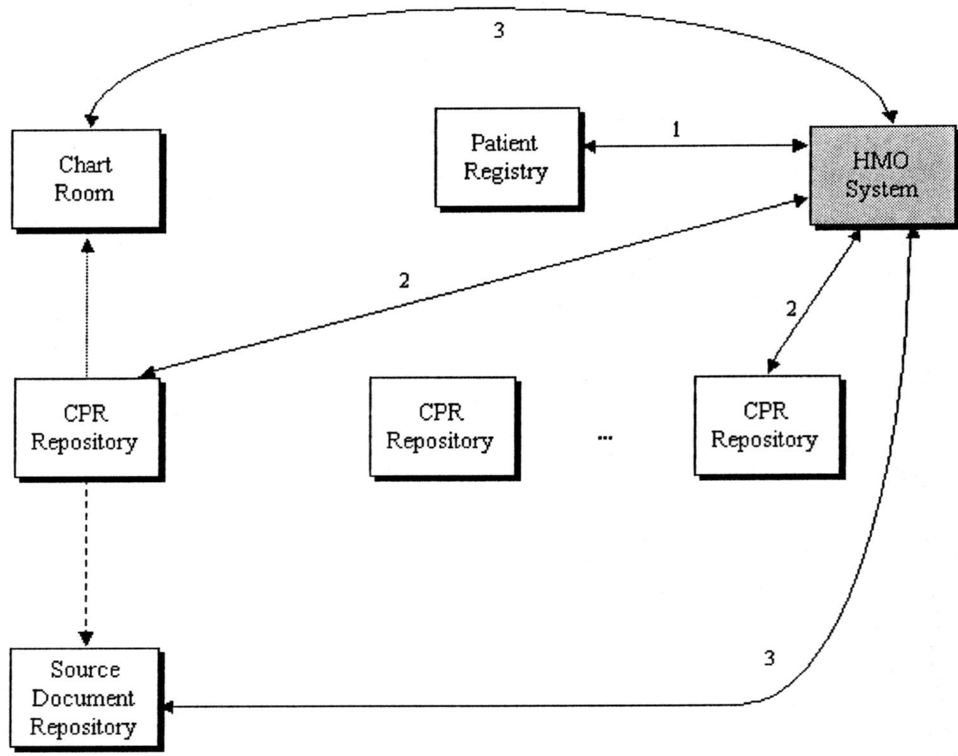

Figure 13.6 Communication within a Universal Patient Record network for an new HMO encounter.

13.6.2 CPR Repository

The CPR Repository contains a summary of patient medical record information. The information in the CPR repository will be stored in national (or possibly international) standard data formats. See figure 13.7.

To produce clinical information to send to a CPR repository, patient chart information input locally must first be converted from the data in local formats to data in the national (or international) formats. There must therefore be information within the healthcare organization to do this translation from the local formats to the national formats.

When CPR repository information is transferred to a healthcare organization via network transmission, it will be in the national standard formats. When it is displayed in patient clinical summaries it will more than likely also be in national formats. One possibility is that pressing a right mouse button over a displayed data element, or button of another pointer device, might show the local value for the data element (e.g., when the right mouse button is pressed when the cursor is over a national patient identifier then the local healthcare organization medical record number would be displayed). This conversion requires information within the healthcare organization to translate national data formats to local formats.

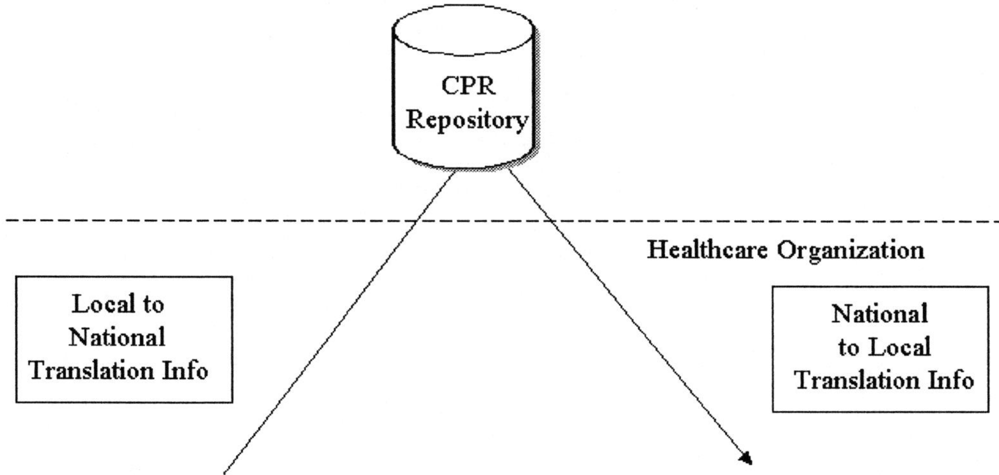

Figure 13.7 CPR repository.

13.6.3 Source Document Repository

The Source Document Repository contains the automated documents created at a healthcare organization during patient encounters. The Source Document Repository will include documents created through the automated patient medical record system, diagnostic images captured through PACS system, and clinical images captured during scanning. See figure 13.8.

In order to preserve the format of a source document as it appears within the healthcare organization where it was input, each source document will be saved electronically as a printed form in the format used by the healthcare organization using the local healthcare organization's data formats. In order for other healthcare organizations to use the source document, saved with each source document data element will be the national format value for the data element.

When a source document is displayed within another healthcare organization, it will be displayed in the form of the printed form at the healthcare organization that created the document so as to present a document that looks the same as seen at that healthcare organization. Pressing a right mouse button over a displayed data element, or button of another pointer device, might show the national value for the data element.

It is expected that HMO source documents in source document repositories will initially be stored in the local format of the HMO. Over time, HMO source documents will probably evolve to use the national data formats contained in the CPR repository, with the HMO using the national data format locally.

13.6.4 Clinical Guidelines Repository

A *clinical guidelines repository* electronically stores clinical practice guidelines. Since a guideline could change over time, a guideline might have several different versions over time, which may all be stored in the repository. A clinical practice guideline might be referenced in a

CPR repository, simply by referencing a clinical practice guideline repository location, an identifier for the guideline and a date or version number for the guideline.

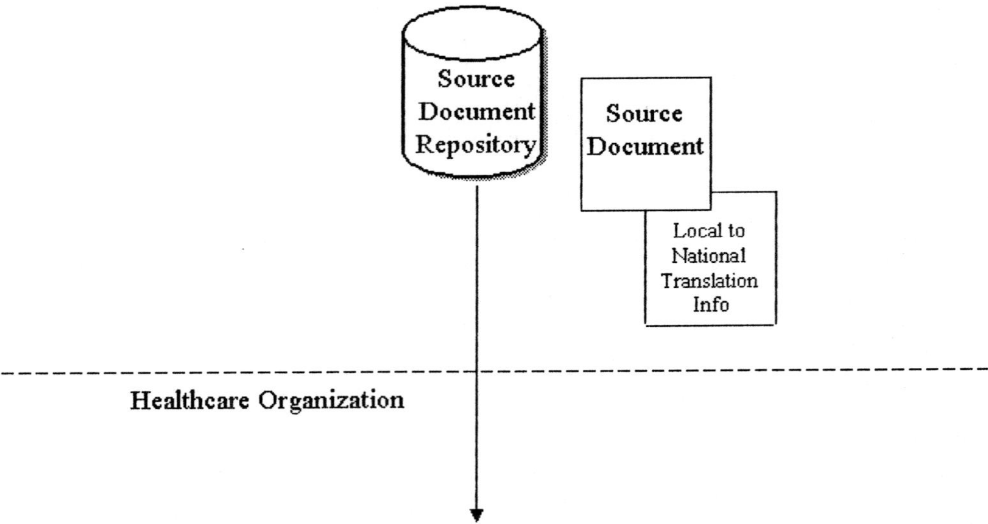

Figure 13.8 Source Document Repository.

13.6.5 Two-Phase Commit, Back Up Data Base, and Archiving

For any database, but especially for the automated patient medical record and its associated databases, the organizations using it do not ever want to lose information due to data being corrupted. In order to protect against such corruption, there are a number of data protection techniques, including *two-phase commit* and *backup* of databases.

Two-phase commit is related to transactions. A *transaction* is a logical set of updates that takes databases from one consistent state to another—see section 13.13. The way this is done is that transactions are structured such that if a transaction fails, then all database updates are backed out, restoring the databases to the consistent state before the transaction. Thus, all database changes associated with a transaction are successfully made or all changes are successfully backed out—this is referred to the *two-phase commit protocol*. The two-phase commit protocol insures that if automated patient medical record information is lost, then it is limited to the last transaction and that the automated patient medical record always ends up in a consistent state.

Backing up the databases is another approach to insuring the integrity of the automated patient medical record. To insure that little information is ever lost, two copies of an automated patient medical record database could be kept. If the working copy becomes corrupted, the backup copy is used instead, and the working copy is ultimately restored from the backup copy. If the backup copy is corrupted, then it is restored from the working copy. When the working and backup databases are collocated, this insures against corruption of the databases due to hardware and software errors. When the databases are in different locations, this additionally insures against natural disasters, such as fires and earthquakes.

For any database, such as the patient medical record, that collects large amounts of information over time where older data is still important but less useful, *archiving* is important. Archiving is storage of patient data or other information on slower, and thus least costly, storage than standard on-line storage; information on the slower storage can be retrieved but may require the requestor to wait a long period of time to retrieve it. Data that is very old may be dropped or put on completely off-line storage.

13.7 STAGING INFORMATION

Staging is transferring patient clinical data from a remote to a local computer before it is needed, instead of at the time needed, so it will be there when it is needed, e.g., at the time of an encounter. This would use similar technology similar to "Internet cacheing" that speeds Internet access by storing popular web pages on computer systems closer to the user, such as is employed by Akamai and Inktomi. Another term for staging is *pre-fetching*.

See figure 13.9. Transferring patient medical record information between platforms (e.g., the CPR repository or source document repository, the central computer, the local computer, another local computer and the workstation) takes significant time. It is thus beneficial to do these transfers ahead of the time that the transferred information is displayed to the caregiver. Often if a caregiver has to wait to receive patient chart information, he will just decide to do without it.

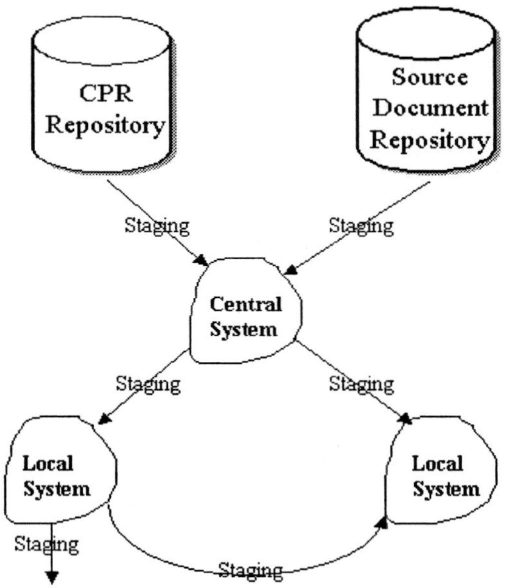

Figure 13.9 Staging.

For example, the clinical summary could be staged (i.e., transferred down) from the central computer to a local computer at the time an appointment or preadmission is made. The clinical summary could be staged from the local computer to a workstation at the time of the patient appointment or registration for the outpatient visit or at the time of the inpatient admission. The clinical summary could then be immediately available on the physician's workstation immediately before the patient is seen.

13.8 DATA AND DATABASES

Databases are places to save information. Databases are composed of either *files* or *tables*. A file is composed of *records*, each record with the same format, and tables are composed of *rows*, each row with the same format. A record or row has a set of ordered *data elements*, for example, medical record number, followed by first name, followed by middlename if any, followed by last name, followed by daytime telephone, etc. Thus a record or row, for example, could identify a different patient or other instance of an *entity*. For a table, because each data element in the same location in the rows is the same time of data element (e.g., a last name), then those same type data element in the successive rows can be viewed as a *column* of the table. Databases can be composed of many different files or many different tables, for example, files or tables for appointments, physicians, medical centers, etc.

This section describes data and databases needed by the automated patient medical record system. It primarily uses *entity-relationship (E-R) diagrams* to describe this data. Creating an E-R diagram is a form of *data modeling*, creating a model of the logical data content of a system.

The system analyst works with a *database analyst* to do the logical design of the database, generally using E-R diagrams, with final results being stored on a *data dictionary* describing the structure of *database tables* and the relationships between these tables, matching those relationships in the E-R diagram; this process is called *logical database design*. The database analyst then maps the tables to disks or other storage devices; this is called *physical database design*.

Indexes may be defined to retrieve rows quickly based upon these index values (a set of data elements) and thus improve the speed of retrieving data from the physical databases. Indexes may be defined either in the logical or physical design phase. *Views*, restricting data elements for view to particular users of the database thus looking like the original tables with fewer data elements, may be defined in both phases; views are made either for security reasons or for hiding information so there are not so many data elements making the data easier to use.

Entities in E-R diagrams are business objects (e.g., bed, user, member, patient, etc.), which may correspond to records on the database and object classes within programs. The *relationships* between these entities are shown in the E-R diagram (e.g., is-a, is-part-of, works for, was seen by, etc.)

E-R diagrams presented here use a notation, United Modeling Language (UML), agreed upon by three computer software professionals, Grady Booch, James Rumbaugh, Ivar Jacobseon (Fowler 2003), who each advocated use of object-oriented design, but who each previously had his own notation for object models. The meanings of various notational elements are presented in figure 13.10.

Basic types of *relationships* between entities are *generalization*, where one entity is a sub-type (e.g., dog) of another entity (e.g., animal)—also referred to as *inheritance* or an "is-a" relationship; *aggregation*, where one entity (engine) is "a part of" another entity (e.g., car); and *association*, where a relationship exists between instances of entities (e.g., a company has a number of offices, a person works for a company).

Associations may be a one to many or a many to one relationship (e.g., a company has many offices), a one to one relationship (e.g., an HMO physician has one primary work location), or a many to many relationship (a patient may be scheduled to be seen by many physicians today, and a physician may be scheduled to see many patients today) or other *multiplicities.* '*' means many. x..y means from x to y instances (e.g., 0..1 means 0 or 1 instances).

Association classes allow you to add data to describe formal associations. For example, a person could be an employee of a company with the relationship between them described by employment information or a contract.

Database design should begin early in the business analysis step and continues on to the development step. Database design consists of two parts: *Logical database design* and *physical database design.*

Logical database design consists of two parts: (1) the identification of business objects whose information is to be stored on the databases, and the identification of the relationships between these objects, and (2) the identification of sets of data ("tables", or "records") making up the database and the format of data elements making up each set of data.

The objects and relationships can be described by the E-R diagrams. Identification of business objects begins in the business analysis step. The E-R diagrams with objects and relationships between them occurs in the Business Analysis and the system analysis steps.

The sets of data—tables for relational databases—are determined in the system analysis step. See section 13.13.

Physical database design consists of defining how the databases will be stored on disks or other storage media. Physical database design is part of the system analysis and development steps. See section 13.13.

13.8.1 Operational Databases Versus Data Warehouses

It is useful to distinguish *operational databases*, those used on-line during day-to-day operations of the business, and analytic or research databases, those used by researchers or executives for analysis. Analytic or research databases have been termed *data warehouses.*

Whereas operational databases are often distributed, i.e., are fragmented, existing at many locations, data warehouses almost always exist at one location. Data warehouses are most often created by collecting information from many operational databases on a periodic basis (e.g., daily, weekly or monthly) and storing them in one location usually through off-line processing at night (i.e., during batch processing). Reference (Gardner 1998) presents the following definition of data warehousing: "Data warehousing is a process, not a product, for assembling and managing data from various sources for the purpose of gaining a single, detailed view of part or all of a business". The structure of data warehouses and operational databases are indistinguishable-- They both are often relational databases consisting of tables (see section 13.13 and figure 13.53).

A significant difference between operational databases and data warehouses is that operational databases require quick access by lots of different application programs without any one program locking out the others, while quick access to data warehouses is not as important, as users doing research, analysis or discovery are few and probably are willing to wait a long time for results.

GENERALIZATION

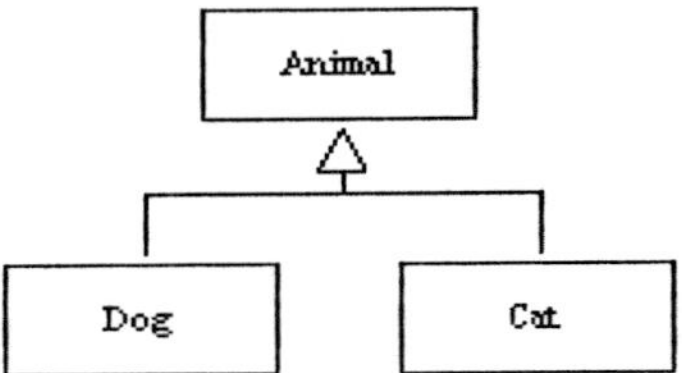

AGGREGATION

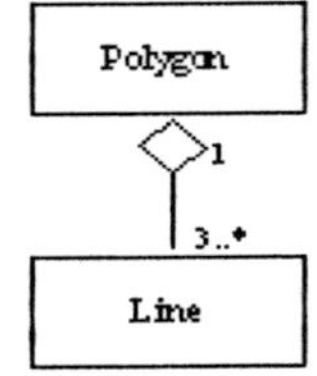

ASSOCIATION

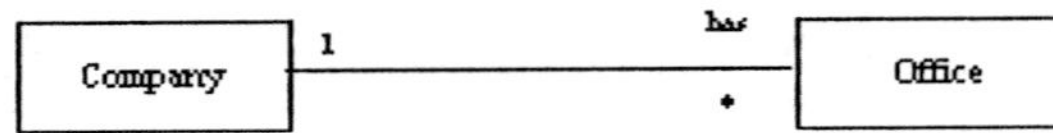

ASSOCIATION CLASS

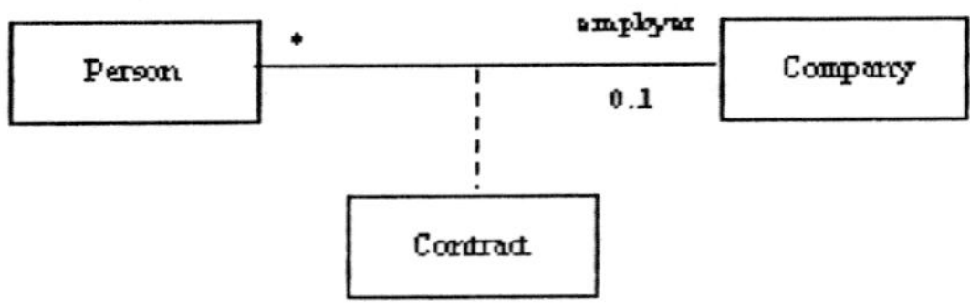

Figure 13.10 E-R diagram constructs.

Operational databases are optimized for a specific set of relationships, those relationships that are most commonly used during operations, while data warehouses are used to discover useful (possibly previously unknown) relationships that could provide useful information for running the organization or doing medical research. Thus E-R diagrams are much more applicable to operational databases.

Again, a transaction is a logical set of updates that takes databases from one consistent state to another. Accessing operational databases on-line is done through system software referred to as *on-line transaction processing (OLTP) systems* (see section 17.3.1), while access to data warehouses is through system software referred to an *on-line analytic processing (OLAP) systems.* OLTP is the processing of transactions by computers in real time for day-to-day business operations, while OLAP is the processing of transactions to analyze data relationships to discover patterns, trends and exceptions. Table 13.1 identifies the differences between OLTP and OLAP.

Table 13.1 OLTP Versus OLAP

Criteria	*OLTP*	*OLAP*
Activities	Supports a business' day-to-day activities.	Analyzes data from previously occurring day-to-day activities.
Time Scale	Current data.	Historical data for trend analysis.
Transaction Length	Short database transactions.	Long database transactions.
Type of Access	Online update/insert/delete.	Batch update/insert/delete.
Update Rate	High update rate.	Low update rate.
Normalization	Normalization is promoted.	Denormalization is promoted.
Volume	High volume transactions.	Low volume transactions.
Recovery	Transaction recovery is necessary.	Transaction recovery is not necessary.
Database Location	Possibly scattered among a variety of databases.	Usually centralized in a single database.
Indexing	Update performance is maximized by limiting the number of indexes to those important for on-line activities.	Optimize ad hoc query performance by including lots of indexes to discover previously unrealized relationships.

13.8.2 Operational Databases

Operational databases are those used on-line during day-to-day operations of the business.

It is useful to distinguish an operational database as a *corporate database* or *application database*. A *corporate database* is a database you want all automated systems in the organization to use that need a particular type of data so that that data can be shared between automated systems and has a consistent format. When data is not specific to a particular automated system or set of closely related automated systems, then it should, in general, be in a corporate database. A corporate database can be stored in one location or replicated in multiple locations with an update at one location distributed to all other locations.

An *application database* is any database that is not meant to be used by all automated systems in an organization. It contains data specific to a single automated system or to a set of related automated systems.

Data in healthcare databases, especially corporate databases, may potentially be shared nationally or internationally. It is thus beneficial to use national or international standards for data in databases where these standards exist. See the appendix.

13.8.2.1 Locations

The following are applicable terms related to locations in an HMO:

- **organization**: the HMO
- **region**: an administrative region within an HMO
- **facility**: a medical center, or a satellite of the medical center, a Medical Office Building (MOB)
- **distributed facility group**: a group of facilities which use the same (local) distributed system
- **administrative facility group**: a medical center and its satellite facilities under the same administration
- **facility department**: an administrative department within a facility (e.g., Medicine, Pediatrics, Emergency Department)
- **subdepartment**: a breakup of a department for some purpose (e.g., appointment booking)
- **performing area**: a location where an order can be sent to be put on a work list or to be transferred to another computer software system, another clinical system, for execution of the order (see work list description under patient lists in section 13.8.2.3)
- **delivery location**: a location where a paper chart or order can be sent
- **nursing unit**: an area of the hospital serving a specific purpose (e.g., ICU, MED, etc.)
- **nursing station**: a nursing station within the unit
- **room**: a room handled by the nursing station
- **bed**: a bed within the room.

An entity relationship (E-R) diagram of these locations is pictured in Figure 13.11. This is likely to be a corporate database.

13.8.2.2 Caregivers and Other Resources

There are various types of human and non-human *resources* that use the system or can be scheduled within the system:

- **caregivers**: A caregiver is an individual who delivers care to patients. Examples are a physician, nurse, lab technician, unit assistant or social worker
- **(system) users**: caregivers, system maintenance personnel and other persons who are allowed to use the system
- **resources**: caregivers, rooms, equipment and other things that may be scheduled.

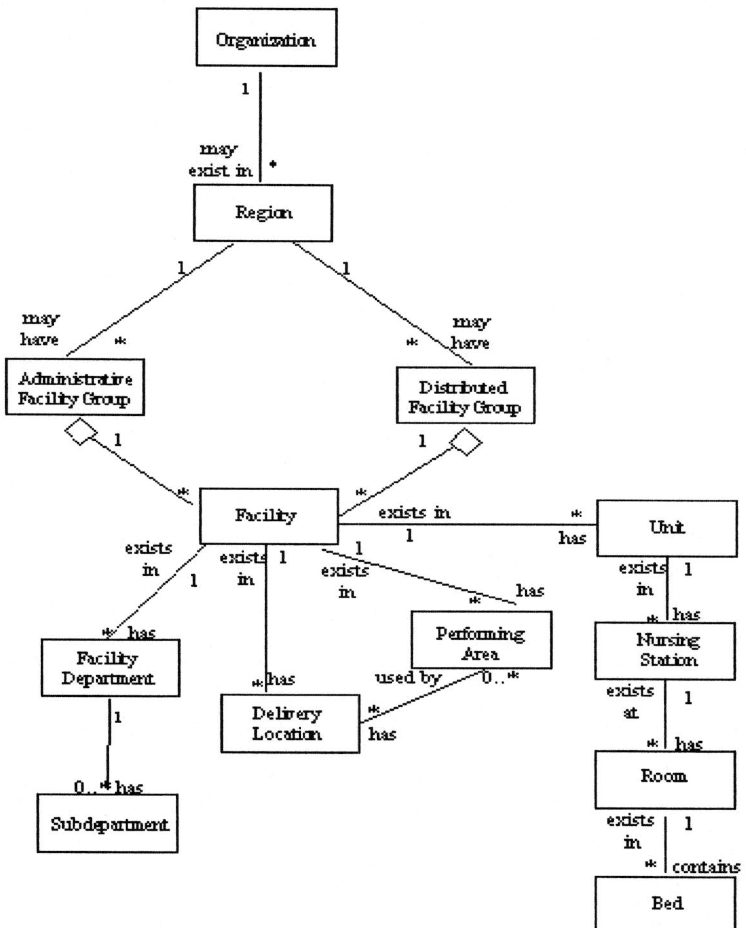

Figure 13.11 Locations.

For a caregiver who is allowed to do ordering, an *ordering caregiver*, ordering capabilities might be described by information associated with this entity and a printer location to send *alarms* on STAT or abnormal results might be identified.

Job categories of a user, e.g., an inpatient nurse, outpatient physician, etc., may be identified by the *job category* entity. This may control how agents work—see section 13.8.2.8.

See Figure 13.12 for an E-R diagram. This is likely to be a corporate database.

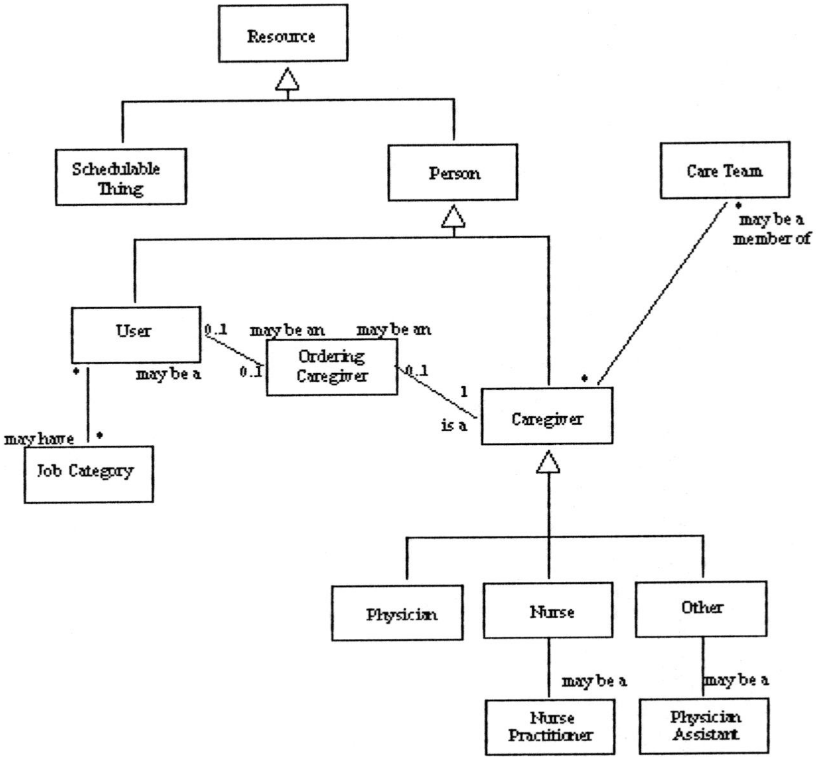

Figure 13.12 Resources.

Care teams are a group of caregivers who work together in care of patients. (See section 12.14.) Members of the care team may be informed of returning STAT or abnormal diagnostic test results via an "alarm" if an ordering caregiver associated with the care team is unavailable, or in addition to the ordering caregiver. A care team could also share clinical messages or e-mails associated with a set of patients and share responsibility for acting on these messages. Associated with the care team may be printer location(s) to send alarms. Characteristics of care teams could vary according to whether they work in the hospital, in an outpatient clinic or the ED. Sometimes order results and messages for a caregiver might more appropriately be sent to an *associated caregiver*, rather than a care team, for example, when the results for an outpatient come back the next day or when an outpatient care team has left for the day. See figure 13.13 for an E-R diagram.

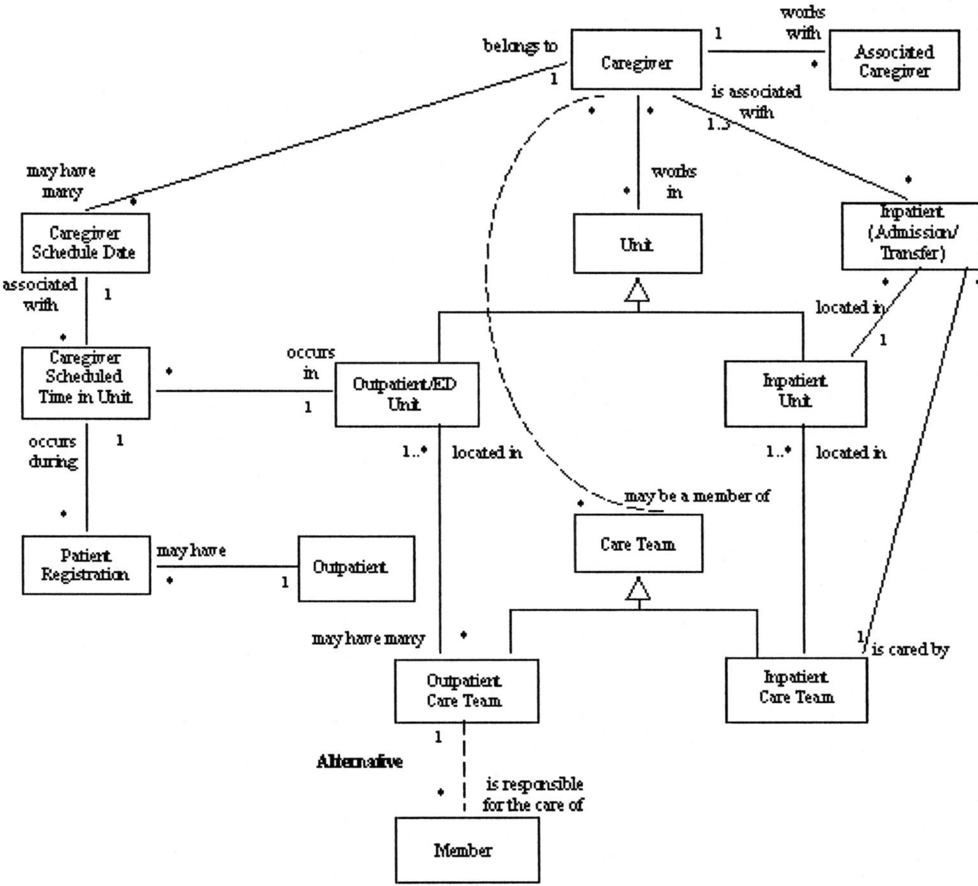

Figure 13.13 Care teams and associated caregivers.

There may be many care teams working in the ED or an outpatient unit. The outpatient or ED patient registration might identify the unit where the patient will receive care. The particular care team for the outpatient would be the one in the unit to which the patient's caregiver belongs. The caregiver's order results or clinical messages for the patient would be sent back to the patient's caregiver if the caregiver was available, and if the caregiver was not available, STAT or abnormal results and clinical messages coming back the same day could be sent to the caregiver's care team if they were still scheduled; otherwise, they would be sent to a colleague, an associated caregiver.

In some HMOs there is an alternative description of an outpatient care team: Each member is permanently assigned to a care team for primary care, generally to the care team of the patient's primary care physician. Whenever the patient comes in for primary care, there is an attempt to have the patient see his/her primary care physician or a member of his/her primary care physician's care team.

Inpatient care teams are always non-permanent. Apart from the physician's seeing the patient, the nurses and other caregivers are assigned to the unit, with each care team generally assigned for a separate shift within the unit. Through an admission or transfer, a physician may be associated with an inpatient as the admitting physician, attending physician, consultant, attending resident, hospitalist or personal physician. Associated with the inpatient may be an assigned care team, which includes nurses and physicians directly caring for the patient--the physician may or not be a member of this care team. STAT or abnormal test results for the patient are appropriately sent to this care team if the physician is not available so that members of the care team can take immediate action if required.

13.8.2.3 Patients, Encounters, and Patient Lists

An encounter is a face-to-face meeting between a patient and a healthcare provider. Patient lists are patients of interest to a particular healthcare provider, often scheduled future encounters between the healthcare provider and patient.

Patients Patients are identified by a patient identifier such as a healthcare organization medical record number or national unique healthcare identifier. Information on the patient including addresses, phone numbers, birth date, sex and patient identifier are referred to as *patient demographics* information (see section 4.4.1.2). This should be a corporate database.

Encounters An *encounter* is a patient coming to a healthcare organization to meet with a caregiver or a phone call which takes the place of an outpatient encounter. Types of encounters include an *inpatient stay*; *outpatient visit*; *emergency department (ED) visit*; a *surgery*; a *phone call encounter*; and a *consultation* where a second caregiver is asked to consult with a caregiver about a patient. A *pre-admit* will be considered to be a category of inpatient stay; an *appointment*, a scheduled outpatient visit for a patient with a resource, will be considered to be a category of outpatient visit. An *observation visit* where the patient comes in and is observed (such as for an impending delivery of a baby) and may be admitted or may return home; this will also be considered to be a category of inpatient stay.

In this book, an encounter is an important organizational entity relating patient visits, admissions, etc. and associated events such as orders. There are some events that should be recorded in the patient medical record which do not result in a formal encounter, or at least do not fit into ASTM's definition of an encounter; see section 7.3.1. One example is a phone contact which does not take the place of an outpatient visit or result in a visit but for which documentation is generated and put in the patient medical record. For such events, it still might be useful have an encounter record on the database so events can be tied to it.

Encounters will have statuses. For example, statuses for inpatient stays include the following: pre-admitted, observation visit, admitted, discharged, transferred, case abstracted; while statuses for outpatient visits include the following: wait-listed, appointed, canceled, no-show, registered, visit completed. For more detailed information on encounters and encounter statuses, see section 7.3.1.

A set of encounters, orders and clinical pathways identified by caregivers as related to the same patient condition or medical problem (e.g., all outpatient visits, clinical lab tests, medications, labor and delivery, etc. related to a pregnancy) is called an *episode*. Encounter(s) leading up to an inpatient admission (e.g., an ED visit where the patient is discharged to the hospital) together with the inpatient admission can be identified as related and will be called a *stay*.

Patient Lists A list of patients associated either with encounters, orders or phone calls is called a *patient list*. A patient list can be for a caregiver (a *caregiver list*) or for an area of a facility (an *area list*). See the E-R diagram in Figure 13.14.

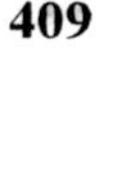

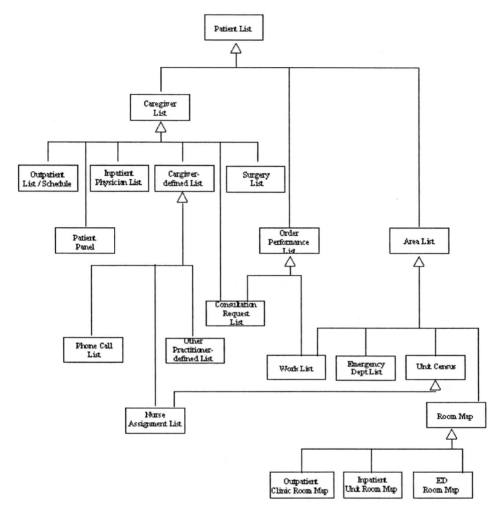

Figure 13.14 Patient Lists.

Types of patient lists include the following:

- *Unit Census* (or *Inpatient List*) that includes all admitted patients in a nursing unit,
- *Outpatient List* or *Schedule* that includes all patients with appointments or registrations for outpatient visits for a given caregiver or non-human resource. A schedule would also identify time where the caregiver is not seeing patients or a non-human resource is unavailable. Ideally, a schedule for a caregiver is for all locations in the healthcare organization where a caregiver works; for efficiency reasons, it may only be for the distributed facility group, with time outside the distributed facility group only showing that the caregiver is outside the distributed facility group.
- *Emergency Department Census* that includes all patients registered in the Emergency Department.

- *Inpatient Physician List* that lists all admissions for which the physician is either the attending or admitting physician, a consultant, a hospitalist or attending resident.
- *An Outpatient Clinic*, *Inpatient Unit* or *Emergency Department Room Map* that is a diagram of all rooms in an outpatient clinic, in an inpatient unit or in the ED that identifies the patient, if any, currently in the room and the room status (e.g., clean, dirty).
- *Patient Panel* listing all patients for which a caregiver is the principal primary care or other provider.
- *Work List* that lists for an ancillary department patients having orders to performed by the ancillary department (e.g., a clinical laboratory test to be completed, blood to be collected), together with details on the order.
- *Surgery List* listing surgeries for the attending caregivers (primary surgeon, assisting surgeon, co-surgeon, consulting surgeon, anesthesiologist, nurse anesthetist and nurse midwife).
- *Caregiver-defined Patient List* that is a list created by a caregiver user from selecting patients from other Patient Lists. A label may be attached to a Caregiver-defined Patient List.

Patients can be selected off a unit census to produce *Nurse Assignment Lists* assigning inpatients to nurses in the unit. These are types of Caregiver-defined Patient Lists, but are also types of Lists because they are composed of lists of inpatients.

Orders may be sent from one caregiver to a second caregiver for a consultation, in which case the order will be put on a *Consultation Request List* for the second caregiver. Orders may be sent from a caregiver to a performing area, in which case the order will be put on a *Work List*. A Consultation Request List or Work List can be set up so that requests could automatically be transferred over to the resource scheduling system wait list, with the wait list request either being either accepted, later resulting in an appointment with the consulting physician, or denied.

Patient Lists may be for a specific date (i.e., **date related**) or for all dates (i.e., **non-date related**). Patient Lists may **show** or **hide** completed encounters. Some Patient Lists allow adding, deleting or modifying patient entries. See table 13.2 for the default characteristics for the various types of lists.

It is expected that the unit census will include the patient identifier and bed location. Entrance of an additional patient identifier and bed location will be equivalent to a *quick admission*, creating an inpatient admission encounter. Other admission information is required to be entered by the ADT clinical system. Once the admission is returned from the ADT clinical system, the admission will be matched up with the quick admission encounter by patient identifier, with ADT information merged in with the quick admission information.

An Emergency Department List can be modified. It allows entrance, deletion and modification of any displayed caregivers associated with a registered patient.

A caregiver can put patients that he will call on his *Phone Call List*. After the caregiver calls the patient dispensing advice, a patient on the list can be identified as having a phone call contact with the caregiver, and, if applicable, having a "phone call encounter" with the caregiver. Patients can also be "removed" from the list.

Patient lists within a local system will only display encounters occurring at facilities in the distributed facility group. An exception is an outpatient schedule that will show patients for the caregiver in all HMO facilities the caregiver works in.

Table 13.2 Characteristics of Patient Lists

Patient List	*Date-Related/ Non-Date Related*	*Show/Hide*	*Add/Delete/ Modify*	*Other*
Outpatient List/ Schedule	Date related always	Show appointments and outpatient registrations in the healthcare organization always. Show cancelled appointments upon request.	Not allowed. (Information comes from the appointment system.)	Besides appointments and registrations, the schedule will show (1) time where the resource is outside the clinics, (2) time where the resource is in a clinic seeing patients but where patients cannot normally be appointed (e.g., drop-in time), and (3) time in a clinic where the resource can have an appointment but none is scheduled. Time that is in transition from appointed to non-appointed will also be shown with either (1) appointments remaining or (2) appointments cancelled. This is the only patient list recommended to go beyond the distributed facility group.
Inpatient List (Unit Census)	Default is non-date related	For non-date related, show all admissions excluding those discharged or transferred. For date-related, show all admissions including thosel discharged and transferred on that date.	Allows "Quick Admission" by adding a patient by entrance of patient identifier and bed; otherwise, add, delete and modify not allowed.	
Inpatient Physician List	Default is non-date related	For non-date related, show all admissions excluding those discharged or transferred. For date-related, show all admissions including those discharged or transferred on that date.	Not allowed. (Information comes from ADT system.)	The caregiver can also select to see only discharged or transferred patients on a date in order of most recently to least recently discharged or transferred.

Patient Panel for Primary Care Provider	Always non-date related	Show patients currently on panel.	Add allowed. Delete allowed to correct those added incorrectly. Removal from panel allowed.	Allow display and search of those removed from panel and primary care provider, if anyone, they were next paneled with.
Emergency Department Census	Default is non-date related	For non-date related, show all patients in the ED not yet discharged. For date-related show all patients in the ED that day, whether still there or discharged.	Allow entrance or modification of the caregivers seeing each patient.	
Practitioner Defined List	Always non-date related	Show all encounters whether complete or not.	Add, delete, modify allowed.	The caregiver can assign a label to the list.
Surgery List	Always date related	Show all encounters, whether completed or not.	Not allowed. (Information comes from surgery system.)	Show time and completion status of surgery.
Phone Call List	Always date related. For patients, not yet called carry over to the next date.	For current date, hide patients contacted by phone and deleted patients, leaving patients to be phoned; optionally, upon show, also show patients contacted. For previous dates, show only patients contacted on that date.	Allow addition and deletion; allow identification of a phone call contact as an encounter.	The caregiver can identify those phone call contacts that constitute phone call encounters. The caregiver can assign a label to the list.
Consultation Request List	Non-date related	Show all consultation requests until they are	Add and delete allowed.	A Consultation Request List entry can be set up to be automatically sent to the schedule system to book an appointment or put the

		appointed, put on the wait list, or deleted.		patient on a wait list for the associated caregiver.
Room Map	Non-date related	End the out-patient encounter for a deleted patient.	Add and delete a patient.	System user can enter a patient identifier or drag over the patient's name from another Patient List for start of exam to put patient in room. Deletion results in ending the encounter.
Work List	Non-date related, but the date and time that the Work List request is created is recorded.	Show all work list requests, hiding those deleted. Show those deleted upon request by date.	Add and delete allowed. When work is completed work request is deleted.	Ordering systems can be set up to add a patient to a Work List for a particular type of order to a designated department or provider. A label, and a department or caregiver can be assigned to the list.

Most patient lists are generated from encounters transmitted from other HMO clinical systems. A schedule also includes identification of time when a caregiver is not seeing patients. Methods of transmission of non-encounter information to the automated patient medical record system from the appointment system, such as schedule time not seeing patients, must be developed.

Selection of Patients A patient can be selected by entrance of a patient identifier, by a Soundex search (a search for a patient based upon the sound of the patient's name, possibly along with other information such as sex and birthdate), by selecting the patient from a patient list, from a displayed e-mail or from a message associated with the patient, or from a displayed alarm or reminder associated with the patient.

Messages Related to Patients A phone message or other message about a patient can be sent via a messaging system as described in section 7.7.3 from one caregiver to another (e.g., from an advice nurse to a physician). With the message, the sending caregiver can set a priority or "importance level" to be reported to the receiving caregiver along with the message (e.g., urgent, normal) that could also signify the maximum length of time given for caregivers to respond to the message and/or get back to the patient. The message can optionally be made part of the automated patient medical record, either by the sending or receiving caregiver. A message a caregiver receives associated with a patient can be selected by the caregiver with the same effect as having selected the patient from a patient list (i.e., selected so the caregiver can bring up the patient's medical record without typing in the patient identifier). The receiving caregiver can respond to the message and close it out, or send the response to another caregiver to call back the patient; the caregiver calling the patient could then close out the message.

Normal e-mail should also be supported but with the additional capabilities to be able to also associate an e-mail with a patient and to be able to optionally include the e-mail in the patient medical record.

13.8.2.4 Patient Medical Record Documents

See figure 13.15. The principal part of the paper or automated medical record for a patient are source documents (those entities in gray) such as history and physicals (H&P's), progress notes, vital sign documents, clinical pathways, etc. and may include orders, results of orders, or addendums. In the automated patient medical record system many relationships may be set up, which may be useful in retrieving these documents.

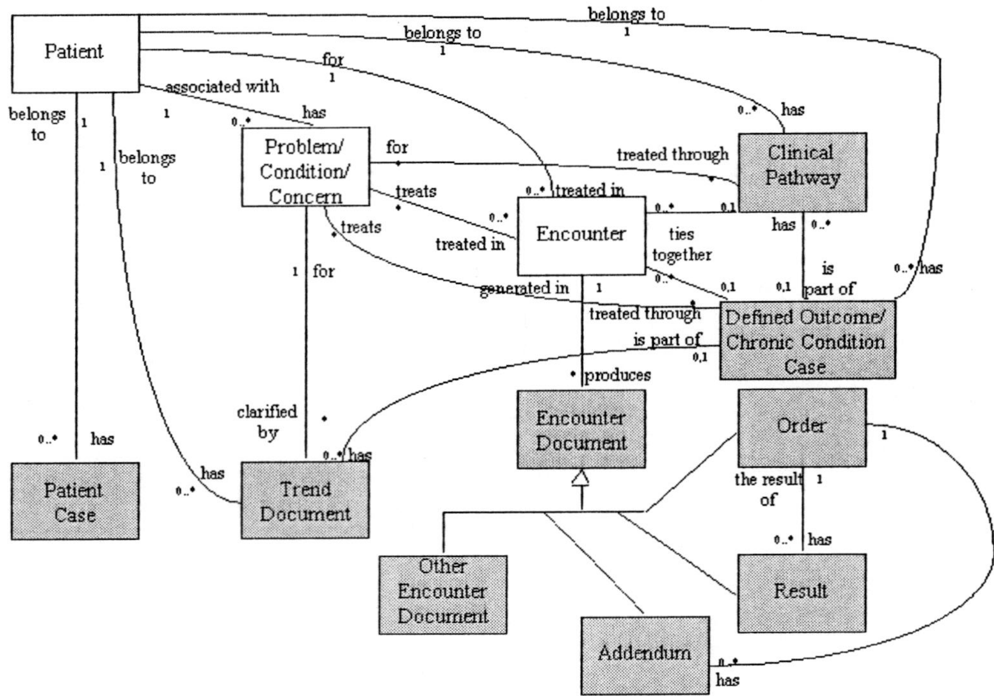

Figure 13.15 Patient medical record documents.

Source documents will be categorized by the encounter they occur in. Encounters may be related by the type of problem, condition, or concern they deal with.

Five types of documents can span encounters: defined outcome cases, chronic care management cases, patient cases, clinical pathway and trend documents. Defined outcome cases and chronic care management cases may include clinical pathway and trend documents.

Externally, *document lists* will tie together encounters and encounter documents. Document lists—see figure 12.16 in the previous chapter—will identify the type of each document, the facility location of the document, whether or not the document is in electronic or paper form, whether or not the document is archived, and other information to allow selection or filtering out of the document. Selection of an encounter, say from a clinical summary, could display (*drill down* to) a document list for a single encounter.

13.8.2.5 Orders, Results and Statuses

Orders The system will provide ordering capabilities for caregivers listed in 7.7.2. It is expected that ordering capabilities would be provided for the following clinical systems:

- clinical lab orders through the clinical laboratory system (which will include microbiology, blood bank, standard and some anatomic pathology lab tests)
- outpatient and inpatient medication orders through the pharmacy system
- anatomic pathology orders through the anatomic pathology system
- consultation requests (referrals) to other caregivers and to performing areas inside and outside the ordering facility
- diagnostic imaging orders through the radiology system
- durable medical equipment (DME) through the DME system.

Besides simple orders ordering a single test, "complex orders" will be handled. Such orders will include repeating orders (e.g., q4h, every 4 hours), conditional orders (e.g., p.r.n., "as needed") and order sets (e.g., CBC, "complete blood count", which generates a series of blood tests).

Orders can be given order priorities, with priority from highest to lowest, for example, life and death, STAT, priority, routine.

Order Profiles For each type and performing area location of an order, there must be information to interpret and validate the order, address the order to send it to the correct location, and to control the types of caregivers who can initiate the orders. It is proposed that for each type of order and performing area location of such an order there be an "order profile".

Control of the caregivers and types of caregivers who can initiate orders is one of many forms of security connected with orders. See section 13.9 for security as related to orders.

Order profiles will exist within each distributed facility group system to identify how to handle orders to and from the distributed facility group system and within the distributed facility group. There will be two types of order profiles, *remote order profiles* and *local order profiles*. In order to identify how to address orders to outside the distributed facility group, remote order profiles will exist for medications, clinical lab tests, etc. to outside systems and to all caregivers outside the distributed facility group for whom consultation requests can be made. There will be a local order profile for each local performing area and for each local caregiver who can receive consultation requests. The local order profile for a performing area identifies the associated work list; the local order profile for a caregiver identifies the associated consultation request list. A local order profile can optionally identify to automatically transfer over work list or consultation request list entries over to the resource scheduling system for automatic scheduling of appointments.

Associating Orders with Encounters Each order, where possible and applicable, will be associated with an encounter—either an inpatient admission, outpatient visit, ED visit, surgery, observation visit, or phone call encounter with a practitioner. During the order, the ordering caregiver will identify the associated encounter. The system will pass the order key to the ancillary system performing the order; it is the ancillary system's responsibility to return the order key with an order status or order result.

Order Statuses, Results, and Addendums *Results* and *order statuses* will be returned by the ancillary system to the ordering facility and will be associated with the order. Statuses for an order and returning results for clinical laboratory orders, radiology orders and clinical pathology orders, are the following: unknown status, service scheduled, service started, preliminary result, result final, result changed/amended, service canceled, service on hold, service continued. Results may be returned with various result statuses: panic or crisis, abnormal, out of range, normal.

The ordering caregiver and/or other identified caregivers or specific printers will receive a notification called an *alarm* if the results meet certain conditions (e.g., being abnormal, panic results, STAT, not being responded to by the ordering caregiver in a given amount of time, results not being reported back within a given amount of time). Caregivers who work together will be defined within the *care team* entity; the caregivers and printers to be alarmed for a particular ordering caregiver and location will be identified along with the situations under which they will be alarmed (see section 13.8.2.2).

The caregivers and printers receiving the alarm could be in the ordering facility or in other facilities. For example, the ordering caregiver could be alarmed in any facility where the caregiver is logged on. If the ordering caregiver is alarmed in a non-ordering facility, the caregiver will be *re-alarmed* when the caregiver logs on again in the ordering facility. From the alarm in the ordering facility, the caregiver could select the patient to see the detailed results.

The printer/caregiver alarm protocol would be controlled by code called an *agent* (see section 13.8.2.8 for a discussion of an *order results agent*). The protocol could include an escalation procedure to inform other caregivers or printers if the ordering caregiver or other caregiver does not respond in a given period of time, or the protocol could inform the ordering caregiver and other caregivers and printers simultaneously of the alarm. The protocol would also identify when alarmed results are not viewed within a given period of time and inform the ordering or other caregiver.

For medication orders, what may be considered equivalent to results are the recording of the administration of medications, for example, of medications administered in an inpatient unit as recorded on a medication administration record (MAR), or administered in an outpatient clinic.

13.8.2.6 Clinical Summaries

A *clinical summary* is a summary of clinical information about a patient, which may include demographics information, significant health problems, past encounters, primary care physicians and other significant caregivers, and medications. See figure 13.16 for an E-R diagram for clinical summaries.

A clinical summary is a summary of clinical information for a patient. In our system, or any real-life system, the clinical summary at any point is likely not to be a incomplete one. For example, there is an *HMO (regional or interregional) clinical summary* for a patient which will continually exist after initial creation at the central (e.g., HMO) level and summarize all the clinical information for a patient within the region. If there are CPR repositorie(s) with the HMO as a subscriber, an *outside clinical summary* for the patient might instead exist with summary information collected from outside healthcare organizations included. *Local clinical summaries*, one for each distributed facility group system, that summarize all the clinical information for a patient within the local distributed facility group will exist after a patient encounter at the facility (and may continue to exist thereafter but not be up to date), and an *inpatient clinical summary* will be created upon the patient's admission, summarizing clinical information during the patient stay and, but last only as long as the inpatient stay. The regional or interregional clinical summary will automatically be copied to the distributed facility group system of the facility where there is an encounter and will be available to caregivers in all the facilities in the distributed facility group; a *patient locator* at the central level will be updated upon encounters and identify the location of the current/next encounter and thus the location of the regional or interregional clinical summary.

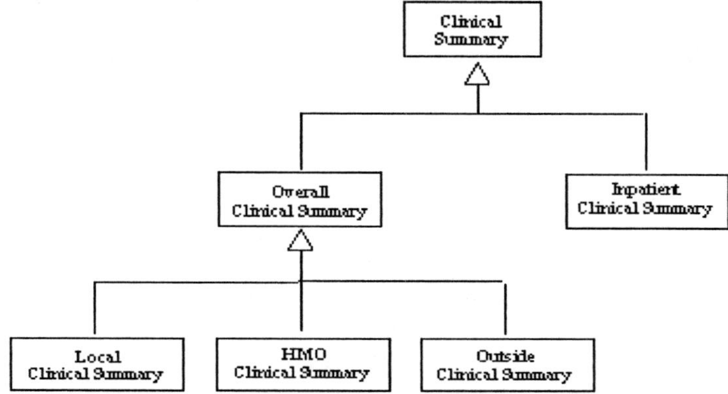

Figure 13.16 Clinical summaries.

Previous to download of the regional or interregional clinical summary, the local clinical summary will be up-to-date up to the last encounter in the local clinical summary. Therefore, only information on encounters beyond that date need to be downloaded. If a local clinical summary does not exist for some reason (e.g., its space was reused), then the whole regional or interregional clinical summary would be copied down.

A local clinical summary will tie together all *documents* generated within a particular distributed facility group, including detailed orders and results, History and Physical, vital signs, SOAP notes, etc., with all documents being immediately available for display. The local clinical summary will also have available the locations of all documents generated by other HMO facility group locations, and if there is a CPR repository, it will also have the locations of all documents from other healthcare organizations, up to the last encounter the local clinical summary has recorded. Documents also may consist of summaries of encounters, called *encounter synopses*, either developed automatically by the system from other chart information or input by caregivers.

The regional clinical summary will tie together all documents in the healthcare organization making up the automated patient medical record with identification of the facility locations of these documents; an interregional clinical summary will locate documents in and outside the healthcare organization. Each of these documents would be stored at the facility and healthcare organization where it was created, and, if outside the distributed facility group, may be copied upon caregiver request or upon protocol to the distributed facility group of the facility where the regional or interregional clinical summary currently exists for an encounter. Synopses outside the distributed facility group will be automatically copied.

For a particular patient, the display of the patient's clinical summary may be optionally tailorable by facility, unit, department, or individual caregiver (via agents, see Section 7.6). Information on the screen would contain enough information to identify the patient plus information selected from the following where available:

- patient demographic information
- a list of all encounters, each with diagnoses, provider and facility and department location, with drill down to associated clinical information, including orders and results
- all orders and procedures, and results and alarms from orders, which will drill down to detailed information
- allergies and adverse reactions, allowing modification and addition*

- immunizations, skin tests and reactions, allowing deletion and addition, as while as recording when administered*
- significant health problems and date captured, allowing deletion, modification and addition*
- potential health problems to be studied and date captured, allowing deletion, modification and addition*
- family/genetic history, allowing modifications and additions*
- biomarkers and identified risk factors for diseases*
- medications with date, dosage, frequency and quantity, allowing modification and addition to identify all medications that the patient currently takes, including those dispensed at facilities outside the organization and including OTC medications, differentiating temporary from stable (long term) medications*
- *alerts* or *reminders* to identify specific patient conditions (e.g., wheelchair, difficulty speaking or comprehending English, visually impaired, violent patient, etc.)*
- a list of defined outcome cases and chronic care management cases for the patient with a drill down to a list of treatment plans, defined outcome notes, clinical pathways, trend documents and other items related to the case and drill down to a list of encounters associated with the defined outcome case*
- a list of clinical pathway documents with drill down to care activities including orders and follow-up visits that may be automatically initiated or scheduled by the system*
- active patient cases*
- active trend documents
- referrals*
- assigned providers / case managers*
- a picture of the patient.

The item's with *'s may be entered and updated by caregivers either through the clinical summary or other sources (e.g., problems, allergies, etc. may also be entered by the caregiver through the SOAP note).

All clinical summary windows can be increased or decreased in size at any time.

The inpatient clinical summary would consist of enough information to identify the patient and areas containing information related to the inpatient stay, which may, for example, include

- patient demographics information
- working diagnoses
- significant health problems
- list of documents, including flow sheets, and nurses' and physicians' progress notes, with drill down to view of these document
- on a temporary basis, important notes within nurses' progress notes (notes within nurses' progress notes that nurses consider important for the attending physician to not overlook)
- orders, procedures, results for the inpatient stay
- medications for the inpatient stay, including identification of inpatient medications actually taken as recorded in the medication administration record (MAR)
- directives
- dietary requirements

- *alerts* related to the inpatient stay, such as an advance directive identified for the admission
- active cases
- active clinical pathways
- active trend documents.

During either outpatient or inpatient care, the encounter physician can make a request for a consultation with another physician. The regional or interregional clinical summary could be copied for the consulting caregiver and combined with the consultation request; the system would later automatically merge back any *remote consultation* encounter to the regional clinical summary in the encounter facility. Through this mechanism, the patient could have remote access to specialized medical expertise at any location within the organization.

As a method to minimize network communication outside the region, an approach would be for the HMO to save chart summary information for a patient received from CPR and source document repositories on a designated local system, referred to as a *virtual system*, that handles out of region information for HMO patients. When CPR repository information is received for an encounter, associated source documents from source document repositories would be automatically ordered and when received, but stored on the virtual system.

When a clinical summary or associated documents are copied into a distributed facility group system for the encounter facility by caregiver request or by protocol, then they will be immediately available for all facilities in the associated distributed facility group.

Within a local system, copies of the regional or interregional clinical summary and associated documents from other regions or organizations are always subject to deletion by a janitor agent (see section 13.8.2.8) based upon least recently accessed. Local documents and the local clinical summary, or the part of the regional or interregional clinical summary listing the local documents, are never deleted, but local documents and parts of the local clinical summary can be archived.

Within a central system, the regional or interregional clinical summary is never deleted, although, with a CPR repository, it could potentially be recreated.

During an encounter, documents would be tied to the local clinical summary via the encounter. The encounter and documents locations would be downloaded for inclusion with the regional clinical summary, where the documents would be associated with the encounter, and, if there were a CPR repository, they would be downloaded to the interregional clinical summary where, again, the documents would be associated with the encounter.

13.8.2.7 Case Documents, Clinical Pathways, Episodes and Stays

Defined outcome cases, patient cases, chronic care management cases, clinical pathways, episodes and stays are all documents or entities spanning multiple encounters.

Defined Outcome Cases See figure 13.17 and section 12.7.1 in the previous chapter. A *defined outcome case* identifies care decisions and encounters related to a treatment. A defined outcome case is composed of a *treatment plan, addendums to the treatment plan and treatment notes*, optional identification of *clinical practice guidelines* followed, *clinical pathways* to identify the treatment plan in detail, or *trend documents.* A defined outcome case occurs across multiple encounters. Each treatment plan, treatment plan addendum and treatment note is associated with the encounter where it is generated. At the beginning of a defined outcome case, *expected outcomes* are identified. After the treatment is complete, the final, *actual, outcomes* of the treatment may be identified and explanation of *variances* between the expected and actual outcomes.

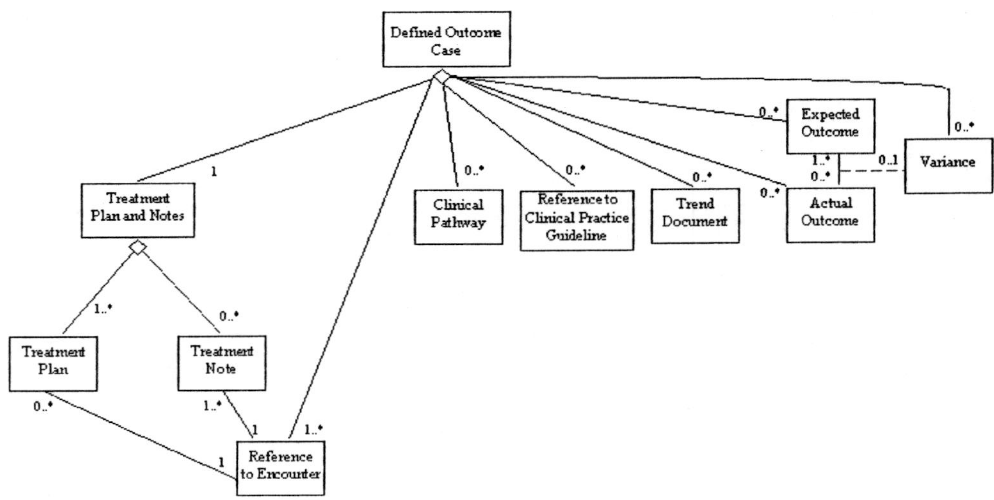

Figure 13.17 A defined outcome case.

Patient Cases See figure 13.18 and section 12.7.2 in the previous chapter. A *patient case* are notes and other information for a case manager, making decisions on how to provide the most cost effective and appropriate care for the patient, including decisions based upon Medicare benefits. A patient case can consist of *case notes*, describing patient care decisions, zero or more *clinical pathways*, and possibly many other documents related to the patient's case.

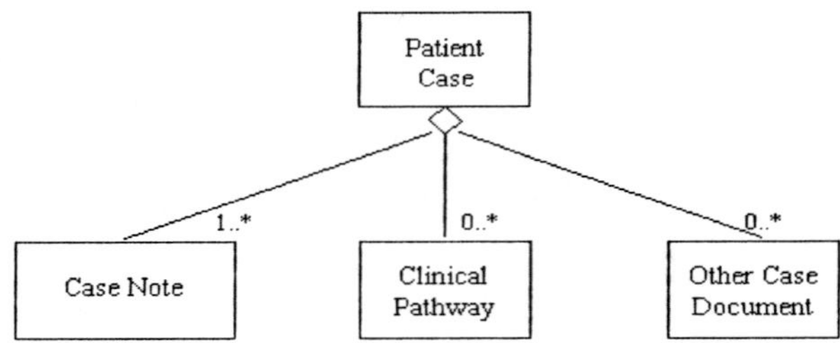

Figure 13.18 A patient case.

Chronic Care Management Cases See figure 13.19 and section 12.7.3 in the previous chapter. A *chronic care management case* describes care for a chronic condition. A chronic care management case can consist a *treatment plan, treatment plan addendums and treatment notes*, and optional identification of *clinical practice guidelines* followed, *clinical pathways* to identify the treatment in detail, *trend documents*. It can include *case notes* for the case manager and possibly many other documents for the case manager. A treatment can include a *treatment plan* and addendum(s) to treatment plans. It can have one or more treatment notes. Each treatment plan and note is identified during a particular encounter and thus must be associated with that encounter. Intermediate *expected outcomes* of the treatment can be identified. Intermediate *actual outcomes* of the treatment may be identified for periodic evaluation of the treatment of the chronic condition. Any *variance* between intermediate expected outcomes and actual intermediate outcomes can be identified.

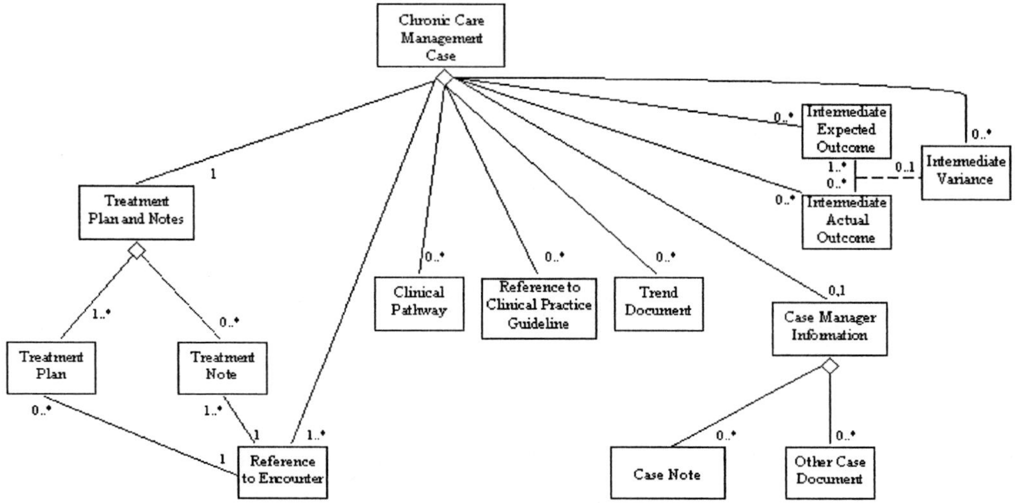

Figure 13.19 A chronic care management case.

Clinical Pathways (a.k.a. Critical Paths) See figure 13.20 and section 12.7.6 in the previous chapter. A *clinical pathway* identifies a *standard of care* for caregivers for a particular *patient problem or condition* with consideration of *risk adjustments* that also may be based upon patient psychological, health and social factors, family/genetic history, patient age, race and sex. Clinical pathways may exist for outpatients, inpatients or both. Clinical pathways may be used for treating illnesses or for managing health and wellness (and may then be known as *health paths* or *life care paths*).

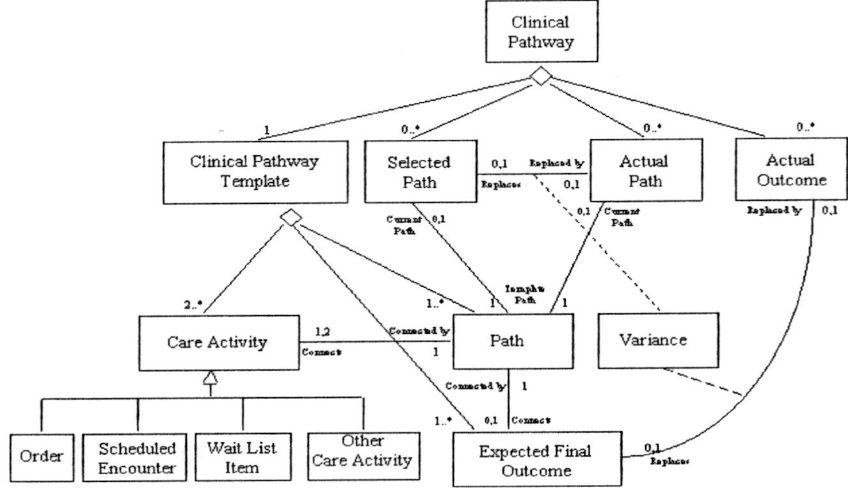

Figure 13.20 A clinical pathway.

A *clinical pathway* consists of a network-like structure, a *clinical pathway template* that consists of *care activities* ordered by various *paths.* A care activity may optionally involve on-line *ordering*, the *scheduling* of an encounter, or *wait listing* of an encounter. Paths may take an *expected* amount of time that may be expressed in terms of a *probability distribution function*, a mathematical function or set of tabular values identifying possible time values based upon analysis of similar care situations. *Expected* or *final outcomes* may replace care activities for the end nodes of the *clinical pathway.*

Caregivers seeing patients may select paths and connected care activities as *actual paths* through the template, after optionally modifying the clinical pathway template, adding paths and connected care activities. Future *expected paths* may be selected along with connecting expected care activities after optionally adding new expected paths and connecting care activities.

When an actual path and expected path differ with different care activities, a *variance* is recorded, identifying why the difference occurred. When an *actual outcome* does not match an *expected final outcome*, a *variance* is also recorded.

Episodes *Episodes* are one or more healthcare services received by an individual during a period of relatively continuous care by healthcare practitioners in relation to a particular clinical problem or situation. They are used to relate *encounters, orders, clinical pathways* and other documents to a particular *patient problem* or *condition.* For example, this might include all outpatient visits, medications, procedures and lab test orders, and labor and delivery related to a particular pregnancy.

Episodes, in the case of this book, are not usually explicitly identified but are related via defined outcome cases or chronic care management cases.

Stays A *stay* is a series of encounters that leads up to an inpatient stay. Examples are the following:

- the patient coming into the ED and consequently being admitted

- the patient coming in for an outpatient surgery that leads to complications that require the patient to enter the hospital
- a pregnant woman coming in for observation, but being admitted for labor and delivery.

Stays, in the case of this book, are not usually explicitly identified but are related via defined outcome cases.

13.8.2.8 Agents Implementing Business Policies

An Agent is code or tables, databases, interfaces between systems, or user interfaces that incorporates business policies into the system. An *agent* is a way of categorizing and separating out such a set of independent business policies so it can be easily changed. These business policies can be business policies related to the organization, region of an organization, distributed facility group, facility, department type, department, unit, caregiver job category or the individual caregiver. An *agent* performs a very specific function (i.e., service) and is triggered based upon a particular event or triggered to run at a particular time. As business policies change, agents are meant to change. Agents also include the administrative procedures of employees in implementing the business policy.

As stated in section 8.7, this book proposes that agents in some ways be treated like employees. An agent should be assigned a manager who understands the business policy and who, with other managers, periodically evaluates the business policy and determines if the agent should be changed.

Each such business policy and agent should be documented. See section 7.6 for more details.

The agent may be a *company agent* performing that function for the entire healthcare organization (a *organizational agent*), for a region (a *regional agent*), for a particular distributed facility group system (a *distributed facility group agent*), for a facility (a *facility agent*), for a department (a *department agent*), for a particular unit type (a *unit type agent*, for example, CCU), for a particular facility department type (a *department type agent*, for example, Pediatrics), for a nursing unit (a *unit agent*), or for an employee job category such as "inpatient nurse" or "outpatient physician" (a *job category agent*). A job category agent can be for the region, distributed facility group, facility, a unit or a department. Finally, an agent may be a *caregiver agent*, a type of agent set up for a particular caregiver, rather than for the company. See figure 13.21 for an E-R diagram for agents.

See table 13.3 for a complete list of the relative priorities of agents. A caregiver agent has priority over all company agents. Thus a caregiver agent written for a particular caregiver performs a duty for that caregiver (e.g., identifying the patient lists available to the caregiver) while that same duty for all other caregivers in the facility might be handled by a facility agent that performs the same duty, but in a different way, as all these other caregivers do not have a caregiver agent for that duty.

Examples of agents are the following:

- **archive agent**—an agent that controls archiving of documents. Documents older than an identified date would be archived, perhaps along with audit information on who accessed the document, and clinical summaries and patient lists would identify the associated documents as being archived and unavailable unless requested.
- **order result agent**—an agent that determines which results to alarm, the caregivers and printers who should receive the alarm, and any escalation procedure (e.g., the alarm is only sent to caregiver B if the ordering caregiver does not respond to the alarm in a given period of time). The order result agent will also keep track of whether or not the result

associated with an alarm was viewed in a given period of time and if not, will apprise the appropriate caregiver(s).

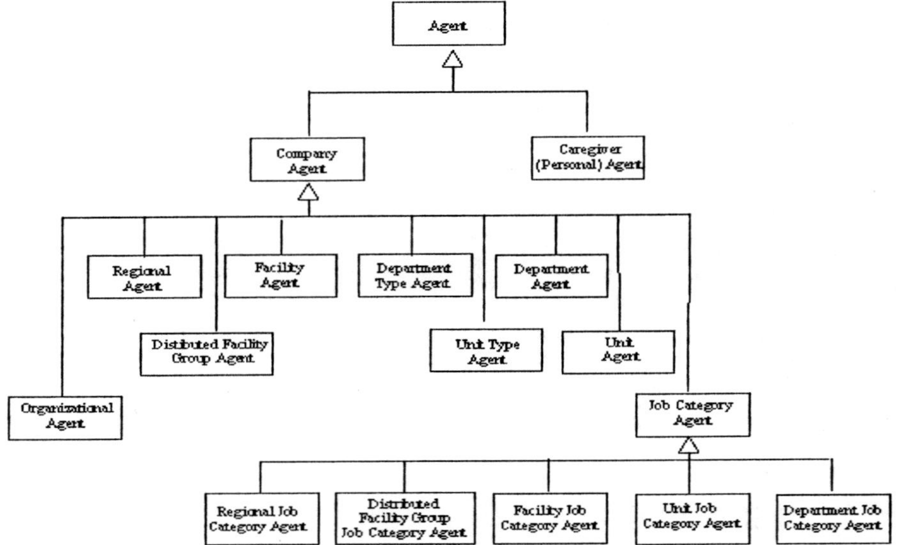

Figure 13.21 Types of agents.

- **admission agent**—an agent to control admission activities such as creating the Inpatient Clinical Summary and copying documents for the admission facility.
- **discharge agent**—an agent to control discharge activities such as destroying the Inpatient Clinical Summary.
- **appointment agent**—an agent to control appointment activities such as copying documents for the appointment facility.
- **outpatient visit completion agent**—an agent to control outpatient visit completion activities such as recording the completion of the encounter in the data base.
- **electronic commerce agent**—supports recording of medical services and orders for purposes of electronic commerce with outside vendors and with insurers.
- **monitoring system filter agent**—Filters out information from a particular monitoring system for inclusion in the chart--(However, it is uncertain whether this corresponds to business policies and where the filtering should occur, within the automated patient medical record system or within the monitoring system, {}).
- **consultant agent**—an agent to control copying of the overall clinical summary and/or documents located at another facility for a purposes of a referral and consultation.
- **backup agent**—an agent to control backup of the entire system.
- **janitor agent**—cleans up copied data and Regional and Interregional Clinical Summary information from a distributed facility group system, removing it when it is considered no longer useful. For example, the least recently used information may be removed, allowing more disk space for other information.

Table 13.3 Priorities of agents

Priority	*Agent Type*	*Suggested System Location*
1	Personal agent	Central
2	Unit / department job category agent	Local
3	Unit / department agent	Local
4	Unit / department type agent	Local
5	Facility job category agent	Local
6	Facility agent	Local
7	Facility group job category agent	Local
8	Facility group agent	Local
9	Regional job category agent	Central
10	Regional agent	Central
11	Organizational job category agent	Central
12	Organizational agent	Central

- **patient list agent**—identifies the types of patient lists available to a caregiver, facility, department, etc.
- **clinical summary agent**—identifies the format of the overall clinical summary and the Inpatient Clinical Summary for a caregiver, facility, department, etc. The format can be determined by the characteristics of the patient, with the format determined by factors such as patient age or sex (e.g., immunizations may only be displayed for children under 13).
- **document location agent**—an agent that controls the names of folders in the chart metaphor and what documents go in what folders.
- **reference document agent**—an agent that controls the health organization documents available to a caregiver (e.g., hospital policies, protocol and procedure manuals).
- **data structure agent**—an agent to control the relationship between a patient list or entrance of a patient's identifier, patient demographics, the clinical summaries and the documents. For example, a regional or personal agent could be written to allow a caregiver to select a patient from an Outpatient Patient List and immediately display (i.e., drill down to) the Regional Clinical Summary. (Other connections would be determined by the system; for example, selection of an encounter on a clinical summary would in all cases drill down to the set of documents associated with the encounter.)
- **security agent**—a company agent to control access to organization information and specific documents as identified in section 13.9. The Security Agent would provide security against unauthorized access and disclosure, maintain the integrity of the data, and confirm the identities of the originators and requesters of the data. The security agent might also provide greater access to information to specific types of caregivers or caregivers in specific departments (e.g., ED physicians and nurses might have access to psychiatry information on the patient, while caregivers in other departments, other than psychiatry, may not).
- **remote security agent**—another security agent to control which documents may be copied and sent to other organizations with business policies determined by agreements of the organization and its (outside organization or region) trading partners. See section 13.9.

- **anonymous order agent**—an agent to control the ability of caregivers to do ordering anonymously and to control view of such orders.
- **public health agent**—an agent to alert the organization and public health officials of usual increases in the incidence of influenza, specific bacterial infections or other public health problems.
- **trending agent**—an agent to identify persistent patient problems to a caregiver based upon information in the automated patient medical record (e.g., a cluster of respiratory infections, signs of potential cancer, etc.).
- **QA / costing agent**—an agent to inform the caregiver of lower cost equally effective procedures or medications and possible drug interactions based upon previous medications and patient medical history. The agent could also check for other quality assurance issues such as compliance with recommendations from JCAHO or other professional organizations, with state or federal regulations, or for possible duplication of orders.

An agent may either run in the background or present a window to the caregiver to collect (parameter) information to control the agent. An agent may consist of code executed in one or in many different servers and in middleware.

Because agents may apply either regionally for all local systems or locally for all or part of a single local system, implementing agents via distributed objects may be applicable. CORBA and DCOM are such specifications for distributing objects across multiple nodes in a network (e.g., in the central system for organizational and regional agents and some job category agents and in the local system for other agents). See section 13.11.3.

13.8.3 Data Warehouses

Business analysis and research databases are referred to as *data warehouses*. In this section a medical research data warehouse is presented and a financial data warehouse is presented. Each data warehouse is mostly or partially generated from patient medical record information.

Whereas relationships in on-line databases are structured to provide optimal on-line access, relationships in data warehouses, if any, are usually structured to either facilitate the most significant on-going reporting or to facilitate research. What is presented in this chapter are E-R diagrams identifying some relationships that could be useful for medical research within a medical research data warehouse and some relationships that could be useful for financial research in a financial research data warehouse in an HMO.

Being made for research and analysis, data warehouses allow the analyst or researcher to find new relationships (e.g., the most useful medications for a particular medical condition). Discovering useful new relationships in data warehouses is referred to as *data mining*.

13.8.3.1 Medical Research Database

Figure 13.21 describes a database that can be generated from patient medical records and can be used for medical research. It excludes patients' social, family, environmental and genetic history that could be added to find associations between diseases and genetic and environmental factors.

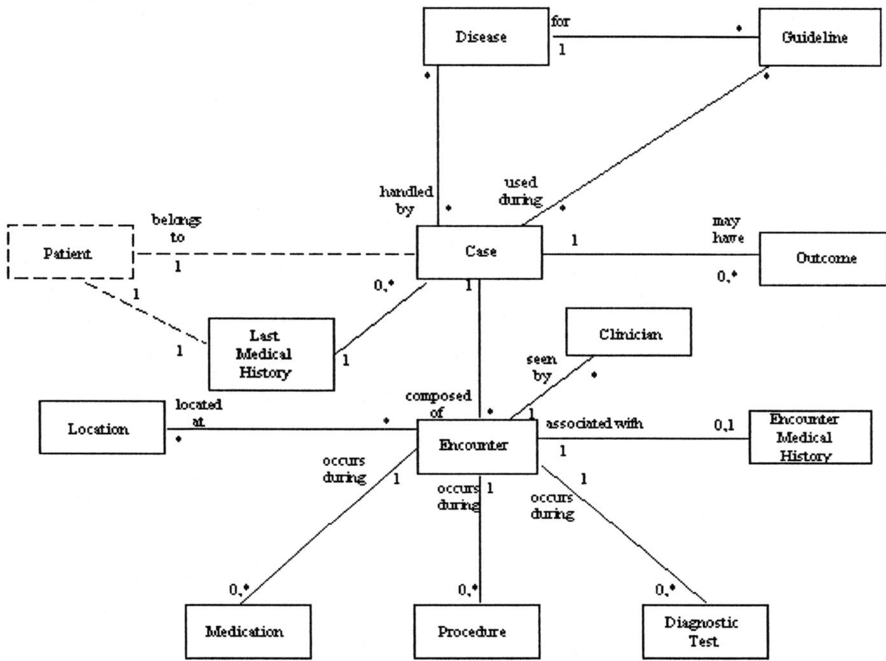

Figure 13.21 A data warehouse for medical research.

Cases dealing with a specific *disease* or *guideline* can be identified. For each case, the *outcomes* can be determined, and the *encounters* making up the case can be identified. The *patient* associated with the case can be determined by selected users. The *last medical history* for the patient of the case can be determined.

For each *encounter*, the geographic *location* of the encounter can be determined and the *medical history* at the time of the encounter can be determined. For each encounter the *medications*, *procedures*, and *diagnostic tests* ordered during the encounter can be determined; alternatively, the *encounters* associated with a *medication*, *procedure*, or *diagnostic test* can be determined. For each encounter, the *clinicians* see the patient can be identified.

The E-R diagram implies that only the relationships shown are ones that analysts and researchers care about. Researchers care about all useful relationships. For example, outcomes of a particular disease using a specific medication can be compared against outcomes for the same disease and a different medication. As another example, outcomes for each physician performing a particular procedure, for example a coronary bypass operation, can be compared (e.g., patient mortalities).

13.8.3.2 Financial Database

Figure 13.22 describes a financial database to determine HMO costs and trends effecting costs, such as changes in membership growth and service costs. For example, identifying capitation fees that are consistent with changes in revenues, changes in membership, etc., can be determined.

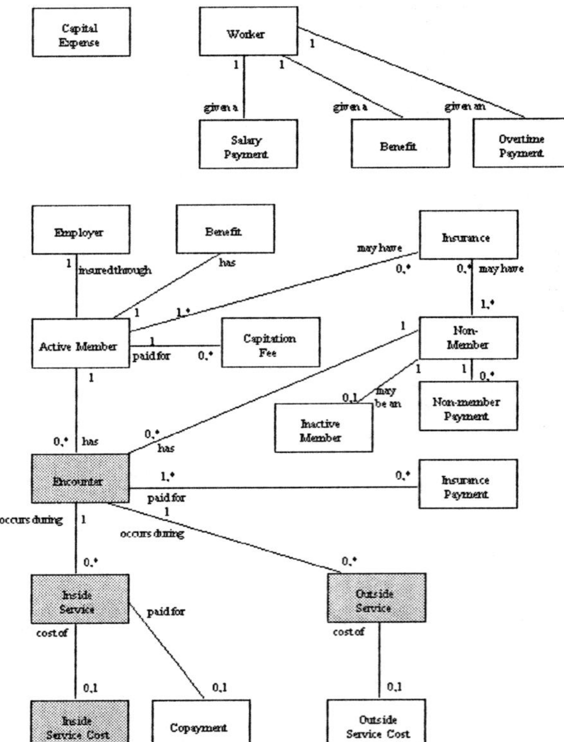

Figure 13.22 A data warehouse for HMO financial affairs.

Part of this information comes from the automated patient medical record system. This information is identified by the shaded entities. The remainder comes from other HMO systems, in particular from HMO financial systems.

Expenses and capital requirements (*employee salaries* and *benefits*, *capital expenses*, *service expenses* inside and outside) can be compared against revenues (*capitation fees*, *co-payments*, *insurance payments* including *Medicare*, *non-member payments*).

Again the E-R diagram describes a very limited number of relationships that analysts and researchers would care about. Many other relationships might be used or discovered. Such a financial data warehouse for a healthcare organization will likely collect information from more financial, clinical and other systems than mentioned here. See reference (Finkler and Ward 1999) on cost measurement and cost management in healthcare organizations for more information.

13.9 SECURITY

A computer and a software system is secure "if you can depend upon it to behave as you expect" (Garfinkel 2002). And thus this book defines *security* as "safeguards applied to an automated system to insure that it behaves as expected".

The next section describes security concepts in general for electronic medical record systems. The second section describes the concept of *protected health information.* The third section describes additional more specific security and security-related requirements this book proposes for our particular automated patient medical record system.

13.9.1 Security Concepts for Electronic Medical Record Systems

The first comprehensive source of requirements for security in electronic medical record systems is the *Health Insurance Portability and Accountability Act of 1996 (HIPAA)*, a law governing the security of electronic medical record systems, is now being implemented by healthcare organizations (CMS 2004).

HIPAA requires that various technical, physical and administrative security measures be combined to protect the privacy, integrity and availability of patients' medical records. Together, these security measures would

- govern the transmission and accessibility of patient medical record information to individuals, organizations and to Medicare, disallowing access to those not authorized to view it
- protect against destruction of medical record information, and
- protect against the unavailability of systems providing access to medical record information.

Security concepts relevant to the implementation of HIPAA requirements, or to any comprehensive implementation of security in an automated patient medical record system and associated clinical systems, are listed in table 13.4. For each security concept, (1) the security concept is described, (2) examples of techniques that may be used to implement the security concept are presented, and (3) a description of how the security concept applies to the automated patient medical record is presented.

Table 13.4 Security concepts

Security Concept	*Description*	*Examples of Techniques to Implement*	*Use in the Automated Patient Medical Record System*
Person Authentication	For a person using a system, is that person who that person says he or she is?	Passwords, smart cards, biometric identification devices in comparison to stored information on each user; sign-on/sign-off, automatic logoff, digital certificates (server certificates) and digital signatures, firewalls	User sign-on and sign-off to system.

Application Authentication	For an application making a request for a service controlled by another application, possibly in another computer and organization, is the application the one identified and in the system and organization identified?	Kerberos, digital certificates (server certificates) and digital signatures, application to application controls (SSL/TLS), host to host controls (IPSec), IP/network address, firewalls	Communication between system and clinical systems, and especially between the system and the CPR and source document repositories.
Terminal or Other Hardware Device Authentication	The terminal or other hardware device together with its location are identified.	Recording hardware identification of terminal, associated type of terminal, and allowable locations, DLC (Data Link Control) or MAC (Media Access Control) address, logical unit, firewalls.	Terminals and other devices in public areas vs. secured areas.
Authorization / Access	The information and services within an application system a person, another application system or device is allowed to access.	Access lists, LDAP	Access to information, secure terminals in secure departments (psychiatry, genetics), ordering capabilities (especially for narcotics), access to remotely located records.
Visibility	The functionality in an application system provided to a person.	Role-based access, person-based access	Functionality provided for meet caregiver's role or individual needs.

Administrative Procedures	Contingency plans for system emergencies; business policies on access control, employee termination procedures, physical protection of data, and consent for use and disclosure of information.	Overall site and organizational security policy based upon assess of risks, including documentation, data backup plan, disaster recovery plan, emergency mode operation, record of access, inventory, employee termination procedures (locks changed, user id removal, cards returned), new personnel clearance procedures and agreement signing, security incident procedures, user education, visual identification of patients, need to know procedures, procedures for loss of a computer or PDA, protection against social engineering, identification of why a system went down.	Operational policies supporting security.
Physical Safeguards	Security of physical computer systems and other equipment.	Overall site and organizational Equipment in secure locations, access badges, cabinets with keys, physical attachment of terminals, identification of terminals and allowable locations, assessment of risks.	Protection of computers and other equipment.
Integrity of Data	The receiver has assurance that data sent is not altered and is from the said user or system.	One-way hash with message digest, digital signature, replay checking, encryption / decryption, virus checking, intrusion detection systems, authorization and access control.	Communication between systems and/or people, including with the CPR and source document repositories.
Encryption / Decryption	Conversion of plaintext to ciphertext / conversion of ciphertext to plaintext; may be combined with compression.	Encryption algorithms, PKI, SSL/TLS, IPSec.	Same as PKI.

Public Key Infrastructure (PKI)	A set of capabilities to allow secure communication across a line by one party with a private key and the other with a public key.	Digital certificate, assymmetric and symmetric encryption, certificate authority, registration authority, public key, private key, digital signature, cross certification, time stamping, certificate revocation, trust mode., secure storage of private keys.	Communication between caregivers caring for a patient. Communication with CPR and source document repositories. Communication with insurers, including the federal government.
Confidentiality	The organization is assured that the data can only be seen by someone who has authorization to see it.	Authorization and access control to a document and to elements within a document when necessary, encryption, PKI, firewalls, intrusion detection systems.	Privacy of medical record information of a patient.
Chain of Trust	For EDI, in which trading partners have specific agreements with each other, this chain of trust can be controlled by contractual agreements. For communication with outside healthcare organizations and medical providers, this chain of trust may have to be governed by laws and healthcare industry standards.	Contracts, service request authentication, cross certification, laws and industry standards.	Communication with insurance and financial systems via EDI; communication with CPR and source document repository; request and granting of permission to copy or disclose patient records.
Identity Verification	The organization has assurance of the legitimate identify of each person, application, local device, and organization involved.	Registration authority; assignment of provider and patient identifiers by HCFA, biometric devices; hardware card identification of a device and a location.	Recording passwords and unique identifiers of humans especially from biometric devices for later authentication; this information could be stored on smart cards secured by the user. Intelligent procurement of hardware. HCFA identification of healthcare organizations and of providers and patients.

Electronic signature	Identification of caregiver who created document that is equivalent of caregiver's signature.	Undetermined, but most likely candidate is biometric information. See references (HIPAA 2000-2003) for requirements for an electronic signature.	Signing source documents; identifying caregivers doing ordering.
Nonrepudiation Evidence	The sender cannot deny sending the information or an electronic signer of a document cannot deny signing the document.	Electronic signature, digital signature, biometric system, smart card, intrusion detection devices, firewalls.	Signing source documents; identifying caregivers doing ordering. Communication of medical information.
Availability of Service	The system is available for use when needed.	Load balancing, firewalls, fail-over recovery, clustering, parallel disk arrays, multi-processors, on-line backups and logging, intrusion detection systems, virus checkers, service level agreements, firewalls, ups (uninterruptible power supply).	Availability of automated medical record system and all clinical systems. Protection against bugs and other unintentional errors. Protection against attacks on systems.
Disaster Recovery	Information is available after a fire, earthquake, a major criminal act, or other major disaster.	Off-site duplication of information for backup. Backup computer systems.	Off-site duplication of medical record information for backup purposes. Backup computer systems for access to the medical record.
Auditing / Recoverability	Security-critical operations are recorded and information is recoverable.	Backups of information; log files; recovery system software; a procedure for emergency access to encrypted information.	All systems.
Remote Access	Secure access from outside the healthcare organization; protection against theft.	Remote access authentication and/or authorization systems that may include encryption and certificates, and logging (RADIUS, TACACS+), Virtual Private Networks (VPN), local system sign-ons, encryption of data on local databases.	Remote terminals. Any access to the automated patient medical record system from outside the organization.

Request / Grant Permission for Medical Records	The creator (HMO or physician) and/or owner (the patient) of a source document can grant permission to an authorized party to copy or disclose the document, and authorized parties can request permission to copy medical documents, perhaps with certain categories of permissions granted by policy.	To be determined.	Requests for medical records and their sending.

Authentication is the system knowing that a user, a terminal or other hardware device, or an application requesting a service of another application is who she, he, or it says it is. *Authorization* is the information and services within an application system a person, device, or another application system is allowed to access, which could be based upon the location of the device, while *access controls* determine how this information and these services can be accessed (e.g., this user can read, add, and replace this information, and this other user can only read it). Authentication and authorization for a person happens when the user logs on. Authentication of another application system requesting a service of the application system could occur just before the request or at log on of the user. Authorization for a terminal or other hardware device could occur every time it is used. Access control could be determined either at the time a resource is accessed or at log on of the user.

Visibility is the functionality provided to a person using the system, the *user* of the system. This visibility may differ depending upon the user's role as a physician, nurse, medical assistant, etc. and may be tailored for a particular user.

Certain aspects of security occur outside the automated systems. *Administrative procedures* and *physical safeguards* must be set in the healthcare organizations using or having access to information in the system.

When communication occurs between two systems, two people, a person and a system, the receiver must have insurance that the data in the communication was not altered and is from the entity it is supposed to be from—that there is *integrity of data*. Such secure communications require a large set of technologies; one such set of technologies is called the *public-key infrastructure (PKI)*. Part of this secure communication is *encryption* of data to change *plaintext* into *ciphertext* that cannot be easily read and can be *decrypted* back to plaintext; encryption is often combined with compression and decompression of the information to reduce the amount of data that needs to be transmitted.

Confidentiality is insuring that information, especially of medical records and other patient information, is only seen by the people authorized to see it. Medical records are both available inside the healthcare organization and outside the healthcare organization; therefore, confidentiality must be assured both inside and outside the healthcare organization. Within the healthcare organization, confidentiality is assured by access controls. Confidentiality externally is assured by keeping unauthorized people out of the system and by secure communication of the medical record to outside the healthcare organization.

Once a medical record has been sent outside the organization, then the healthcare organization no longer has direct control over the information. Confidentiality is dependent upon a *chain of trust*. For EDI, in which trading partners have specific agreements with each other, this chain of trust can be controlled by contractual agreements. For communication with outside healthcare organizations and medical providers, this chain of trust may have to be governed by laws and healthcare industry standards.

For authorization purposes and also for identification within medical records, system users, devices, computer applications, healthcare organizations, medical practitioners, and patients must be uniquely and conclusively identified. This requires *identity verification* that requires an infrastructure governed by trust, technology, laws, and industry agreements, that currently does not completely exist. HIPAA mandates unique physician and healthcare organization identifiers and has proposed unique patient identifiers.

Currently, paper medical records and medical orders must be signed by a physician and/or other authorized medical practitioner. The electronic equivalent of a physical signature is an *electronic signature*. Although an electronic signature for an electronic medical record has not been standardized and is no one particular thing (HIPAA 2000-2003), an electronic signature must insure that the signer cannot deny signing the document, referred to as *nonrepudiation*. Nonrepudiation also applies to other senders of communications within the automated system, in that the sender cannot deny that he or she sent the communication.

Another aspect of security in automated systems is the insurance of the *availability of service*, that systems do not go down and that complete functionality of the system is available. This is particularly important for our system, where availability of the system is required at all times, for 24 hours 7 days of the week (24 x 7). Unavailability of the system or of parts of the functionality of the system may occur because of overloading of the system, program bugs, attacks by hackers, hardware failures—these and other causes of failures must be protected against.

Related to availability of service is *disaster recovery*. If there is a fire, earthquake, a major criminal act, or other disaster that destroys a chart room or computer systems, then there is a backup of this medical information and backup computer systems located off-site to the disaster. Disaster recovery is more feasible with an automated patient medical record, where the duplicate information is on kept on computer storage media, than it is with paper medical records, where medical records must be manually copied to paper or microfilm.

Security-critical events must be recorded so the causes of failures can be identified and recovered from. *Auditing* is recording security-critical events on a log file so an audit trail of these events can be recorded so the causes of the failures can be determined. When an automated system does go down under normal operations, then the system must be recovered to resume operation where it left off; this can be done by *recovery procedures*, such as restoring the system from backups or using a log fail to back out operations that caused a failure. For cases where an employee is unavailable and the employee has encrypted information, such as on disk, there must be a way for the healthcare organization to access the information in emergency situations.

To enable caregivers and others to better perform their jobs, *remote access* to the automated systems may be required. This requires attention to security threats. If a terminal is stolen, you do not want the thief to have access to patient information on the system; information can be protected by requiring sign-ons to use the system and by encrypting database information so a disk cannot be removed and read on another machine. Secure remote access to the automated patient medical record system for dial-in connections or direct connections can be assured by use of remote access authentication and/or authorization systems that may include encryption and certificates, and logging (RADIUS, TACACS+); the Internet could be used as the network with encryption of transmissions through use of virtual private networks (VPNs).

When it comes to medical records, special consideration must be given to both administrative and technological methods of *requesting permission* to copy medical records or disclose information in medical records, and of *granting permission* to do so.

Security measures for an automated patient medical record must provide a balance between many things, including the following: patient privacy; healthcare organization privacy; caregiver access to medical records; government and regulatory organization requirements; and costs and cost savings to the healthcare organization and patient.

13.9.2 Protected Health Information

HIPAA has introduced the term, *protected health information*. This is any information in any media that relates to "an individual's past, present, or future physical or mental health status, condition, treatment, service, products purchased, or provision of care", and in any way identifies the individual (e.g., combines medical information, gender, and geographic location to identify an individual).

HIPAA establishes a disclosure policy for this information, including the following (HIPAA 2002):

- **to the individual:** An individual has a right to his or her healthcare information.
- **required for medical treatment of the individual:** Medical practitioners need to have the information to provide care.
- **to entities based upon HIPAA regulation:** Entities might be able to receive information based upon regulations, subject to *need to know*, *minimal disclosure necessary*, *de-identification* of the individual, confidential use of information, legal status of the recipient, and/or consent.

The *need to know* means that if a caregiver is authorized to see certain protected health information as part of her work responsibilities and needs to see the protected health information of a particular patient to perform her job, she is allowed to do so. Even doctors and nurses don't have the right to look at all the health information about every patient; for example, a physician caring only for children has no right to look at the medical record of adult patients unless that physician is also helping to care for them.

For disclosure of healthcare information—other than for treatment, for disclosure to the patient, or as a result of government regulation—the *minimum* amount of information *necessary* should be disclosed.

De-identification means removing patient identifiers so that patient information can be distributed without breaking federal privacy rules. Reference (HIPAA 2002) explains how to de-identify protected health information.

HIPAA mandates that health organizations track the disclosure of PHI and maintain records that will, on demand, supply reports and disclosure statements on a patient's PHI to any patient who requests such a report. An individual has the right to receive an accounting of disclosures of PHI made by the health organization in the six years prior to the date on which the accounting was requested. This is referred to as *disclosure accounting*.

13.9.3 Wireless Security

Section 12.3 describes wireless communication that could occur between point-of-care computers and servers. Because wireless signals are "out in the open", they require a special kind of security. Some approaches to wireless security are technical and are described in reference (Dismukes 1998-2003). An example is *WEP (Wired Equivalent Privacy)* that describes how wireless signals can be encrypted.

(The Chinese have adopted the WLAN standard for wireless that is similar to IEEE's 802.11b wireless standard but it uses a different security protocol, *WLAN Authentication and Privacy Infrastructure (WAPI),* rather than WEP. IEEE is exploring the possibility of incorporating WAPI into 802.11. (Lemon 2003))

Within a hospital or medical office building, *access points*, antennas, are set up that allow point-of-care computers to communicate via wireless with servers. These access points should be set up so the signals cover an area of the hospital or medical office building (for example, a number of rooms), but do not go outside the hospital and do not go outside the floor.

13.9.4 Additional Security Concepts for Our Proposed System

This section identifies additional security concepts that may be appropriate for our proposed automated patient medical record system.

Identifying a user, as stated in the previous section, is called authentication and what information a user can access is called authorization. A user would be able to sign on to the system at each distributed facility group computer at which the user has a *user account*. In the proposed design, a caregiver will have a user account for every distributed facility group that includes a facility where the caregiver works.

One business requirement stated earlier was to provide quick log-on and sign-off of the system, so the caregiver spends very little time logging on and off the computer. Possible log-on approaches, in addition to the usual on in most systems now—the keying in of a password on the keyboard, are scanning of the caregiver's identification badge or *smart card*, or use of a *biometrics* recognition device, such as a fingerprint reader or voice recognition device (see section 17.2.6 for more discussion of this subject). A *smart card* is a credit care size plastic card containing a microprocessor. *Biometrics* is the utilization of an anatomical or behavioral characteristic in order to verify the identity of an individual.

It is proposed that there be a time-out period after non-use of the terminal, with blanking of the screen. The system would continue where the user left off after the user logged back on.

Associated with a terminal would be a *terminal profile*. The terminal profile might define a *logon group*, a group of users associated with the terminal who are allowed to log on.

Associated with all user accounts will be security information in an area called a *user profile* with other user information coming from a database on caregivers. The user profile is expected to contain the user's password and security codes that identify which special security access the user has. The secure codes will be used to control the visibility of information by department, unit or by individual document, with one or more secure codes optionally associated with each department in each facility, each unit in each facility and each document in patient clinical information.

Also the user profile would identify the job category(-ies) of the caregiver, thus identifying standard ordering and other activities. And the user profile might contain information to enable automatic system logon to other HMO clinical systems when the user logs on to the automated patient medical record system.

Associated with a physician may be a *DEA (Drug Enforcement Agency) number* to identify that the caregiver can order narcotics. Alternatively, the DEA number may come from a *credentialing system* that records HMO information for the credentialing of a provider, including licenses (such as the DEA license), medical school and other degrees, insurance, board certification, certificates, hospital privileges, specialties and sub-specialties.

Associated with a nurse practitioner may be a drug "furnishing number" that allows the NP to order drugs and devices in accordance with standardized procedures and protocols approved by a supervising physician. Alternatively, this could come from the credentialing system.

A secure code within a user profile may also be used to control a caregiver's ability to order a specific test or specific procedure that will be done anonymously (e.g., Alzheimer's testing, HIV testing, therapeutic abortions). Only caregivers that the caregiver has pre-identified will be able to identify the patient associated with such a test or procedure. Such an order will be referred to as an *anonymous order*.

If a user logs on to a second distributed group system concurrently with logon to the first on the same computer, he will not have to re-enter his password. The previously entered password will be carried over.

At any time including user logoff, the system will optionally allow the user to set a *bookmark* related to a user account to identify where he left off and to return to that exact location—patient list, clinical summary for a particular patient, or document list with selected documents for a patient—upon user logon. This is similar to a *snapshot*, which allows return to information for a particular patient.

The system will also audit viewing of all documents, results and alarms, recording who saw them.

Further, an *electronic signature* mechanism (HIPAA 2000-2003) will be provided for all documents where the equivalent paper document requires a caregiver signature. This electronic signature must be legally valid in all states in which the associated document could be viewed; the electronic signature will be transmitted with the document. Control over which documents can be copied outside the organization or region will be controlled by agreements between the trading partners and other regulatory rules and laws, such as HIPAA in the United States.

The system will enforce the *data integrity of a completed document*: after the editing process and/or electronic signature, no information in the document may be lost or altered in any way.

Mechanisms for handling caregiver collaboration on the same patient encounter may exist. This may include two or more caregivers seeing the patient one after the other or together. It may also include a caregiver being consulted during the patient encounter, which may involve a caregiver who does not work within the distributed facility group of the patient encounter—this is a case where the consulting caregiver may not have a user account within the distributed facility group of the patient encounter. This latter situation will be referred to as a "remote consultation" and is discussed in section 13.10.

Based upon the existence of a central system and local systems, table 13.5 identifies a proposed scope of *visibility* of various types of information within the proposed system. Patient lists, clinical summaries and documents are available for concurrent view by multiple caregivers.

During a patient encounter in a facility in one distributed facility group, clinical summaries and documents may be copied to another distributed facility group system to enable a consulting caregiver to provide advice on the patient. See the next section on interfaces under the title "remote consultation".

Table 13.5 Proposed scope of visibility of information

Data Item	*Scope of Visibility*
Patient Demographics	Stored centrally. Available within each distributed facility group.
Patient Lists	Distributed facility group of the associated encounters, except for schedules that are centrally located and exist whereever the caregiver works.
Local Clinical Summary	Distributed facility group.
Overall / HMO Clinical Summary (dependent upon whether the HMO keeps track of outside HMO encounters or not)	Central system and distributed facility group for the facility for an encounter. The Overall / HMO Clinical Summary will automatically be transferred over from the central system to the distributed facility group of another facility based upon a later encounter taking place or upon a future encounter scheduled with the previous encounter being identified as being complete. Also, as a "consultant", a caregiver with another distributed facility group or an Agent can request a copy of the Overall / HMO Clinical Summary.
Inpatient Clinical Summary	Distributed facility group.
Source documents, including order and results documents	Distributed facility group. If an encounter occurs at a facility within another distributed facility group, a caregiver or agent can request a copy of a non-local source document referenced in the associated Regional or Interregional Clinical Summary.
Encounter synopses	Encounter synopses will be within the distributed facility group and copied after the encounter to the central level. Upon a new encounter, the synopses, if necessary, will be sent down to the distributed facility group of the encounter.
Translation information	Translation information, information to translate patient data elements from local to regional data and back, will be sent over with a copied source document from another healthcare organization.
Data Dictionary	Stored at the central level. Available at each distributed facility group system. (The data dictionary identifies the meaning and format of each data element and can also be used to identify *protected health information.*)
User Profile	The distributed facility group where the caregiver user has a user account.
Terminal Profile	The distributed facility group of the facility where the terminal is located.
Order Profile	Are specific to a distributed facility group. Remote order profiles for a remote order in the distributed facility group of the ordering facility must be matched by a local order profile at the performing area distributed facility group.

13.10 INTERFACES

Networks enable different computer systems to communicate via wire or radio connections. The hardware and software that enables information to be passed between any two computer systems are called *interfaces.*

This section describes the interfaces that might be needed for an automated patient medical record system that has the network configuration described in section 13.4. For the automated patient medical record system in our HMO, we have chosen to have a central HMO computer system tied to smaller distributed (facility) group systems—local systems--which each handle automated patient medical record processing for a set of HMO facilities. Ancillary departments, such as clinical laboratories, the pharmacy, and radiology are handled by their own clinical computers connected to the central system or to a distributed group system. Inpatient and outpatient encounters are recorded through other clinical computers connected to the central system or to a distributed group system. This section describes proposed interfaces for this set up of connected computer systems.

Interfaces for our automated patient medical record system include the following: (1) interfaces with other clinical systems within the healthcare organization, (2) interfaces between the central system and distributed group systems, and (3) interfaces with systems outside the healthcare organization. Where possible, all network communication of information should be accomplished through messages in HL7 format, a standard for network communication between healthcare systems.

Section 13.11 describes the basics of healthcare network communications and interfaces, identifying techniques that can be used to build these interfaces, or any other interfaces.

13.10.1 Interfaces Between the Automated Patient Medical Record System and Other HMO Clinical Systems

Clinical information received from centrally-connected clinical systems through the central system Centrally-connected clinical systems may send an encounter or a change in encounter status, return a result and/or an alarm associated with a previous order, send back an order status change, send back a clinical system generated order as a result of another order (e.g., the clinical laboratory may redo a test with results way out of range assuming a piece of equipment is malfunctioning), or send a patient demographics update to the central system. Communication is via HL7. See figure 13.23.

An encounter or encounter status change will be sent to the encounter facility and any other local system computer having a facility with an outstanding encounter for the patient. Outpatient appointment or outpatient visit encounters are sent to every facility where the associated caregiver potentially works in order to generate the outpatient schedule within the associated distributed group systems.

A "discharge" encounter status will close the associated outstanding encounter, and will inform the central system to expect the complete patient medical record encounter information.

An order, change in order status or results will be sent to the ordering facility. Any change to patient demographics will be updated in all local systems.

Clinical information is sent to a distributed group system from local clinical systems within the facilities Local clinical systems directly connected to the distributed group system may send an encounter or encounter status change, send a result and/or an alarm from a previous order sent to the clinical system, send back an order status change, send back a local clinical system generated order as a result of another order (e.g., a facility clinical laboratory may redo a test with results way out of range assuming a piece of equipment is malfunctioning), or send a patient demographics update. Communication is via HL7. See figure 13.24.

An encounter or encounter status change will be sent to any other local system with a facility with an outstanding encounter for the patient. Outpatient appointment or outpatient visit encounters are sent to every facility where the associated caregiver potentially works in order to generate the outpatient schedule with the associated distributed group systems.

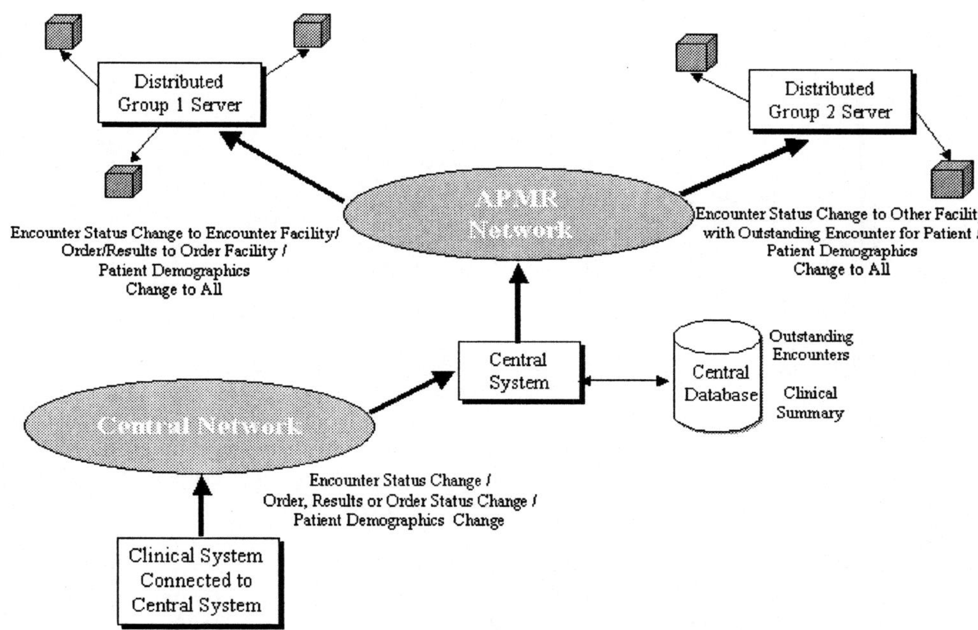

Figure 13.23 Clinical information from clinical systems connected to the central system.

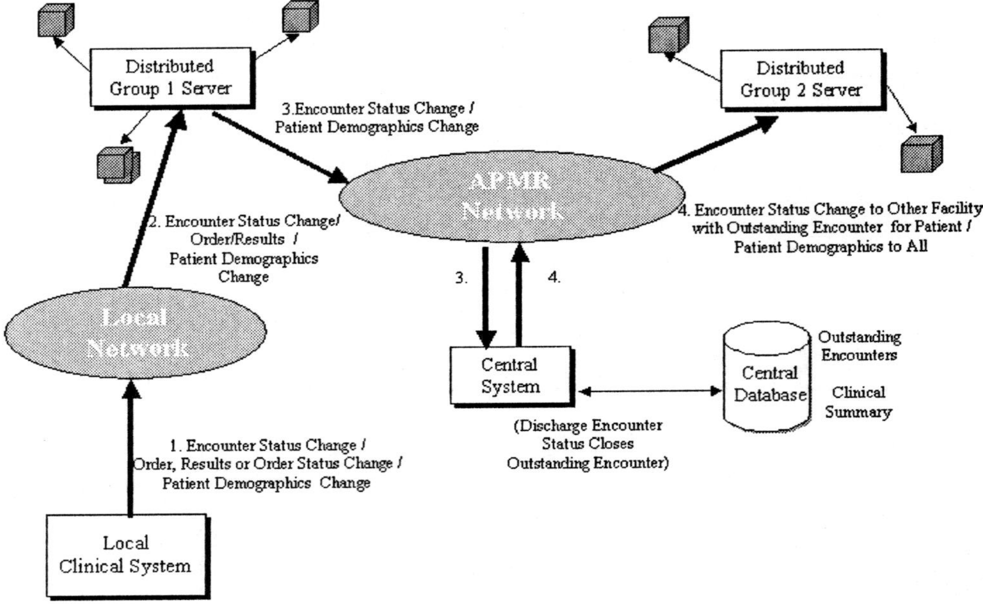

Figure 13.24 Clinical information from clinical systems connected to a distributed group system.

A "discharge" encounter status will close the associated outstanding encounter, and will inform the central system to expect the complete patient medical record encounter information. Any change to patient demographics will be sent to the central system and updated in all local systems.

Distributed group system systems connected to the central system Instead of an admission being identified through the ADT system, an admission, a "quick admission", can first be identified through the automated patient medical record system through adding a patient to an inpatient census, patient list or inpatient unit room map. In such a case, ADT would be informed of the admission after which further information on the admission would be collected through ADT.

A completion of an outpatient visit will mark the outstanding encounter as closed, and will inform the central system to expect the complete patient medical record encounter information.

A change in patient demographics in a local system will be sent through middleware to other HMO clinical systems. (The patient demographics change in turn will be sent back to the local systems from the other clinical systems; see figure 13.23.)

See figure 13.25 for the case where the clinical system has an interface through the central system. See figure 13.26 for the case where the clinical system is directly interfaced with the local system.

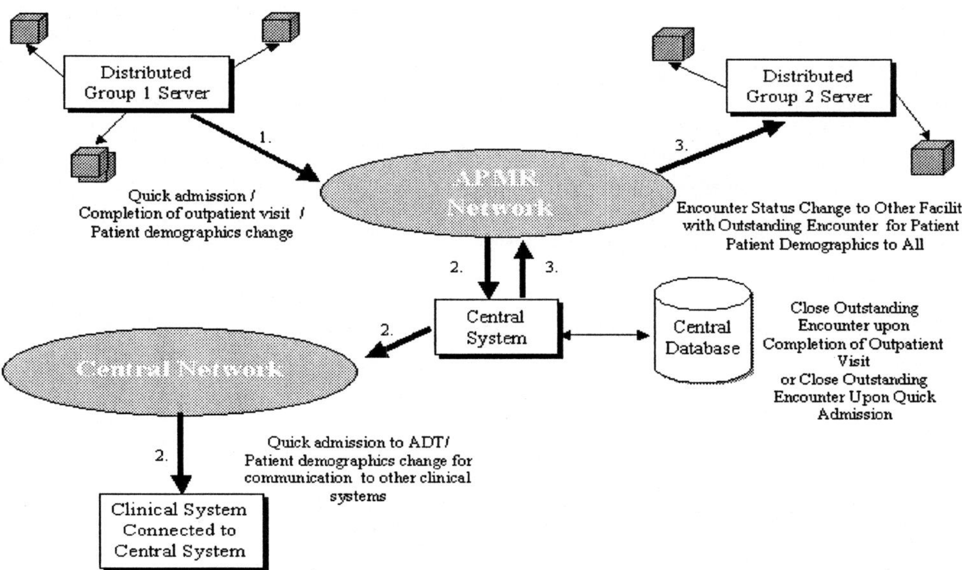

Figure 13.25 Clinical information from distributed group system to clinical system connected to the central system.

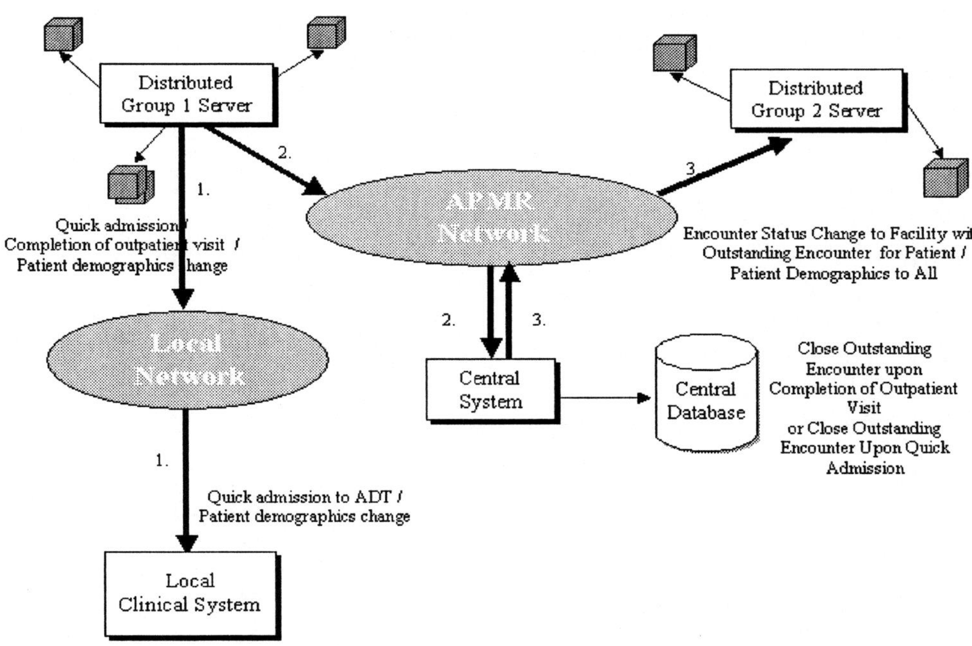

Figure 13.26 Clinical information from distributed group system to a local facility clinical system.

An order being made via the central system A caregiver can send an order to be executed to an ancillary system via the central system, such as a medication order to the pharmacy system; see figure 13.27. One caregiver can also make a consultation request to a second caregiver in a facility in another distributed facility group, placing the order on a consultation request list for the second caregiver, or the caregiver can send an order to a performing area in another distributed facility group, placing the order on a Work List in the performing area; see figure 13.28. Orders might also be saved in the central database, including those internal to a local system.

A completion of an outpatient visit will mark the outstanding encounter as closed, and will inform the central system to expect the complete patient medical record encounter information.

An order being made through a local clinical system A caregiver can send an order to a local ancillary system to be executed, such as a medication order to a local pharmacy system; see figure 13.29.

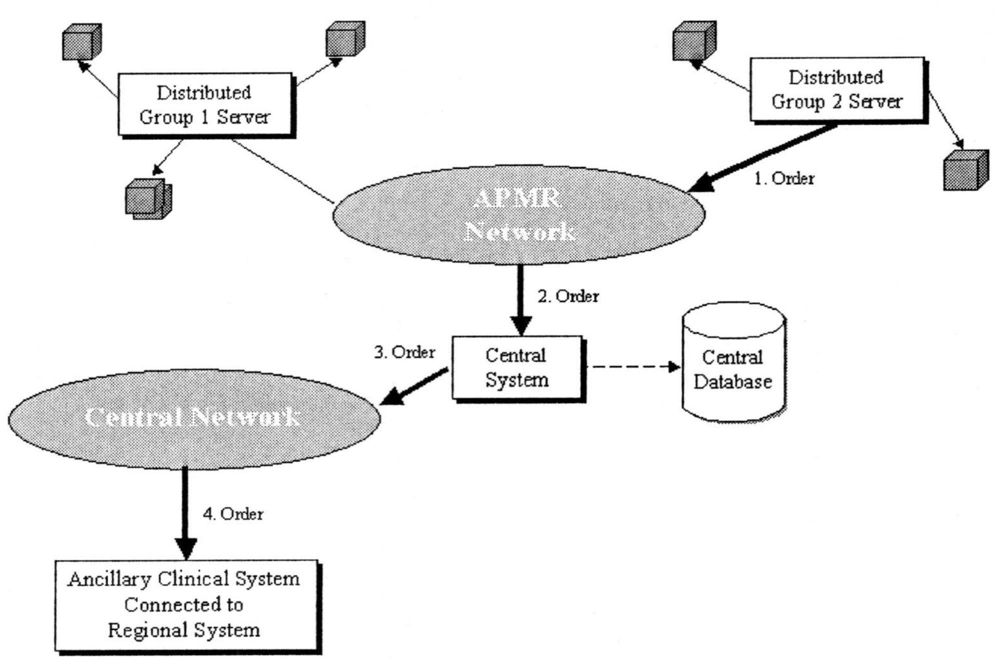

Figure 13.27 Order to an ancillary system connected to the central system.

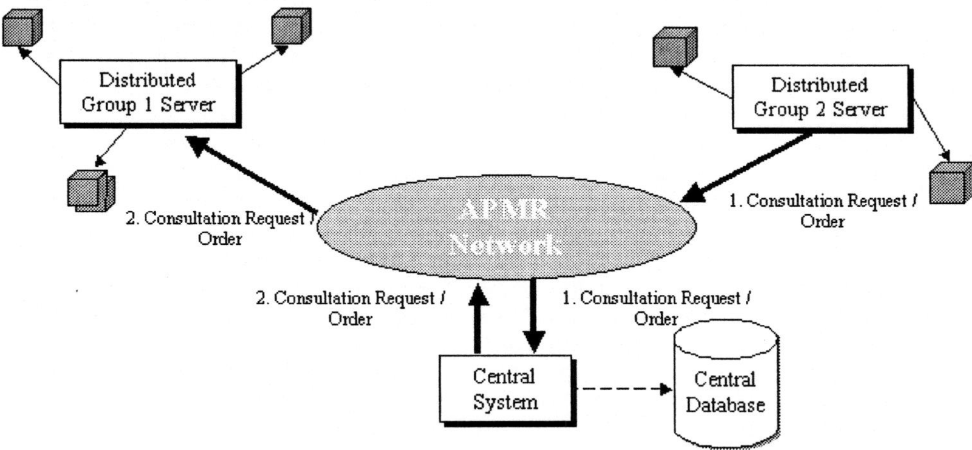

Figure 13.28 Order through another distributed facility system.

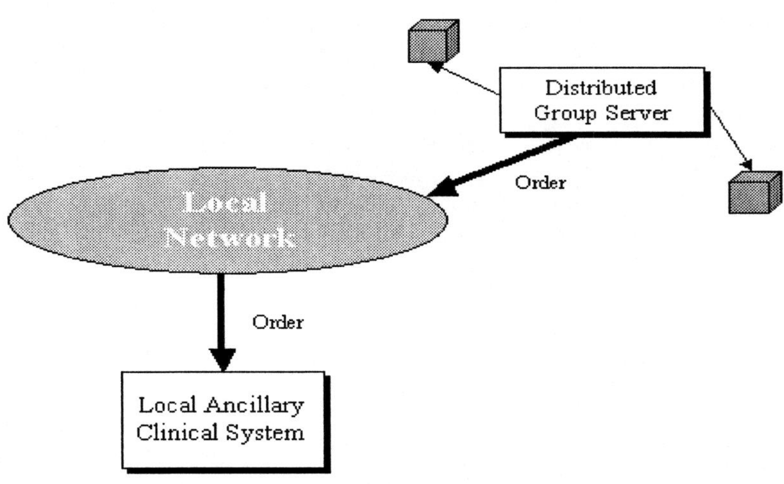

Figure 13.29 Order from distributed facility system to local clinical system.

Interfaces to load and update local HMO translation/validation information In order for local systems to do ordering, they must have information to validate or translate the ordering information including clinical lab test directories and drug formulary information. Note that there are three potential alternatives for storage of HMO validation and translation information from other clinical systems.

Alternative one would have the information only reside in a clinical system, and not the automated patient medical record system, in which case the clinical system, rather than the automated patient medical record system, would be doing any translation or validation of automated patient medical record information; this would save on costs of shipping the information to the automated patient medical record system but require information to be translated or validated to be shipped to the clinical system with a response back.

Alternative two would have the information duplicated in each applicable distributed facility group system; this would have the greatest efficiency in doing translation and validation of automated patient medical record information but would require the shipping of the checking information to each of the distributed facility systems.

Alternative three would be to have the clinical information reside in the central system; this would allow the information to only reside in the central system and not each of the distributed facility group systems, but would require shipping down of clinical information and would provide somewhat less efficiency than alternative two in doing any translation or validation of automated patient medical record information. Alternative three is assumed in figure 13.30.

Interfaces to load and update this translation/validation information may either be on-line interfaces shown by Path (1) or off-line batch interfaces shown by Path (2). These interfaces may include the following: (1a) on-line initial load of information; (1b) on-line update of information, such as downloading a newly identified caregiver in the other HMO clinical systems; (2a) initial load through a batch job, such as one to read the First Databank Tape for medications in a drug formulary, or one to load resource information. (2b) Periodic update through a batch job, for example updating CPT4 and ICD9 code lists at the same time they are updated in the other HMO clinical systems. See figure 13.30. **So that current and historic clinical information can be translated properly, translation/validation information must be kept up to date at all times with the same information in the other HMO clinical systems and historic translation/validation information must be kept.**

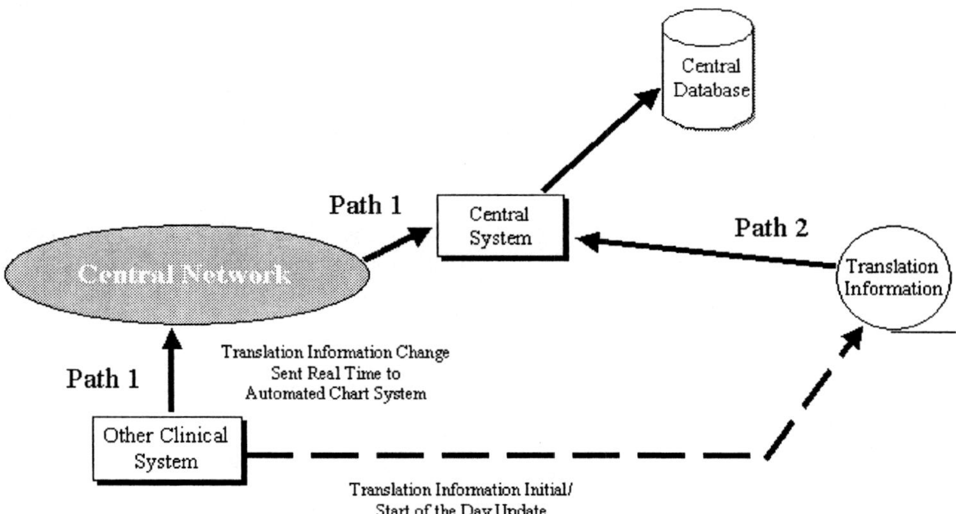

Figure 13.30 Translation information loads/updates.

Schedule updates or changes sent from the appointment scheduling system Because the patient list for outpatients should consist of a schedule not only including a list of patients with appointments and registrations for a date but also time when the caregiver is unavailable, still open for appointments or outside the HMO, there must be an interface to the appointment system to retrieve this caregiver time information. These processes could be similar to validation/translation information updates and changes shown in figure 13.30.

Whenever there is maintenance of the schedule, the changed schedule information would be sent to the central system from the appointment system. See figure 13.31. A distributed facility group system could use this schedule information and merge it in with appointments and registrations in each distributed facility group where the caregiver could potentially work. A schedule would exist at any facility where the caregiver would potentially work.

A request for an appointment, returned appointment times and booking selection Whenever a caregiver books an appointment through the automated system, this appointment request would be sent to the appointment system. Appointment time that is available, if any, would be locked by the appointment system and returned to the automated system for display. The caregiver would select one of the available appointments, with the selection being returned to the appointment system and notification to unlock the other selections. Optionally, the search could be continued for further appointment selections from which the caregiver could make a choice of which one to book. See figure 13.32.

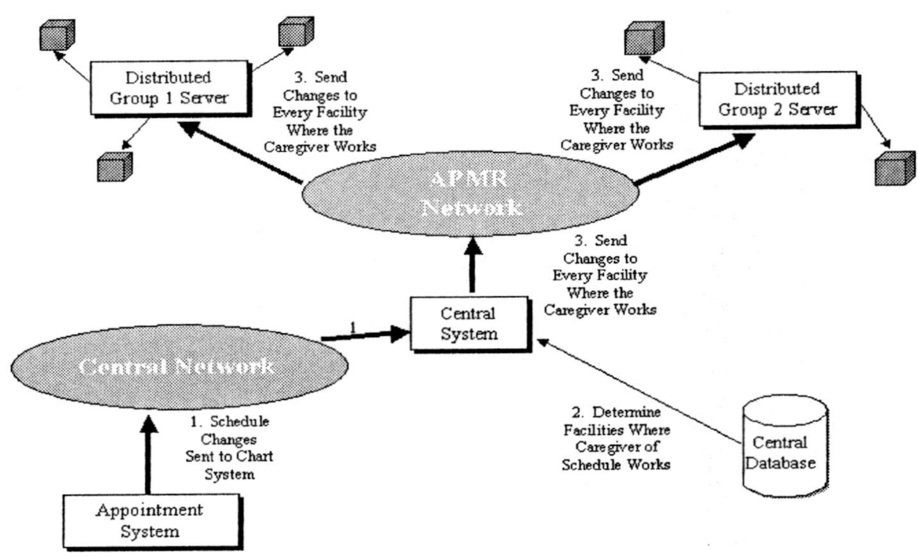

Figure 13.31 Schedule changes.

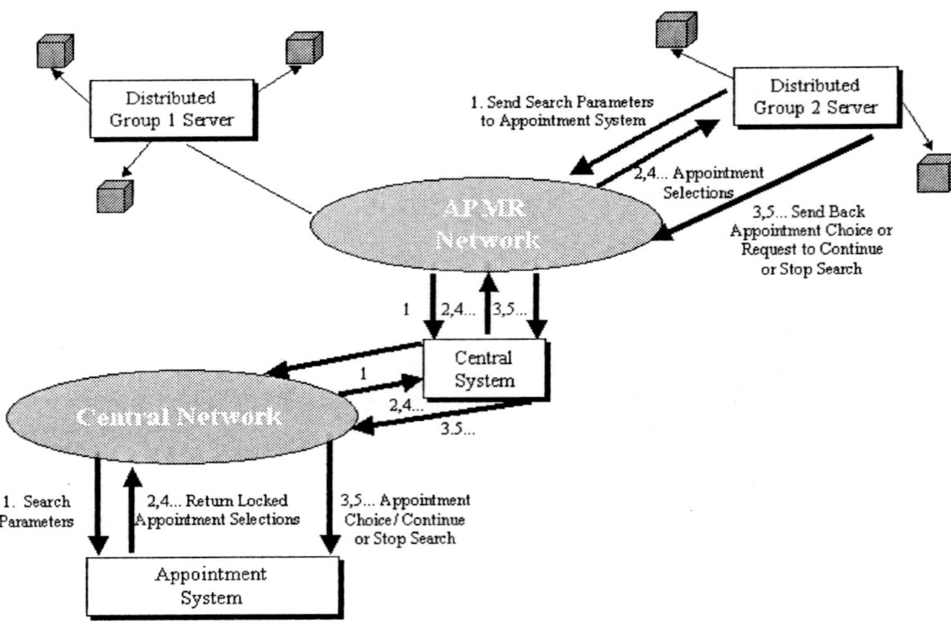

Figure 13.32 Appointment booking.

13.10.2 Interfaces Between the Distributed Facility Group Systems and Central System

A clinical summary transfer request upon a new encounter sent to the central system Upon receiving notification of a new encounter (such as an appointment, preadmission, admission without preadmission) from an HMO encounter clinical system, the central system will cause the clinical summary for the associated patient to be sent to the system handling the encounter facility and mark the encounter as an "outstanding encounter". See figure 13.33.

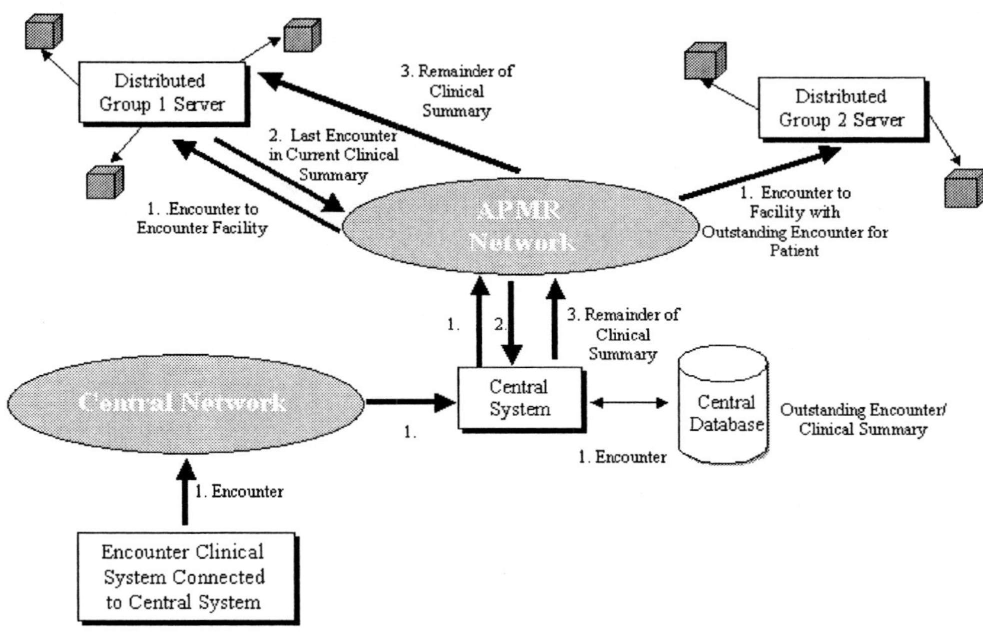

Figure 13.33 Clinical Summary sent to the central system upon an encounter.

Note that the distributed facility group of the encounter facility may already have a copy of the clinical summary together with associated documents. Only the encounters of the clinical summary that the local computer does not already have will be sent. The local computer must inform the central computer of the last encounter it has for the patient. Note that source documents for previous encounters may be resident in the local system or previously requested from another system and already exist. Also agents on the local system may also automatically request source documents.

A Clinical Summary transfer request upon a new encounter sent to a distributed facility group system Upon receiving a new encounter from an HMO encounter clinical system, a local system will send the encounter to the central system along with the last encounter in its current clinical summary for the patient. See figure 13.34.

The central system will send the clinical summary for the associated patient to the computer of the encounter facility. The central system will mark the encounter as an "outstanding encounter" in the central database. And the encounter will be sent to any other local system with a facility having an outstanding encounter.

Note that the distributed facility group of the encounter facility may already have a copy of the clinical summary together with associated documents. Only the encounters of the clinical summary that the local computer does not already have will be sent. Note that source documents for previous encounters may be resident in the local system or previously requested from another system and already exist. Also agents on the local system may also automatically request source documents.

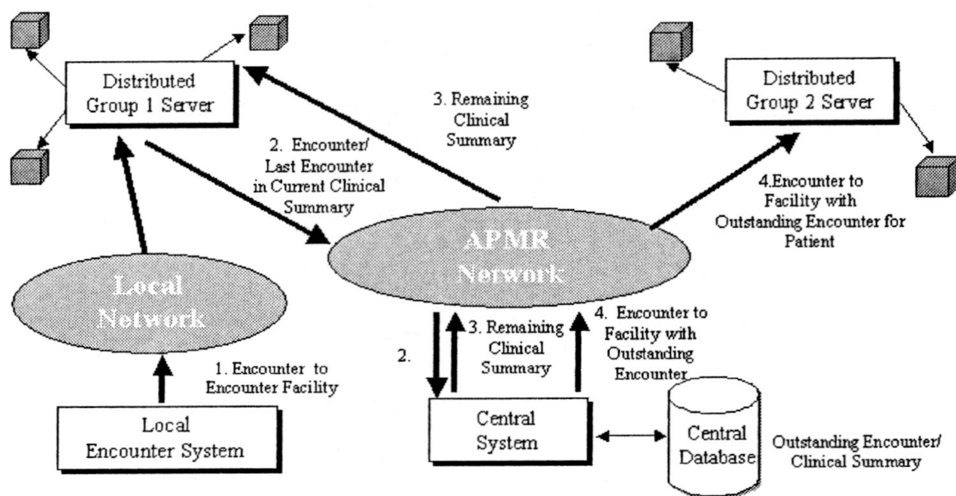

Figure 13.34 Clinical Summary sent to a distributed facility group system upon an encounter.

A remote consultation A caregiver at another facility in a different facility group of the encounter can provide consultation advice for another caregiver who is seeing the patient—this will be referred to as a "remote consultation". The consulting caregiver can request a copy of the clinical summary from another distributed facility group system for purposes of providing consultation advice to the caregiver in another facility. See figure 13.35. The consultation will be identified as an "outstanding encounter" with the encounter being recorded on the central and consulting facility clinical summary.

A document copy request This is a request to receive a copy of a document referenced through the (inter-) regional clinical summary but located at an HMO facility handled by another distributed facility group system. (Translation information might be copied over with the document, especially, when the document comes from a system in another region or from an outside organization, such as from a reference laboratory.) See figure 13.36.

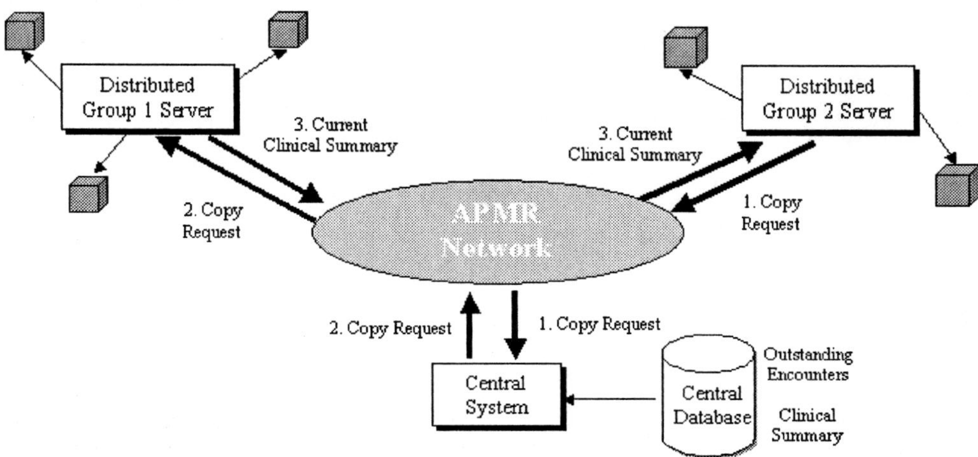

Figure 13.35 Remote consultation.

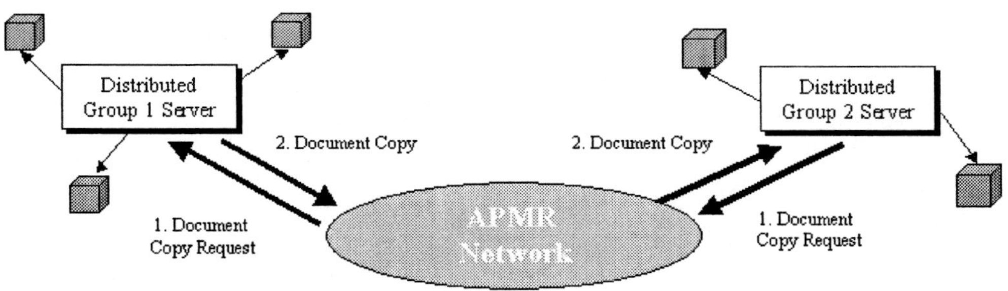

Figure 13.36 A document copy request.

Creation and updating of data warehouses Batch processing could collect new information, perhaps daily, from local system clinical summaries and source document databases and from other HMO systems. This information could be merged and loaded to create or update the data medical resource and financial warehouses identified in section 13.8.3.

13.10.3 Interfaces with Systems Outside the HMO

The HMO being informed of a visit outside the HMO Upon HMO subscription to CPR repositories for HMO patients, possibly via a patient registry, the HMO is informed of an HMO member's outside healthcare visit. See figure 13.37.

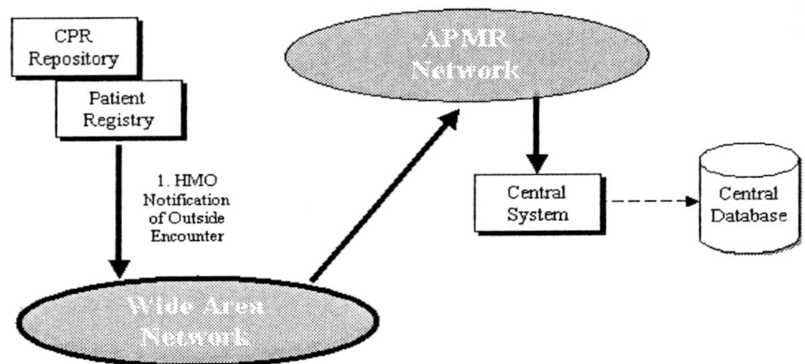

Figure 13.37 HMO notification of an outside HMO patient encounter.

An HMO requesting CPR repository locations for new HMO member or a visiting non-member Upon HMO identification of a new member (perhaps from the HMO membership system) or upon identification of a non-member visit to the HMO (perhaps from the HMO appointment or registration system), the HMO makes a request of the patient registry for CPR repository locations containing patient encounter information. See figure 13.38.

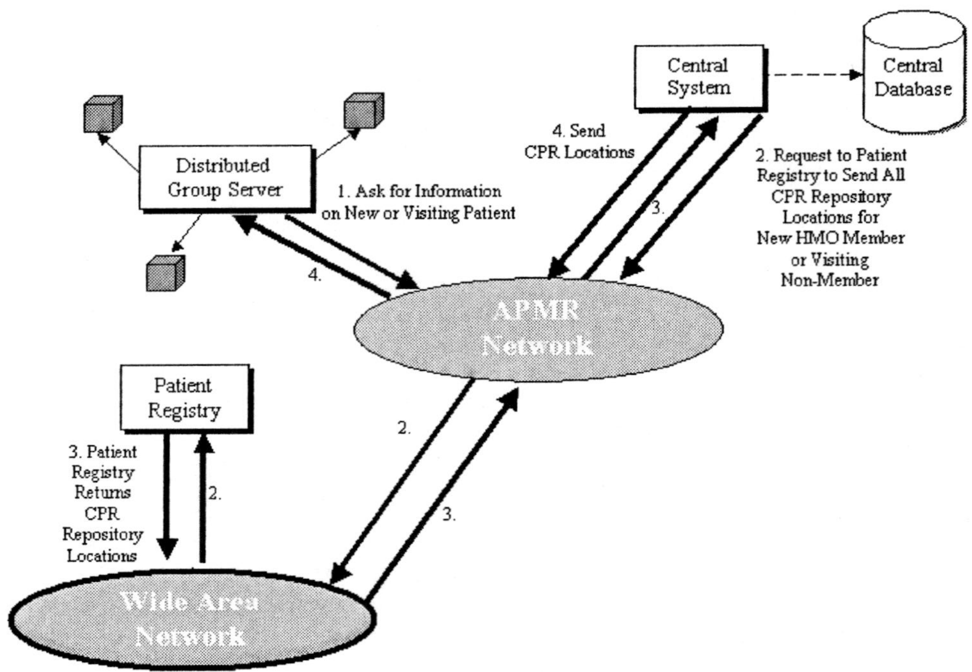

Figure 13.38 CPR request for new HMO member or non-HMO member.

An HMO requests and receives CPR repository information Upon locating the CPR locations of a member's or non-member's encounter, the HMO requests and receives this information merging it with clinical summaries, possibly sending it to distributed facility group systems where there are outstanding encounters. See figure 13.39.

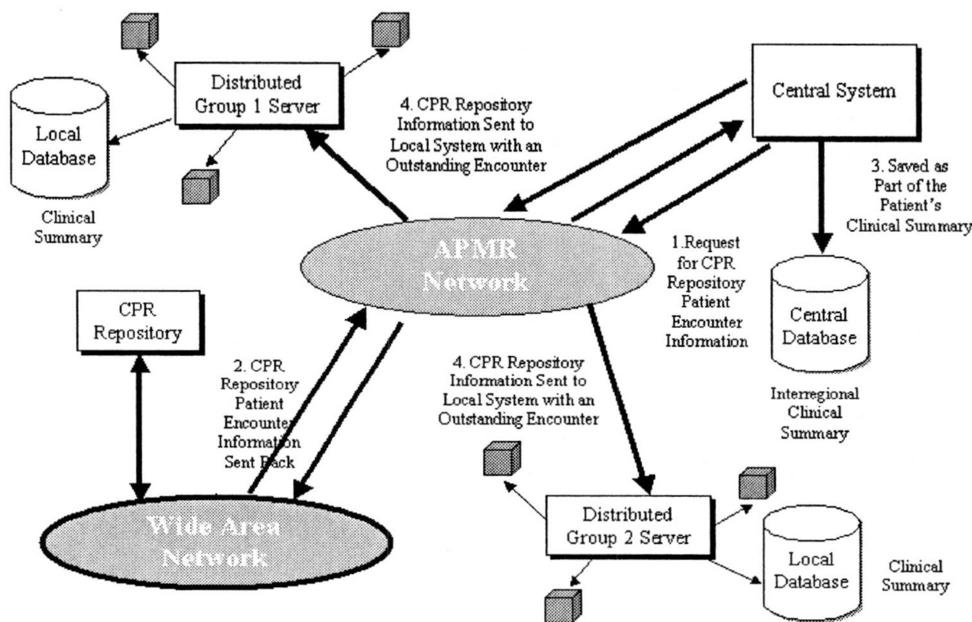

Figure 13.39 CPR encounter information sent to HMO upon HMO request.

An HMO requests and receives source document repository information Request source documents for an encounter from a source document repository. Save source documents on the central system or on a virtual local system. See figure 13.40. Note that a medical document that is in some other healthcare organization's chart room, rather than a source document repository, may have the capability of being electronically ordered; either a mechanism to transfer the chart information electronically or to send a copy of a paper chart by mail may be set up by the other healthcare organization; see subsection labeled "An interregional document copy request".

Patient encounter information sent to the CPR repository and other local systems with outstanding encounters after an encounter After an encounter, the CPR summary of encounter information, patient demographics information, and the locations of medical documents created during the encounter should be sent to the CPR repository. Information is stored in a queue and possibly resent if acknowledgment is not received. See figure 13.41. This information should also be sent to all distributed facility groups where there is an outstanding encounter to keep (Inter-) regional clinical summaries at these locations up-to-date.

As stated in earlier chapters, it is proposed that patient encounter information put into the CPR (and into clinical summaries) be translated to data in national standard formats.

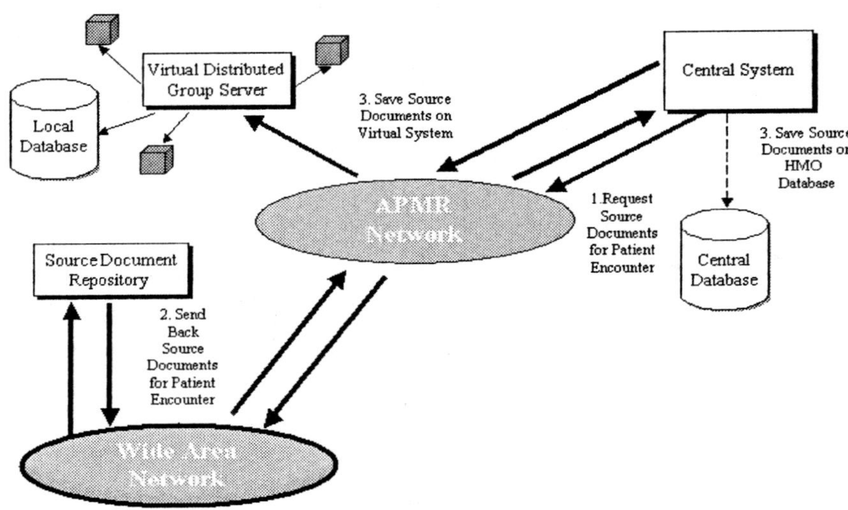

Figure 13.40 Source documents information sent to HMO upon HMO request.

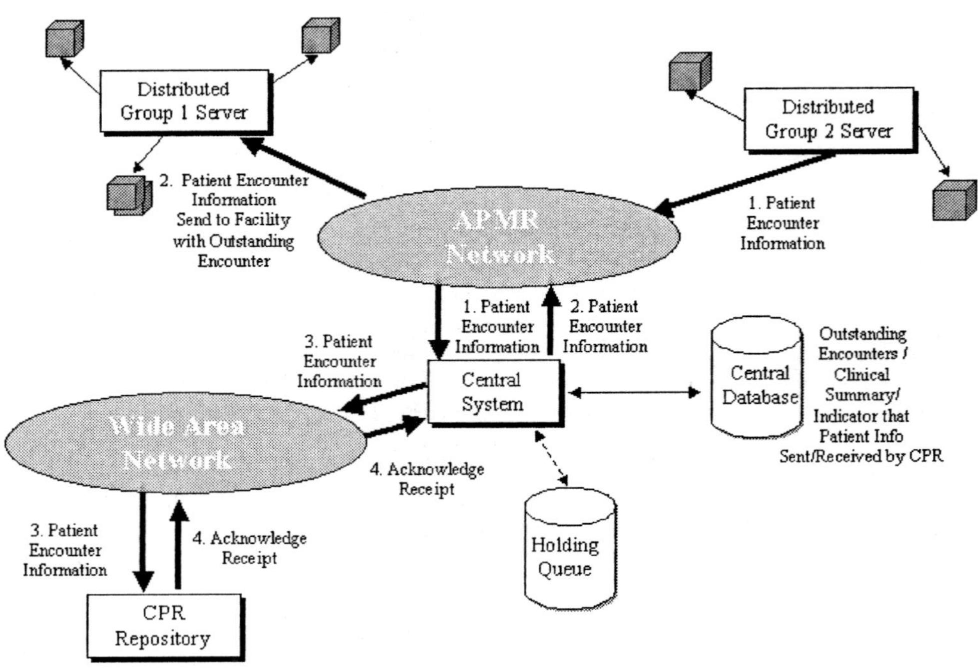

Figure 13.41 Patient encounter information sent to the CPR and distributed facility group systems with outstanding encounters.

A request for a source document outside the HMO Request a copy of a source document outside the current region of the HMO or outside the HMO referenced in an overall clinical summary. (Translation information might be copied over with the source document, especially, when the source document comes from outside the HMO.) See figure 13.42.

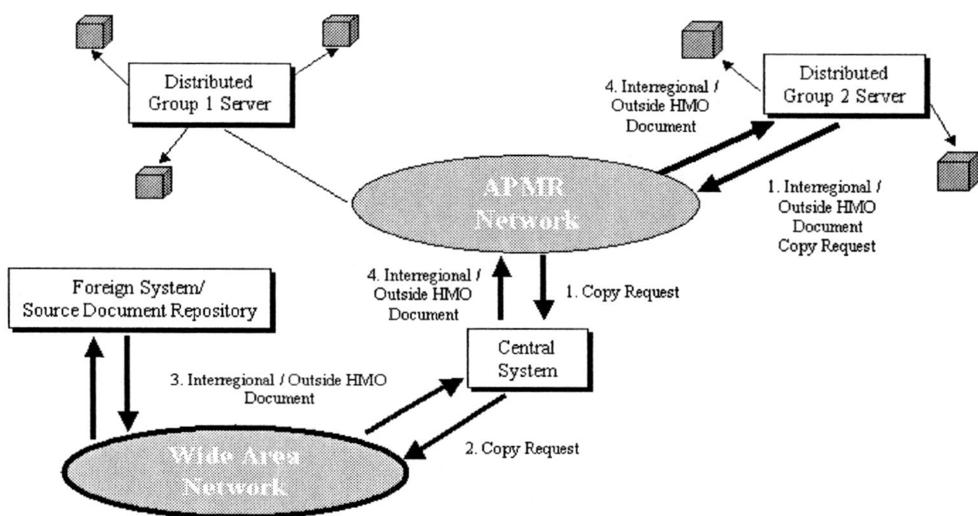

Figure 13.42 A request for a document outside the HMO.

An interface to an outside agency to assign or look up a universal patient identifier for a patient or another identifier such as one for a healthcare provider; interfaces to periodically download and update standard identifiers The CPR repositories and source document repositories, as well as possible clinical summaries, will reference a patient by a universal patient identifier. A universal patient identifier for EDI has been mandated by law. A possible mechanism for looking up and assigning such a Universal Patient Identifier is presented here.

If there is a new patient to the HMO, the HMO should have the ability to do an inquiry through a remote "assigning authority" organization who assigns such identifiers to determine if the patient already has a patient identifier and either return a newly assigned identifier or return the existing identifier (see figure 13.43). Transmitted to the assigning authority will be a set of patient identifiers that together could uniquely identify the patient (e.g., last name, date of birth, sex, mother's maiden name, etc.); although other organizations use the term in a different way, I will refer to this set of identifiers as the "master patient index" for the patient.

Other national identifiers have also been mandated will require similar on-line inquiry and assignment. These include a healthcare organization site identifier or healthcare provider identifier. Other standard data elements not requiring immediate update might be handled by tapes sent from assigning organizations.

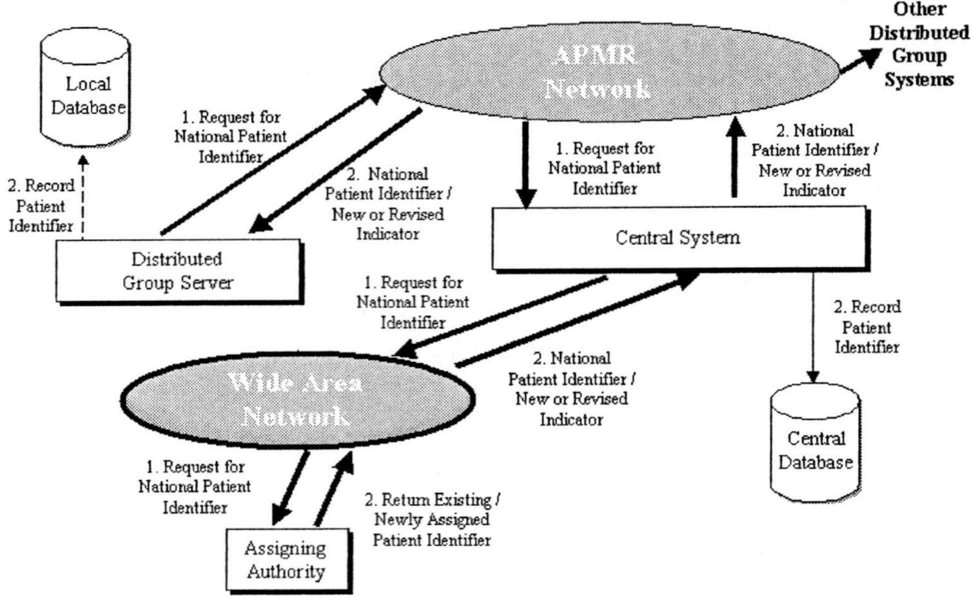

Figure 13.43 National patient identifier request.

Source documents periodically archived to the source document repository As described in earlier chapters, it is proposed that, after an encounter, that source documents and associated encounter information be sent to a source document repository. See figure 13.44. The (new) location of the source document would also be recorded in the CPR repository and central system to be store with the encounter information. The source document could be saved in a queue and possibly resent if acknowledgment of receipt is not received. Agents within the HMO system could schedule and control archiving of source documents. Translation information, to translate from the local to national data standards, would be created during the documentation or ordering step and included with a source document sent to a source document repository.

Clinical practice guidelines from clinical practice guideline repositories New clinical practice guidelines for the HMO could be saved in an HMO clinical practice guideline repository; a clinical practice guideline might later be updated with the previous version also being kept. National Clinical Practice Guideline Repositories might also exist. The automated patient medical record might reference a clinical practice guideline-by-guideline identifier, repository location and document creation date. A guideline could then be later retrieved using these keys.

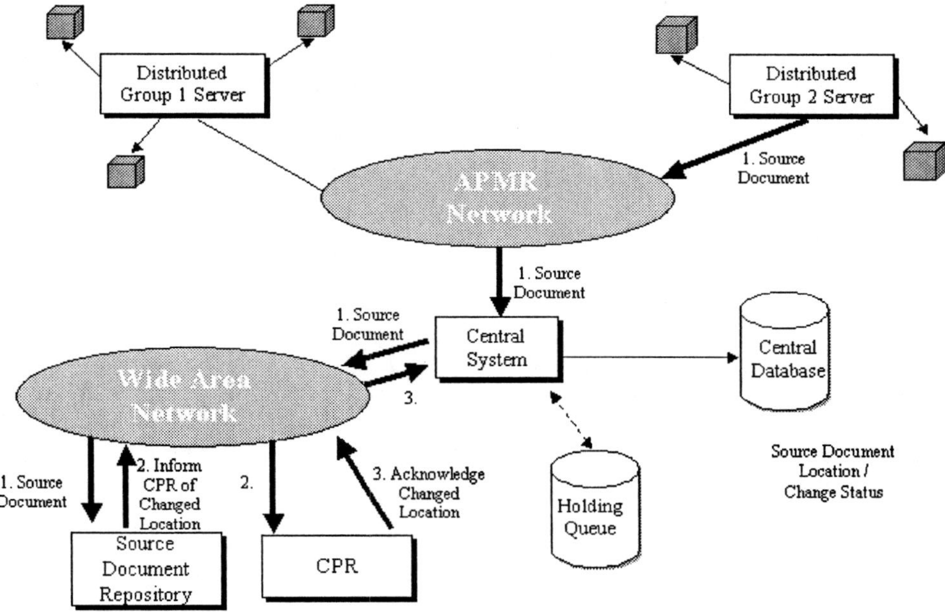

Figure 13.44 Archive source documents.

13.11 NETWORK COMMUNICATION TECHNIQUES: MIDDLEWARE

This section describes network communication techniques that may be useful for implementation of interfaces in the automated patient medical record system. These techniques include the following:

- *message queues*
- *remote procedure calls (RPCs)*
- *object request brokers (ORBs)*
- *mobile code*
- *interface engines*
- *clustering.*

System software that handles such network communication is termed *middleware*. Figure 45 provides an illustration to discuss some of these middleware concepts.

A standard format for network communication within healthcare computer networks is HL7. HL7 is one network layer in a set of seven possible layers. HL7 and other network layers are also explained in this section.

13.11.1 Message Queues

See Figure 13.45(a). Rather than requiring a receiving computer system to be up in order to send a message, a message could be put on a queue on the sending system and sent to a queue on the receiving system when the receiving queue is available. The receiving system could either periodically check the receiving queue for messages or be informed by the queuing system of a message and then pick up the message.

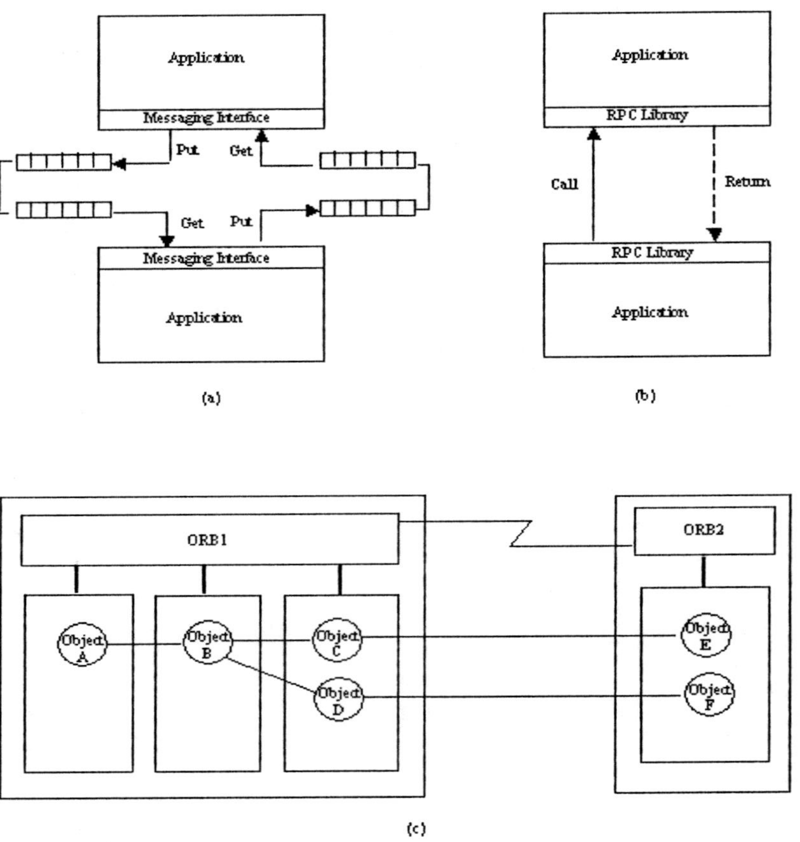

Figure 13.45 Network communication.

Message queues are particularly applicable when it is extremely important that a communication between two systems not be lost. This applies to orders sent from the automated patient medical system to ancillary systems.

The most used message queuing system software is IBM's MQSeries (Gilman and Schreiber 1996).

13.11.2 Remote Procedure Calls (RPCs)

See Figure 13.45(b). A procedure is a block of code that may be initiated (called) from many different programs with return to the next location in the calling program after completion.

Remote procedure calls (RPCs) behave like local procedure calls except that code may be in two or more different computer systems in a network, rather than on one. RPCs insulate the application programmer from the details of the underlying network. RPCs require synchronous connections between systems (i.e., they require the other system to be up).

If the system initiates an on-line query where the information comes from a clinical system other than the automated patient medical record system, an RPC would be the appropriate vehicle. For example, the system might initiate an on-line query via an RPC to receive a provider schedule from the resource scheduling system, pick up patient benefits information, or locate or request patient charts.

13.11.3 Object Request Brokers

See Figure 13.45(c). Object request brokers (ORBs) permit objects to transparently make requests to, receive responses from, other objects, which may be local or remote. The client making the request does not know or care about how this communication happens, how the objects are activated or where the objects are.

The concept of an object is presented in section 13.14.2.

Once a client makes a request for a service on an object, the ORBs are responsible for all the tasks required to find the object implementation in the network, to prepare it to receive the request and to finally transmit the request. It is also responsible for communicating the results to the requester. ORBs can be implemented (transparently) via RPCs or even by messaging queues.

Objects and ORBs would be particularly suited to handle *agents*. Agents apply at different levels (e.g., an agent may apply organizationally, regionally, for a facility, for a particular caregiver). The agents could be stored centrally or locally depending upon where they apply.

Commercial methods for implementing ORBs are CORBA (Bolton 2001) and DCOM (Thai and Oram 1999).

13.11.4 Mobile Code and Mobile Agents

Mobile code is a program traveling on a heterogeneous network from one computer to any other, executing on the destination computer (Thorn 1997). The most well known programming language for such programs is Java.

Such a program is usually run under a *browser* or a *virtual machine interface* with the program being interpreted rather than being run as a compiled program. This allows the same program code to be run on any computer without consideration of the type of processor being used (Intel, IBM 360, Sun Solaris, etc.). Also, the program code does not have to be permanently stored on the computer where it is run, but can be shipped down when needed, alleviating problems of having to copy the program to many different computers when there is a new version of the program. Such "add-on" pieces of software that enhance the capabilities of a browser application are termed *plug-ins*.

The principal disadvantage of mobile code, such as an automated system written in Java, is that the code has to be shipped down over the network from a host computer permanently storing the system to the computer where it is run, with a resulting long wait by the user until the automated system is loaded. Loading of the programs making up the automated system on a local computer is likely to be done each time the user logs on, and thus a user would have to wait a significant period of time after he logs on to his computer before he could run the system.

Another disadvantage of mobile code is that *interpreted* programs generally run much slower than compiled ones.

Rather than using mobile code for an entire automated system, mobile code could be used for execution of small programs. For example, mobile code could be used for implementing an *agent*, producing a "mobile agent". For example, one copy of a regional agent could be stored on the central computer and shipped down when necessary to any local computer when needed to execute the associated business rule on the local computer. In such a case, the time to download the program on the network would not be a factor.

13.11.5 Interface Engine

Interface engines have been developed for the healthcare industry. An interface engine is a middleware product, usually implemented on a dedicated computer, that receives, logs, optionally translates and forwards messages between application systems running on different systems, guaranteeing their delivery even though the receiving system may be temporarily down. Since interface engines are developed for the healthcare industry, a protocol almost universally supported is HL7.

For example, the ADT system might send admissions to the interface engine in HL7 format. The interface engine could send the admission on to both the pharmacy system and clinical laboratory system, also in HL7 format, so these systems could later match up paper orders with the admission and patient's bed location. At the same time, the interface engine might translate the HL7 admission message and put the admission on a database for the automated patient medical record system, so the automated patient medical record system could match up a later order with the admission.

13.11.6 Health Level 7 (HL7) Network Protocol

The International Organization for Standardization (ISO) and other organizations have defined models for network communication. Various *network layers*—a set of data in a network message with a header and trailer for a particular purpose—are used for different purposes, description of hardware, routing, connections, data integrity, etc. Layers are striped off at various points. Layers, except for the innermost layer, consist of header and trailer data. Seven layers are defined by the ISO. Usually, not all layers are used; for example, TCP/IP uses 4 layers.

The innermost layer is called the application layer and provides the data for the software application using the network communication. For health care communications, especially between commercial clinical systems, *Health Level 7 (HL7) application messaging protocol* has been defined.

Version 2.3 of HL7 supports messages in the following categories:

- Patient Administration (e.g., admission, discharge, transfer, register)
- Order Entry (e.g., diet order, supply order, pharmacy order)
- Financial Management (e.g., diagnosis, procedures, guarantor, insurance)
- Observation Reporting (e.g., narrative reporting, waveforms reporting)
- Master Files/Shared Dictionaries (e.g., clinical test directory update, drug formulary update)
- Medical Records/Information Management (tracks documents or entries that have been or will be transcribed)

- Scheduling (e.g., appointment making and inquiry about scheduled activities)
- Patient Referral (identifies referrals from one healthcare practitioner to another)
- Patient Care (tracks acute or chronic medical problems and associated goals, roles, clinical pathways and variances).

An example of a series of HL7 messages between an ordering system and a pharmacy system are as follows:

- a new reoccurring medication order for an inpatient is sent to the pharmacy system from the ordering system
- a filler ID is passed back from the pharmacy system to the ordering system
- a message is later passed back to the ordering system that the medication has been administered
- the ordering system later sends a message to discontinue the order.

13.11.7 Clustering: Fail-over Recovery and Load Balancing

There are two potential problems with network connections: (1) A connection can go down, thus potentially causing the system to fail, and (2) a connection can be overloaded, thus potentially causing the system to slow down. In section 13.12.1 we presented one approach to handling a connection that goes down, a message queue. In this section we explore an approach that handles both connections that go down and those that are overloaded, *clustering*.

A *cluster* is a group of computers working together to share resources or workload. Figure 12.22 in the previous chapter shows an example of clusters and the use of clustering. A cluster enables *fail-over recovery*, meaning that when the primary computer (server) goes down, a backup computer (server) automatically takes over. A cluster enables *load balancing*, distributing processing and communications activity evenly among computers in a cluster so no computer is overloaded. Clusters also allow one computer to be brought down, with the other computers taking over the load of that computer that is brought down.

Clustering should be used anywhere where there is the possibility of a *single point (of) failure* (i.e., where there is a network connection that, if it went down, would cause the system to fail in some way), and where it is critical that the system does not fail.

As examples, clustering applies to web servers and to interface engines, with information being sent to a secondary web server to handle a web connection when the primary web server goes down, or to a secondary interface engine to handle an HL7 connection when the primary interface engine goes down.

Clustering could apply to pharmacy systems receiving medication orders. If a pharmacy system went down, the order could automatically be sent to a different pharmacy system to fill the medication order.

13.12 COMPONENT ADAPTABILITY

Component adaptability is use of various strategies to procure, develop or structure a system or component of a system so that the system or component can more easily be replaced in the future by an improved system or component. These strategies include the following: (1) following an open architecture for software and hardware and following healthcare data processing standards so an improved system that follows the same standards can replace the previous system using those standards; (2) using a system that is independent from other systems (e.g., an e-mail system that can be replaced by another independent e-mail system); (3) designing a component of a system—say Component A, a user interface—such that it shares data with the remainder of the system but is otherwise independent from the rest of the system, thus allowing Component A to be replaced by Component B, a different user interface, if the replacing component (Component B) produces the same data as Component A; and (4) using periodically renewable, instead of very long term, contracts for vendor systems, thus not being monetarily forced to use a vendor system that should be replaced.

For example, the use of HL7 as a healthcare network communication standard opens up the possibility of having replaceable systems and supports component adaptability—see figure 13.46. If each of the clinical systems connected to the automated patient medical record system uses a standardized HL7 connection with the automated patient medical record system with very specific standards for the type of system (clinical laboratory system, ADT system, resource scheduling system, etc.), then replacing such a system with an improved one could "potentially" be as simple as plugging another one in that uses the same protocols. Such a level of clinical system inoperability does not yet exist.

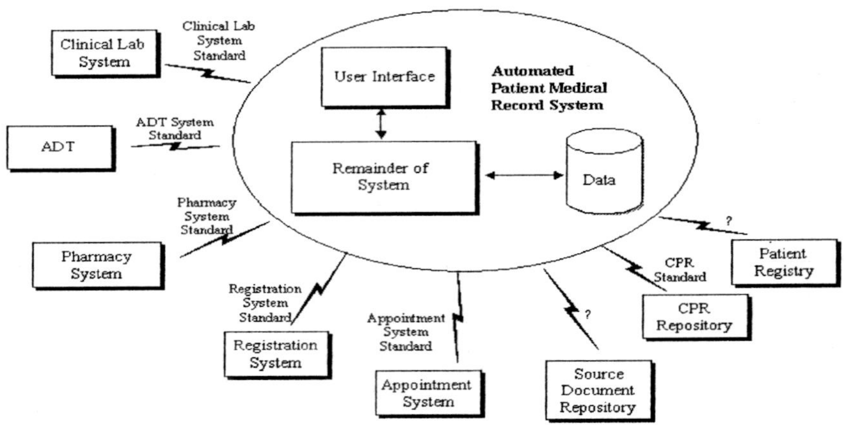

Figure 13.46 Component adaptability.

Component adaptability with the use of HL7 or other standards can also apply to the automated patient medical record system in its communication with the CPR repository, source document repository and patient registry. As long as automated patient medical record system follows strict standards with respect to its communication with the CPR repository, source document repository and patient registry, the automated patient medical record system itself can potentially be replaced by another equivalent system (although this might be traumatic for the healthcare organization).

The automated patient medical record system can itself be viewed as multiple separate systems. In particular, as mentioned in chapter 12, the user interface can be considered to be a separate system from other parts of the automated patient medical record system, such as from its data components and communication with other clinical systems and with the CPR and source document repositories and patient registry. The user interface can thus potentially be changed without effecting the underlying automated patient medical record system--as long as a new user interface provides the exact same data as before, a new user interface can easily replace the new. For example, one user interface could be based upon selection from lists while a replacement one might require more textual input. A user interface could be changed to support caregiver workflows in a different fashion without change to the underlying system. (Because user interfaces should be viewed as being "replaceable", they should not be the primary reason for selecting one automated patient medical record system over another.)

13.13 DATABASE DESIGN

Databases are a way of structuring and storing data, including patient lists, encounters, documents, patient demographics and caregiver information. For example, information in the automated patient medical record system described in section 13.8 can be stored on the automated patient medical record system's databases. Databases connected with mainframes, central databases, are usually on one platform (i.e., one computer), while *distributed databases* are usually on many.

Most databases today, whether centralized or distributed, are *relational databases*, with a paradigm of *tables*, where there may be a patient table, a patient encounter table, etc. See figure 13.47. (There are other types of databases that are stored in formats other than table structures, but these are only common on older mainframe systems, so this section will address the table paradigm only.)

Each *row* in a table is an *instance* in the table; for example there be a row for each patient in the patient table, a row for each patient encounter in the patient encounter table and a row for each diagnosis during a particular patient encounter in a patient encounter diagnosis table. Each instance is composed of *data elements*; for example, a patient table instance may be composed of data elements of patient identifier, patient first name, patient last name, etc. Because each data element in the same location in the rows is the same time of data element (e.g., a last name), then those same type data element in the successive rows can be viewed as a *column* of the table. A set of data elements in a row in combination are usually set up with this set of data elements uniquely distinguishing one instance from another; for example the patient identifier uniquely distinguishes one patient from another; this unique set of data elements is termed a *primary key* in the table. In distributed databases, these tables (or entities) could be stored on different platforms.

Primary keys allow a particular instance of a table (i.e., a particular row) to be retrieved based upon the key, and allow consecutive retrieval in an identified order. Relational databases also allow retrieval based upon any other set of data elements in a table, some of these combinations of data elements can be specifically identified via *indexes*, allowing the database system to structure a table for quicker retrieval based upon that index.

A language that allows an application programmer to create a table, add a row to a table, select a row for a table and/or select data elements from a table, is called *Structured Query Language (SQL)*. Some standard type SQL statements are SELECT (to select data), UPDATE (to change data), INSERT (to add rows) and DELETE (to delete rows).

For example, a SELECT statement might be "SELECT First_Name, Last_Name FROM Patient WHERE Patient_Identifier = '118386390';", where First_Name and Last_Name are data elements (columns) within a Patient table and Patient_Identifier is another data element (column). The row with the Patient_Identifier '118386390' would be selected and First_Name and Last_Name would be returned.

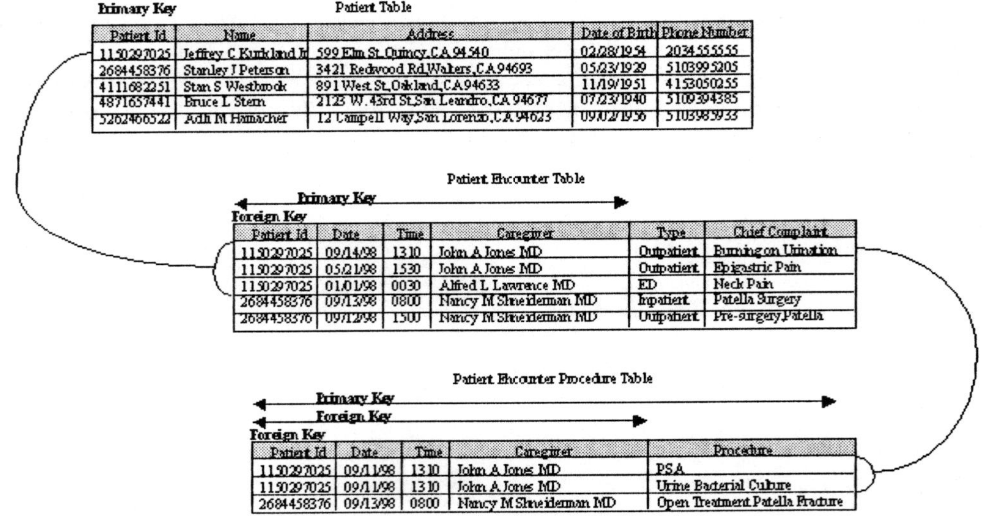

Primary Key

Patient Table

Patient Id	Name	Address	Date of Birth	Phone Number
1150297025	Jeffrey C Kirkland Jr	599 Elm St, Quincy, CA 94540	02/28/1954	2034555555
2684458376	Stanley J Peterson	3421 Redwood Rd, Walters, CA 94693	05/23/1929	5103995205
4111682251	Stan S Westbrook	891 West St, Oakland, CA 94633	11/19/1951	4153050255
4871657441	Bruce L Stern	2123 W. 43rd St, San Leandro, CA 94677	07/23/1940	5109394385
5262466522	Adh M Hamacher	12 Campell Way, San Lorenzo, CA 94623	09/02/1956	5103985933

Patient Encounter Table

Primary Key

Foreign Key

Patient Id	Date	Time	Caregiver	Type	Chief Complaint
1150297025	09/14/98	1310	John A Jones MD	Outpatient	Burning on Urination
1150297025	05/21/98	1530	John A Jones MD	Outpatient	Epigastric Pain
1150297025	01/01/98	0030	Alfred L Lawrence MD	ED	Neck Pain
2684458376	09/13/98	0800	Nancy M Shneiderman MD	Inpatient	Patella Surgery
2684458376	09/12/98	1500	Nancy M Shneiderman MD	Outpatient	Pre-surgery Patella

Patient Encounter Procedure Table

Primary Key

Foreign Key

Foreign Key

Patient Id	Date	Time	Caregiver	Procedure
1150297025	09/11/98	1310	John A Jones MD	PSA
1150297025	09/11/98	1310	John A Jones MD	Urine Bacterial Culture
2684458376	09/13/98	0800	Nancy M Shneiderman MD	Open Treatment Patella Fracture

Figure 13.47 Simplified database tables.

Based upon parameters, SELECT statements could return entire tables if the condition selects multiple rows. Actually, this is the approach that relational databases used to create "virtual tables" from one or more tables. These "virtual tables" are called *views*. A common reason for creating views is to hide from a user information the user is not allowed to view.

Different tables of the database may have *relationships* with each other. Through a process to help create these tables called *data modeling*, these relationships can be expressed by *entity-relationship (E-R) diagrams*—see section 13.8. *Entities* are tangible objects, such as organizations, caregivers, patients, charts, encounters, procedures, etc. In general, each entity corresponds to a table. For example, there might be a relationship between a "patient encounter" entity and a "encounter procedure" entity of "occurs during". Thus the relationship addresses all encounter procedures occurring during the patient encounter. To express this relationship, the encounter procedure entity (or table) would likely contain the patient encounter primary key as a data element. When a primary key of a table instance is stored in an instance in another table, this key value is termed a *foreign key*; for example, the patient key that is stored in an patient encounter table instance and the patient encounter key that is stored in an encounter procedure instance are foreign keys (see figure 13.47 again).

Now with one table referencing another table, there are potential problems in keeping the two tables in synch. For example, if the encounter is deleted and the associated encounter procedures are not deleted, then the encounter procedures are referencing an encounter that no longer exists. *Referential integrity* is a rule that states that every foreign key value in one table must either match a primary key value in some other table, or it must be null.

Some database systems allow *stored procedures*, essentially processing code, to be stored along with the data in a database. Such stored procedures can be *triggered* based upon a set of rules. For example a stored procedure could be automatically executed when an "encounter" instance is deleted in order to delete all referenced instances in the "encounter procedure" table first.

Applications updating databases are usually written in terms of *transactions* where each transaction either *commits* database updates or *backs* them *out*, in either case leaving the database in a consistent state. This technique is called a *two-phase commit.*

The main purpose of a two-phase commit is to stop other applications that are running on other workstations from writing on the same part of data your application is writing to, and thus creating garbled or inconsistent data. A part of the two-phase commit process, but of more general use, is to allow an application to *lock* parts of a database (e.g., several tables) for a time period, disallowing other applications from updating those parts of the database until the application issues an *unlock*.

In order to ensure the stability of tables, a technique called *normalization* can be used. Normalization is a procedure for placing data elements in tables in databases according to a set of dependency rules so as to create stable data structures that minimize *data redundancy* (duplicated data) and maximize *data independence* (changing data or data relationships within the database without having to make major changes to software that use the database). Normalization includes doing the following:

- *First Normal Form (Eliminate Repeating Elements):* Elements in a table that repeat for each row should be moved to a separate table with one repeated item per row of the new table. For example, the encounter procedures should be a separate table and should not be made part of the patient encounter table, as the one table approach requires that the designer assign a maximum for the number of encounter procedures, creating for a badly structured table.
- *Second Normal Form (Eliminate Redundant Data)*: Data in a table that is not directly related to the primary key should be moved to another table. For example, a department name and department number in a physician table should not both be in the physician table; these should, instead, be stored non-redundantly in a department table.
- *Third Normal Form (Eliminate Many to Many Relationships)*: Separate tables should be created to get rid of many to many relationships in E-R diagrams. This enables relationships to have more definite meanings.

There are 5 accepted normal forms, but the above 3 are the ones most commonly followed.

Although normalization removes some forms of data redundancy, sometimes *data redundancy* is necessary for efficiency reasons, especially in a distributed database system. For example, the clinical laboratory system directory of tests (a type of master file) might exist in the clinical laboratory system, and might be *replicated* in the automated patient medical record system so clinical laboratory systems orders could be made in the automated system. Such replicated parts of the database usually must necessarily consist of fairly static information; such information might, for example, only be updated nightly in *batch*, and thus potentially be somewhat out of date for a while.

Data integrity is another desirable characteristic of databases. Every table, row and data element within a table must be used precisely for what it was intended. For example, an appointment table must not be used to store a visit, as these are two different things. In order to insure later integrity of information, a data element to store the height of an object must not be used to store the width of the object, even though both may use the same units of measurements. To insure this *data integrity*, a *data dictionary* is often created to describe the structure and use of each table, each row, and each data element, and describe the relationship between tables identical to corresponding relationships in E-R diagrams.

A data dictionary contains *meta-data*, data about data. For example, a data dictionary description of a prescription (medicine order) table might include the following meta-data for each row and data element (only selected information is shown):

- patient = Unique Healthcare Identifier (key field)
- date = date of prescription (key field, in form MMDDYYYY, where MM is numeric month, DD is day of month and YYYY is the year)
- time = time of the prescription (key field, format: 999999 where 999999 is military time including hours, minutes and seconds with values from 000000 to 235959)
- priority = urgency of prescription (values: "STAT", "routine", "rush")Master Files/Shared Dictionaries (e.g., clinical test directory update, drug formulary update)
- encounter date = date of encounter when prescription was made
- encounter time = time of encounter when prescription was made
- prescriber = Unique Physician Identifier Number identifying the clinician ordering the medication
- drug name = brand or generic name of the drug and manufacturer
- dosage = quantity, units
- route = route of drug
- schedule = times per day.

Database design in the system analysis step involves database analysts working with system analysts (who represent the automated systems which will use database), and domain experts and domain analysts (who understand the business—e.g., the healthcare business—and thus understand the meaning of the data in the database); the database analyst serves as a facilitator to gather information to design the database. Database design consists of *logical database design* and *physical database design*. Logical database design identifies sets of data (called "tables", "records" or "entities") making up the database, the format of data elements making up each entity, and the relationships between the entities. A way of defining sets of data (called "entities") and relationships between these entities are entity-relationship (E-R) diagrams, as previously discussed in section 13.8. A standard way of defining the data elements making up each entity (or table) are data dictionaries. *Physical database design* uses the logical design information to map the data in the database to physical files. The actual database is created in the implementation step.

Database administration is an important organizational duty during the design and after the implementation of the database. Database administration are the tasks necessary to insure data integrity including referential integrity, non-redundancy of data, immediate up-to-dateness of data, integrity of the meaning of data as recorded in data dictionaries, security, and database software installation and upgrades.

A word about our example tables in figure 13.47: The tables are unrealistic in that unique alphanumeric identifiers would probably be kept for caregivers (e.g., NPI identifier), rather than names that may occur in many different forms; for example, when names are used, "Jonathon" might be stored one place for the first name, "John" in another place and an initial in another place. And these tables are also unrealistic in that a CPT or other definitive procedure code is likely to be stored for a procedure, rather than a vague textual procedure description.

This section presents the briefest of introductions to database systems. There are many comprehensive books on databases, such as (Martin and Leben 1998).

13.14 SOFTWARE DESIGN

Programs are instructions coded in a computer language. Another term for a program or programs is *software*. A *computer language* is the vocabulary and syntax of a set of symbols that may be used to tell a computer what it is to do. The computer language can be used to write programs than can be *compiled:* converted to sets of on and off switches that are in a machine language that a computer could use to execute the program.

The previous parts of this chapter, in essence, dealt with establishing an infrastructure for the programs constituting the application. For example, the programs constituting the automated patient medical record system would use the databases defined in this chapter, would implement the interfaces defined in this chapter, would requires coding of the agents defined in this chapter, and would implement the staging and security techniques in this chapter.

Programs are created for the central system, local system servers and local system workstations. If there are patient registries, CPR repositories and source document repositories, there is additional code and programs for these.

The central system must keep a complete clinical summary for all patients in the HMO and pass the clinical summary down to a local system when there will be an encounter to occur at a facility associated with the local system. The central system is responsible for handling communication with the outside world, including patient registries, CPR repositories, source document repositories. It is responsible for communication with ordering systems, sending results and alerts to the local system of the order.

The local system must handle the user interface described in Chapter 12, alerts to a caregiver, and downloading of clinical summary information and document locations after an encounter; it handles communication with local clinical systems. For the user interface in Chapter 12, there are functions for each of the icons shown in figure 12.6 and described in section 12.2.2 (functions for patient lists, patient identification, clinical summaries, patient chart, searching, cases, encounter synopses, ordering, documentation, appointment making, e-mail and messaging, medical references, recording the position, making a note, providing help to the user) and an overall function for the main program that displays the icons and controls menus and over parts of the main screen, in essence, tying all the other functions together.

There are a number of different software design strategies available for defining the necessary programs in each system. There are quite a few books on software design, including (Sommerville 2000). Two major categories of software design are *structured design* and *object-oriented design*.

13.14.1 Structured Design

Structured design is a way of designing an application system by breaking the system's program code into *subsystems*, by breaking subsystems into *functions*, by identifying *programs* making up the functions, and identifying *routines* used by the total of programs and subprograms. A *subsystem* is a set of *functions* that are logically grouped together, with the subsystems, together, making up the system. A *function* is the smallest discrete, complete set of code of an automated system that can be initiated by the user and run to completion to produce a single purpose set of results (e.g., a stand-alone function to look up patient demographical information about a patient, a function to issue an order for medication, or a function to make an appointment for a patient). *Programs* are logical combinations of code specific to the subsystem functionality. *Routines* are general-purpose code that may be used in many different programs, generally including the passing of data via input and output parameters associated with a routine name.

For example, for the automated patient medical system, there might be subsystems that include a Patient Lists, a Patient Identification, Patient Chart, Searching, Ordering and Documentation subsystem, among others. For the Patient Identification subsystem, there might be two functions, one to search for the patient's identifier based upon patient characteristics (e.g., last name and birth date), and another to display patient demographics information, such as full name, sex, birth date, phone numbers, address, based upon the patient identifier. For each function, there might be one or more programs providing the code for each function. Routines to support the Patient Identification subsystem and its functions might include various routines, for example, one to get the patient identifier based upon the characteristics, one to retrieve patient demographics and patient benefits based upon the patient identifier, and one to do a Soundex search for a patient identifier for patients whose names sound like an entered name. For example, a routine with parameters, "Get-Patient-Name (Patient-Identifier, Patient-Name) " with input parameter of "Patient-Identifier", and output parameter "Patient-Name" might return the patient's name given the patient's identifier. In the past, such routines were put together into "subroutine libraries", groups of related routines.

Real-time systems are often built using *on-line transaction processing (OLTP)* systems. A module within an OLTP system is called a *transaction.* Structured design also applies to OLTP systems. In real-time systems, there are many users competing for the same databases. A *transaction* is code that makes logical updates to databases, taking the databases from one consistent state to another; in other words, if the transaction for some reason fails to complete, then the databases are backed out to the previous state.

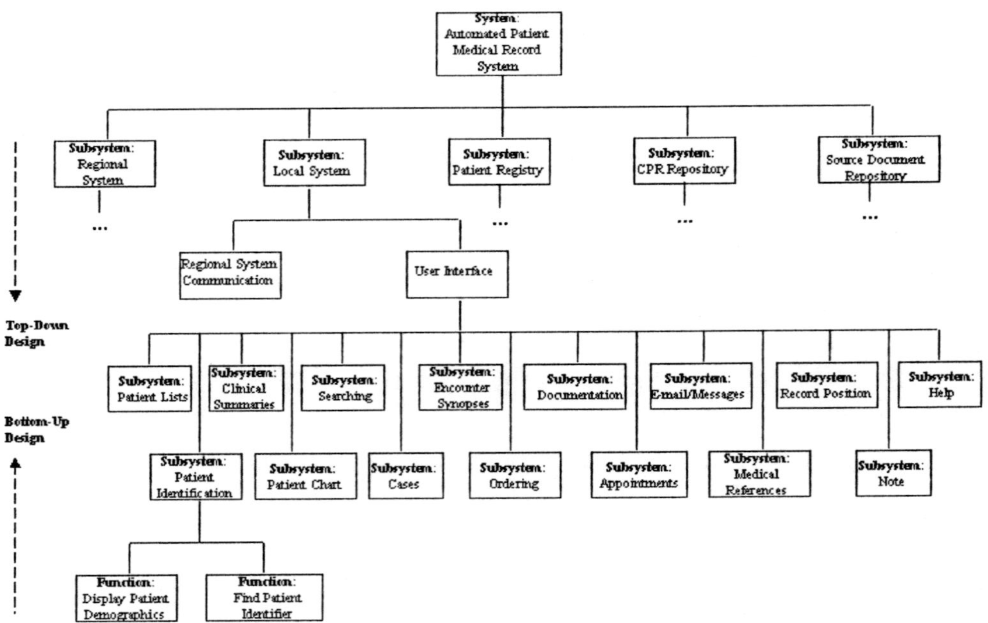

Figure 13.48 Structure chart.

A *structure chart* might be set up to identify the system, show the breakup of the system into subsystems, show the breakup of subsystems into programs, and identify routines. See figure

13.48 for a structure chart for the automated patient medical record system. For each program and routine, *program design language (PDL)* to describe in structured English what the program or routine does could be later used to create the program or routine in a programming language.

Defining the high level modules first is called top-down design; modules not yet defined in terms of code or PDL can be replaced with a place-holder that performs nothing or much less than the full function of the module, called a "stub". Bottom-up design is defining low-level modules first and then combining them together into higher-level modules.

13.14.2 Object-Oriented Design

Object-oriented design is a way of designing an application system by breaking the system program code into objects. Objects are abstract or real-world entities. Examples of objects in the automated patient medical record system are patient, chart, order, appointment, and e-mail. Examples of objects appearing in windows are windows, bitmaps, drop-down menus; message and dialog boxes, group boxes, static text boxes, scroll bars, input fields, single-selection lists, radio buttons, check boxes, and tabbed structures.

An *object class* can be created for an object, that

- defines *data* associated with the object
- defines routines called *methods* associated with the objects
- defines what data within the object class is available to programmers using the object class (usually all data is hidden and methods are used to provide the data)
- defines what methods are available to programmers using the object class and which are not.

For example, figure 13.49 shows an object class for a mail message. The data is shown at the top of the object class, being marked "private" meaning that the data is not available for retrieval or setting by programmers using the class. Methods available to outside programmer use are "Mail Message", "Send Message", "Forward Message" and "Delete Message". The "Format Message" method is "private" and not available to outside programmers. Hiding data and methods within the object class from outside programmers is called *encapsulation,* which is an example of the more general concept of *information hiding.*

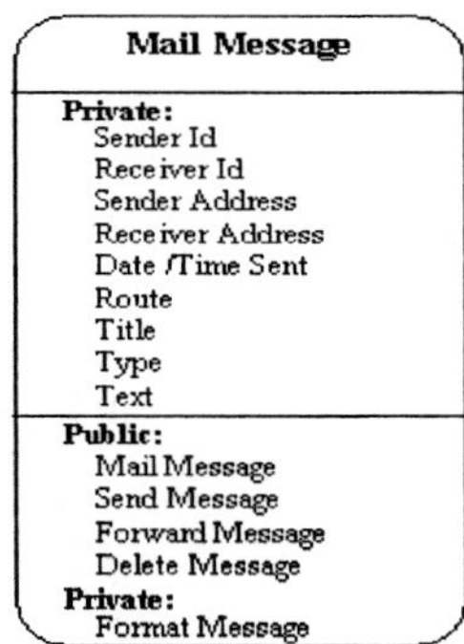

Figure 13.49 Example (object) class.

A programmer using the object class can create an *instance* of the "Mail Message" class, causing the "Mail Message" routine to be executed, probably setting up a new mail message with the programmer passing the text, sender, receiver and other information. Use of the "Send Message" for the instance could send the message off to the receiver.

The automated patient medical record system programs can be defined through use of objects; however, a more common use of object-oriented design is to create object libraries that can be used in place of subroutine libraries. For example in the last section it was mentioned that a set of routines all connected with handling patient information could be combined into a "subroutine library". These routines can be more elegantly combined into a "patient" object, together with other objects in an object library.

An important concept for objects and object classes is *inheritance*. One object class can be inherited from another. For example, figure 13.50 shows the object "inpatient" and "outpatient" being inherited from the object class "patient". When an instance of "outpatient" is created or an instance of "inpatient" is created, then an instance of "patient" will be automatically created. Any public method within the object class "patient" will be available through the object class "outpatient" or "inpatient"; thus, any method which applies to both outpatients and inpatients can be defined once for "patient".

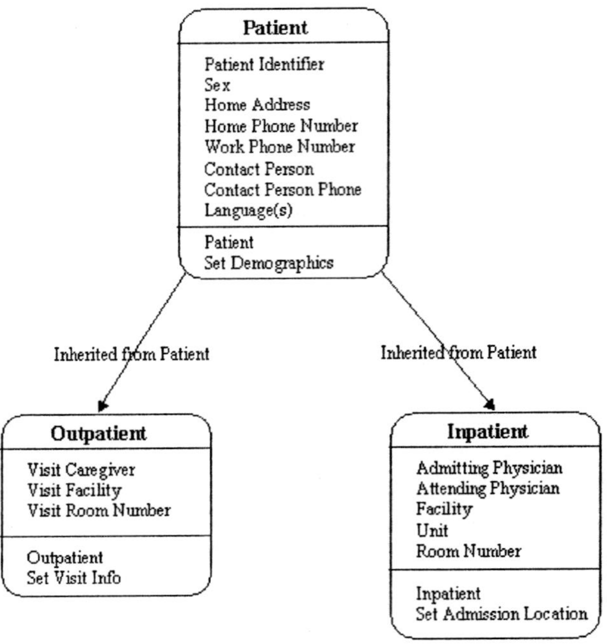

Figure 13.50 Inheritance.

The object class from which other object classes inherit characteristics (e.g., patient) could be identified as an object class which the outside programmer cannot use to create an instance. Such a class is referred to as an *abstract data type*. An abstract data type allows the same data and methods to be used by all inherited objects.

13.14.3 Aspect-Oriented Design

Object-oriented design requires that methods be associated with objects. This gets in the way of defining general-purpose "methods" that cross the boundaries of many objects, applications or computer systems.

A new programming paradigm is *aspect-oriented programming* (Miller 2001). In aspect-oriented programming parlance, "methods" are referred to as *units* and units providing this "crosscutting modularity" are called *aspects*.

Aspects are useful in providing some capabilities of use by agents, which, as we pointed out in a previous section, can cross applications or computer systems:

- logging
- error and failure recovery
- distribution of information among computers
- security strategies
- resource sharing
- synchronization policies.

Aspects can be used to implement what one article (Filman et al. 2002) calls the *-ilities*:

- reliability
- availability
- responsiveness
- performance
- security
- manageability.

13.14.4 Use of Techniques in Combination

Structured design, breaking the system into subsystems and modules, can be used in combination with creation of object libraries, which can substitute for subroutine libraries. Aspects can be used in place of objects when there is functionality that crosses subsystems.

Key Terms

abstract data type
access controls
access point
administrative procedures
ADT system
agent
aggregation
anatomic pathology
ancillary system
anonymous order
application database
appointment
appointment system
aspect
aspect-oriented programming
association
auditing
authentication
authorization
back out
backup
biometrics
black box view
bookmark*
Caregiver-defined Patient List
chain of trust
ciphertext
clinical data repository (CDR)
clinical guidelines repository
clinical laboratory
clinical laboratory test directory
clinical system
clustering
component adaptability
confidentiality
consultation
Consultation Request List
corporate database
credentialing system
data dictionary
electronic signature
emergency department (ED) visit
encapsulation
encounter
encounter system
enterprise architecture,
entities
entity-relationship (E-R) diagrams
fail-over recovery
granting permission
Health Insurance Portability and Accountability Act of 1996 (HIPAA)
Health Level 7 (HL7) application messaging
protocol
identity verification
IEEE's 802.11b
index
information hiding
inheritance
inpatient stay
instance
interface
interface engines
interpreted
load balancing
local order profile
lock
logical database design
logon group
master file
message queue
meta-data
methods
middleware
minimal disclosure necessary
mobile code
multiplicity
need to know
physical database design
physical safeguards
pre-admit
pre-fetching
primary key
program design language (PDL)
programs
protected health information
public-key infrastructure (PKI)
radiology
recovery procedures
referential integrity
registration system
relational database
relationships
remote access
remote consultation
remote order profile
remote procedure calls (RPCs)
requesting permission
resource
results
routine
row
Second Normal Form (Eliminate Redundant Data)
single point (of) failure
smart card
software
staging
stored procedure
structure chart
structured design
Structured Query Language (SQL)
subsystem
surgery
Surgery List
system architecture
system analysis

data element
data independence
data integrity
data modeling
data redundancy
data warehouse
database administration
database
DEA (Drug Enforcement Agency) number
decrypted
de-identification
disclosure accounting
distributed databases
distributed system
DME formulary
First Normal Form (Eliminate Repeating Elements)
function
generalization
drug compendium
durable medical equipment (DME)
network layer
nonrepudiation.
normalization
Nurse Assignment Lists
object request brokers (ORBs)
object-oriented design
observation visit
on-line analytic processing (OLAP) systems
on-line transaction processing (OLTP) systems
order profiles
order statuses
outpatient visit
Patient Panel
Performance and Scalability Plan
pharmacy
phone call encounter
Phone Call List
table
terminal profile
Third Normal Form (Eliminate Many to Many Relationships)
transaction
triggered
two-phase commit
unit
unlock
user profile
view
virtual system
visibility
WEP (Wired Equivalent Privacy)
white box view
WLAN Authentication and Privacy Infrastructure (WAPI)
Work List

Study Questions

1. For a single automated system, what is system analysis? What parts of a system is a system analyst responsible for designing? What else is system analysis?
2. What part of designing a watch is system analysis most like? In order to design that part of a watch, what must the designer know? What is a black box view? What is a white box view?
3. Name the two major types of clinical systems to which the automated patient medical record system must be interfaced. Give examples of each. In order to run these systems, what master file information must be loaded? What is a master file?
4. This book proposes that there be a clinical practice guideline repository and there be a patient identifier assigning authority. What would these do? What must happen before these could become realities?
5. What are interfaces?
6. How does a two-phase commit and backing up data protect against data corruption in databases?
7. What is staging? What does this do?
8. Creating an E-R diagram is doing what? What do the two letters stand for, and what are these? What is data modeling? Is data modeling a part of logical database design or physical database design? What are each of
13. How do WEP and WLAN protect security of wireless communications? What are access points and how does setting access points correctly protect the security of wireless communications?
14. What are the following network communication techniques: message queues, remote procedure calls (RPCs), object request brokers (ORBs), mobile code, interface engines, clustering. What are network layers?—What is HL7 and what is the network layer for it?
15. Component adaptability allows one component of a system to be replaced by a similar (and better) component. Give an example of component adaptability in the automated patient medical record system and what measures enhance component adaptability.
16. The principal components of relational databases are tables. Name the components of tables. What are views? What are distributed databases? What would happen if a table is deleted and another table has data elements with the key of that table?—What are these types of keys called? Why would one of the keys shown in the tables in figure 13.47 never occur?—Why?
17. What is normalization? A table of dogs has dog

these? Does a system analyst normally participate in both logical and physical database design?—Who participates in both? Name some types of relationships. Draw an example E-R diagram and explain. When logical design is complete, what structure is often used to save the metadata for entities?—What is metadata? In the book text example of this structure, what is missing?

9. What are operational databases and OLTP? What are data warehouses and OLAP? What are two types of operational databases? Name two types of data warehouses and give examples of each might be used. Is setting up relationships ahead of time more important for operational databases or data warehouses?

10 What are resources? What are patient lists and some possible characteristics of patient lists? An agent?

11 Name some technical aspects of security. Name some administrative aspects of security. What is HIPAA?

12 What is protected health information? How does this relate to the concepts of need to know, minimal disclosure necessary, and de-identification? What is disclosure accounting?

name, favorite food 1, favorite food 2, and favorite food 3—Why is this bad and what normal form does it violate? A table of physicians for each physician has the physician's department number and department name—What normal form does it violate and how do you correct it? Each member "may go to many" medical centers and each medical center "may have many" members who go to that medical center—What normal form does this violate?

18. What is a program? What is another term for a program or programs? What is the term for the hardware to run programs?

19. What are two main ways of designing software? What is the difference between a routine and method. What is the purpose of a structure chart? What is the purpose of an object? How can structured design and object-oriented design be used together?—Why are methods within objects better than libraries of routines (called "subroutine libraries")?

20. How does aspect-oriented design differ from object-oriented design?

CHAPTER 14

Breaking the Project Into Phases

CHAPTER OUTLINE

14.1 PROJECT CONTEXT: PROJECT PLAN BREAKING THE PROJECT INTO SUBPROJECTS, OR PHASES

A large-scale complex project (such as improvement of patient care through automation of the patient medical record) involves completing many interrelated subprojects or *phases*. The phases for the project are determined in the project plan step in the overall project design phase, and may be changed any time the overall project design phase is redone. See figure 14.1, previously shown in figure 2.8.

From the phases, a project plan for the project is developed by ordering the phases in a network, determining how they overlap in time in their execution. The ordering of phases is dependent both upon technical and managerial considerations, with those phases dealing with infrastructure being done early on in the project—see section 14.4. Each phase could then be treated like a project, being assigned a phase project manager, with the identification of all the tasks in the phase project plan. The results of this process are thus an overall project plan scheduling phases, and project plans for each of the phases, each scheduling tasks for the phase.

For tasks and then phases, time, costs, resources, and performance parameters are assigned based upon project constraints from management. Obstacles to the completion of the project (risks) are identified, and contingency plans may be developed for obstacles should they occur.

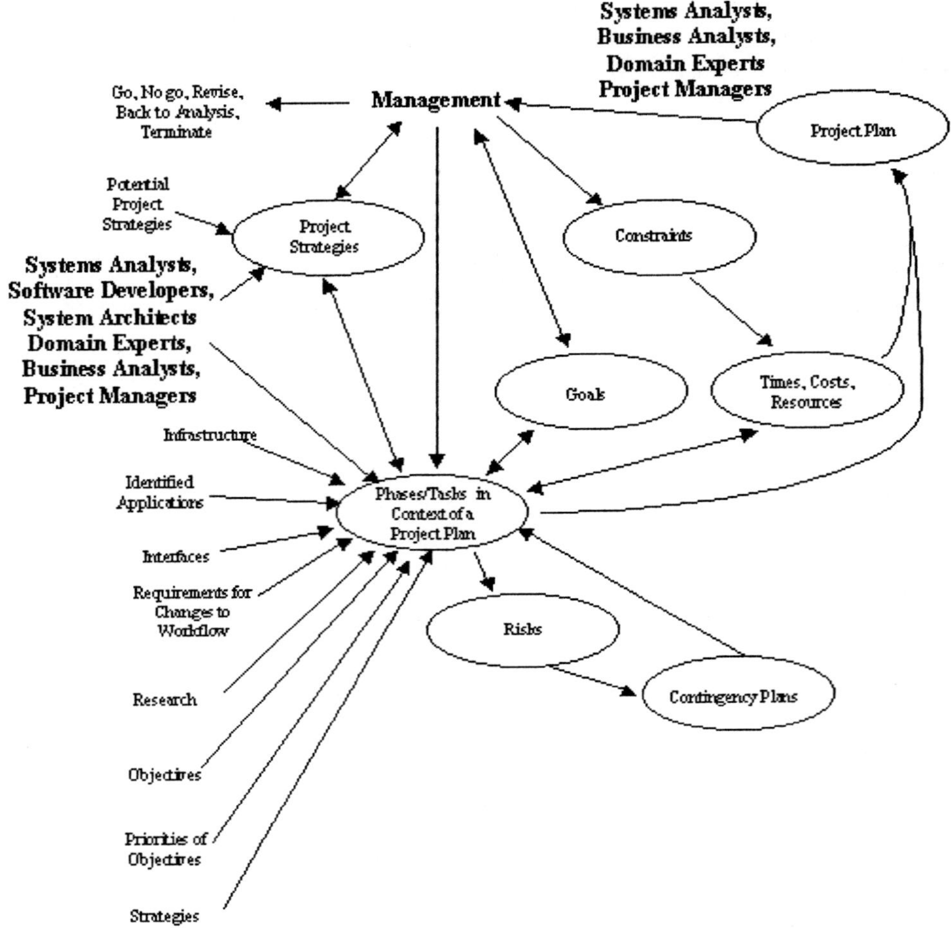

Figure 14.1 Project plan step: breaking the project into phases or a phase into tasks.

At the end of the project plan step, the overall project plan and various phase project plans will have been determined in detail, including the estimated costs of each task and each phase; because of this, at the end of the project plan step, upper management will have better information on the true costs of the entire project and of each phase than in the evaluation step where the initial estimation of costs was done and the initial determination to go ahead with the project was done. At this point, upper management can determine again, based upon costs, whether to go ahead with the project or not, or whether to pare down the project.

The success of the project from management's point of view is that the project meets certain project objectives. Because these objectives are normally not all reached until the end of the project, it is useful to develop goals that lead to the objectives (e.g., for 50% of patient visits in the HMO, the medical record will be automated by end of the third year.) The project plan can be used to determine the best points in the project to measure these goals to measure the progress of the project.

Note that in many project management books, the term *program* is used in place of what this book calls a *project*, and the term *project* is used in place of what this book calls a *phase*. When used in this sense, *program* has the more specific meaning: loosely coupled but tightly aligned sets of projects aimed to deliver the benefits of part of a business plan or strategy. For example, the NASA space program includes many projects, such as the International Space Station project and the project to send the rover Opportunity and rover Spirit to Mars.

14.2 PROJECT MANAGEMENT

Project management is "a systems approach to development and implementation of a defined set of inter-related products with the development and implementation described by a project plan breaking the development and implementation into tasks stated in terms of *time*, *costs*, *resources*, and performance parameters" (Gouse 1988). A *project plan* is "a description of events to come" (Wysocki and McGary 2003). The end product of the project is a change to the organization that must work together with all the other parts of the organization. *Resources* to do a project may include workers, equipment and rooms.

Project management involves a project manager. Through the process of planning, organizing, directing, controlling and monitoring, the project manager coordinates the application of resources to the project with the objective of completing tasks within the project plan, with the final task being the implementation of the project.

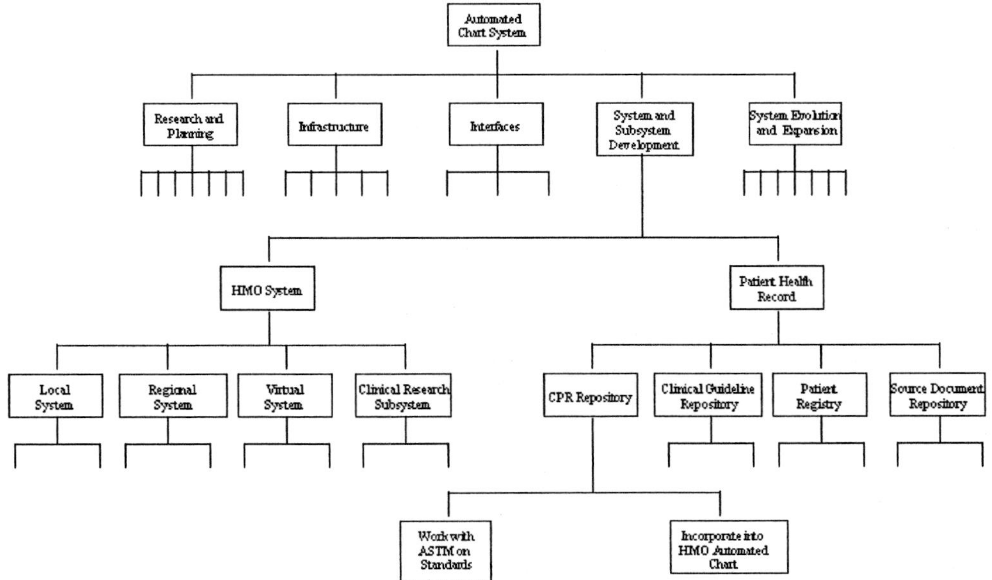

Figure 14.2 Work Breakdown Structure (WBC).

For a complex project, the project plan for the overall project would have *phases* of the project in place of the tasks. Each phase would have its own project plan with tasks being activities within the phase, and would likely have its own phase project manager.

Both phases and tasks, which can then be scheduled, can be determined by an approach such as a *Work Breakdown Structure* (WBS). The project can be broken down into phases for the overall project and to tasks for a phase of the project. For example, figure 14.2 illustrates a WBS for the overall automated patient chart system project.

The project and phase plans should include *milestones.* A milestone is a marker for a major event in the project.

As we noted previously, in particular after each phase and before the next, an evaluation should be done by management to determine if goals are being met and objectives are in the process of being fulfilled, and a decision is made on whether or not to change or continue the project. Such a decision point has also been called a *gate* (Buttrick 1997). A gate is one of a number of decision points in the project where an evaluation is made to revise or terminate the project. In order to get upper management to commit a significant amount of time at the appropriate time to evaluate the progress of the project, it might be useful to schedule gates in the project plan.

Anticipated project risks should also be considered, along with *contingency plans* for handling these risks if they indeed occur. One approach is to schedule a task in the schedule to do the contingency plan; this task would start at the time the risk is expected to occur. For example, a risk might be that national standards for the automated patient medical record have not yet been established; a task would be put into the project just before standards are needed to determine if standards exist, initiating a contingency plan if not.

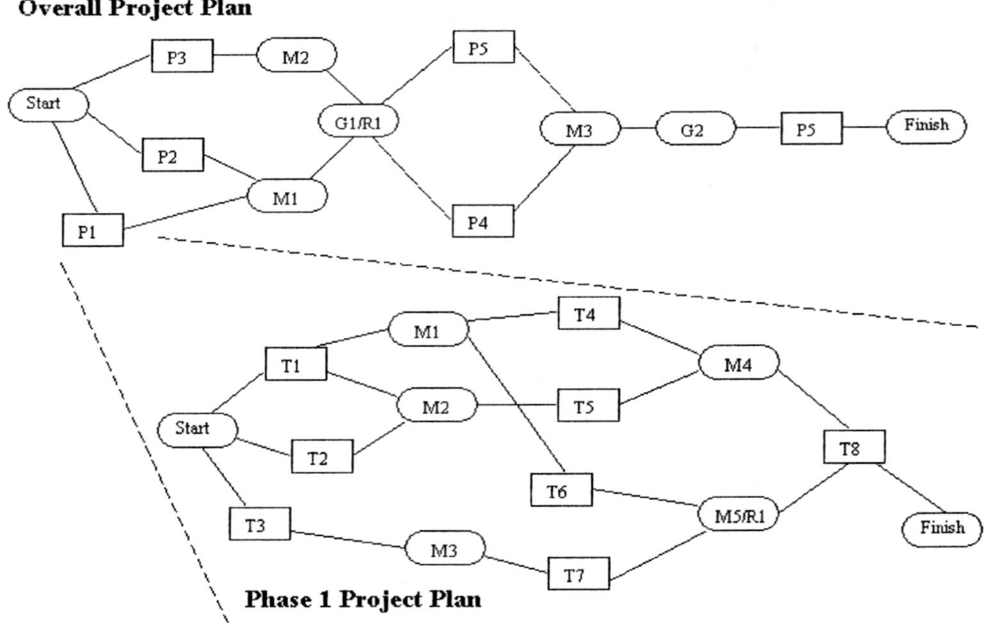

Figure 14.3 Project plans: phase/task network.

The overall project plan can be viewed as a network of phases. See figure 14.3. Each phase, itself has a project plan, which is a network of tasks. 'P' represent a phase, 'T' a task, 'M' a milestone, 'G' a gate, and 'R' a risk consideration point. Each task is assigned time to accomplish, costs, personnel and other resources (e.g., equipment) to accomplish, and performance parameters. From these, time, costs and resources for each phase can be determined; from this, the time, costs and resources for the overall project can be determined.

14.2.1 Gates

Initially in the initial evaluation step and thereafter in evaluation steps occurring at predetermined points in the project, management will reevaluate the project for adherence to objectives and to determine if the project should be changed or should move forward. See figure 2.3.

These evaluation points are the same as what we have termed here as *gates*. Compare the evaluation step presented earlier in figure 2.5 to this chapter's description of a gate, presented in figure 14.4.

A large program or project such as the automated patient medical record system program must be evaluated periodically by management for adherence to current company objectives, business strategies and goals, monitored as to ROI and compared to other projects. *Gates* are decision points where these evaluations occur. This evaluation determines the following (see figure 14.4):

- Can the project be simplified or improved?
- Does the project still fulfill company objectives, further the goals of the company and implement business strategies?
- Does the current ROI of the project justify its costs? Will there still be funding?
- Is it better to implement another project or other projects with higher priority instead?

Termination of the project might be considered if any of three latter questions is "no".

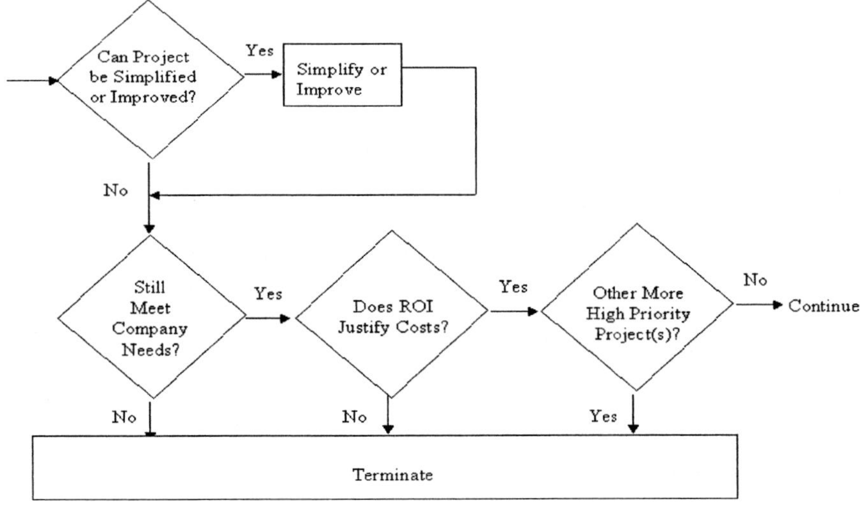

Figure 14.4 Decisions made at a gate.

14.2.2 Risks, Contingency Plans, and Mitigation

Risks can be identified at any time during the project. Some risks can only be identified when the occur—see the next chapter. Other risks can be anticipated at this stage, with decision points and contingency plans built into the schedule just before the risk would occur.

For example, a phase may require that an event takes place first (e.g., standardization of medical vocabularies in the healthcare industry). There must be a *contingency plan* if this doesn't take place.

Within a project plan, a risk could involve the choice of two phases, with a contingency plan resulting in one phase being done instead of the planned one. See figure 14.5. For example, there may be a phase to replace all HMO clinical systems with a common system for each type of clinical system, with inclusion of HL7 interfaces for each to the automated medical record system(s). Such an approach may prove to be too costly, so a contingency plan might be to substitute a phase simply implementing HL7 interfaces between existing clinical systems and the automated medical record system(s), if the other approach turns out to be too costly for the corporation at the time of the start of the risk determination.

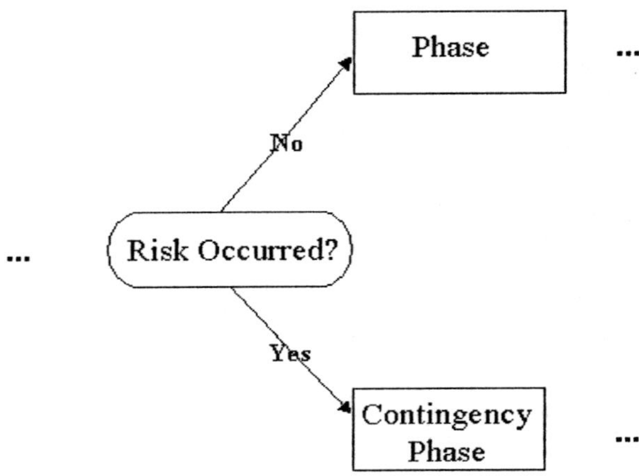

Figure 14.5 A contingency phase.

To *mitigate a risk* is to take whatever actions are possible in advance to reduce the effect of an identified risk in the project. In general, it is better to spend money on mitigating a risk than it is to include a contingency plan for a risk.

The expected project time delay of a risk can be measured by multiplying the probability that a risk will occur times the time delay that would occur if the risk did occur. An expected value for the delays in the project due to the risks can then be calculated by including these expected values as additional times within the project plan diagram at the times of the expected risks. Of course, there will likely be additional delays in the project due to unexpected risks.

14.3 DETERMINATION OF PHASES FOR THE AUTOMATED PATIENT MEDICAL RECORD PROJECT

The determination of the phases (the sub-projects) of a large project and their order is an important and difficult task. The governing principles for breaking the project up into phases are that

- Phases should be small enough to be manageable by a single project manager assigned to the phase, but not so small that the phase project manager does not have control over resources and decisions that determine the success of his phase.
- Every phase of the project must be done with a clear understanding of how the phase fits into the overall project. Phases are developed with an understanding of the logical dependencies between phases, such as this phase must precede another one as it supplies the information needed in the following phase.
- Phases that incorporate the overall infrastructure to tie the phases together should be done early on (a security system).
- Phases might be determined based upon achieving management goals (e.g., such and such a capability should be completed by such a date, or such and such phase will make money for the corporation and should thus be done first).

In order to start off this process, it is useful to break up the project into logical project categories. A phase might either be defined to be the same as a logical project category, cross project categories, or be one part of a project category. This process can, as stated in section 14.2, be facilitated by a Work Breakdown Structure.

The automated patient medical record project, if initiated by a single HMO, might consist of the following interrelated project categories:

1. **Planning and Research**—Plan the overall project. Plan the necessary research areas (see chapter 17) so they could be completed before their scheduled implementations.
2. **Infrastructure**—Implement hardware and software infrastructure within medical centers. Install wiring, networks, computers, printers and other peripherals, and system software, including operating systems. Infrastructure should generally be installed only as needed, such as hardware and software for diagnostic imaging (PACS) systems. Maintenance personnel to support changes and corrections to hardware, to released software and to controlled documentation could also be considered part of the infrastructure, or could, alternatively, be considered to be a separate project category.
3. **Interfaces**—Implement interfaces between the subsystems as described in section 13.10. Develop an implementation plan for the HMO, CPR repository, patient registry, and source document repository hardware and software infrastructure as necessary to implement the interfaces.
4. **System and Subsystem Development** Design, develop and install the necessary systems and subsystems for the HMO (initial local system, regional system, CPR repository, source document repository, patient registry, virtual local system, and clinical research subsystem). Integrate HMO clinical systems with the regional and local systems.
5. **Reengineering the HMO** Workflows of caregivers must be redefined radically, at least to the extent that the automated patient medical record system is included in their workflow.
6. **System Evolution and Expansion** Create additional local systems, if applicable. Create additional local and regional systems in other healthcare organizations. Create additional CPR repositories and source document repositories for Patient Health Records for patients outside the HMO.

Let us look at each of these project categories individually.

14.3.1 Planning and Research

Project planning is required to coordinate development, including the following:

- a plan for development of the various subsystems including their order of development based upon dependencies between the subsystems
- a plan for development of interfaces between the subsystems
- plans for incorporation of hardware and operating infrastructure both within the HMO and external to the HMO
- plans for incorporation of new technology and research ideas into the system
- plans for incorporation of national or international standards into the system as they are agreed upon
- plans for evolution of the subsystems, especially of the local system as new capabilities and chart documentation is added and as additional local systems are added.

As research of different areas becomes complete, the new ideas or technologies must be integrated into the automated patient medical record system (e.g., group communication capabilities, voice recognition, monitoring systems, etc.). Chapter 17 describes many of these research areas.

14.3.2 Infrastructure

Infrastructure is the underlying foundation or basic framework of a system which must be done before the functional part of the system can be done. Before the automated patient medical record and universal patient record can be implemented, computers and system software, networks and peripheral devices must first be installed in medical centers. Space requirements must be taken into account, such as how the computer system could fit into a small room. Rewiring may have to be done, possibly making it difficult, for a short time, to work at the work site during installation of the wiring. New buildings might even be necessary.

System software and new hardware may have to be installed, including, for example, hardware and software for networks. work stations, pen computers, voice recognition, etc.

Installation of wiring, networks, computers and system software including operating systems, and peripherals in medical centers is a major effort that must be coordinated with the development and installation of the system so the installation of hardware and system software installation occurs before installation of the application software. Likewise, the hardware and software for the CPR repository, source document repository, and patient registry must be installed before it is needed in the development plan. However, it is also useful to follow the reverse philosophy also: to delay as long as possible the procurement of hardware and system software such as operating systems so that the newest technology can be employed or so that the technology has been around long enough to decrease in price.

Having the correct personnel at any point of time during the project is part of the infrastructure. For example, maintenance staff to support hardware and software installation and updates, and to manage controlled documentation is part of the infrastructure.

14.3.3 Interfaces

An interface is the connection between any two components of a computer system and the protocols of information passed between the components. As subsystems of the automated patient medical system are being developed, the necessary interfaces between the subsystems such as described in section 13.10 must also be developed and implemented as they are needed. Before an interface can be implemented, the associated hardware infrastructure must be implemented.

14.3.4 System Development

The systems and subsystems that will be developed for our project assuming the design in chapter 13 are the following:

1. **HMO and affiliated healthcare organization systems**

- initial local system
- central system
- other local systems
- clinical research subsystem
- virtual system

2. **Universal Patient Record**

- source document repository
- CPR repository
- clinical guideline repository
- later, the patient registry.

14.3.5 Reengineering of the HMO

Caregivers must be trained in use of the system. They may have to change their prior work patterns. See chapters 11 and 12.

14.3.6 System Evolution and Expansion

The system must be developed so it could evolve over time. For example,

- additional local systems could be added to a healthcare organization system
- the universal patient record network might be implemented and expanded over time from that shown in figure 6.3 to that shown in figure 6.4, as described in section 6.3.
- systems in additional healthcare organizations to handle the automated patient medical record could be added and integrated with the universal patient record over time
- higher bandwidth networks could be integrated into the universal patient record
- higher bandwidth interfaces could be added within a healthcare organization
- advanced systems, such as research projects or diagnostic imaging systems (PACS) could be added.

The HMO system could be expanded to other HMO regional locations and other alliance and outside healthcare organizations. The universal patient record could be expanded to add additional CPR repositories, source document repositories; see sections 6.3 and 17.2.1.

14.4 SEQUENCING PHASES

The phases (or tasks) of the project must now be ordered and possibly be done concurrently dependent upon constraints. Phases are ordered based upon three types of constraints (Wysocki, Beck, and Crane 2000):

- **infrastructure is done first:** infrastructure is the foundation for everything else
- **technical constraints:** imposed by the logic of the system
- **managerial constraints:** imposed by management for a particular reason.

The same approach can be used for ordering tasks within a phase project plan.

14.4.1 Infrastructure is First

There is an unequivocal answer to what to do first on a project—That is *infrastructure.* Infrastructure is the underlying foundation or basic framework that must be done before the functional part can be done. Or a definition I like: All those things you don't see.

The problem with doing infrastructure first is that there are often no results that are apparent to upper management of the organization. A useful analogue is the building of a house. The infrastructure of a house is the engineering design and drawings of the house together with the foundation and structural elements of the house that hold the house together and keep it from falling (the foundation, the beams, trusses, joints, the side walls). But immediately after the infrastructure is finished, the occupants still cannot live there.

The infrastructure in the automated patient medical record system includes all the following:

- the analysis and design documents for automated patient medical record system—the controlled documents
- the automated patient medical record databases and programs
- the medical center and medical office buildings and wiring in these buildings
- the workstations, servers and networks within the medical centers and medical office buildings, and the support personnel for them
- the data center and the software and hardware systems, including operating systems, networks, data storage and file sharing mechanisms, data and file backup procedures, system logon and security systems, and the people who run these system
- the people who do the project
- the people who maintain hardware systems and programs, and the software and people who control new software releases
- the trainers, the user documentation and the training classes
- the reliability and performance requirements and the performance evaluation team
- the network connections to other software systems
- etc.

The infrastructure is time-consuming to do, requires a lot of thought, is costly, and is absolutely necessary. But upper management may not understand why the organization has spend so much money and time without receiving any tangible results.

Lots of people think that Microsoft does well because its software is so good. This may be true, but other companies have good software also. The one plus that Microsoft has over everyone else is that **it controls the infrastructure!** It makes the operating system for most of the computers in the world—some of the things you don't see.

When building the automated patient medical record system, a health care organization must concentrate on one thing first—the infrastructure—for it holds everything else together!

Infrastructure should never be overlooked. PR (public relations) is important in this respect to inform people of infrastructure. PR is only important when you want people to be aware of something they don't already know, and only often enough so they don't overlook it when they need it!

14.4.2 Technical Constraints

Technical constraints are logical constraints. Examples are the following:

- One phase (or task) requires input from another phase (or task) and thus must be done later (e.g., for legal and technical reasons, the log-in and other security parts of the automated patient medical record system should be implemented before other parts of the system).
- A critical resource or resources, or one-of-a-kind piece of equipment, must be available for each of two phases full time and thus only one phase may be done at a time.
- A phase in the project is required to be done by a particular date (e.g., by government mandate).
- Research is required to be done before a phase can be done, thus delaying it (For example, research is required into best methods of searching through the automated patient medical record for relevant information before this capability can be implemented).
- The company does not get specialized personnel to do the project at the time needed.

14.4.3 Managerial Constraints

Managerial constraints are management imposed. Examples are the following:

- The project must demonstrate success early—thus a phase producing a high return on investment is done first.
- Management wants to finish a particular phase by a certain date.
- The project manager might want to do some easier parts of the project first so he gains a modicum of comfort with the project work.

Management constraints can be reversed while technical ones cannot. If circumstances require changes in the order of phases or tasks, then the project manager might consider negotiating with management to change a managerial constraint.

14.5 INCORPORATING GOALS WITHIN THE PROJECT PLAN

Goals for project objectives and business requirements can be determined for the end of the project or strategically determined for intermediate points in the project. The *intermediate goals* can be evaluated in the overall project plan at a gate (e.g., those places marked with a 'G' in the example project plan in figure 14.3—with the 'G' standing for "gate" rather than "goal"). Gates, and goals, could also be included within the project plan of a phase.

Key Terms

contingency plan
cost
gate
goal
infrastructure
interface
intermediate goal
managerial constraint
milestone
phase
project management
project plan
resource
risk
task
technical constraint
Work Breakdown Structure (WBS)

Study Questions

1. In this book, what is a "phase"? In many project management books, what terms do they use for "project" and "phase"? For discussion: Is the term "project" in this book really the same as the term "program" in other books? Is development of the automated patient medical record a project or a program? Is development of the universal patient record a project or a program?
2. A project plan is defined as "a description of events to come". One type of event is a "task". What are three items that may be associated with a task? Name some types of "resources". According to this book, what are other types of events? Can these events occur at the same time? In what type of event would one test to see if a goal had been reached?
3. What is the difference between a Work Breakdown Structure (WBC) and a structure chart? How are they similar?
4. What is the purpose of a gate? What over thing in this book is most similar to a gate?
5. How are risks and contingency plans related? How large can a contingency plan be?
6. If a phase is too small or too large, what are some of the problems?
7. In order to do a project, there must be communication between the project members. Name some reasons why there must also be communication with personnel in other groups.
8. Why should infrastructure be done early on? Why might management not realize the importance of infrastructure?
9. Give examples of technical constraints and managerial constraints in the automated patient medical record project. What category of constraints is discretionary?

CHAPTER 15

An Example Phase to Develop a Clinical Data Repository (CDR)

CHAPTER OUTLINE

15.1 PROJECT CONTEXT: A PROJECT PLAN FOR A PHASE

A *phase* constitutes a subproject within the overall project. Phases can completely or partially overlap in time. Phases can be done concurrently, or they can have dependencies upon each other, with a particular phase requiring the completion of a prior phase before it can be started.

This chapter presents an example phase in the automated patient medical record project. In this phase, HMO clinical systems will be interfaced with the automated patient medical record system. The current healthcare industry standard for interfacing these clinical systems is HL7 network protocol.

Information from the clinical systems needed by the automated patient medical record system would be stored on a database. In the healthcare industry, such a database that stores information from clinical systems is referred to as a *clinical data repository (CDR)*.

For our automated patient medical record system, the CDR is a major portion of the information making up the patient medical record (e.g., encounters, orders and results). The CDR would later be expanded to include other patient medical record information (e.g., progress notes and other such documentation, orders made through the automated patient medical record system rather than the clinical systems, the complete on-line medical record including CPR and source document repositories).

Like for the total project, a phase is a project consisting of project steps. Project steps that can occur in a phase, and more specifically, in the CDR phase, are the following:

- **Business analysis step:** Determine business requirements for the CDR, required changes to the organization when the CDR is completed.
- **Business reengineering step:** Determine how employees will function differently due to the CDR. Determine how information from the CDR (medications, clinical laboratory orders and test results, appointments and outpatient registrations, inpatient stays) will be displayed through the automated patient medical record system, and how printed reports from the CDR will look.
- **System analysis step:** Determine technical requirements for the CDR database, for the interfaces with the other clinical systems to gather data for the CDR, and for code to support display and reporting of CDR information.
- **Development step:** Based upon the system analysis step, create the CDR database, interfaces between the clinical systems and automated patient medical record system, and the screens, dialogs and reports. (Note: This step only occurs within a phase, as phases are where actual products are created.)
- **Implementation step:** Implement the CDR in the organization. (This step also only occurs within a phase.)

The CDR will eventually be expanded to include the full capabilities of the automated patient medical record system. Thus, the Business Analysis, Business Reengineering and system analysis steps for producing the CDR must be consistent with the equivalent steps for the overall project. In other words, the CDR must be able to evolve into the fully-automated patient medical record system.

15.2 A PHASE TO CREATE A CLINICAL DATA REPOSITORY

The CDR is a collection of clinical information—encounters, orders and results—from various clinical systems. This clinical information might include the following and more:

- Hospital stays from ADT (i.e., information on inpatient encounters)
- Appointments from the appointment system (information that could be used for outpatient encounters)
- Members registering for an outpatient visit (i.e., information on outpatient encounters)
- Laboratory orders and results from the clinical laboratory system
- Medications requested, medications picked up, and drug allergies from the outpatient pharmacy system
- Medications ordered and taken from the inpatient pharmacy system
- X-ray orders from the radiology system.

In section 13.2, as shown in figure 13.1, it was stated that building a software system is like designing and producing a watch: The externals are usually designed by a group who look at the system from an external or black box view, unconcerned with how the internals work. On the other hand, the internals are built by a group that needs to match up the internal subsystems with the external functions they need to support, thus requiring a white box view of the system. Figure 15.2 illustrates this black box / white box view as related to development of the CDR.

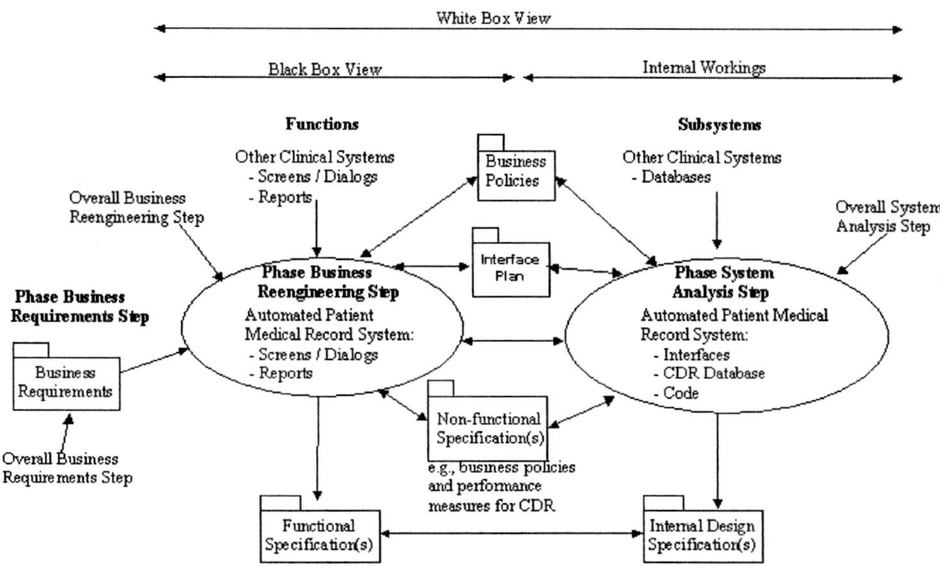

Figure 15.2 White box / black box view of a phase to create a CDR.

In the business analysis step of the CDR phase, a set of business requirements for the CDR would be developed. These business requirements would describe the business rationale for creating clinical system interfaces and the CDR. These phase business requirements must be consistent with the overall system business requirements for the total automated patient medical record system.

The phase business reengineering step would identify how the CDR information would be displayed within the automated patient medical record system. The phase system analysis step would identify the CDR databases and system interfaces sending the information from the clinical systems to the automated patient medical record system.

The interfacing clinical systems would identify encounters and information that would provide a large part of the automated patient medical record: clinical lab orders, tests, and results; outpatient and inpatient medications; x-ray and interpretation of results; etc. The organization of some of these parts of the automated patient medical record—clinical lab tests and results, for example—could probably be determined by looking at screens and dialogs or reports within the originating clinical systems. And the organization of the CDR database within the automated patient medical record system could be partly determined by the organization of similar information in the clinical system databases.

The various clinical systems might have individual databases such as are shown in figure 15.3. In the hospital (ADT) system, admissions, discharges and transfers could be organized by the medical center facility where they occur. In the appointment system, appointments could be identified for each patient. In the outpatient pharmacy system, medications at a pharmacy could be in the order patients and physicians request the medications. In the inpatient pharmacy system, inpatient medications could be identified by hospital unit where patients are located. In the clinical laboratory system, clinical laboratory orders might be ordered by time received, with results being connected to orders, with possible amended results being attached as addendums.

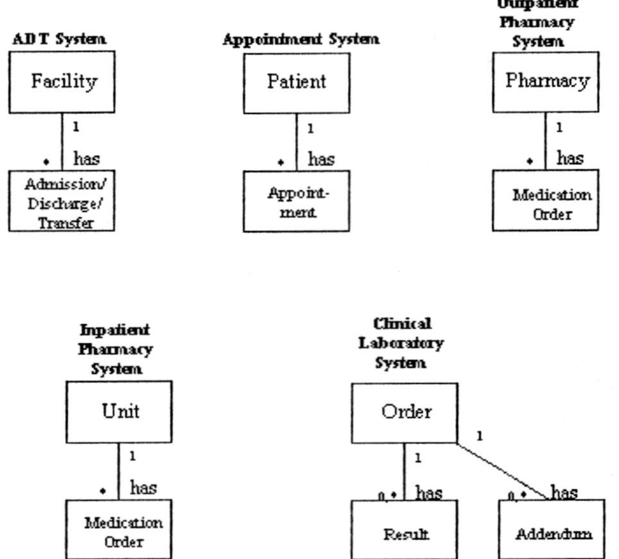

Figure 15.3 Clinical system databases.

From the overall business reengineering step and system analysis step as described in previous chapters, it is clear that the automated patient medical record system will require a different organization for this clinical information—see the database in figure 13.16. Organizing this information by patient and encounter as if figure 13.16, we get the database shown in figure 15.4 combining encounters with orders and results.

The business reengineering step for the CDR phase would identify how the CDR database information would be displayed in the automated patient medical record system: the screens, dialogs and reports.

In the development of systems, screens and dialogs that logically function together are referred to as *functions*. For example, the screens and dialogs displaying clinical laboratory test orders and results could be one set of functions. A specification is written for each function, a *functional specification*. A functional specification should be written so that requirements for a function can be tested after development to verify that that the resulting function in the developed system works correctly. Functional specifications would be the products of the phase Business Reengineering and development steps. Information that goes across functions such as required response times for all functions and business policies as they apply to the CDR are recorded on *non-functional specifications.*

The CDR database, clinical system interfaces, and the code to support the functions would be defined in detail in the phase system analysis step, resulting in written specifications for this code, these interfaces and the CDR database. These written specifications are referred to as *internal design specifications.* These internal design specifications would be products of the phase system analysis and development steps.

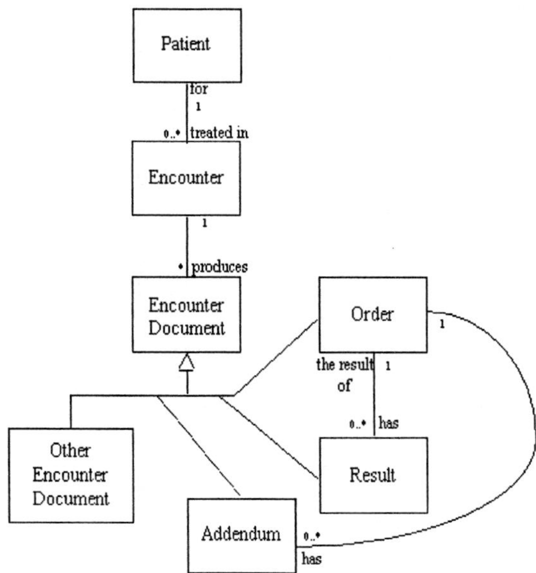

Figure 15.4 Proposed clinical data repository database.

Interfaces between the clinical systems and the future automated patient medical record system would be recorded in an *interface plan.* The interface plan would be determined within the Reengineering, system analysis and development steps.

The functional specifications and internal design specifications would be used in the phase development step to create the physical CDR system. In the phase implementation step, the system would be installed in one or more healthcare organization locations for actual use. A phase project plan step would create a project plan for tasks in the development and implementation steps.

Organizational *business policies* that apply to the CDR need to be incorporated. Since organizational business policies can cross many automated systems and business processes, the business policies should be recorded in a document that applies to the total organization. How these business policies are incorporated within code and databases needs to be recorded with the business policies so non-technical personnel can manage these policies. Example business policies that apply to the CDR phase might include the following:

- **Security policies:** Implement security consistent with organizational security policies, such as described in section 13.9.1. This might include physician or caregiver only access to the CDR patient information, smart card logon, automatic logoff in non-secure areas where patients are examined.
- **Access to psychiatry and genetic information**: Restrict the display of patient psychiatry and genetic information to appropriate subsets of physicians or caregivers.

- **Assignment of primary care physicians for HMO members**: Within CDR displays, the primary care physician assigned to a patient would be displayed.
- **Quality of information**: All data will be verified for correctness and adherence to business rules for it.

At the end of a phase or at any other time in the project, there could be an evaluation step that could be prescheduled in the project plan. Such an evaluation step is referred to in this book as a "gate", a point where a project is to be re-evaluated for costs, feasibility and adherence to the goals of the organization. See section 14.2.1.

15.3 A BUSINESS ANALYSIS STEP FOR A PHASE

The business analysis step of a phase differs somewhat from that of the overall project. There are two differences:

1. During the business analysis step of a phase, obstacles are evaluated—For the initial overall project, this evaluation of obstacles is done in the evaluation step because it must first be determined if there are significant enough benefits to do the project.
2. During the business analysis step of a phase, there is a determination of whether or not the overall design of the system should be revisited.

Compare figures 15.5 and 2.3.

In the business analysis step for the initial overall design, evaluation of obstacles is not included unlike other instances of the business analysis step. Evaluation of obstacles could be very costly, so during the initial overall project analysis this evaluation is deferred until after the evaluation of objectives (benefits), because the project might simply be rejected due to not providing enough benefits to the organization. On the other hand, a phase of the project is not started until there is a significant commitment by the organization of doing the project; thus, in such a case, there is no question that the evaluation of obstacles should be done in its entirety. Also in later overall analyses, the business analysis step also includes an evaluation of obstacles as, likewise, at this point there is also a signficant commitment to doing the project.

Part of the business analysis step of a phase is identifying that the overall design of the project needs to be re-done due to the impact of the phase on the project. Some examples of reasons for revisiting the overall design during a phase are the following:

- The phase was defined by a research project and little was known about the phase at the start of the project; thus the phase was not included in the initial overall design--see example research phases in chapter 17.
- It is learned in the phase that the phase requires information that is not available.
- The new phase takes over the functionality previously in another part of the system, and thus that other part of the automated patient medical record system must be changed.
- The phase does something better than other parts of the project (e.g., has a better user interface) and the overall system should be changed to conform to the ideas of the new phase.

The extent of this revisiting of the overall design is dependent upon how much was known about the phase at the beginning of the project. For a complex phase where little was previously known about the phase at the beginning of the project (e.g., a phase done after research), this new overall design process may be as involved as the initial one.

For the CDR phase, for example, the business analysis step might discover that the clinical laboratory system or pharmacy system is incapable of identifying the encounter in which the clinical lab test or medication was ordered. In such a case, the clinical laboratory and pharmacy systems might have to be changed to include encounter information before the CDR phase begins. One way to insuring match-up of orders with encounters is to have all orders be done through the automated patient medical record system, requiring the caregiver doing the ordering to match up the order with the encounter before the order is sent over to a clinical system to be filled.

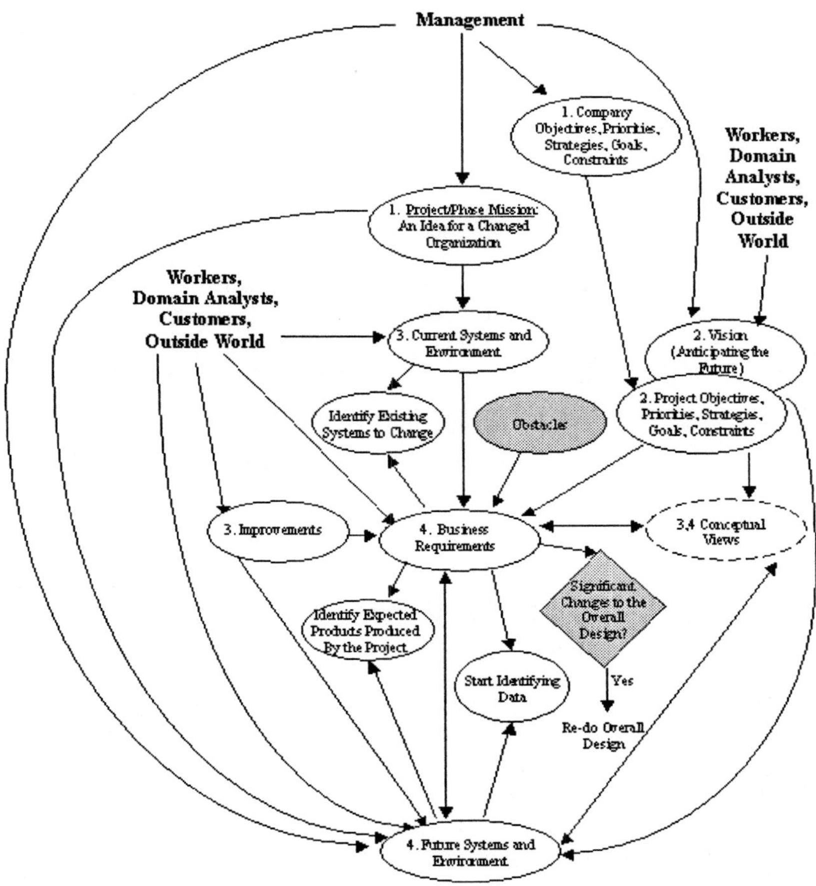

Figure 15.5 Business analysis step for a phase.

15.4 THE PROJECT PLAN FOR THE PHASE BREAKING THE PROJECT INTO TASKS

The project plan for a phase will be a standard project plan consisting of a network of interrelated tasks, rather than a network of phases as was the case for the overall project. Chapter 14 discusses project management, both for phases and the larger project. Many good books exist on project management including (Wysocki and McGary 2003) and on project planning for software development including (Futrell, Shafer, and Shafer 2002).

In order to do the initial overall project plan, the project plan for each phase must be done to some extent, so the project plan step for a phase can use and refine this earlier phase project plan, in particular refining tasks for the development and implementation steps of the phase.

15.5 THE DEVELOPMENT STEP

The development step may only occur in a phase, not as part of overall design of the project. This is so because the overall design is done to pre-plan or re-plan the project, whereas a phase creates the products of a project. See figures 2.3.

A development step only occurs if there is a new automated system or a change to an automated system in the phase. There are both in our example phase. There is likely to be many changes to existing clinical systems to interface them with the CDR, and there would be a new automated system, part of the automated patient medical record system, to collect the clinical information and store it on the CDR. (There also could be a new clinical system to replace an old one so it could interface with the CDR, but this would probably be done as a separate project outside the automated patient medical record project.)

The development step takes two different forms dependent upon whether the automated system is developed in-house or procured from a vendor. In our example phase, implementing HL7 interfaces for clinical systems to send information to a CDR, some of these systems could be organizationally developed, while others are likely to be vendor systems.

15.5.1 The Development Step for an Organizationally-Developed System

The development step for an organizationally-developed system (or subsystem), involves developing program specifications for the functions and programs making up the system, programming the automated system from these specifications, and testing the resulting automated system. On the other hand, changes to existing systems would involve changes to existing program specifications. Figure 15.6 identifies the parts of the development step that are applicable for organizationally developed systems.

The phase to create the CDR would probably involve organizationally developed systems in the following ways: (1) creation of a new subsystem to record information gathered from clinical systems to the CDR, and (2) changes to existing clinical systems to develop HL7 interfaces (e.g., collecting hospital admissions in ADT, clinical lab results in the clinical laboratory system) to send the information over to the new subsystem, besides (3) possible new organizationally developed systems or vendor systems to replace existing clinical systems which have HL7 interfaces.

The development step for an organizationally developed system is described in more detail in section 15.7.

15.5.2 The Development Step for a Vendor System

The development step could alternatively involve newly installed or changed vendor systems. Such vendor systems have been termed *commercial off-the-shelf (or COTS) software* (Voas 1998). Using COTS may produce significant savings in time and money over the initial creation and installation of a system within the organization. There are also many potential problems with using COTS systems, however, including the following:

- no control of upgrades that may cause significant changes from the originally planned system, including unwanted ones
- other customers could disagree with any requested changes and thus the changes may never be implemented
- dependence on the vendor to make changes; as a result, changes could be implemented more slowly than required by the organization

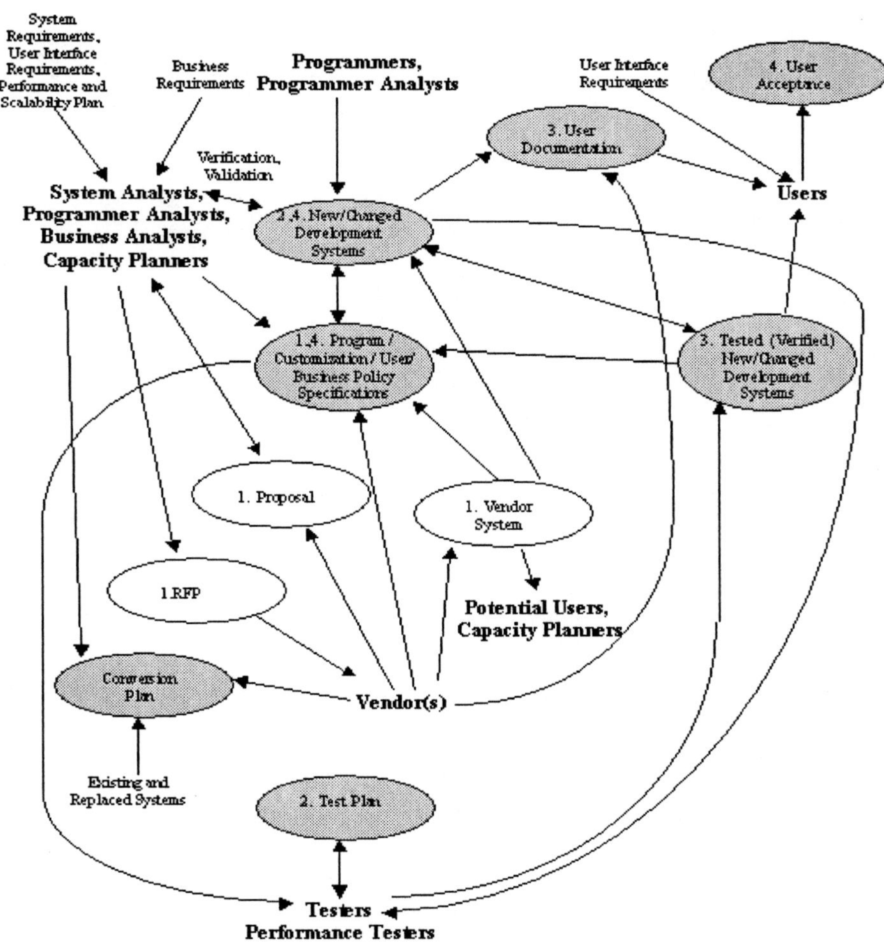

Figure 15.6 In-house development of an automated system (dark bubbles).

- COTS are like black boxes and thus it is hard for system analysts to verify that the COTS perform safely, securely and reliably—a seeming "must" for an automated patient medical record
- for a COTS system, building a system to meet business requirements may not be possible; in fact, the reverse may be required, the business requirements might be dictated by the COTS system
- unless you are able to do performance testing, you will have to rely upon the vendor's statements that their system can handle the transaction and database volumes needed by your organization
- the vendor company could go out of business.

Reference (Kuver 2004) describes strategies for the selection and installation of COTS (vendor) systems in detail, with an emphasis on systems that are used for an entire enterprise, such is the case with our automated patient medical record system.

Now, let's consider the development step for a vendor system. Figure 15.7 identifies those parts of the development step applicable to vendor systems.

15.5.2.1 Procuring a Vendor System

The organization may decide to buy a new vendor system for a phase, e.g., a vendor clinical system that has an HL7 interface for a clinical laboratory for a region of the HMO that interfaces with the automated patient medical record system.

The process of procuring an appropriate vendor system for such a clinical system might involve the following sequence of events: The organization talks to organizations that evaluate the particular type of system (e.g., a clinical system) and speaks to people in organizations that use such systems to identify possible vendors. They match vendors against requirements gathered in previous phases of the project. The organization may send out a *request for information (RFI)* to gather additional information from vendors on their products.

The organization may pare down the number of vendors. The organization sends out a *request for proposal (RFP)* to each of the selected vendors, identifying necessary business and system requirements for the clinical laboratory system. Interested vendors would respond with a proposal describing how their system would satisfy the requirements, including how the vendor system would be customized. System analysts, business analysts and users would test out the vendor systems, evaluate vendor proposals determining how closely they meet system and business requirements, and compare vendor system costs. A *solution alternative analysis* document might be created that compares the various systems based upon requirements. A vendor is selected based upon the comparison of systems.

A contract for the vendor system is created, identifying agreed upon customization specifications. The vendor system with customizations is developed. Testers would produce a test plan for the customized vendor system according to system requirements, vendor documents and customizations. The vendor program would be tested, if there were any errors, the customizations would be changed and/or specifications would be updated. Retesting would occur until there were no errors detected in the developed system or specifications. Users would compare the tested system and user documentation supplied by the vendor against the previously agreed upon user interface requirements produced in the business reengineering step.

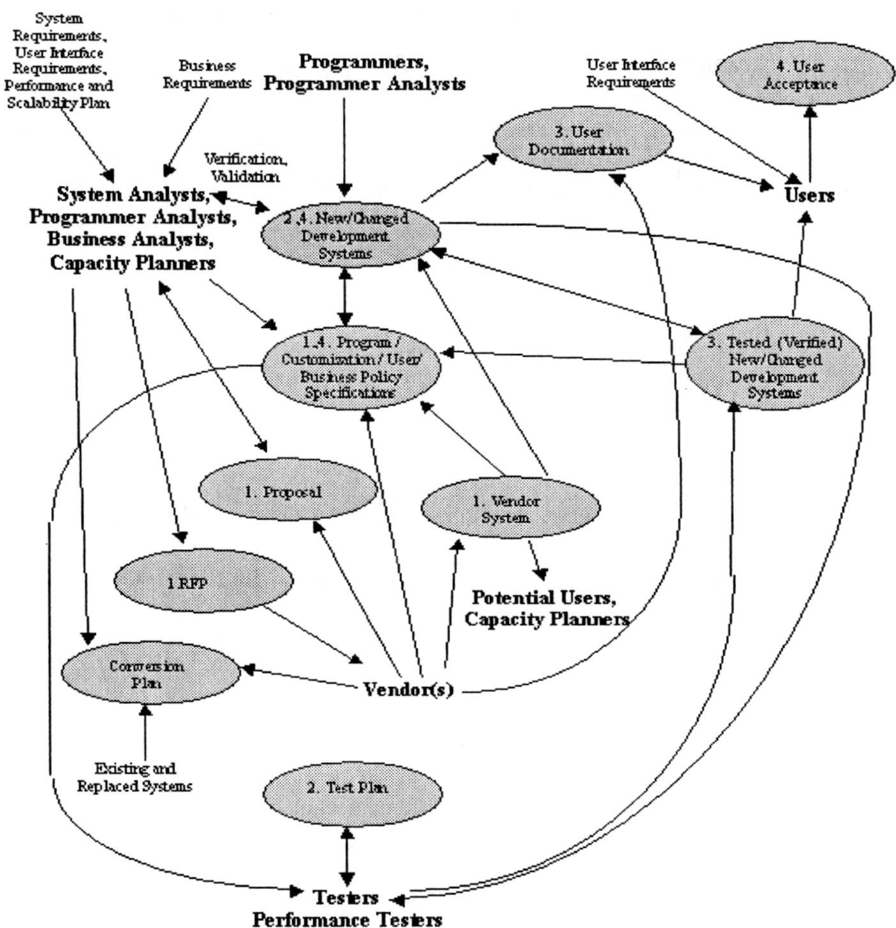

Figure 15.7 Vendor procurement of an automated system.

15.5.2.2 Changing a Vendor System

Changes to an existing vendor system, such as a clinical laboratory clinical system, would, on the other hand, involve negotiations between the vendor and the organization. A contract involving the new customizations would be developed, with business and system analysts verifying that the system met systems and business requirements, including business policies. Thereafter, a test plan would be created and the system tested and revised until there were no errors in the system or specifications. If applicable, users would verify that the user interface is as expected.

15.5.2.3 Replacing a Vendor System

Where possible, vendor systems that follow existing industry standards both for systems and healthcare should be used (e.g., a clinical laboratory system that follows HL7 interface standards and clinical laboratory device standards as identified in the appendix). This enables a vendor system to be more easily replaced by another vendor system or by an internally developed system that follows those same or similar standards.

Replacement of a vendor system is also facilitated by having a vendor contract that is flexible, which allows for change if there are unanticipated changes that require the system to be replaced. For example, periodic licenses offer more flexibility than very long term ones.

These ideas to facilitate the replacement of a vendor system with another vendor system or an organizationally developed system again fall under the concept of *component adaptability*.

15.5.3 Planning for Availability, Capacity and Performance

Important in developing an automated system or purchasing a vendor system is that the system be able to handle the current and future capacity of users, transactions and network traffic. Performance testers should provide advice to developers on how to develop systems that meet such capacity requirements, in particular on selection of the correct hardware, networks and system software. Performance testers should test vendor systems to see if they meet capacity and performance requirements before they are purchased.

Either for an organizationally developed system or for a proposed vendor system, performance testers could set up a *test bed* computer system for the new automated system, stressing the system with the expected future number of transactions and network traffic, mimicking the future system, to determine if the system will adequately function in the future.

Systems such as the automated patient medical record system must be available on a virtual 24 hour times 7 days a week basis. This requires thorough testing prior to release of the system to insure that there are no bugs in the system that cause the system to go down, as well as planning ahead for the future so the system does not reach capacity in terms of required disk storage, CPU and other requirements.

For (hopefully rare) situations where the system does become unavailable, it is important that there be a back-up mechanism to later input the information that was not input when the system was down and to later receive input from other systems that could not be received because a system or systems were down. Data input during this back-up process should also be sent to all interfacing systems that would have received it if the system was up, with the results of the input being identical to what it would have been if the system was up.

15.5.3.1 Service Level Agreements

In order to insure that the availability and performance of the system is adequate, a *service level agreement (SLA)* could be written. This is a contract between the end users of the system and the group running a system and/or the vendor providing the system that makes an agreement upon a predefined level of service (Lee and Ben-Natan 2002), in particular availability and performance levels. For example, the system must be up 99.5% of the time on a 7 x 24 basis, the system will support 'x' simultaneous users during its peak hour of a week, with 95% of users receiving a response time of 2 seconds or less during the peak hour. Application time-outs will occur less than once in 50,000 sessions. If the agreed upon service is not reached, or periodically falls below a certain level, the group running the system or the vendor would be penalized, e.g., monetarily.

Source Level Agreements are often made between a company's information technology group running the system and the end users within the company using the system. Usually monetary penalties are not actually incurred in such a case.

If a vendor is contracted to not only provide but also run a system, then the SLA could occur between the company and that vendor. In such a case monetary penalties usually incur upon performance or response times differences with the SLA contract.

An SLA could also potentially occur between a vendor who provides an application system and the company, who both has end users using the system and who also runs the system. Such a situation could be very complicated as the company provides some services (running the system) that could influence performance, while the vendor provides the product that also has an influence on system performance. An SLA may then have to differentiate the services that the company is responsible for and the services that the vendor is responsible for. For a vendor, additional agreements could exist to turn over vendor code to the organization if the vendor should fold.

A service level agreement, in any case, is sort of like an insurance policy for performance problems, but does not make the performance problem go away. Like an insurance policy, it is best that it never be used. If performance does degrade a system significantly, even if all lost revenues could be recovered through the service level agreement, the prestige of the organization could be effected, employees could be demoralized, and lawsuits could ensue. It could take a very long time to correct the performance problems.

15.5.3.2 Service Management Systems

System software, called *service management systems*, can measure system performance and record when it goes below a certain level (e.g., response time is too long). Such systems could be used to evaluate compliance with service level agreements.

15.5.4 Planning for Data Conversion

During the development phase, a *data conversion* plan could be created to convert existing information on databases to the format of data required by new databases, such as the CDR. The data conversion plan would be executed during the next phase, implementation.

15.6 THE IMPLEMENTATION STEP

Like for the development step, an implementation step only occurs during a phase, not as part of overall design of the project. The implementation step implements infrastructure for the project, an automated system, a change in an automated system, or other changes in the organization.

See figure 2.10. Implementation could include installing the infrastructure for a system, such as computers, wiring and networks for an automated system; this should occur very early in this phase. Information in existing systems could be converted according to the conversion plan developed in the development step to the format required by new databases. A tested development system could be installed. In coordination with the installation of the automated system, the users could be trained in the new systems and workflows, then the system would be used within the work environment using the changed workflows.

Our example phase might involve installing new wiring, computers, terminals and networks, replacing and changing clinical systems, which include HL7 interfaces, and installing the program and computer system(s) to interface with the clinical systems, including the program which puts the information on the CDR. If new clinical systems are required, because existing ones are inadequate, training of users of the new systems would also be required.

If a new clinical system replaces an old one, then conversion of existing data from the format of the old system to the format of the new system may be required with transfer of the data from the old to new system. Thereafter, and users would eventually have to stop using an old system and start using the new system.

15.6.1 Approaches to Phasing Out an Old System

Reference (Lozinsky 1998) identifies a number of different approaches for phasing out an old system and phasing in a new one:

- ***direct cut over***: turning off the old system the day the new system goes into operation—usually a very risky approach
- ***parallel operation***: running both the old and new system concurrently and comparing results to verify both systems function alike
- ***phase in***: running the new system in a portion of the enterprise first, adjusting the way it works if necessary, and incrementally replicating it in other parts of the enterprise
- ***limited parallel operation***: running the new system with real data to test and verify functionality, but the new system does not completely parallel the old system
- ***retroactive parallel operation***: using the old system for running the business and entering the same data in the new system whenever the day-to-day operations permit.

15.7 MORE INFORMATION ON IN-HOUSE DEVELOPMENT OF AN AUTOMATED SYSTEM

This section describes the Development step for an automated system developed inside the healthcare organization.

15.7.1 The Development Step in the Software Development Life-Cycle

The technique chosen by this book is to show the life cycle of an entire comprehensive project to change an organization. The project could include, or could be primarily, the development of software (e.g., the automated patient medical record system).

The *software development life-cycle* shows the life cycle of the development of software alone in an organization. The software development life-cycle is shown on the right in figure 15.8. This can be compared against the corresponding project steps shown to the left of the software development life-cycle steps.

The conception of the automated system occurs as the first part of the software development life-cycle. Correspondingly, in the business analysis step of the project, the mission for the project is determined.

Requirements are the next step in the software development life-cycle. In the project steps, business requirements are determined during the business analysis step and user interface requirements are determined in the business reengineering step.

The next step in the software development life-cycle is the design step. In the project steps, the design of the user interfaces may be part of the business reengineering step, with the initial design of the programs within the automated system being done in the system analysis step.

The next steps in the software development life-cycle are the implementation and test steps, programs are created, interfaced and tested. These steps together are equivalent to the development step of a project, which is based upon the system design in the system analysis step and user interfaces from the business reengineering step.

Project Steps	Software Life-Cycle Steps
Business Analysis	Concept
	Requirements
Business Reengineering	
	Design
System Analysis	
Development	Implementation (Code)
	Test
Implementation	Operation and Maintenance
Maintenance	

Figure 15.8 Comparing project steps with software life-cycle steps.

The final steps in the software development life-cycle are operation and maintenance. The project steps include an implementation step to do user training and reengineering of the organization prior to operation and maintenance, which would exist as part of the software life-cycle, but are not usually broken out as a separate step in the software life-cycle.

Maintenance is the process of changing a system after it has been delivered and is in use.

Although the diagram is figure 15.8 may not be true to the time scale of each step, some references note that testing can take up 50% of the development effort (Sommerville 2000), while maintenance could take 50-80% of the total costs of an automated system, including all the costs from conception to retirement. This emphasizes the importance of automated system testing and maintenance, which will be discussed further in the following sections.

15.7.2 The Development Step in More Detail

As is implied by figure 15.8, the development step includes coding of the automated system and testing of the automated system. Figure 15.9 expands on these coding and associated activities and upon the testing activities, which together make up the development step.

Code Code is the programming content of an application.code. Coding an automated patient medical record includes writing specifications upon which the code is based. The subsystems and functions making up the automated system, which would be identified and described in the system analysis step (see section 13.14.1 and figure 13.48), are described in detail during the development step through program documentation. This program documentation includes functional specifications, each describing a subsystem or function making up the automated system, and internal design specifications, each describing a program making up the subsystems and functions.

Databases and interfaces identified in previous project steps that are used within a function are referenced within the functional specification. Those that are used within a program are referenced within the internal design specification.

The programs are then coded based upon the functional specifications and the internal design specifications. As the automated system is developed through the coding of the functions and programs, the resulting system is used to simulate production use of the system, with user review of the system.

Testing Testing involves *validation* at the end of development to run the resulting code to show that it functions as identified by the functional specifications and internal design specifications, and *verification* that involves "human comparison" of the requirements for the system with the resulting functions and programs. **(Kit 1995)**

Validation involves first validation of individual functions and programs (*unit testing*), validation of these functions and programs working together into subsystems and in the entire automated system (*integration testing*), and validation of interfaces between the automated system and other automated systems (*interface testing*).

During development, the automated system should be tested by users during a simulation of production use of the system (*usability testing*). *Acceptance testing* is the process of comparing the end product of development with the current needs of its users; acceptance testing often involves operating the system in production for a pre-specified period.

During the creation of the program specifications, these specifications should be *verified* as matching the requirements. Whenever there is a mismatch, then the inconsistencies should be corrected by changing the program specifications or code to match the requirements, or sometimes, by reviewing and possibly changing the requirements for the system.

System testing is the process at the end of development to validate that all the requirements have been satisfied by the automated system. Requirements include requirements of all sorts identified so far: business requirements, user interface requirements, security requirements, performance requirements, volume requirements, reliability requirements, etc.

For example, one form of system testing is testing the system for bottlenecks that could cause the system to take a long time to respond to users when many users are using the system (*performance testing*). Because of the expense of performance testing, it is not often done until problems in response time are found; however, this book identifies how cost-effective performance testing can be done prior to production. See sections 10.12 and 11.7.

Whenever inconsistencies or errors are found through validation or verification, the code or documentation should be corrected, with subsequent retesting, which should include testing of all the parts of the automated system.

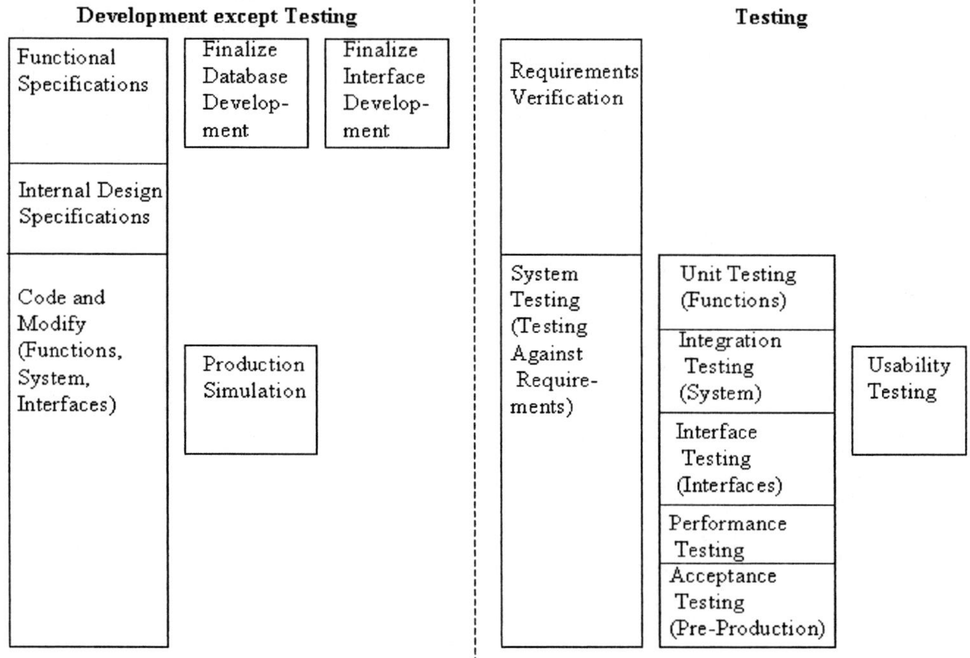

Figure 15.9 In-house development.

Functional specifications and internal design specifications should be maintained along with the program into the "operation and maintenance" step in order to make later changes to the automated system easier. The requirements for the automated system should also be preserved; this is best done by including the business and user requirements associated with a function within the functional specification. When there is a change made in a function during maintenance, the functional specifications and internal design specifications would be changed along with the program, with testing insuring that the changed program matched up with changed specifications and requirements.

After maintenance changes are made, tests done during development or previous maintenance could be re-done to insure that parts of the system that should not be changed continue to function as before. This retesting after a maintenance change using previous tests is called *regressive testing* or *regression testing*.

15.7.3 Building for Maintainability of the Automated System in the Development Step

As stated in section 15.7.1, maintenance could involve 50-80% of the total costs of an automated system, including all the costs from conception to retirement. *Maintenance* is the process of changing a system after it has been delivered and is in use. *Maintainability* is a measure of how easy or hard it is to change the system without introducing new errors in the system or inconsistencies in the requirements.

Part of the maintainability of a system is dependent upon things that are done in the coding part of the development step. Figure 15.10 describes some things that could be done during coding to make the system more maintainable or less maintainable.

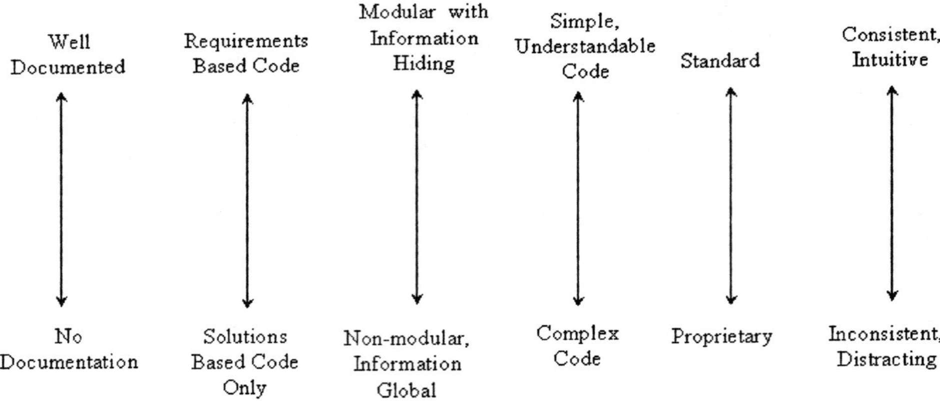

Figure 15.10 The development step and elements of maintainable systems.

15.7.3.1 Documentation

Maintenance changes, like the original software design itself when it replaces an existing system, are based upon either correcting errors or upon changes to requirements.

Requirements should be clearly recorded for the system in documentation and when there is a change to a requirement, the associated documentation should be updated to incorporate the changed requirement. The maintenance change can then be based upon this documentation.

Without any documentation on the system, no one in the automated system's maintenance group really knows how the automated system, functions or programs are supposed to work. Without documentation, knowledge of the system is dependent upon key employees; if these key employees go away, then the system becomes unmaintainable. Additionally, unknowledgeable members of the maintenance group have no checks on changes they will make, introducing unintended features which have little or no relationship to the original requirements of the system.

On the other extreme is having a complete set of documentation as is shown in figure 2.11, with each item in each document being traceable to the sections in each other document. Although this would describe the system and its requirements in complete detail, doing this would be cost prohibitive. The best approach is something in between these two extremes.

This book suggests that, for the maintenance phase, keeping functional specifications for the subsystems and functions in the system and internal design specifications for each of the programs, with the functional specifications including the requirements related to the functions.

15.7.3.2 Requirements-Based Code Versus Solutions-Based Code

In order to match code back to requirements, it is useful to relate variables and data back to requirements-based concepts rather than solutions-based concepts.

Requirements represent "what" was done, and sometimes also "why" it was done. Solutions represent "how" something was done. There are most often many solutions for a requirement.

For example, a requirement might be "if appointment is considered critical and patient does not show up for the appointment, put the patient on a list to call the patient". Code in the form, "**if** appointment-critical **and** patient-not-seen **then** ..." relates to requirements-based concepts. Code in the form "**if** (appointment-priority = 3) **and** (appointment-status = 4, 5, 9, 21, 23 or 64) **then** ..." in replacement doesn't.

The latter code suffers from a number of problems that make it difficult to later relate the code back to the requirements: (1) "appointment-priority" and "appointment-status" are solutions-based concepts rather than a requirements-based concepts. (2) "appointment-priority" and "appointment-status" address concepts at a lower, finer level than that of the requirements concepts "appointment-critical" and "appointment-no-show". (3) "appointment-priority" and "appointment-status" use solution-based values (3, 4, 5, 9, ...) instead of more descriptive ones (e.g., critical-appointment, appointment-canceled, patient-no-show, etc.).

15.7.3.3 Modularity and Information Hiding

Modularization and information hiding are two ways of simplifying programs. *Modularization* is breaking up code into blocks of reusable code. *Information hiding* is hiding data or code from a programmer that the programmer does not need to know about.

The most useful way to modularize a program is to create routines, functional common code which can be used many times within a single program or by many different programs. Routines are described by "what" they do and the information provided to the routine, the inputs, and the information returned from the routine, the outputs.

Consider the following: A very large subsystem of the automated patient medical record system is written as one large program and all the data within the program is in global storage (i.e., the data in storage can all be read or updated at any point in the program). Further, "goto" statements appear liberally throughout the program, with the "goto" jumping to any point in the program.

This is a very difficult program for a maintenance programmer to maintain for a number of reasons: Firstly, the programmer has to comprehend, and take into account, the entire large program and all of its data to make changes. Secondly, the programmer has to consider that data can be corrupted at any point during the program. Thirdly, the program does not take into account there being any common code used repeatedly within the program, which there often is in many programs.

Some ways to make the program simpler are the following:

- **Modularity:** break code into smaller and, ideally, re-useable modules (less complex) versus a single continuous program (more complex)
- **Getting rid of GOTOs by use of *structured code*:** use structured code constructs (less complex) versus non-structured constructs such as goto (more complex, possibly producing "spaghetti code"). Figure 15.11 identifies *structured coding constructs* (Baker 1977). (Note: Many computer languages only support structured coding constructs.)
- **Information hiding via restricting scope:** hide information from the programmer that he does not need to know about by restricting the scope of a variable to a particular program or routine (less complex) versus making the information global (usually more complex)

- **Information hiding via object-oriented techniques:** hide information and routines from the programmer that he does not need to use via object-oriented techniques of making data elements and methods private instead of making all of it public.

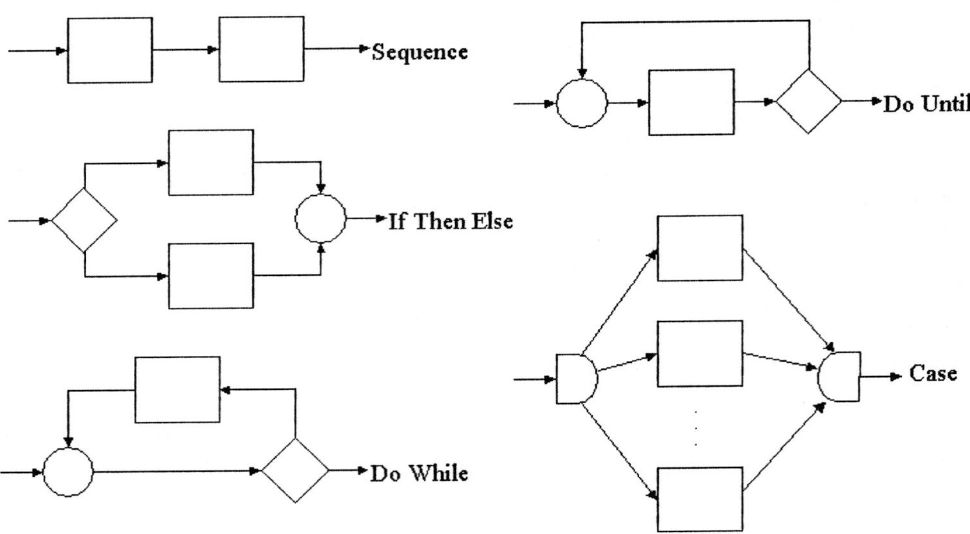

Figure 15.11 Structured programming concepts.

Modularization, including use of object-oriented methods, is itself a form of "information hiding", as the modules can be considered to be "black boxes" as the programmer using them needs to know "what" the module does and what are its inputs and outputs, but does not need to know "how" the module does what it does. As long as the "what" and inputs and outputs remain the same, the "how" can change without the program using the module needing to be changed.

Use of structured code to eliminate "GOTOs" facilitates the break up of programs into modules.

15.7.3.4 Simple, Understandable Code

Because a program is likely to later be maintained, a program, besides being functional, should be a form of communication, providing the future maintenance programmer with sufficient information on the program to easily maintain it. Thus, all means should be used to make the program understandable.

Examples of ways to make a program simpler or more understandable are the following:

- When the programmer has a choice between a "clever" way of doing things in code versus a "simple" or "commonly used" way of doing things, the programmer should always choose the latter.
- Ideally, a simple, straight-forward style of programming should be agreed upon at the start of development step and used in the entire project.
- When a maintenance programmer makes changes to a program, he or she should follow the same style used in the program.

- Conventions that are commonly used in the industry should be enforced. For example, for Microsoft Windows programs in C and C++, the convention is to differentiate different types of variables by a prefix to the variable depending upon type of variable, called the "Hungarian Naming Convention" (McConnell 1993). This may simplify the code.
- As stated earlier, code should be requirements-based, rather than only solutions-based. See section 15.7.3.2.

15.7.3.5 Standards

For a large-scale complex project in a healthcare organization involving automated systems, there are at least two sets of *standards* that are important:

1. General computer-related standards
2. Healthcare standards.

For maintenance reasons, it is important to have standards because

- There is a greater number of maintenance programmers and programmer analysts who are available to be hired, and thus inability to maintain the system due to unavailability of appropriate personnel is less likely (e.g., the C++ programming language is a standard and thus many programmers who use this language can be found, while MUMPS has not reached this level and thus there are many fewer programmers who know this language).
- The automated systems can be more easily interfaced with outside automated systems in the future, in particular with the universal patient record. (Interfacing with HL7 is the standard for healthcare systems.)
- Industry-wide standards are produced by a large number of experts meeting together, thus producing a standard with wide applicability. For example, the largest hardware companies might have gotten together to establish a standard thus making hardware components from these companies interchangeable.
- Code upon which an industry- wide standard is based is most often maintained outside the company using the standard, thus, saving on development and maintenance costs for the company using the standard.
- Industry-wide standards are likely to be very well defined, thus reducing the chance for errors.

Healthcare standards are described in the appendix.
There are many computer-related standards, including those for

- programming languages or platforms (There are many standards, but the most common are C++, .NET, COBOL, and Java)
- database management systems (IBM's DB2 and Oracle are more used than other systems)
- database query language (SQL is the standard)
- network communications (TCP/IP; IEEE and ANSI have compatible standards)
- distributed code (CORBA, RMI, and DCOM are the standards)
- operating systems (UNIX, LINUX, IBM MVS, and the current versions of the Microsoft Windows operating systems)
- Internet scripting language (HTML, and XML in the future).

15.7.3.6 Consistency and Intuitiveness

There are two levels of consistency and intuitiveness that are important in the development step: consistency and intuitiveness in the code, and consistency and intuitiveness in the user interface.

Consistency in code—for example, using the same set of modules throughout, such as modules for user input editing—allows one programmer to copy and reuse the code of others. Consistency and intuitiveness in the code makes it easier for one programmer to understand the code written by other programmers.

Consistency and intuitiveness in the user interface allows the user, in this case the caregiver, to concentrate on his job, caring for the patient. For example, doing the exact same thing differently on three different screens—say selecting an encounter—forces the caregiver to stop and think about what the screen does. Selecting the encounter the same way on all screens—the most intuitive approach that is consistent with other parts of the system and meets standards—enables the caregiver to give greater concentration to caring for the patient.

Key Terms

acceptance testing
business policy
clinical data repository (CDR)
coding
commercial off-the-shelf (or COTS) software
component adaptability
data conversion
direct cut over
function
functional specification
information hiding
integration testing
interface plan
interface testing.
internal design specification
limited parallel operation
maintainability
maintenance
modularization
parallel operation
phase
phase in
regression testing
regressive testing
request for information (RFI)
request for proposal (RFP)
retroactive parallel operation
service level agreement (SLA)
service management system
software development life-cycle
solution alternative analysis
standard
structured coding constructs
system testing
test bed
testing
unit testing
usability testing
validation
verification

Study Questions

1. What is the difference between information in the CDR and information for the total automated patient medical record system?
2. What project steps identified in this book only occur in a phase? Why?
3. Is the CDR database part of a black box view or only a part of the white box view of the CDR? What about functions?
4. Name some clinical systems that provide information for the CDR?
5. Does a project manager have more control over implementing a functional specification or an
10. An automated system can be either developed in-house or can be purchased from a vendor. What is software purchased from a vendor called?
11. What does SLA stand for? What is it? It is a contract between what groups? What system can monitor compliance with an SLA?
12. Name some ways a new automated system can be implemented given a previous automated system. Why is data conversion often necessary in such a situation?
13. What is the software development life-cycle?
14. What does coding mean? Name some systems that

interface plan?

6. Name some business policies that could be associated with the CDR.
7. In the initial overall design, obstacles are looked at in a later step than for a phase. Why?
8. Why does the overall design of the project sometimes have to be revisited?
9. The initial overall design breaks a project into phases. A phase project plan breaks a phase into what? What other events could occur either in the project plan of a project or phase?

support coding.

15. What is validation and what is verification? What is another name for validation? Name some types of validation.
16. For an automated system, what does maintenance mean? Name some ways an automated system can be made more maintainable.
17. What are the two main types of standards for a CDR or automated patient medical record system?

CHAPTER 16

Monitoring and Control of a Project

CHAPTER OUTLINE

16.1 PROJECT CONTEXT: MONITORING AND CONTROL OF A PROJECT

This chapter deals with unplanned events that can occur at any point during the project Subjects covered are

- controlling changes to insure the stability of project products
- monitoring the project to anticipate, identify and control risks
- incorporating changes to the organization during the project.

16.2 CONTROLLING CHANGES TO INSURE STABILITY

In order to provide stability to the project, project agreements must be recorded, and any changes to agreements must be evaluated for their effects upon other agreements. These agreements should thus be recorded in *controlled documentation* (Whitten 1995), and when an agreement is changed, then all other agreements that are based upon that agreement must be reevaluated.

In order to appreciate the importance of controlling documentation, the reader should look at figure 2.11 showing possible documentation in a project. Assume that system requirements are being developed for a project and there is a change in a business requirement. Since the system requirements document and various other documents are written based upon the business requirements, then all sorts of documents, and later on project products, may need to be changed to account for the change in the business requirement. Therefore, especially later on in a project, you want to incorporate changes only when they are necessary, as there may be lots of work to do to incorporate the change.

In order to manage controlled documents in a very large project, there is often a *change control board* (Whitten 1995) for the project to review changes. The change control board would include the overall project manager, phase project managers, representatives of workers, users, the data processing group and business policy management, and usually a change control administration manager to update schedules and provide unbiased advice on business, technical and administrative decisions. Problems of interest to upper management, such as budget issues, would be escalated up to them for resolution.

Thus a *controlled document* is an important document created during a project that cannot be changed without approval of a change control board within a change control process.

As the project progresses, the responsibilities of the phase managers might be consolidated and the change control board might grow smaller, eventually just handling maintenance changes rather than monitoring the project.

When a phase is completed, resulting automated systems should go into *maintenance* mode. Changes to an automated system agreed upon by the change control board would be sent to a business group for design and to a maintenance group for implementation in the automated system. The maintenance group is often part of the group that did the development of the automated system.

Once a phase is implemented, a help desk should take telephone calls from users of an automated system. The help desk would give advice on the use of the system and report on errors and suggested enhancements to the maintenance group who would go through the change board for review.

As the automated system matures, a user group might take over the change control board in reviewing changes.

16.2.1 Controlled Documents

Collectively, controlled documents could include the following information:

- organizational objectives, priorities of objectives, strategies and goals
- project objectives, priorities of objectives, strategies, goals and constraints
- business requirements
- workflow requirements
- system requirements
- organizational business policies
- interface plans
- functional specifications
- internal design documents (programming specifications)
- vendor customization specifications

- programs and program code
- databases and data dictionary
- test plans
- performance and scalability requirements (a "performance and scalability plan")
- user documentation, including descriptions of user interfaces.

Controlled documents apply not only during the development of the system, but after the system has been implemented. After an automated system has been completed, it goes into "maintenance mode" to make *fixes* and *enhancements*. Documents should be kept up-to-date with both development and maintenance mode changes to the system.

Fixes are changes to an automated system to make the system consistent with existing business and user requirements for the system, while *enhancements* are changes to make the automated system correspond to changed business or user requirements. Fixes and enhancements are usually prioritized as to how significant they are to proper running of the system. Documentation on business and user requirements is important here to differentiate between fixes and enhancements, as most often significant fixes are prioritized over enhancements and enhancements usually require more money and time to implement, as they often change the overall design of the system.

As indicated in chapters 13 and 15, documentation that describes an automated system for the system analysts and programmers based upon business and user requirements are functional specifications and internal design specifications. Insuring that any changes in the automated system also be recorded in the functional and internal design specifications provides reference documents from which system analysts and programmers can use to develop or maintain the software making up the automated system.

Technical items from which an automated system can be built—program code, network structures, and database definitions—are also controlled. Program code, hardware setups, and database definitions for previous versions of the automated system are also kept in case a severe problem occurs that requires a changed automated system to be backed out, returning to a previous version. This process, called the *release process* or *version control* is described in detail in section 16.2.4. This process insures that if two programmers or analysts are making changes to the software or database, that they do not override the other's changes.

Controlled documents can be used

- to control changes that may seriously harm a project
- to distinguish an error in the project from a change in the project.

An *error* is an inconsistency between how an agreement, workflow or automated system is implemented and how it is documented—this is either an error in the implementation or in the documentation. A *change* is a modification in the way an agreement, workflow or automated system is implemented when the implementation matches the documentation of it—for a change, both the agreement, workflow or automated system and the documentation should be changed.

Put another way, if controlled documentation says something should work a particular way and that was the agreement and that something does not work that way, then this is in *error* in the way things were implemented. If the controlled documentation says something should work a particular way and that was not the agreement and that something works the way agreed upon, then this is an *error* in the controlled documentation. If the controlled documentation says something should work a particular way and that was the agreement and that something works that way, and now there is an agreement that things should work a different way, then this is an *change* for both the controlled documentation and the implementation.

A *fix* is a correction of an error in an automated system, while an *enhancement* is implementation of a change in an automated system.

Other documents than those listed above are usually less tightly controlled. Often these documents are not controlled because they require frequent changes. Examples are project plans, risks and contingency plans, and discussion ("working") documents. However, all documents should only be changed with careful consideration and consultations.

16.2.2 Change Control Board

Questions the change board might ask are the following:

- Is the change necessary? When?
- What groups are impacted by the change? How will dependencies and schedules be impacted?
- Is there a more effective and preferred change to the one that is proposed? Can changes be consolidated?
- How and when can the change be best made with the least negative impact?
- Will the change also change the overall project?
- After approved: What is the priority of the changes with respect to other approved changes?

If the change would change the overall project or change other phases in the project, then the overall design will have to be re-visited to determine the change's effect on other phases of the project.

16.2.3 Maintenance of an Automated System

Once a function has been completed in an automated system, changes must be introduced in a very disciplined fashion. Changes to existing functionality in an automated system is called *maintenance*. Figure 16.1 illustrates the process of maintenance in an automated system using the UML concept of an *actor*, a stick figure either representing a user of a system or an external system that needs information (Fowler 2003).

A change is proposed by the business group, management or users. A change document describing the change is written. (A change could result from a change in a business policy.) The change is reviewed and approved by the change control board or a user group for the automated system.

The change is discussed with the technical development group who will implement the change and the *quality assurance (QA) group* who will test the change. The function or functions to be changed are analyzed by the business group and the changes are incorporated into the function(s) through updating functional specification(s) describing the functions from an external view. Non-functional specifications may also be updated, for example, for changed performance or business policy requirements.

The development group uses the functional and non-functional specifications to identify the internal changes to the system. The development group makes changes to the internal design specifications and the interface plan, and makes changes to a development version of the automated system or interfaces with other development systems.

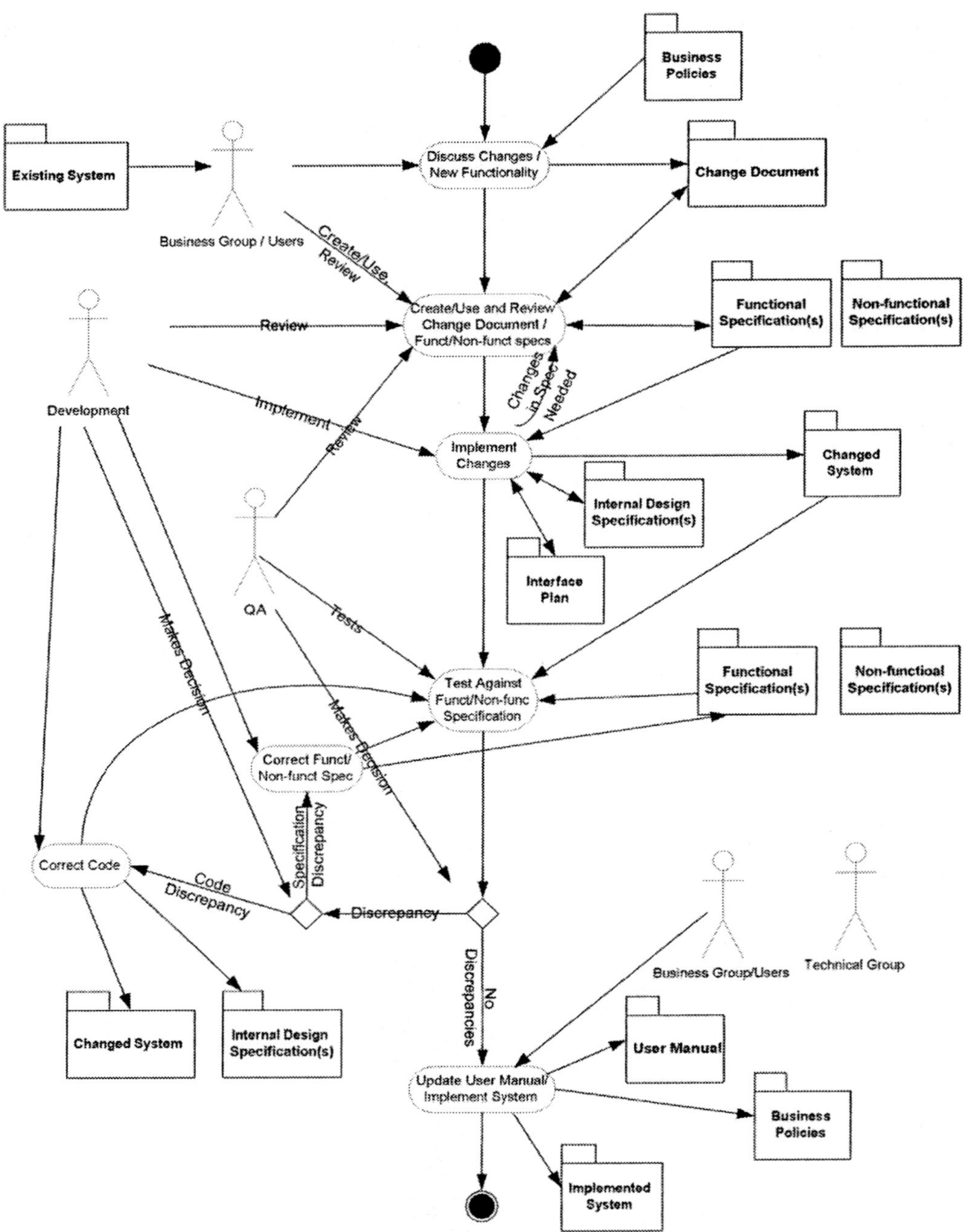

Figure 16.1 Maintenance in an automated system.

QA tests the development version of the automated system and compares the way it works as compared to the functional and non-functional specifications. If there are any discrepancies between the automated system and specifications, it is determined whether there is an error in the changed system or in the specifications. The errors are corrected in either the changed system or specifications. The automated system is then retested against the functional and non-functional specifications.

When no discrepancies are found, user manuals describing the function are updated and any changes to business policies are recorded. Changes to automated systems are implemented in the healthcare organization. Technical documents (program code, data dictionaries, interface descriptions) are updated within release control, with old versions kept to back out the changes if necessary.

16.2.4 The Release Process

A fully functioning automated system or set of automated systems that is delivered to the customer is called a *release* (Whitten 1995). Subsequent releases could fix program errors or introduce changes in the automated systems. Such a release is created from program code, hardware, and databases which together can be used to build or rebuild the automated system.

The release process is also a controlled process. Although new and changed code, databases, etc., should be heavily tested before the release, unexpected problems sometimes occur just after a release. If the release fails, the changed code, databases, etc., should be backed out with return to a previous version of the system (i.e., return to the previous release).

Because the release process generally involves keeping each successive version of the automated systems, the release process is also referred to as *version control.*

Control of software changes—program changes—is called *software configuration management*. Software configuration management is the discipline of managing the evolution of large and complex software systems, through control of different versions of the software, changes back to a previous version, variants of programs, and cooperation (Conradi and Westfechtel 1998).

Variants of a program are two programs that function the same or nearly the same but differ slightly in some way; for example, two variants work exactly the same, but work under two different operating systems. *Cooperation* is allowing multiple developers to work on the same program at the same time, then merging changes—This cannot always be done successfully.

16.3 MONITORING THE PROJECT TO TAKE CARE OF RISKS

Monitoring here means to observe a project or the results of a project in order to change the direction of the project when necessary.

16.3.1 Monitoring the Project

The project manager *monitors* the overall project. A phase project manager monitors his phase. The phase project manager reports to the overall project manager of any risks.

Jointly, phase project managers and overall project manager should

- identify risks, potential project problems, as early as possible
- identify when goals may not be met
- identify when constraints may be violated

- ensure that contingency plans occur before problems occur
- provide and receive project status for the phases and total project.

When there is a significant chance that the goals of the project will not be met, this risk should be reported to upper management. Also, when the constraints of the project may be violated, specifically, costs being overrun and schedules significantly slipped, these risks will be reported.

When there are disagreements between the phase project manager and overall project manager, then resolution will be escalated to the change control board. Lack of resolution there could escalate to upper management.

Figure 16.2 from reference (Hall 1998) lists types of risks, identified and not identified. Of the identified risks, these can be separated into those that the project managers consider to be important and those not considered to be important; of these, the important risks can be built into the schedule as discussed in section 14.2.2. Of these identified important risks, some will be actual problems and contingency plans in the schedule would be initiated.

Of the identified risks, some will be considered not important. These risks considered to be unimportant may, as expected, not become problems, or they may indeed become problems.

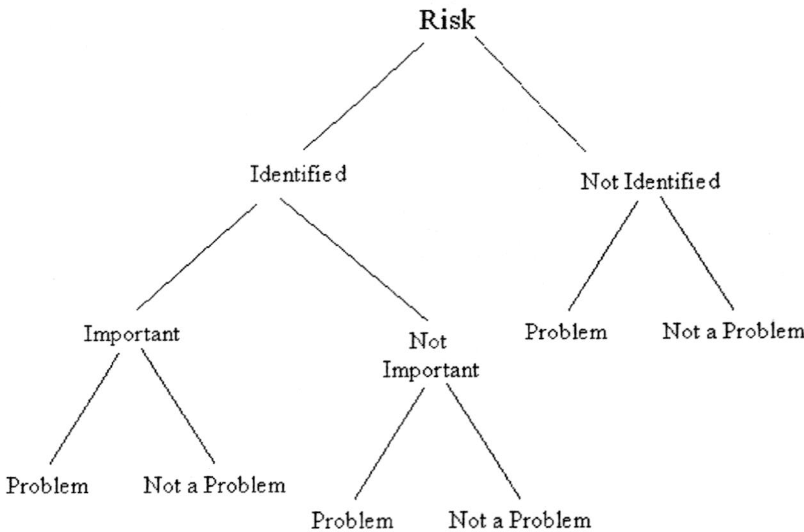

Figure 16.2 Categories of risk. (Hall 1998)

The other category of problems, unidentified problems, have a higher likelihood of being overlooked. Of these, some will become problems and others will not.

Thus, as shown in figure 16.2, there are three paths that result in problems:

1. Those risks that are identified as important and you do nothing about them
2. Those risks that are identified as unimportant and later change into a high risk
3. Those you do not identify and later become problems.

Risks in 1 should never become a problem because the project managers would build contingency plans for them into the schedules. Risks in 2, although probably not built into the schedule, should be recorded and remembered and periodically revisited by project managers to determine if they are now turning into problems. Unidentified risks (3) require constant monitoring by project managers to identify and resolve.

In this book, we discuss complex projects where a lot is likely to be unknown, and thus it is likely at points in the project that the project will be ahead of technology and ahead of standards, resulting in risks involving these areas. There are also likely to be many generic project risks; table 16.1 from reference (Cule, Lyytinen, and Schmidt 1998) identifies the top ten project risks, ranked from most important down to least important, as compiled from studies in three different countries, the USA, Hong Kong and Finland. The results were very much the same in each country.

Table 16.1 Generic software project risks (Cule, Lyytinen, and Schmidt 1998)

Project Risk	*Importance*
Lack of top management commitment to the project	9
Failure to gain user commitment	8
Misunderstanding the requirements	8
Lack of adequate user involvement	7.5
Failure to manage end user expectations	7
Changing scope/objectives	7
Lack of required knowledge/skills in the project personnel	7
Lack of frozen requirements	6.5
Introduction of new technology	6
Insufficient/inappropriate staffing	6
Conflict between user departments	5.5

16.3.2 Monitoring System Performance

A potential problem when automated systems are involved is the potential of the systems not being able to handle initial volumes or increased volumes of data in the future. To take care of this, *performance monitoring* should be a part of all automated systems, especially those that are likely to grow in size, identifying potential future *bottlenecks* in the system, including lack of disk space, lack or processing power, approaching transaction limits, long before they become a problem, so corrective action can be taken.

This process is very complex because automated systems will grow in size due to systems being installed incrementally (e.g., they may be installed at a pilot location first) and due to future increases in number of customers over time. It is also complex because new technology may become available that handles greater capacity but that will incur additional costs to the organization to implement. In this book, it is proposed that information required for this planning be kept in a *performance and scalability plan document* that identifies required response time and other required performance characteristics, future projections of increases in number of customers handled by automated systems, bottlenecks identified so far, and contingency plans for resolving anticipated future performance problems. The performance and scalability plan document would be used by business planners who would project increases in numbers of customers, performance monitors who identify bottlenecks in systems, and capacity planners who would identify requirements for changes to hardware and system software.

16.4 INCORPORATING CHANGES IN THE ORGANIZATION IN A PROJECT

Changes in *business policies* could result in changes to employee workflows, and changes in automated systems, including automated system workflows, databases, code and user interfaces. Ideally, the business policies would be defined as agents (see section 7.6); this could make changes much easier to implement.

Changing business policies is not a "one shot" deal but should involve ongoing process management and improvement. Once business policies have been implemented or change, they should be monitored for actual improvement in business operations or for their intended effects. The employees should be heavily involved in changes to business policies, as such changes are a social process in addition to a business and technical process.

For example, it is likely that there would be many changes in business policies occurring during our project. The following are two examples:

- To compete with lower cost health insurance companies, our HMO has allowed members to buy policies with much lower capitation fees but with a large deductible amount.
- A business policy was to associate every source document for a patient with an encounter and every result with an order. This was found to not always be possible.
- The U.S. Government passed a law that requires emergency departments to give each patient showing up for treatment a *medical screening exam* to determine if the patient does indeed have an emergency condition.

A Large *Deductible* To compete with lower cost health insurance companies, our HMO has allowed members to buy policies with much lower capitation fees but with a large deductible amount. The member, for example, might have to pay for the first three thousand dollars of medical care each year and then pay a co-pay per visit after the deductible has been paid. Because of this, this has changed some aspects of demand management: members are now much more reluctant to come in for care now than they were previously, as member's would have to pay for the care until the deductible was reached. As a result, advice nurses now more often need to encourage members to come in for care when it is medically necessary.

Advice nurses were informed of this change in members' attitudes. To assist advice nurses in the identification of such members, a new automated function was given to advice nurses to identify a member's benefits and remaining deductible.

In addition, the connection between the automated patient medical record identifying services and the billing system billing for these services become more important. As a result, completion of this connection was moved to an earlier phase in the project.

(Note that after the deductible, some PPO insurances, unlike our HMO, pay a certain percentage of costs, typically 70-80%. The remainder to be paid by the patient (20-30%) is called *co-insurance*.)

Encounters, Orders and Results The HMO expected that source documents created during an encounter for a patient could all be associated with with the encounter and that all source documents dealing with results could be associated both with an order, with the order associated with the patient encounter. However, in practice, a number of exceptions were found, including the following:

- Sometimes unsolicited results are returned.
- Sometimes it is too time-consuming to associate a scanned documents to be included in the automated patient medical record with the exact encounter or with the order.
- Some documents, such as the advance directive, are associated with the patient rather than any single encounter.

To account for such documents, (1) a document that could not be associated with an encounter was associated with a dummy encounter including date, time and caregiver, and (2) a result that could not be associated with an order was associated with a dummy encounter including date, time and caregiver, and an associated dummy order. Additionally, a patient's source documents over possibly a span of dates can be selected from a document list, with the documents being placed under agreed-upon selectable tabs such as encounters, clinical lab results, letters, etc. with the assumption that all documents are related to the same episode of care.

Emergency Department Medical Screening Exam A U.S. law, the *Emergency Medical Treatment and Active Labor Act (EMTALA),* was passed to discourage emergency departments from turning away or transferring patients who were in need of services but were unable to pay for these services (EMTALA Online 1994-2003). Its key provisions are the following:

- An emergency department is required to provide a *medical screening exam* to any person who comes to the emergency department requesting an examination or treatment for a medical condition.
- If the emergency department determines that the patient has an *emergency medical condition*, the emergency department must provide further examination and provide treatment to stabilize the patient's medical conditions. An emergency department can transfer such a patient to a more appropriate facility only if it cannot provide the patient with the necessary care.

As a result of this new law, to accommodate the medical screening exam, the HMO changed the way the automated patient medical record worked in the emergency department and changed employee workflows in the emergency department. The screens as shown in sections 12.11 and 12.12 were changed to collect information for the medical screening exam.

The medical screening exam is begun by an RN upon the patient coming to the emergency department and continues through the treatment phase for the patient. The medical screening exam serves as the main part of the history and physical (H&P). The HMO has decided to also use the results of the exam to support demand management: through the medical screening exam the RN determines whether the patient needs to be seen in the emergency department or can be seen in the less costly outpatient clinic.

Note that the following is one definition of an *emergency medical condition* consistent with EMTALA: A medical condition that with the absence of immediate medical treatment could be expected to (1) place the patient's health (or for a pregnant woman, the unborn child's health) in jeopardy, (2) seriously impair bodily functions, or (3) create serious dysfunction of any bodily organ or part.

Key Terms

bottleneck
business policy
change
change control board
controlled document
deductible
emergency medical condition
Emergency Medical Treatment and Active Labor Act (EMTALA)
enhancement
error
fix
maintenance
medical screening exam
monitoring
performance and scalability plan document
performance monitoring
quality assurance (QA) group
release
release process
risk
software configuration management
variant
version control

Study Questions

1. Why is it important to control documentation in a project? Name some documents that may be controlled. What group is usually responsible for this process? What groups of people are often included? When is upper management involved? After a project completes, what usually happens to this group and what happens to automated systems?
2. How do you tell the difference between an error and an enhancement? To correct an error you implement a what? To implement an enhancement you make a what?
3. What is the "release process" and "version control"? What is it used for? What documentation is controlled? What is control of software changes called? What are "variants"? What is "cooperation"?
4. What is "monitoring" a project? Name some of the things project managers might monitor. When monitoring a project, a project manager monitors risks—what kind of risk requires the most vigilance?
5. What is "performance"? Why is it important?
6. If an organization changes, what effect may it have on a project? What has the same effect on a project as a change in the organization?
7. What is EMTALA? What is an "emergency medical condition"? What is a "medical screening exam"? How did our HMO use the medical screening exam for "demand management"?

CHAPTER 17

Incorporating Research and Advances

CHAPTER OUTLINE

17.1 PROJECT CONTEXT: INCORPORATING RESEARCH AND ADVANCES IN A PROJECT

Creation of an automated patient medical record system goes beyond development of a software and hardware system. It requires research in the areas of new technology and medicine. It requires the development of national (or international) standards for medicine and new technology. It may require new laws.

See figure 17.1. In a research phase, after the research is done, there is an evaluation that determines whether to continue the research. A decision might be made to continue the research step, discontinue the research, or to proceed with incorporating and implementing the research into the project systems.

Incorporating the research into the project produces a new phase. Like for other phases, as part of the business analysis step of the phase, a determination should be made as to whether the overall design needs to be redone to incorporate the research ideas into the overall project.

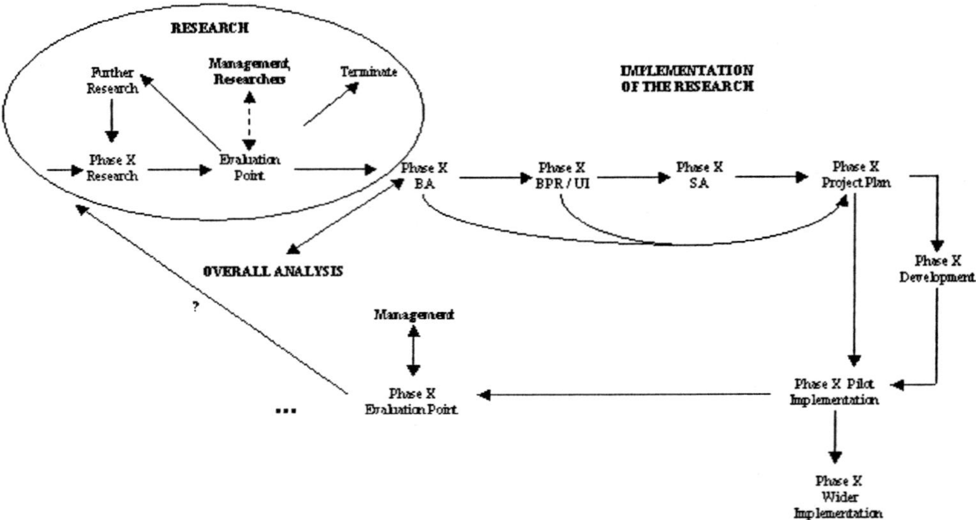

Figure 17.1 A research phase.

17.2 HARDWARE TECHNOLOGY

Hardware technology is changing at a rapid pace, with increases in speed, storage capacity, portability, battery life and battery size, and other capabilities. New technology is continually being introduced, becoming less expensive as it matures. Some new technology, which existed in the past but was impractical, now is practical (e.g., biometrics).

17.2.1 Universal Patient Record Network and Telecommunications

The CPR and source document repositories are dependent upon there being high bandwidth networks.

Chapter 6 speculates on the main external network connections required for a universal patient health record. Figure 6.3 identifies what an initial network for an HMO and alliance healthcare organizations or for different regions of an HMO might look like. Figure 6.4 identifies what a network might look like after the system evolved into one handling unaffiliated healthcare organizations also.

In both cases, it is assumed that broadband connections would be required for a healthcare organization's connections to its own CPR repository and source document repository, probably using *dedicated lines*. For the extended network in figure 6.4 it is assumed that lower bandwidth connections, such as over an Internet, might suffice for connections to outside CPR repositories and source document repositories, as universal patient record information in outside healthcare organizations in the future could potentially be in many different possible locations, and thus dedicated network connections would not be feasible. In the future, with higher bandwidth public networks such as *Sonet* optical networks using *WDM (wave length division multiplexing)*, dedicated lines may not be necessary (Clark 1998).

In any case, network communications involving patient medical records are likely to require a larger amount of information than other types of network communications as

- **Diagnostic images:** Some information may be voluminous, especially *diagnosticl images* such as digitized MRIs, x-rays and cat-scans.
- **Security:** Extra information is required in the communication to insure secure and reliable communications. For example, for connections that require high security, encryption of information is needed, necessitating transmission of more information and thus higher bandwidth than non-encrypted data, and reliable communication requires two-way communication with the receiver of the information acknowledging correct receipt of the information.

In order to determine the network requirements for an automated patient medical record system, application analysts should work together with network analysts to identify the size and frequency of messages and the network bandwidth needed to handle these communications. Only through such an analysis can it be determined whether existing networks are adequate for the healthcare network required, or if network structures based upon future hardware, and software, advances are required.

Part of such a network likely will include the Internet or a similar such network, perhaps one dedicated to healthcare. It should be noted that typical Internet communications are much slower than direct connections between computers. Figure 17.2(a) shows a possible connection over the Internet. A workstation might make a request for information from a Web server, establishing a path connecting these computers. The Web server sends back the requested information, through the same or another path. Usually, both the workstation and Web server are connected to the Internet through *Internet service providers (ISPs)* from whom they buy time. ISPs may buy time from other ISPs or be connected to computers or routers called *network access points (NAPs)* from whom the ISPs buy time. The NAPs interconnect, providing paths between ISPs.

Compare this Internet path with two computers that are directly connected. See figure 17.2(b). Such a bi-directional direct connection is referred to as a *point-to-point connection*, with equality of the capabilities of the computers it is referred to as *peer-to-peer connection*. Such a direct connection should be much faster than the Internet connection. Internet-type connections obviously have much higher security risks than direct connections.

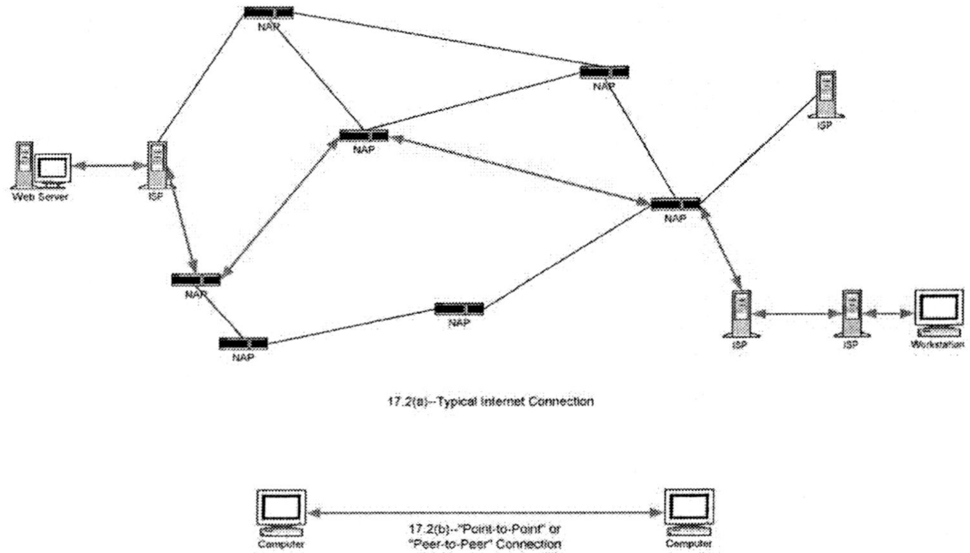

Figure 17.2 Some types of Internet network connections.

17.2.2 Computer Architecture

Computer architecture is the structure and interaction of the hardware components of a computer. Some current changes in computer architecture that could have a very positive effect on the development of the automated patient medical record system are the following:

- **Lighter weight computers with increased battery life:** decreases in size and power consumption of computer systems, making for very lightweight, portable, but easy to use, computer systems that are mobile and can be carried around or easily picked up, and have a very long battery life (e.g., a thin, lightweight, clipboard size computerized equivalent to the patient chart)
- **Greater use of multimedia:** computer architectures that support multimedia processing, including speech, voice recognition, high density images, and video encode and decode and databases that support multimedia
- **More processing power:** Many computers can be executing a single problem, or a single computer can support many processors:

  Grid computing is concurrently applying the resources of many computers (with at least one processor in each) in a network to a single problem that requires a great number of computer processing cycles or access to a large amount of data. The most well known use of grid computing is the SETI (Search for Extraterrestrial Intelligence) @Home project searching for life in outer space (Berman, Fox, and Hey 2003)

  Multiprocessing is using multiple processors in the same computer, allowing multiple parts of one or more programs to run at once. Multiprocessor scalable computers (also known as parallel processors) with anywhere from 2 to 100 processors that can be used as servers and that can also support simultaneous multithreading—*multithreading* is executing parts of one or more programs at the same time, e.g., in two different processors. This multiprocessing capability could be used to execute programs for multiple workstations concurrently, while the multithreading capability could be used to execute the same program code (e.g., agents) concurrently. Multiprocessing capability is particularly important for very large databases (e.g., data warehouses) and by operational databases that can be used by a large number of users. Most multiprocessors fall into three categories: Symmetric Multiprocessors (SMP's), clusters, and Massively Parallel Processors (MPP's). This architectures are said to support scalability of large databases.

17.2.3 Computer Storage

The CPR and source document repositories are dependent upon there being high capacity storage media. Such storage media can store information and retain it when the system is turned off. Existing technologies include

- **rigid or *hard* magnetic *disks:*** relatively high-speed and high-volume storage using electromagnetism to store data.
- **disk arrays:** hard disks tied together by connections between them. This arrangement allows relatively inexpensive disks to store a large amount of information redundantly so if data is lost, it can be recovered. One version is RAID.
- ***optical disks:*** high-volume, slower speed and less costly storage than hard disk, using laser rather than electromagnetism to read and write data. Examples are CDs and DVDs.
- ***magnetic tape:*** relatively inexpensive storage with very large storage capacities, but they provide serial access, rather than random access, to data.
- **autochangers**: racks of tape cartridges or optical disks that can be moved by robotics, the most common of which is a *jukebox* for optical disks.

Using these storage technologies, there are a number of different types of storage architectures using these technologies, including the following (Intel 2002):

- **direct attached storage:** a disk drive directly attached to a server for clients. This is the most common means of transferring data over Local Area Networks (LANs). It has a high cost to manage, and is expensive to scale.
- **network attached storage (NAS):** storage is directly attached to the network, much like a server. Storage traffic is transmitted over the LAN also. Can be easily supported by network personnel. Not scalable because storage traffic could swamp other network traffic.
- ***storage area networks (SANs):*** networks dedicated to connecting servers to storage devices that doesn't interfere with other network traffic in the enterprise LAN. Flexible and scalable but expensive. Uses fiber channels and thus expertise in the personnel who support it.
- **Internet SCSI:** encapsulating SCSI commands into TCP/IP packets enabling network communication to a storage unit to be treated like communication between computers on the Internet. A high-cost, low-cost, long-distance storage solution. Standards for Internet SCSI are now being established.
- **MAID (massive arrays of idle disks) systems:** Disk backup systems that use massive arrays of idle disks—Advanced Technology Attachment disk subsystems—could displace magnetic tape libraries for archival data functions. (Mearian 2004)

- **COLD (Computer Output to Laser Disk):** a system for archiving data to one or more optical disks in a compressed form, which is slow but easily retrievable. Over one million pages of print could be stored on one 5 ¼" optical disk. Optical disks often are stored on jukeboxes. COLD is often used for scanned documents. This strategy has replaced microfiche. (TechTarget 2000-2004),
- **content-addressed storage:** a magnetic high-volume disk-based WORM (write once, read many) device. It insures that the content does not change and allows search for documents given a set of associated indexes. (Pastore 2003)

More and more data is being stored on its own network apart from the LAN, on "storage area networks", SANs, using fiber channel technology (light waves). A SAN links storage devices, including disks, disk arrays, and magnetic tape, to create a pool of storage that users can access directly. With SANs and fiber channels, data can be transmitted at higher speeds over greater distances than other methods. With the volume of medical information and need for speed of access to this information in our HMO, SANs may be an appropriate way to pool storage devices within our HMO.

The basic rule of storage of medical records electronically is that as documents age they will be accessed less often. Thus, as documents age they can be put on lesser cost storage devices—Usually this equates to slower access devices. For example, final archiving of medical documents might be output to COLD.

17.2.4 Workstations, Including Portable Computers and Wireless Networks

Both lightweight and desktop computers are needed for an automated patient medical record.

In order for a computer to be used at the "point of care", it must not get in the way of communication between the caregiver and patient. Thus it must be portable and unobtrusive. Ideally, it would be connected to servers via a wireless network, so it would not be attached by wires and be carried from location to location, and so it need not have a hard disk, which adds weight and consumes energy in its use. It must be light, especially so it could be carried around without strain. A very portable computer is especially necessity for home health care.

As previously discussed in section 12.2.3, a number of different types of "portable" computers currently exist, including the following:

- *Laptop computers*
- *PDAs (personal digital assistants)*
- *Tablet computers.*

Laptop computers are increasingly becoming excellent substitutes for full-size PCs, with adequate screen sizes, full size keyboards, with multi-GigaByte+ disks and wireless network connections. But such computers are 6 pounds and over, still too heavy to carry around all day, and are not unobtrusive, with keyboard input.

Small computers are available, referred to as PDAs or personal digital assistants, but they are way too small—especially screen size—to be useable for recording patient care and have a less powerful operating system than larger computers, although they have been used by a few nurses in inpatient care and physicians in recording prescriptions.

A type of "portable" computer that may be of use in the future is a tablet-size pen computer, perhaps the size of the current patient chart. With future technology, such a computer could possibly be made very lightweight; it could possibly be so lightweight, that it could be portable, or it could stay in the patient's room, being treated identically to the current patient chart. (Note that some laptop computers convert into pen computers, sometimes removing keyboards or hard disks, making them lighter.)

The advantage and also possible liability of the pen computer is that there is either no keyboard, or the keyboard can be detached making the computer less obtrusive, and the computer can be used like a chart pad when being used in the care of a patient. This then requires that input be by pen, rather than be keyboard. Input then as described in section 12.2.4, more by selection than character input, is thus necessary to use a pen computer efficiently, with the pen computer being able to recognize the caregivers printing or handwriting.

Handwriting recognition software in pen computers is often not very good. In the future it may, hopefully, much improve.

Current versions of pen computers are made lightweight by not having a keyboard, and, when having a wireless connection to a server, not even having a hard disk. For the current really lightweight pen computers, those without keyboards or off-line storage, everything input to the pen computer is saved in memory. Loss of power, for example, a battery going dead, could lose all information—the answer to this problem is having data input immediately transmitted through a wireless network to the server, so the data would never be lost. For other heavier pen computers having hard disks, information could be saved to the hard disk and not lost.

In any case, current battery technology is a limitation for all portable computers. For pen computers without permanent hard disks, battery technology needs to be improved so that loss of data could not occur. For pen computers with hard disks, battery technology needs to be improved so constant recharging becomes unnecessary, although if a pen computer is kept in a docking station when it is not in use, say in the inpatient's room or in an outpatient exam room where it can be recharged, then this may not be a problem.

In all cases, to insure true portability, wireless networks should be used. In that regard, there is some concern about wireless networks that use radio waves in wave lengths that interfere with medical instrumentation. Wireless communication that extends outside the medical building, as stated earlier, also poses security concerns of being intercepted.

For any portable computer, theft or loss is another potential problem. Valuable medical record information could be lost and patient information privacy could be compromised.

17.2.5 Diagnostic Image Storage and Monitors

Storage of diagnostic images requires special hardware because of storage to display them monitors to display them.

Diagnostic images, also called *medical images*, are a number of technologies producing digital images of the internal body that can be used for diagnosis. Digitized computerized diagnostic image systems are sometimes called *PACS (Picture Archiving and Communication System).*

Diagnostic images are different than *clinical images* that are scanned medical documents producing images that can be stored on the automated patient medical record system along with completely automated documents.

Diagnostic images must contain significant information to be of use. As mentioned earlier in this section, storage and transmission of such information requires very high capacity and quick storage and requires very high bandwidth network connections.

What is also needed is a monitor with a very high resolution, a high refresh rate, and which is probably quite large in physical size. Each pixel (or dot) must be able to either display a great number of colors or a great number of gray scale values. Monitor resolutions are measured by a dot matrix array of points, expressed in terms of number of horizontal pixels (or dots) in length by the number of vertical pixels in height (e.g., 1048 x 1048). Refresh or scan rates must be high enough for the screen not to flicker (e.g., 60 Hz). Each pixel (or dot) may be a different color or gray scale value; stored for each pixel would be a binary number, or set of on and off switches, to identify the color or gray scale value (8 bits to represent colors or shades of gray). Standard or typical values for VGA are 640 x 480 pixels with a refresh rate of 60 Hz supporting 16 different colors per pixel. Typical values for super VGA are 1024 x 768 pixels with 256 colors or 1280 x 1024 with 16 colors.

Although diagnostic images on a screen can be scrolled, full size display is much easier for a caregiver to use for diagnosis. Full size display of diagnostic images for a representative PACS system generally requires higher resolution than VGA.

There are concerns with high-resolution monitors. High-resolution monitors often cost a lot of money, and further, such monitors may take up lots of space. Further, such monitors may not be able to also substitute for the lower resolution monitors for other purposes; thus, space would be required both for the high-resolution monitors and the lower resolution ones. Therefore due to cost and space considerations, it is unlikely that every physician ordering a diagnostic image would have such a monitor available to view the diagnostic images. Unless a copy of the diagnostic image is passed back to the ordering physician like it is in many cases now, the ordering caregiver would probably not be able to see the diagnostic image—he would only be able to read the interpretation. In such a case, a PACS system might not be of much benefit to many of a healthcare organization's physicians.

Despite these issues, the Kaiser Permanent HMO is building a new hospital that will have digital diagnostic images in place of analog ones. In the future, more and more healthcare organizations are likely to move to digital diagnostic images.

Digitization of diagnostic images is a necessary requirement for the up and coming field of computerized assistance in diagnosing diagnostic images. Only when diagnostic images are digitized is this feasible.

17.2.6 Security Hardware: Smart Cards, Biometrics, etc.

A number of technologies are required to support security for an automated patient medical record and universal patient record.

Security and smart cards were previously discussed in section 10.10. A *smart card* is a credit card size plastic card containing a microprocessor. A number of possible healthcare uses for smart cards, more formally called *Integrated Circuit Cards (ICCs),* were mentioned in this paper:

- to enable a caregiver to gain secure access to an automated healthcare system
- to enable a patient to gain secure access to the his own medical record
- to store a patient's medical history, in particular emergency medical data, and insurance information
- to store condition-specific information on a chronic condition or pregnancy.

Many European countries use smart cards for healthcare. The European Union has developed a specification for the inoperability and security of smart cards in the EU as well as requirements for future use of smart cards in healthcare as an enabling technology (eEurope 2003). For example, most European countries use smart cards for healthcare insurance purposes. Countries including Austria, France, and Ireland have plans to use smart cards for emergency medical information. Germany also uses smart cards as provider identification cards. Some smart cards have been used for particular health conditions including pregnancy, renal dialysis, and implanted defibrillator devices. NETLINK promotes smart card standards not only for some European nations but also for Canada's province of Quebec.

Smart cards suffer from the potential of loss or theft. Use of smart cards to store information suffers from the potential of inaccurate information, especially medical information, and thus potential liability.

Another method of providing security access for a caregiver to an automated patient medical record system and to a patient to see his medical record is *biometrics*, using a person's physical characteristics to identify the person. Commercially available systems exist that identify caregivers by the following methods (Phillips 1997):

- fingers
- hands
- eyes
- faces
- voices
- keystrokes
- signatures.

Smart card technology can also be combined with biometrics for extra security. Biometric data could be stored on a smart card and compared against that input from the caregiver user.

17.2.7 Caregiver Tracker (Indoor Positioning System)

In order to support outpatient clinic, inpatient unit or emergency department room maps, a caregiver tracker is needed. Such a system is an *indoor positioning system (IPS).*

Each caregiver seeing patients within an outpatient clinic would wear a "tracker". The tracker would be able to identify when a caregiver entered a room or left it. This tracker information could be fed to the automated patient medical record system which could use it to identify that a caregiver has seen the patient and what room he has seen the patient in, updating an "outpatient clinic room map" (see figure 12.22).

If there was a workstation in the room, the caregiver would be automatically logged on to the automated patient medical record system. And as he left he would automatically be logged off. This would insure that confidential patient information for the current patient was not available to a subsequent patient. The practically of *caregiver tracking* should be evaluated for cost and feasibility.

Indoor positioning systems are of two types: gateway systems and mobile positioning systems. A gateway system reads the signal as a tag passes a gate. In a mobile positioning system, a tag periodically sends out a signal that is received by a receiver. (Stahl et al. 2004)

17.3 SOFTWARE TECHNOLOGY

17.3.1 Mainframe Systems Versus Distributed Systems (Including the Intranet)

In order to support a lot of users of an automated patient medical record systems for a large healthcare organization, the organization must either have large mainframe computers or a distributed system consisting of many computers connected in a network, and probably both.

This book describes an automated patient medical record system that is distributed system with interfaces with other clinical systems and interfaces through a TCP-IP, Internet type, network, to a patient registry, CPR and source document repositories. A *distributed system* is implementation of a single application system on multiple computer systems at different locations with the systems usually connected by a network.

IBM Corporation's *Customer Information Control System (CICS)* is a transaction processing system on IBM mainframe systems and is IBM's most popular mainframe system software system. The high use of mainframes using CICS systems, with continuing predictions that they will all be replaced by distributed systems, has shown that there are still many advantages of mainframe CICS systems over distributed systems:

- a single sign-in
- easy release of new and changed programs
- strong support for on-line transaction processing (OLTP) that splits processing into transactions, where a transaction (e.g., entry of an order) is a logical unit of work that usually involves a set of updates to a database that can either all be made permanent at once or all backed out if something goes wrong—Note that transactions are a necessary attribute for high volume systems (Gray and Reuter 1993)
- consistent security
- fail-safe backup of database information to any previous time
- no program failures due to program incompatibilities
- excellent use of multi-processing and multi-threading (multi-tasking), and also multi-programming (with respect to CICS and other mainframe programs running concurrently)
- large disk drive capacities
- spooling (queuing) of printouts on printers
- the ability to have central control of the entire system.

To be successful, distributed systems must also gain most of these capabilities.

Distributed systems in general are composed of many heterogeneous (i.e., different brand or model) computers with distributed databases and operating systems, with the computers connected by computer networks. Computers include servers that run the main software for multiple workstations (client computers), and may include mainframe computers. Each workstation serves a user with the workstation handling the GUI user interface for the particular user and passes information to the server to run the associated program on the server. (Distributed) databases are usually on the server or on connected mainframe (large scale) or minicomputer (medium scale) systems.

Distributed systems have the following advantages over CICS systems:

- GUI user interfaces with windowing
- the ability to distribute processing among workstations, multiple server computers and legacy systems, and thus there is less of a chance of any component getting overloaded and causing poor response time
- independent control of independent systems.

As much as possible, the automated patient medical record system and universal patient record must possess all these positive attributes of CICS and distributed systems. Commercial products are available that provide CICS-like capabilities for heterogeneous distributed systems; some of these products are as follows:

- network communication management products (e.g., SNMP, Simple Network Management Protocol that is a protocol standard that has evolved as a support mechanism for TCP/IP based networks)
- remote control of remote servers or workstations
- *single sign-in* products with security control of multiple systems and all of the data
- OLTP (on-line transaction processing) products
- distributed database products, including data integrity features
- print service (to control and queue printouts)
- time service (to synchronize time among different systems)
- directory services to create a directory of files stored on multiple distributed computers
- software distribution products that allow software in remote computers to be installed, updated or removed without doing it manually
- change management software that keeps a history of changes so the system can be changed back to a previous version of the software, if necessary.

Together, these products support enterprise management of an organization's distributed computer network. Together, these products, if available as a total package, are collectively referred to as an *enterprise management system (or package).* In order for enterprise management system to work, the distributed network must follow standardized technology and structures for hardware, operating systems, data bases, fault tolerances, and network and communications transport, referred to as "open systems architecture" or simply "open architecture". The Gartner Group has stated that of the enterprise management packages implemented so far, after 36 months only 30% have been fully implemented and an additional 10% are partially implemented (Gillooly 1998).

(Note: A proposal for synchronizing the times on computers is to use the U.S. Atomic clock. The U.S. atomic clock, located outside Boulder, Colorado, sends out radio wave signals identifying the exact time. The U.S. atomic clock is operated by the U.S. Department of Commerce's National Institute of Standards and Technology.)

A part of any automated patient medical record system, whether mainframe or distributed GUI system, should be the Internet, for medical reference and potentially for chart information. The Internet is the most successful "distributed system". Its advantages are the following:

- composed of many independent systems
- communication occurs between systems, even when some network paths are down
- consistent network, naming and other standards that work despite systems being independent.

Although the Internet is probably the most successful distributed system, use of the Internet only for the patient medical record has the following problems:

- within the Internet, there is a lack of memory about a user and the previous screens he has seen ("statelessness"), thus making it difficult to develop secure, sophisticated, systems—see section 12.2.3
- the Internet is slow for an operational system

- there are potential major security risks with use of the Internet for the patient medical record; since the Internet is open to the general public, its use potentially opens up access to the patient medical record to the general public.

It should be noted that new standards are currently being developed for the Internet and TCP/IP-like (Internet-like) networks. For example, internet protocol IP version 6 (IPv6) has been identified as the next Internet and a replacement for the current IP version 4 (IPv4) protocol (Hinden 1996). IPv6 would have the following advantages over IPv4:

- expanded addressing—allowing more locations to be uniquely identified within the network
- additional routing techniques—possibly allowing for somewhat higher speed networks and greater redundancy of connections
- greater support for transmission of multi-media
- additional security features.

A future network entity with similarities to the Internet is the "digital library".

From 1994 to 1998, the federal government through the NSF (National Science Foundation), DARPA (Defense Advanced Research Projects Agency), and NASA, funded the Digital Libraries Initiative (DLI) to do research on the study of a distributed library on-line (Svenonius 2000). Although the universal patient record is more homogeneous than such a digital library, it involves many of the same issues of organization, access, security and use of distributed information resources, and thus research on digital libraries may apply to the universal patient record.

17.3.2 Utility Computing

For healthcare organizations that cannot afford to have their own computer systems for the automated patient medical record, *application service providers (ASPs)* with *n-tier systems* are a possibility. ASPs with n-tier systems could support utility computing.

Utility computing is treating computing like an electric utility, telephone company, or other type of utility where computing service for a particular application is paid on a "pay-for-use" basis. For example, the automated patient medical record can be provided to small healthcare organizations and "customers can use a shared infrastructure and pay only for the capacity that each one needs" (Gayek et al. 2004).

An IBM System Journal is devoted to utility computing (Birman and Ritsko 2004). It discusses the need for new relationships for companies using utility computing services and those providing it, about the need for new system architectures, about the need for new pricing policies, about service level agreements (SLA), among other topics.

The model for a utility computing system is the "application service provider (ASPs)" as discussed earlier in this book and "n-tier systems" as shown in figure 12.20. Reference discusses the need for specialized tiers, for example a "metering server"(Gayek et al. 2004).

17.3.3 Agents and Organizational Business Policies

Agents enable business policies to be implemented in automated systems with the control of these business policies by business people rather than technical people.

The word "agent" has been used for many different abstract things, from a special way of writing programs to a program that specializes in a particular job function, similar to a very specialized human worker, to a program that can reason and communicate with other agents (Caglayan and Harrison 1997). With my concept of "agent", either of the first two definitions may apply with agent-to-agent communication also being a possibility, but I have a far less abstract definition of an *agent*: a way of categorizing and separating out a set of independent code or tables implementing an organizational business policy, so that this policy could be easily implemented and as necessary later be changed by the people responsible for the business policy, rather than solely by computer people, without effecting the other code in the system. With this concept, a healthcare organization is not totally dependent upon programmer expertise to change business rules embedded within software systems.

Agents are best handled by distribution of agent code within the various computer systems making up the automated patient medical record system. Code or tables for regional agents should be in a regional computer. Code or tables for other agents might be in local computers. Distribution of this code might be best handled by use of CORBA, or other system software that enables distribution of this code.

Agents are a huge research area.

An agent can assist in incorporation of an organizational business policy in a system. An agent is only part of this incorporation. An organizational business policy should be documented and can implemented through a combination of code or tables (an agent), interfaces between systems, database information used by the agent, user interfaces to control input of the necessary information, and operational policies that users must follow to follow the business policy.

17.3.4 Security Software

Implementation of security within the automated patient medical record and universal patient record system must handle the many levels of security demanded by the system:

- federal regulations controlling access to a patient health record
- multiple state regulations controlling access to a patient health record, where the patient health record, in total, may exist in many different states of the U.S.
- potential international access to the patient health record
- caregiver access to patient clinical information based upon caregiver need to know
- patient access to his patient health record
- control of caregiver ordering
- control of caregiver ordering of controlled substances
- possible special security for some categories of patient clinical information, such as information related to psychiatry and genetics.

Because of these many levels of security demanded of the systems, security may be the "Achilles' heal" that may make it difficult to fully implement the universal patient record.

17.3.5 Searching and Selecting from the Automated Patient Medical Record

Within the last few years, significant research has been done by commercial companies on information retrieval of textual documents on the Internet via "search engines" and related software. Although this may have direct applicability to retrieval of information in medical literature, and perhaps will have future applicability to anonymously searching through the universal patient record databases for patients for medical research, it may not apply to searches through the medical record by a clinician in the care of a patient. The latter, I think, is an area where significant additional research will be needed.

As discussed in section 7.7.6, creating a useful information retrieval (i.e., searching) method for clinicians to find information in the automated patient medical record and universal patient record is closely related to establishing a consistent medical vocabulary and thesaurus of medical terminology (see section 17.4.7). Clinicians must have a common medical vocabulary or the clinician who tries to find information will be searching for different information than the information that was entered by previous clinicians.

17.3.6 Group and Collaborative Communication

Patient care is often a collaborative effort, involving a number of different caregivers all caring for the same patient. Because the automated patient medical record can be available to many different caregivers at the same time, whereas the paper chart is only available at a single location, the automated patient medical record has great potential for enhancing this group, and collaborative, communication amongst caregivers in the care of a patient. *Group communication* is concurrent view of documents by multiple users at the same time and possible updating at the same time. In this book, *collaborative communication* is communication while two or more caregivers have access to the automated patient medical record.

Group and collaborative communication by caregivers may be

1. **same time/same place:** two or more caregivers, located at the same physical location, are looking at, and possibly adding to, the patient chart at the same time
2. **same time/different place:** the telemedicine situation where two or more caregivers, possibly located at different physical locations, are looking at, and possibly adding to, the patient chart at the same time
3. **different time/different place:** the chart is accessed by a single caregiver at a time with communication possible via various means, including e-mail or messaging.

Case 3 is not a problem, as only a single caregiver is accessing the chart or other information at a time.

Cases 1 and 2 are nearly functionally equivalent and they are problematic. These cases must be handled by concurrency, and other, controls such as

- identification of *readers* who can view a part of the automated medical record along with others and *writers* who can view and update that part of the automated medical record when it is being viewed
- file sharing
- locking out of other users (possibly at the document or field level)
- back out procedures if things go wrong
- possible priority of assess of one caregiver over another
- *cooperative editing systems*, "multi-user systems where the actions of one user are instantaneously propagated to all the other participating users" (Ionescu and Marsic 2000)
- other controls.

In order to determine the required concurrency controls and other techniques for cases 1 and 2, the following questions must be answered: Can one caregiver be viewing a document in the chart, while another is adding to the document or changing it? If allowed or not, how does the system control this?

If one user is updating a document and another is viewing the document, will the viewer also see the update? If so, how can this be done?

Can two caregivers, or more, be adding to the same document in the chart at the same time? If so, how does the system control this? An example presented in this book was an emergency department triage document that included an H&P (see figures 12.49 and 12.52).

Can the two caregivers be changing the same fields at the same time? If so, what are the rules for this?

For case 2, same time/different place, where caregivers may be at vastly different geographic locations, the caregivers may work in two different facilities, each associated with a different distributed system. How is the chart concurrently accessed in this situation? What concurrency, and other, controls are required?

17.3.7 Voice Recognition

Voice recognition—computer recognition of voices—is currently practically used in medical care, especially in the radiology department for dictation of radiology results. Various companies have viable systems, including Dictaphone, Kurzweil and IBM .

Voice recognition is increasingly be used directly by physicians who in turn would do their own medical transcription—voice input and then editing—in place of medical transcriptionists. The Garner group in 2001 predicted that "continuous speech recognition will result in a 70% reduction in healthcare transcription staffing by 2004."

Considerations for picking voice recognition systems are the following:

- **speaker dependent versus speaker independent systems**: With speaker dependent systems, each user must go through sessions of inputting his voice so the system can adequately recognize his voice.
- **discrete speech input versus continuous speech input**: Discrete speech systems require the user to pause between words. Continuous speech systems do not.
- **vocabulary supported by the system**: Various available systems have vocabularies for internal medicine, radiology, orthopedic surgeons, emergency medicine, pathology, diagnostic imaging, cardiology.
- **documents supported by the system**: Some systems support particular kinds of documentation (e.g., SOAP notes, radiology reports).
- **RAM memory required**: because systems, especially the more sophisticated systems, require lots of RAM memory to run, the existing computer systems that can currently use them may be limited.
- **languages supported**
- **operating system required**.

Various companies are in competition for the medical speech recognition market, including Dragon, Kurzweil, IBM, Dictaphone, and Kolvox. Any chosen system must have the capability of being integrated into the automated patient medical record system.

Voice recognition is also used in connection with call centers. Interactive voice recognition (IVR), also known as voice response units, or VRUs, is technology connected with a call center that interprets the caller's voice and performs actions accordingly.

17.3.8 Handwriting Recognition

Handwriting recognition—printed or handwriting recognition by computers—is important because, without it, pen computing is not feasible. I feel that pen computers are the only truly portable, unobtrusive, computers. Among all types of computers, a tablet pen computer, alone, can unobtrusively replace the current chart pad.

Considerations for handwriting recognition are the following:

- **printed input versus cursive input**: Can the user use handwriting or must he use printed input?
- **controlled input versus writer dependent input**: Must the user use a controlled input, inputting characters in a specific ("graffiti-type")format, or will the system accept the user's chosen character set?
- **use of dictionary and word relationship techniques:** Does the approach use a dictionary to improve accuracy? Does the approach user probabilities of certain words following others?
- **training:** Does the approach require training (i.e., the user to give controlled samples of input)?
- **obsolescence:** Is there a chance that the system will become obsolete? Many systems using handwriting recognition have disappeared.
- **part of the computer s operating system:** So far, most handwriting recognition programs have been part of the operating system. If the handwriting recognition program is not part of the operating system, then consideration must be made about the capability of the program with specific applications and with the automated patient medical record system.
- **RAM memory required**: Because pen computers are usually limited in memory, but the quality of a handwriting recognition program might be dependent upon the size of the program, RAM memory requirements may be important.

Reference (NICI Handwriting Recognition Group 1995) identifies links for pen and mobile computing and handwriting recognition.

17.4 MEDICAL AREA RESEARCH

17.4.1 Cases and Outcomes Research

Outcomes are the results of care given to a patient. The purposes of treatment cases and chronic care management cases are twofold:

1. continuity of care
2. evaluation of the outcomes of the medical care—with these outcomes based upon the patient, the medical condition of the patient, the treatments given and procedures given—so that different care, procedures and treatments for the same medication condition and similar patients can be compared and evaluated, and **so that patient care can be improved.**

How do you evaluate outcomes? How do you compare outcomes? These are research questions to be answered.

The outcomes of a treatment should be a final part of the treatment case and a part of chronic care management case. In order to evaluate outcomes equitably for various providers, the condition, age, sex and other characteristics of the patient, available from the Patient's Clinical Summary, should be taken into account.

One method to evaluate outcomes is a questionnaire given to the patient after a treatment, SF-36 or HSQ-12 (Health Status Questionnaire). Such questionnaires are currently available for a number of conditions, including knee replacement and hypertension. The questionnaire deals with gathering information on the patient's perception of his quality of life after the medical care. The adequacy of such an outcomes evaluation is an open question, and methods of outcomes evaluations are likely to further evolve in the future.

Some outcomes can be more objective, such as measuring a patient's blood pressure after a treatment to reduce the patient's blood pressure. In fact, the patient may not even notice a difference in his health or quality of life, even if his blood pressure was successfully lowered.

The evaluation of general diagnostic testing for preventive healthcare based upon outcomes, such as sigmoidoscopy, can be evaluated on a statistical basis, comparing those who were given the test versus those who were not. For example, the rates of colorectal cancer and severity can be compared in those who had the sigmoids and those that did not.

The *evidence-based* evaluation of medical tests, treatments and procedures based upon outcomes is crucial for the future improvement of medical care—see references (Sackett et al. 1996) and (Forrest and Miller 2002). Even older medical procedures are coming under scrutiny. Much more research is needed in this area.

Outcomes can be used to evaluate medical care in other ways also

- to evaluate physicians
- to determine any measures taken by a physician—such as how the physician explains a medication condition to a patient or whether the physician is the patient's regular physician—that have a positive or negative effect upon the well-being of the patient and that increase or decrease a patient's confidence in that physician.

How outcomes can be measured and their use will be continuing research areas.

Another research area is the proper use of treatment cases and chronic care management cases in continuity of care. Users of treatment cases and chronic care management cases require a new discipline in patient care. Sometimes a number of different caregivers may see the patient during the period of the treatment or management of the patient's chronic disease. For purposes of continuity of care, the treatment, in general, should be continued according to the current treatment plan. Study should be done to determine how feasible this is and/or how to train physicians to have this discipline.

17.4.2 Determining Best Clinical Practice Guidelines and Best Protocols

The *National Guideline Clearinghouse* is comprehensive database of clinical practice guidelines for treatment of medical conditions based upon the best scientific evidence developed in association with public and private healthcare organizations. Each guideline is supported by a particular medical organization (NGC 1998-2004).

An HMO may require a clinical practice guideline for a medical condition not included in the *National Guideline Clearinghouse*, or the HMO may want to establish its own clinical guideline.

If so, the HMO must establish its own guideline, possibly based upon treatment cases, chronic care management cases and outcomes, or get the guideline from another source.

Research is required to determine how to best establish new clinical practice guidelines. Reference (Starfield 1998) states that patients' needs and biological, social and environmental determinants should be factored in with the standard approach of determining clinical practice guidelines by best evidence as determined by randomized, controlled, clinical trials.

There is also indication that determination of best practices is also somewhat subjective. For example, in a study to determine whether clinical laboratory tests were appropriate or not, estimates of inappropriate laboratory use varied greatly (4.5% - 95%) (Walraven and C. David Naylor 1998).

When cost factors come into play, determination of a best practice may vary from year to year dependent upon changes in costs, even though the consideration of best medical practices stay the same. Because of an HMO's and fee for service world's differing view of costs, an HMO and the fee for service may make very different decisions on what is the best practice.

Once best practice guidelines are determined, they must be communicated to HMO caregivers. ASTM has a specification for the Guideline Elements Model (GEM), a standards for storing and organizing information in a clinical practice guideline (ASTM 2002). Further research needs to be done in the many different subject areas dealing with best clinical practice guidelines.

Similar to a national database of clinical practice guidelines for medical conditions is a national database for protocols for advice nurses, and perhaps appointment clerks, based upon chief complaint. Such a database would standardize medical care at the point where the patient first requests care. Of particular importance is identifying emergent situations.

17.4.3 Predicting Diseases

Section 8.6 describes what are very large new areas of research: Analytic disease prediction, descriptive disease prediction, and disease progression analysis.

Potentially, disease progression analysis could be used to restructure the patient medical record. The book (Tsiaras and Worth 2002) shows that visualization can be used to picture the progressive growth of a fetus before birth. Visualization could also potentially show the progression of changes in a body or a part of the body during aging and/or during a disease. Such a progression of pictures (or visualizations) could be used to identify where a person is in the progression of a disease. Used together with biomarkers, it could be used to identify treatment decision points when disease decisions should be made before the disease gets harder to treat.

Identifying gestation, aging, and progression of various diseases and progressions after treatments via visualization of different parts of the body together with biomarkers, treatment decision points, and possible and recommended treatments for the various types of diseases with probabilities at any point for the future progressions could allow a compendium of aging, disease and treatment progressions to be described. This compendium is termed here to be a *disease map*.

Identifying for a particular individual, the individual's current progression of bodily changes for aging, diseases and treatments identifies particular paths within the disease map. Together with biomarkers for the individual, the set of such paths could be kept for an individual describing the individual's current health and enabling prediction of progression of diseases and aging in the future. Some of the biomarkers could be from the individual's genome while others are measured over time. This visualization of progression of a disease together with associated biomarkers, treatments and treatment decision points is termed here to be a *disease path*.

By analogy, a disease map is like a road map and disease paths are each like routes on the road map that were taken. A disease path facilitates preventive care in that the progression of a particular disease at any point in the disease can be identified, the correct biomarker to identify the current state and predict the future state of the disease can be identified, and treatments can be tailored for the current and future disease state.

Disease maps and disease paths could also be a means for physicians to better communicate with their patients. Patients could visually see what their condition might look like or might progress to. Treatment options could be explained in context.

A model of prostate cancer that is like a disease map is presented in reference (Meng and Dahiya 2002). It shows the pathes of progression from a normal prostate to prostatic intraepithelial neoplasia or prostate adenocarcinoma to advanced prostate cancer or metastatic prostate cancer to hormone-resistant prostate cancer based upon genes and genetic alterations.

As indicated by the example in section 8.6, where "BPH (benign prostatic hyperplagia, enlargement of the prostate) over a number of years causes progressive blockage of urine flow causing a man's bladder to become distended and less elastic", there can be multiple related disease paths for a patient's condition: in the example's case, disease paths for the prostate problem and for a related distension of the bladder. Relationships between diseases and disease paths could be for many different reasons: due to systems biological effects (e.g., interactions between RNA, DNA, proteins, gene expression, cells); due to mechanical reasons as in the example (where one organ physically affects another organ); due to drug interactions (e.g., a drug for a disease causes a side effect); or due to other effects.

Disease maps and paths would combine both visual changes and changes in biomarkers. Research of autoimmune diseases has shown that prior to the visual symptoms of a disease, changes in biomarkers often occur. For example, about half of patients who later developed rheumatoid arthritis had autoantibodies for the disease an average of four and a half years before diagnosis; autoantibodies also often foreshadow the onset of lupus (O'Conner 2004).

The idea of disease progression analysis through disease paths and disease maps introduces many questions: *How reliable is prediction of the progression of a disease?* Biomarkers that precede a disease do not necessarily predict the disease. And certainly there is a degree of randomness that has an effect upon predictions; for example, a change in the retina of an individual's eye could cause blindness, but its effect is dependent upon how close it happens to occur to an area of the eye where acute vision occurs: the macula. *Would prediction of disease necessarily be of benefit to the patient?* Could prediction of disease cause a patient to be uninsurable (Pollitz, Sorian, and Thomas 2001)? What if a disease could be predicted, but there were no risk-free cures for the disease, or no cure at all? As stated earlier, an individual's values must be taken into account when determining if disease prediction is applicable to a particular individual.

The whole of disease maps and disease paths, I think, is a brand new area, which can only be accomplished—if at all—after much thought and research. The first questions to ask are "Is such an approach feasible?" And, again, "Is such an approach useful?"

With genetics and genomes, biotechnology, new technologies, and new drugs increasing the complexity and variability of best medical practices, it is becoming increasingly important to develop a straightforward method to communicate to physicians treatments and the disease states for which the treatments are applicable and most effective. It is equally important to identify individuals who can most benefit from these treatments. Together, disease maps and disease paths have this potential.

17.4.4 Full Disclosure to the Patient

Proper evaluation of treatments and care is dependent upon the accuracy of information in the patient medical record. Accuracy of information in the patient medical record could be enhanced by patient review of his medical record after a visit. The possibility and practicality of patient review of chart information should be studied.

Consider a patient who has a consultation visit with a retinal specialist for previous blurriness in his left eye, which a previous retinal specialist diagnosed as macular degeneration. Figure 17.3 shows the consultation sheet that the patient later received.

From the patient's recollection there are a number of inaccuracies in the consult:

1. Blurred vision 1 month ago was in the left eye, not the right.
2. The patient was never told to use an Amsler grid.
3. The consult never mentions that the patient was told that myopic degeneration usually behaves differently than age-related macular degeneration and is a different disease, and that having myopic degeneration does not mean the patient will get age-related macular degeneration.

Inaccuracy 1 could be catastrophic if there was an operation. Because the patient was given the consultation sheet, inaccuracy 2 is of no consequence, but would be of consequence if the patient has not received it. From the patient's point of view, the most important statement to the patient, point 3, was left off the consultation sheet, whether it was of medical consequence or not.

What this example shows is the following:

- Physicians may have inaccuracies in their reports, which the patient could catch (see 1 above).
- Physicians may think they have told the patient something when the physician hasn't. Patient review of the visit information could convey to the patient this information.
- What a patient perceives as the most important statement to him may not be included in the consultation sheet. Such information could only be gathered by talking to the patient.

Thus disclosure of patient medical record information to a patient may protect against inaccuracies and physician misconceptions. Patient medical record information does not necessarily capture clinical information that the patient considers to be the most important.

Patient review of the patient medical record could also have negative consequences, including possible lawsuits and lesser patient regard for the physician. The usefulness of full disclosure of medical record information to a patient after a visit requires more research to weigh its benefits versus its possible disadvantages.

Now let me return to the point that that the medical record does not always capture what the patient perceives as the most important statements made to him in the interview by the physician. In the above case, there are no, at least immediate, medical consequences in the patient knowing that he has myopic degeneration rather than age-related macular degeneration, but consider another case where a physician's statements, not captured in the chart, could have significant medical consequences.

INITIAL CONSULT

PATIENT'S NAME: John Doe

DATE: 6/6/97

The patient's past medical and ocular histories were taken and reviewed. A full work-up and examination was done.

HISTORY: He developed the sudden onset of blurred vision in the right eye 1 month ago. He has been told about macular degeneration in the right eye. He is here for a second opinion.

VA:	RE: 20/25 LE: 20/50	
IOP:	RE: 20 LE: 20	BP: 130/70

RE: Thre is mild retinal pigment epithelial atropy, lacquer cracks and chorioretinal atropy. No subretinal hemorrhage or exudate is present.

LE: There are moderate laquer cracks. No subretinal hemorrhage is present in the macula.

IMPRESSION: Myopic degeneration, both eyes. Probable old Subretinal neovascularization, left eye.

I discussed the findings of today's exam with him. The vision is improved. No treatment is necessary. It is best to watch this. The natural history of myopic degeneration associated macular hemorrhage is such that is frequently best left alone. Hopefully, this will hold. I have discussed the importance of monitoring the vision and amsler grid at least weekly. I have asked him to call if there is a change in vision or symptoms.

FOLLOW-UP: Return as needed.

Sidney Smith, MD
1000 First St.
Forest, CA 99999
800-555-2345

CC: patient

Figure 17.3 Consultation sheet.

In the early 1980s, a study was done where subjects were given two treatment alternatives (Campanale and Skakun 1997):

- **Surgery alternative**: "Of 100 people having surgery, 90 live through the post-operative period, 68 are alive at the end of the first year and 34 are alive at the end of five years."
- **Radiation alternative**: "Of 100 people having radiation therapy, all live through the treatment, 77 are alive at the end of one year, and 22 are alive at the end of five years."

The subjects were asked to pick the most attractive alternative. Because of the recognition that more patients were alive after 5 years with the surgery alternative, only 18% picked the radiation alternative.

Another set of subjects were presented the same information, but where it focused on mortality rates:

- **Surgery alternative**: "Of 100 people having surgery, 10 die during the surgery or the post-operative period, 32 die by the end of the first year and 66 die by the end of five years."
- **Radiation alternative**: "Of 100 people having radiation therapy, none died during treatment, 23 die by the end of one year and 78 die by the end of five years."

In this case, the 44% choose the radiation alternative! With this restatement of the same information, subjects clearly focused on the number of deaths after the surgery and after the radiation treatment.

Here is where a difference in the physician presentation of information might have a huge influence on a patient's decision, and probably where the patient medical record would not capture how this information was presented! Perhaps a patient's rationale for a decision could be captured by talking to the patient after the encounter and patient education could be introduced where such significant decisions must be made by the patient.

17.4.5 Reengineering for Team Care

Changing from a paper chart to an automated patient medical record system requires that all caregivers learn how to use computers. It requires that caregivers change current practice patterns from individual care to more of a team-centered view of care, no matter whether the team is a formal or informal one. Probably the most significant change will be caregiver adoption of a case management approach for tracking treatments, so treatments can be consistent and followed through, so treatments and their outcomes can be evaluated, and so healthcare given can be evaluated and improved.

Chapter 8 describes how an HMO might be restructured to make best use of the automated patient medical record system.

17.4.6 Telemedicine

Telemedicine is the delivery of healthcare and the exchange of healthcare information across distances using telecommunications technology. It can include viewing the universal patient record, including diagnostic images, clinical summaries, and everything else in the patient medical record, at multiple geographic locations. It could include teleconferencing, using two way televisions.

It could include the remote use of medical instrumentation. At least the following medical instruments which can be used remotely currently have defined ANSI interface standards (Kohli 1996): dermscope (for images of skin), ophthalmoscope (for images on the interior of the eye), otoscope (for images of the middle ear), laparoscope (for structures within the abdominal cavity), nasopharyngoscope (for examination of the sinus cavity and nasopharynx), intraoral scope (for inside the month, usually for dentistry), bronchoscope (for examination of the bronchi), sigmoidscope (for examination of the rectum and sigmoid colon with attachments to allow biopsy), and stethoscope (for heart and lung sounds), with the potential of significant results automatically being recorded in the automated patient medical record. Other currently existing remote instrumentation, without ANSI standards also exist (e.g., tele-ultrasound for OB/GYN and real-time interactive digital diagnostic quality transmission of Echocardiograms).

Telemedicine is already being done, via telephones, radio and also more sophisticated communication. In order for it to become more widespread, higher bandwidth networks must become available, and the group communication/concurrency problems described in section 17.3.5 must be solved.

17.4.7 Medical Vocabularies and Terminology

In order to have a universal patient record—or even an automated patient medical record within an HMO—that all caregivers can understand, steps must be made toward a common *medical vocabularies* and (free text) *terminology* within the chart. See section A.7, "Medical Vocabularies and Terminology Within the Chart", in the appendix.

This common medical vocabulary will result from agreements between healthcare professionals (U.S. National Library of Medicine 1994). The most well known attempt at creating a common medical terminology dictionary and thesaurus is the United Medical Language System (UMLS) developed by the National Library of Medicine.

17.4.8 Patient Medical Terminology

Upon an outpatient visit, a patient should be given a report the patient can take home. This report should use a medical terminology understandable to the patient. As far as the author knows, there is no study to develop a medical terminology for patients—a *patient medical terminology*.

17.4.9 Artificial Intelligence and Assistance in Diagnosis Through Expert Systems

The MYCIN project to use artificial intelligence to do medical diagnosis began in 1972 at Stanford University (Alison 1994). A number of systems, made for very specialized medical areas, e.g., blood infections and heart disorders, do excellent jobs at medical diagnosis, but only in this very specialized areas.

The caregiver is guided through a number of questions about the patient. At intermediate points the system explains its decisions so far. At any point, the caregiver can ask why a question is asked. The artificial intelligence system eventually comes up with a diagnosis or a list of diagnoses with the probabilities of each. Usually, the system will explain its reasoning for selection of diagnoses. Another term for such a system is an *expert system*.

Another type of expert system that has been created (Dankel and Russo 1988), rather than determining the diagnosis, enables a caregiver to verify his diagnosis. The caregiver enters a tentative diagnosis for the patient and the system gives criteria that must be satisfied for the diagnosis to be correct. The system then asks questions to help verify or refute the criteria, and thus the diagnosis. Such an approach requires significantly less input from the caregiver and makes use of the fact that the caregiver probably already has ideas about likely diagnoses.

With the Mycin-type expert system, automatically inputting patient clinical information from the automated patient medical record into an expert system to determine a diagnosis is probably not a realistic idea. However, using a working diagnosis to give the caregiver a set of criteria that must be satisfied for the diagnosis to be correct, the approach of the second type of expert system, is probably realistic. The proposed expert system also supports *differential diagnosis*, identification of the disease by comparison of the symptoms of two or more similar diseases.

17.4.10 Monitoring Systems

As mentioned in section 5.3.2.2, monitoring systems, including *Guardian Angel systems*, are problematic because they produce a constant stream of information. Storage of the total of this information in the automated patient medical record is not feasible and, even if it was, it would probably be counterproductive, as to be useable, it would need to be analyzed and filtered anyway.

Caregiver filtering and analyze of ICU monitor information, or of Guardian Angel system information input by a user, to pick out pertinent information for inclusion in the automated patient medical record would be a very difficult and time-consuming process for a caregiver. Whether or not it is feasible to automate this filtering needs to be determined.

17.4.11 Clinical Decision Support and Cost Containment

While a caregiver enters documentation, or immediately after a caregiver orders, the system could make clinical decision support and cost containment decisions. This is a large research area for the HMO.

For example, during the ordering and documentation process, the system could inform the caregiver of the following:

- choice of better, less costly medications, than the one being ordered
- recommendations based on best practice guidelines
- non-compliance with JCAHO or other professional organization standards
- non-compliance with state or federal regulations
- drug allergies and interactions
- possible duplicate orders.

17.5 MOLECULAR BIOLOGY

The practice of medicine is likely to change in major ways in the coming decades due to greater understanding of the way the human body works. This understanding comes from the field of *molecular biology*, the study of genomes and cells. The business side of molecular biology is called biotechnology.

This change in practice of medicine could increase the need for a universal patient medical record to store information that is costly but valuable to collect, such as information on the individual's genetic information, the *genome*, and the genome's current functioning within the individual, termed *gene expression* with an individual unit of inheritance, of which there are many in the genome, being a *gene*.

In the last ten years, many scientists have entered the field of molecular biology research for development of new medications, diagnostic tests, and treatments. And investors have put billions of dollars into biotechnology companies.

The use of molecular biology for medical purposes is termed *molecular medicine*.

17.5.1 The Basics of Molecular Biology

A principal reference for this section is (Alberts et al. 2002).

At the heart of molecular biology is the genome and proteins in the cells in our body that, among other things, form structural elements and control biochemical reactions. The *genome*, the genetic material in a human, having perhaps 40,000 genes, serves as a template to create *proteins*, with each gene producing a *polypeptide* molecule, which most often singly produces a protein by folding up in a shape distinctive of the protein. Proteins form networks with other proteins and control the biochemistry and thus the functioning of the body. Table 17.1 lists some of the uses of proteins within the human body.

Table 17.1 Uses of proteins in the human body (Alberts et al. 2002)

Use	*Examples or Description*
Enzymes	Speed up reactions in an organism without themselves being consumed; most of the chemical reactions which occur in biological systems are catalyzed by enzymes
Structure	Cartilage and bone; cell membranes; collagen; muscles
Contractile Fibers	Used in muscles
Storage	Hemoglobin stores oxygen; ferritin stores iron in the liver
Transport of particles	Iron transported by transferrin; hemoglobin transports oxygen from the lungs to other tissues while it transports carbon dioxide to the lungs; some proteins form pores in cellular membranes that transport ions
Messengers	Proteins are involved in the transmission of nervous impulses; biological processes can be coordinated between cells in tissues and between different organs via hormones (e.g., insulin)
Regulation	Regulation of gene expression
Antibodies	Defends the body against foreign agents, e.g., bacteria, viruses and fungi.

Although the genome serves as a template to create proteins, there are many regulatory controls turning on and off genes, thus controlling the creation of these proteins. This turning on of a gene is called *gene expression*. Some genes, known as *housekeeping genes*, are active all the time as they are essential for a cell's activity, while others are turned on as needed.

A genome in a human consists of 46 *chromosomes*. Each person has 46 chromosomes in each and every cell in his or her body. He or she has 23 chromosomes from each of his parents. Two of these chromosomes are sex chromosomes. A male has an X chromosome from his mother and a Y chromosome from his father. A female has two X chromosomes, one from each parent. Cells become specialized early in human development, but continue to have the total 46 chromosomes, but with different gene expression.

Proteins are long strings of amino acid molecules, of which there are 20 types in the human body. The *amino acids* are combined together chemically to form *polypeptides* that fold to produce proteins. The folding determines how the protein will function in the human body.

Each chromosome includes a very long molecule of DNA from which these proteins are created. *DNA* is short for deoxyribonucleic acid.

Each DNA molecule in a chromosome contains four types of bases, adenine (labeled A), thymine (labeled T), cytosine (labeled C) and guanine (labeled G). A segment of X base pairs is shown in figure 17.4. Two strands of molecules making up the DNA are arranged in a double helix. The backbone consists of alternating sugars and phosphates. For DNA, a base, combined with a deoxyribose sugar and a phosphate group is called a *nucleotide.*

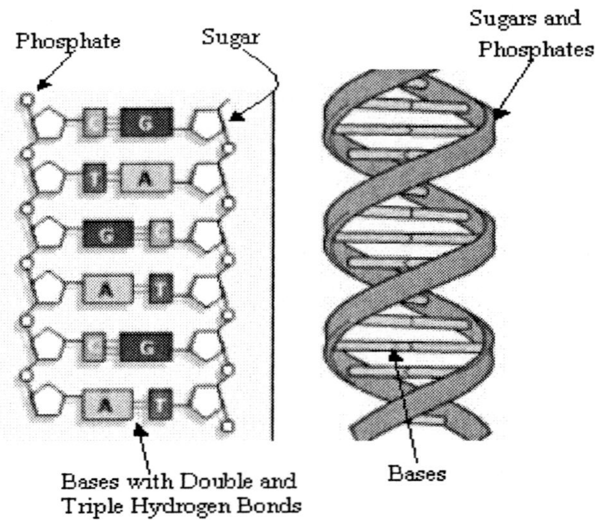

Figure 17.4 Two views of DNA.

The backbone is like the sides of a circular ladder with a set of paired bases serving as the rungs. The bases are complementary in structure, with A always bonding with T and G always bonding with C. Hydrogen bonds, similar to bonds between water molecules holds the double strands together.

In the total of 46 chromosomes, there are 3 billion *base pairs.* Thus in a chromosome, there is an average of 65 million base pairs.

The DNA in each chromosome, and specifically the bases in the DNA molecule, serve as the template for creating the proteins. Strings of bases are copied by means of creation of another long but much shorter molecule, called an *RNA transcript*. *RNA* stands for ribonucleic acid.

There are different types of RNA, but each is similar in structure to DNA except that it is single-stranded with bases but not base pairs and with a similar, but different type of sugar than in DNA. The RNA transcript copies one DNA strand of bases, forming a complementary set of bases in the RNA transcript, except for uracil (U) replacing thymine. The a G in the DNA template produces a C in the RNA transcript, a C produces a G, a T produces an A, and an A produces a U. This process is called *transcription.*

In bacteria, the RNA is then used to create a protein. In humans some sequences of bases are cut out from the RNA (transcript) and the remaining pieces are spliced together—This creates another strand of RNA called messenger RNA (mRNA). This process is termed *splicing*.

The splices that are cut out are called *introns*, and the splices that remain are called exons. Often the *exons* are combined in different ways; thus resulting in many more mRNAs then genes. This process is called *alternative splicing.*

The messenger RNA is then read three bases at time to identify an amino acid to add to a polypeptide molecule. This process is continued to the next three bases and so on, with the peptide produced eventually consisting of a long string of amino acids. The polypeptide folds to produce a protein. This process of creation of polypeptides and proteins from messenger RNA is called *translation*.

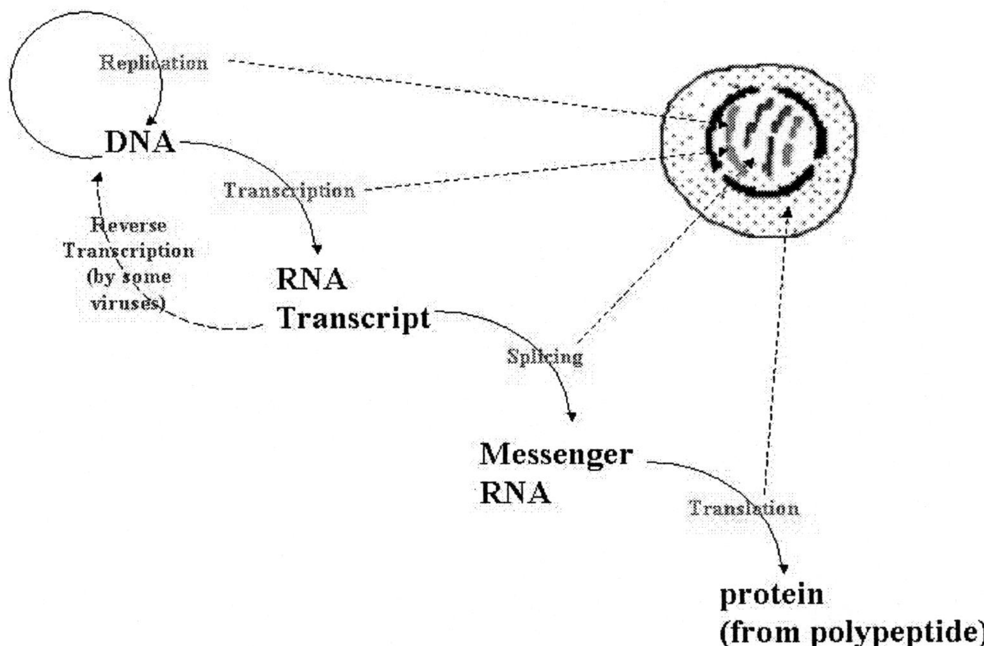

Figure 17.5 Central dogma of molecular biology plus splicing.

The DNA sequence of bases in a strand from which the RNA transcript is created is called a *gene*. Among other things, gene expression governs human characteristics such as eye color and whether the hemoglobin in your blood functions normally.

Before human cells divide, the 46 chromosomes are replicated by each of the DNA molecules and the chromosomes making copies of each other by creating complementary strands. This process of making complementary strands and thus replicating is termed *replication.*

The chromosomes and DNA are contained in the *nucleus* of each human *cell.* Outside of the nucleus is *cytoplasm* that is surrounded by the *cell wall.*

See figure 17.5. Replication of the DNA occurs in the nucleus. Transcription of the DNA creating the shorter RNA transcript occurs in the nucleus. Splicing of the RNA transcript to create the messenger RNA occurs in the nucleus. The messenger RNA is transported through the nucleus pores to the cytoplasm where it is used as a template to create the polypeptide.

There are various means of regulating a gene, controlling gene expression and the creation of proteins. Table 17.2 identifies some of the ways gene expression is controlled.

Table 17.2 Control of gene expression (Alberts et al. 2002)

Description
Controlling how and when a given gene is transcribed (e.g., by regulatory proteins)
Controlling of splicing of RNA
Controlling which mRNA molecules in the nucleus are able to go to the cytoplasm
Selecting which mRNAs in the cytoplasm are translated
Selectively degrading mRNA in the cytoplasm
Selectively activating or inactivating proteins

Mitosis is the part of cell division where the nucleus divides with the pairs of 46 chromosomes and two nuclei with 46 chromosomes are created before the division of the cell into two.

As part of reproduction, sperm and eggs, *germ cells,* are created. Cells divide a second time to half the number of chromosomes—this process is call *meiosis.* Prior to this dividing, equivalent parts of pairs of chromosomes may break and recombine to create chromosomes that are a mixture of the chromosomes of the individual's parents—this process is termed *(general) recombination.* Thus, the chromosome in the sperm or egg is not the chromosome from one parent, but a mixture from both parents.

At time of fertilization, when a sperm fertilizes an egg, a complete cell with 46 chromosomes is created. Since it is not yet differentiated into skin cells, nerve cells, etc., it is called a *stem cell.* During the process of division, the cells communicate with each other and differentiate into specialized cells.

Mutations are changes in the bases in genetic material. The consequence of a mutation is dependent upon whether it occurs in a germ cell or non-germ cell, called a *somatic cell.* Mutations in germ cells do not affect the individual but affects future generations. Mutations to somatic cells cannot be inherited but effect the individual.

Mutations, depending where they can occur,

1. Can have no effect, because much of the genome does not produce genes

2. Can speed up or slow down the expression of a gene
3. Can produce a different polypeptide, one that produces a protein that does not function at all in its original role, one that functions worse, or rarely, one that functions better.

The human genome has about 3 billion base pairs. When the DNA of two individuals are compared, there is about 1 difference per every 1900 base pairs. Generically, *genetic polymorphisms* are differences in DNA sequences between human beings. Single differences in bases are called *single nucleotide polymorphisms* (*SNPs*). SNPs occur in large groups of consecutive bases in blocks called *haplotypes.* The study of these differences in SNPs and haplotypes is expected to be important in identifying differences between humans, especially in disease susceptibility. See references (Human Genome Project 2004) and (The Wellcome Trust 1999).

DNA not only occurs in the nucleus of human cells, but also within *mitochondria*, organelles within the cytoplasm that convert energy for use in a cell. Mitochondrial DNA also produce proteins.

Further, *viruses*, many that can cause serious illnesses in humans, are composed of DNA or RNA wrapped in a protein coat, which is the genetic material of the virus (Strauss and Strauss 2001).

Viruses where RNA serves as their genetic material, mostly members of the *retrovirus* family, have an enzyme called *reverse transcriptase* that produces a double-stranded DNA molecule from a single-stranded RNA molecule. See figure 17.5.

17.5.2 Molecular Biology and Disease

How does this all relate to disease?

Molecular biology can be used in the diagnosis and treatment of disease in many ways. The following are some examples and potentialities:

- **Genetic polymorphisms causing disease can be identified**: A single base difference within a gene is the cause of sickle cell anemia, resulting in abnormal hemoglobin; an error during meiosis can result in an extra chromosome resulting in down's syndrome; errors in splicing can cause thalassemia syndrome, resulting in abnormally low levels of hemoglobin. Amniocentesis enables prenatal diagnosis of genetic diseases. Studying SNPs or haplotypes can be used to identify genetic diseases.(Miller and Cronin 2000)
- **Predisposition to various diseases can be determined:** Women with the BRCA1 and BRCA2 genes have a predisposition to developing breast cancer, while those people with the MLH1 and MSH2 genes have a predisposition to developing colon cancer. These genes can serve as biomarkers for breast and colon cancer respectively (Myriad 2004). Also diseases can be related to mitochondrial genes (Holt 2003).
- **Infectious diseases can be diagnosed:** Identification of bacterial DNA and viral RNA within human cells can be used to identify the presence of viruses, such as hepatitis B and C, HIV and herpes simplex, and of bacteria, such as those causing tuberculous meningitis. (Science Links 2002)
- **Classification of cancer can be made more precise:** Genetic changes can cause cancer. According to a genetics researcher I talked to, classification of cancer by genetic defects may result in more precise classification of cancers than pathology, thus making for more precise treatments and better outcomes.

- **Diseases can be diagnosed earlier:** By analyzing the patterns of proteins in blood serum of people with and without ovarian cancer, researchers were later able to identify the women who had ovarian cancer (Michalowski 2002).
- **Treatments and biopsies diagnosing diseases can be less invasive:** Optical coherence tomography (OCT), based upon fiber technology and laser light, produces a picture of the cross-section of body tissue without requiring a biopsy (Wright 1997). Molecular imaging refers to contrast-tagged molecular agents which bind to target molecules (those keyed to a particular disease) in the human body; the target molecule can then either be diagnosed or drugs can be targeted to these molecules (Currey 2003).
- **Proteins can be made in larger quantities via *recombinant DNA technology*:** Once a gene for a particular protein has been cloned, it can be inserted into the genome of a microorganism, producing large quantities of pure proteins. Insulin is one protein that can be produced in this way. (Iowa Public Television 2003)
- **Drugs can be developed, and developed with fewer side effects:** Overproduced proteins resulting from a disease can be identified; drugs can be designed to block the protein's activity; the drug can then be used to verify that it does not prompt production of possibly harmful proteins, causing side effects (Signal Research Division 1999). Many antibiotics in modern medicine selectively inhibit bacterial protein synthesis by exploiting the structural and functional differences between bacterial and human translation processes, affecting bacterial protein synthesis but not human protein synthesis (Pedersen 2004).
- **Cell migration can be controlled:** Cell migration such as occurs in cancer metastasis and arthritis disease processes can potentially be identified and be controlled (Davis 2001).
- **Defective genes can be corrected:** This is called *gene therapy*. Severe combined immunodeficiency disease, or SCID, also termed "bubble boy disease", can be cured by gene therapy. There are many candidates in the future for gene therapy, including cystic fibrosis and Huntington's disease. New genes are inserted into the genome. (However, gene therapy is not without its risks.) (swisstox.net 2003)
- **Stem cells have the potential to prevent some diseases:** Stem cells have shown promise in use to control Parkinson's and other diseases. One study found that embryonic stem cells transplanted into people with advanced Parkinson's can survive and continue to relieve symptoms for as long as eight years after the transplant. (Kiessling and Anderson 2003)

Clearly, biotechnology and molecular medicine have a rich and varied future. Molecular biology is a major foundation for evidence-based medicine in the future.

The study of molecular biology in its total is called *systems biology*. "Systems biology aspires to connect the dots of all of the body's RNA, DNA, genes, proteins, cells, and tissues, elucidating how they interact with each other to create a breathing, blood-pumping, disease-fighting, food-processing, problem-solving human" (Cohen 2004).

17.5.3 Molecular Medicine and the Universal Patient Record

How can a universal patient record potentially support molecular medicine? There are number of possible ways:

- storing the genomic information of an individual

- recording changes in transitory biomarkers that include changes in gene expression
- providing surveillance information to public health organizations on new and existing viruses, as well as other micro-organisms, causing disease in patients.

The following instrumentation currently exists for identification of genomes and gene expression:

- *DNA/RNA sequencer*: Sequences of bases in human and microorganism DNA and in virus DNA and RNA can be determined.
- *DNA microarray*: Proteins profiled produced as a result of genes (gene expression) can be identified.
- *PCR (polymerase chain reaction)*: Short stretches of DNA can be amplified a million fold to enable easier analysis, either by sequencers or microarrays.

17.5.3.1 Storing the Genome and Recording Gene Expression

The genome for an individual could potentially be stored in the following ways:

- recording an individual's complete genome
- recording alleles that predispose the individual for disease—*alleles* are variants of the same gene that can occur at the same focus
- recording single nucleotide polymorphisms (SNPs) or haplotypes as compared to a reference genome—this is a compact way of recording the entire genome, as only one in 1900 bases differ between humans
- recording disease-related genes in the individual together with current gene expression
- recording the many different biomarkers for a disease, which now could include genes that identify a predisposition for a disease and gene expression—proteins—that perhaps could be used to identify the early stages of a disease.

If the complete genome of an individual could be stored, either by storing the complete genome directly or by storing SNPs, then, together with measurements of gene expression, descriptive epidemiology studies could be done to cross-correlate these genes and gene expression with diseases. This would provide a database for later analytic epidemiology studies to identify gene and gene expressions and other biomarkers that can be used to predict or diagnose diseases.

After such studies, any of the above information could be used to predict and diagnose diseases for the individual patient.

The following is example of how recording of genetic differences can help in control of diseases: Iceland has one of the largest genetics databases in the world, which houses the medical records of Icelandic citizens. By associating genes with disease, they have discovered a gene that may double an individual's risk of developing a life-threatening stroke or heart attack. It has been discovered that the gene ramps up production of an inflammatory protein, leukotriene. An experimental drug is being tested that is triggered by leukotriene that lowers the amount of leukotriene. This drug has the potential for decreasing the chance of stroke or heart disease in the patients with the gene. (Sternberg 2004)

Gene expression is beginning to be used for diagnosis and is considered to be another diagnostic factor that has false positives and false negatives in diagnosing a disease—for example like elevated fasting plasma glucose as a diagnostic indicator of diabetes mellitus. The genome can both be used to definitively identify the future occurence of a disease—for example, purely genetic diseases such as thalassemia and sickle-cell anemia—and to identify a statistical possibility of an individual getting a disease. Use of the genome to identify a statistical possibility of an individual getting a disease presents the new security concern of an insurance company denying care, or an employer denying a job, merely because of this potential.

17.5.3.2 Surveillance of Viruses and Other Micro-organisms

Molecular biology can be used to detect, and recognize or categorize viruses or other micro-organisms in patients (Morse 1996). The automated patient medical record would enable there to be an active *surveillance system* to report viruses and other microorganisms that cause disease to public health organizations. Through this information, public health organizations could identify disease outbreaks and identify new previously unknown viruses. Public health agencies could then stave off epidemics and prepare new vaccines earlier than previously (e.g., for new strains of influenza). They could thus save lives.

17.6 LEGAL/LEGISLATIVE

17.6.1 Security

In order to influence legislation, standards for security of the universal patient record must be agreed upon between caregivers. A number of groups have an interest in this are and have held conferences, as identified in the appendix, section A.8, "Privacy, Confidentiality and Security". The most significant U.S. Government influence on security in medical care has been *HIPAA*.

17.6.2 Laws

Lobbying should be done to insure that state, federal or WHO (World Health Organization) rules and laws regarding the universal patient record are not so restrictive that they disallow caregivers from effectively using the universal patient record. State laws in different states must not be contradictory, allowing inconsistent access to the universal patient record information from one state to another (e.g., only allowing access to caregivers who are licensed in that state, even though the caregiver is licensed in another).

If a physician in one country provides medical assistance to another caregiver in another country does he need licenses for both countries? What if the physician serves as a *mentor* for the caregiver (in this book, mentoring is caregivers randomly or selectively reviewing automated medical records, asking questions about the medical record, and discussing alternative medical practices in order to improve healthcare.)?

17.6.3 Contracts

Certain aspects of the automated patient medical record system may require contracts between healthcare organizations (e.g., an HMO and alliance setting up an initial patient medical record system, as described in section 17.2.1) and contracts between healthcare organizations and trading partners (e.g., in use of EDI for electronic commerce). Again, such agreements should not be so restrictive that they disallow access to the patient medical record information that otherwise would have been allowed by federal and state laws.

17.6.4 Protection Against Bad Laws

In 1966, I drove home from a college class on my motorbike. A car went through a stop sign and turned left into my path. Trying to avoid the car, I turned sharply left, but the car hit the motorbike and the motorbike landed with tremendous force on my left knee. Immediately, I had a dream that I turned on a light switch and was severely shocked throughout my body.

As I lay upon the ground, I could not see. I had a pain in my leg so severe I would have prayed to die. People were holding me down, stopping me from breathing and making the pain even worse as I was pleading to get up to straighten my leg.

An ambulance came and I was given a shot of morphine. The pain immediately went away.

In 1970, the United States passed the *Controlled Substances Act* limiting access to drugs such as morphine. I have always wondered, if my accident occurred four years later, would I have received that shot of morphine that took away that excruciating pain?

How many ill-conceived laws are there that have harmed patient care?

17.7 STANDARDS

17.7.1 Hardware and Software Standards

There are many hardware and software standards, for example for the Internet and XML, network communication, wireless communication, computer languages, database management systems, multimedia, storage and other hardware devices, with standards controlled by many different standards organizations. As hardware and software technology advances, software and hardware standards quickly change.

However, at any one time, an organization has a choice of a multitude of different types of standardized hardware and software, with large organizations often having different needs than smaller ones. In general, the hardware and software standards should be chosen based upon the following factors:

1. Will software handle the organization's business requirements for it with an easily used user interface?
2. Will software and hardware support communication with other healthcare organizations, government and accreditation agencies, and organizations with whom the healthcare organization does business?
3. Will software or hardware handle the current volumes and current bandwidth needed?
4. Is the software or hardware available at a cost the organization can afford?
5. Is the hardware and software adaptable for the future or will it become obsolete in a short time?
6. Will the companies the organization bought the hardware or software from or who support the hardware or software be going out of business?

7. Is there sufficient technical personnel to support the type of hardware or software at an affordable cost if it needs maintenance or change?

Some required standards may not yet exist. For example, for an automated patient medical record, new, more powerful pen tablet computers, and thus more powerful pen computer operating systems, and hardware, are required. Pen computers must become much lighter in weight without sacrificing capabilities. Given the proper operating system and hardware, the pen tablet computer is, I think, the ideal portable computer to be used for caregiver input of patient clinical information. To be accepted, this pen operating system would require a handwriting recognition system that was highly accurate.

17.7.3 Healthcare Standards

Healthcare standards that apply to an automated patient medical record or universal patient record appear in the appendix. Some of these healthcare standards are government mandated (e.g., HIPAA) while others are so commonly used that it is important that healthcare organizations follow them (e.g., HL7), while others are dictated by the nature of the business of the healthcare organization (e.g., accreditation agency and biomedical instrument standards).

17.8 INITIAL AND FINAL OUTCOMES: BIRTH AND DEATH CERTIFICATES

When an individual is born, a birth certificate is filled out. When an individual dies, a death certificate is filled out.

In order to promote uniformity in birth and death certificates in the various states of the United States and thus to enable sharing of vital statistics and health information, the United States has produced a model birth certificate and model death certificates: the *U.S. Standard Certificates of Birth and Death, and the Report of Fetal Death* (NCHS 2003).

Medical information in birth and death certificates together with information in the automated patient medical record could provide valuable information for medical research. Death certificates often identify immediate and underlying causes of death and contributing factors, Further, after a person's death, together with the death certificate information, an autopsy may be done, more completely identifying the causes of death and diseases at time of death.

In the future, the individual's genomic information may be collected at birth or death and thus could be a future addition to the birth certificate or death certificate. Including genomic information in the birth certificate may bring up fears that a person's destiny would be determined by his genetics rather than by his efforts—This was the subject of the 1997 American movie *Gattaca* (Niccol 1997)—but the genome may become so important in medical care in the future that inclusion in the birth certificate and subsequently in a universal patient record may be the only logical thing to do.

Key Terms

agent
alternative splicing*
amino acid*
application service provider (ASP)
biometrics
caregiver tracking
cell
chromosome*
clinical image
collaborative communication
component adaptability
Controlled Substances Act
cooperative editing system
Customer Information Control System (CICS)
dedicated line
diagnostic image
DICOM
disease map
disease path
distributed system
DNA (Deoxyribonucleic Acid)
DNA microarray*
DNA/RNA sequencers*
EDIFACT
enterprise management system
evidence-based
exon*
expert system
gene
gene expression
gene therapy*
genome
germ cell*
grid computing
group communication
Guardian Angel system
handwriting recognition
haplotype*
hard disk
Integrated Circuit Card (ICC)
Internet service provider (ISP)
HIPAA
intron*
laptop computer
magnetic tape
medical image
medical vocabulary
meiosis*
mentor
mitochondria*
mitosis*
molecular biology
molecular medicine
multiprocessing
multithreading
National Guideline Clearinghouse
network access point (NAP)
n-tier systems
nucleotide*
nucleus*
optical disk
outcome
PACS (Picture Archiving and Communication System)
patient medical vocabulary
PCR (polymerase chain reaction)*
PDA (personal digital assistant)
project
project plan
peer-to-peer connection
point-to-point connection
polymorphism*
polypeptide*
protein*
reader
recombinant DNA technology*
recombination, (general)*
replication*
retrovirus*
RNA (ribonucleic acid)
RNA transcript*
single log-on
single nucleotide polymorphism (SNP)*
smart card
somatic cell*
Sonet
splicing*
stem cell*
storage area network (SAN)
surveillance system
systems biology
tablet computer
telemedicine
transcriptase*
transcription*
translation*
U.S. Standard Certificates of Birth and Death, and the Report of Fetal Death
utility computing
voice recognition
WDM (wave length division multiplexing)
writer

*=These molecular biology terms do not appear in the glossary.

Study Questions

1. After research is completed there is an evaluation point to do what?
2. What technologies can make networks very fast? Why do medical networks require greater bandwidth than other networks? What are advantages and disadvantages of using the Internet for medical networks?
3. What types of workstations are available for the automated patient medical record? What makes some of them more useful for using at the point-of-care?
4. For storage of documents that are used less and less frequently as they age, e.g., source documents, you want to migrate them to slower and less costly storage as they age. In section 17.2.3, rank the computer storage methods as to applicability to older documents.
5. Why do diagnostic images require special hardware? What is this hardware? What are diagnostic images, medical images, and clinical images?
6. How can smart cards be used for the automated patient medical record? What is biometrics?
7. In the past, distributed system were heterogeneous computers tied together by a network. In what ways should a distributed system for the automated patient medical record instead be more like a mainframe system?
8. What is utility computing?
9. How so agents support business policies?
10. Name the various broad types of security that the automated patient medical record and a universal patient record must handle?
11. What is the relationship between medical vocabularies and searching?
12. What is "group communication" and what is "collaborative communication"? Discuss the need for an automated patient medical record of having two readers at the same time, a reader and a writer at the same time, two writers at the same time? What system would help the latter?
13. When is discrete speech input okay and when is continuous speech input required?
14. For what kind of computers is handwriting recognition required?
15. Why is it important in medical care to measure outcomes?
16. You are a physician in an HMO. From what sources are you likely to get clinical practice guidelines? What are these?
17. This book proposes the use of "disease maps" and "disease paths". What are they? What are they analogous to? Why might there be multiple disease paths for a single medical condition?
18. What are the benefits and dangers of having the patient read his or her medical record? Discussion items: How can a physician be sure that a patient makes the correct decision on a treatment? Should there be two versions of the automated patient medical record, one for clinicians and one for patients?
19. Discussion items: How would an automated patient medical record change the relationships between caregivers?
20. Discussion item: Why have expert systems such as MYCIN not been used more in medicine? How successful would the alternative presented in the text be?
21. In order to usefully record information from a Guardian Angel System or a monitoring system for inclusion in the medical record, what must be done?
22. Name some ways in which an automated patient medical record system could check what a physician enters. Discussion item: What are the benefits and dangers of such an approach?
23. What is the human genome? What are genes? What is their relationship to polypeptides and proteins? What is the usefulness of proteins in the body? What is gene expression? Discussion item: How does molecular biology relate to medicine and how might it change medicine?
24. What mechanism changes genes?—If a gene changes in a germ cell and in a somatic cell whose health might it affect? Do genes normally change? Does gene expression change? Discussion items: Why might it be useful to record the human genome in the patient record in the future? Gene expression in the patient record? Genes or other base sequences?
25. In medicine, what is a surveillance system?
26. What is the most recent U.S. law affecting security of medical record?
27. Discussion: Will conflicting laws, regulations, and agreements make the universal patient record unfeasible? When do contracts apply and when do laws apply?
28. What is the "Controlled Substances Act".?
29. Discussion: What is the importance of software, hardware, and healthcare standards?
30. What do birth certificates, death certificates, and fetal death certificates provide to medicine and public health? Why is it important to have a national model for these when each state determines their content?

CHAPTER 18

The Automated Record and Universal Patient Record in Perspective

CHAPTER OUTLINE

18.1 A PERSPECTIVE

The automated patient medical record system may seem to be for physicians, but it is really for patients. With its extension to a universal patient record, these patients could include virtually anyone in the world.

And because there never could be enough physicians in the world, and healthcare is essential, then something else must be tried to provide quality medical care to more people. Hopefully, the automated patient medical record system and universal patient record are part of this. The universal patient record can help patients receive better, quicker and more effective medical care, even in remote locations, through telemedicine, where medical care is now impossible, with general physicians and nurse practitioners being the consultants to nurses or other less trained caregivers who care for the patients. Patient care can be improved by experienced caregivers mentoring less experienced ones, reviewing medical records, asking and answering questions, and making suggestions for improvement of care.

The automated patient medical record system and universal patient record will be very difficult to develop, requiring contributions from many, many people and the cooperation of many people.

The only remotely comparable system to the automated patient medical record system and universal patient record is the Internet! Like the Internet, the implications of developing a universal patient record may go far beyond anything that was originally imagined.

18.2 PROMISES OF A UNIVERSAL PATIENT RECORD

Western medicine is oriented toward short-term treatments of medical conditions.

Recently, my sister-in-law died at age 56 of the many complications of type II diabetes, including kidney and heart failure. I asked the doctor whether her illness, and her ensuing blindness, could have been avoided. He said yes, if she had only taken better care of herself as a young woman.

A medical article I once read said that of 100 people who get hepatitis C, 20 recover on their own and 80 develop chronic infections. Of the 80 who develop chronic infections, 60 remain clinically well despite chronic infection, while 20 develop cirrhosis. Of the 20 who develop cirrhosis, 5 die of liver failure while 5 die of liver cancer (Harvard Medical School 2000). If patients with hepatitis C were tracked over their lifetimes and given proper care—with the knowledge of what lifestyle and environmental factors influenced hepatitis C—could these results be improved? If my sister-in-law was given preventive care for type II diabetes, could she have lived a healthier, longer life?

Besides identifying a patient s medical conditions, a universal patient record could collect genetic, lifestyle, and environmental factors influencing the health of the patient. The universal patient record would thus serve as a database to associate diseases with genetic, lifestyle, and environmental factors. Patients could then be identified as having greater risks of a specific disease, with caregivers informing the patients of how the disease could be prevented. Patient care could then become more long-term oriented, preventing, as well as treating, diseases.

Western medicine is the province of physicians, often working individually in the care of a patient, who are usually restricted to work in one very specific geographic location of the world.

One billion people in the world lack even the most basic medical services (Franco 2000). A book, *Where There is No Doctor*, is a manual for village healthcare workers, informing them on how to give first aid and emergency care to patients and on how to administer public health to the community, such as educating the community on how to have clean drinking water (Werner, Thuman, and Maxwell 1992). The healthcare worker is taught to recognize conditions that absolutely need near-term care by a physician; a patient report document appears in the back of the book for a village healthcare worker to communicate a patient's medical condition to a physician. Could the patient report document of the village healthcare worker be automated to communicate it via handheld computer directly to a physician for review and identification of critical medical situations?

There are too few physicians in the world, too few nurses, and too few other healthcare workers. The world must make better use of all its healthcare workers.

An innovative Web site in India that made specialty care available to a larger population is DoctorAnywhere.com (Express News Service 2000). It afforded communication over the Internet between physicians caring for a patient and specialty physicians geographically located anywhere, including communication of x-rays and other medical documents. Could this communication of medical documents be enhanced by a universal patient record?

A universal patient record could foster team care of patients, serving as a communications vehicle about the patient and his medical conditions between caregivers and a communications vehicle over a long period of time between any one caregiver and any other caregiver (including the same caregiver).

A universal patient record changes medical care from only being short-term care oriented to long-term, preventative-care, oriented. It removes patient care from being the province of the single physician to that of the responsibility of many different healthcare care providers, possibly located anywhere in the world.

With a universal patient record:

- Communication between caregivers of all types would be enhanced, whether the caregivers worked on a single treatment for a patient, over many treatments for a patient (say for a chronic condition), or over a patient's lifetime.
- There would be a single patient medical record, rather than many fragmented ones.
- The genetics, lifestyles, and environmental conditions that resulted in diseases could be better determined as a result of a research database derived from universal patient records. There would be greater emphasis on preventative care—patients could then be told how they could prevent diseases before they occurred.
- Better patient care could be provided that avoids medical mistakes due to lack of information.
- Healthcare workers would work across borders and provide healthcare even when they were located remotely from the patient, or remotely from each other. There would be greater sharing of information on uncommon and emergent diseases.
- Public health agencies, caregivers and the public can be more quickly informed about public health problems.
- Healthcare would become more universal and less costly.

Would there be untoward effects of a universal patient record?

Do we risk loss of the personal contact between the physician and the patient? Do we risk overworking physicians or having them lose their prestige? Would healthcare suffer for the people who can afford the very best healthcare? Would there be enough financial incentives to bring healthcare to the underserved in the world? Would other factors, such a patient privacy, doom the effort to produce a universal patient record?

Can such a universal patient record revolutionize patient care? Or must patient care be revolutionized first to make use of a universal patient record?

All things change, with foresight they improve.

18.3 CREATION OF AN AUTOMATED PATIENT MEDICAL RECORD AS A PATIENT CARE DECISION

Any large-scale complex software project, including the automated patient medical record and universal patient record, is more complicated than the sum of its par be designed as a whole like a building, with significant parts that are hidden, constituting the system's *infrastructure*. Here is part of an **old** article that very much applies to the **new** automated patient medical record system, and proposed universal patient record (Wasserman 1977):

"

THE NATURE OF DISCIPLINE

Discipline, which may be defined as behavior or order maintained by training as behavior or order maintained by training and control, takes many forms. Discipline for Olympic athletes, for example, involves a regimen including extensive conditioning, competition, and a controlled diet. The mental disciplines followed by a chess master involves study and memorization of many games, along with in-depth analysis of board positions and possible moves and countermoves.

A different form of discipline can be seen in engineering fields, depending upon conformance to a set of rules and procedures. An engineering effort involves a specific sequence of steps beginning with a general plan, proceeding through detailed design, and concluding with implementation of the design. At each stage of the process, it is essential to carry out a series of activities in order to guarantee the success of the effort.

In constructing a building, for example, one must begin with artistic renderings, proceed to more detailed architectural design, and finally to blueprints prior to the beginning of construction. Also, the building site must be tested and prepared, checking for things such as drainage characteristics, soil quality, and stability. The various aspects of a building -- the plumbing, the electrical system, the heating -- must all be designed in harmony in order to assure that the finished building will be of the desire quality and will function properly. Furthermore, all of these design steps precede the construction.

The steps involved in the design and construction of buildings are well understood; it is possible to impose a specific methodology on the entire process. At the same time, however, there is adequate room for individual creativity and innovation, since detailed design and blueprints can serve to validate the ideas.

DISCIPLINE IN SOFTWARE ENGINEERING

The premise that an engineering type of discipline should be applied to the process of software design and development resulted in the coining of the term "software engineering" in 1968 (Naur and Randall 1968). It was recognized that software creation was a hit-and-miss business, based largely on ad hoc techniques. A large number of major software projects had failed completely or had been subject to severe time delays, cost overruns, or other serious problems. Many of the software systems exhibited unpredictable, hard-to-correct errors, were poorly documented, and fell short of user requirements such as measures as response time. In addition, these systems were often difficult to maintain, since the code was incomprehensible as a result of poor programming practices.

It became painfully apparent that there was a need to improve the quality and dependability of software production. The techniques being used did not work consistently and had a disturbing tendency to fail whenever a new or complex problem was attempted. The development of suitable programming methodologies presented a number of potential benefits, including the following:

1) improved reliability,
2) verifiability, at least in an informal sense
3) adaptability of programs
4) comprehensibility
5) effective management controls
6) higher user satisfaction.

Now, as in 1968, however, software engineering remains more of a wish than a reality. In the intervening years, however, there has been a great deal of investigation. into the nature of programming and the process of software development. The result of this effort has been the recognition that a form of engineering discipline can be applied to software construction with considerable success.

As with the construction of buildings, the construction of software can be separated into a design stage and a construction stage. If we are given a complete and consistent design for a piece of software (software blueprints), then the process of constructing a program which implements that design is generally straightforward.

One of the problems that has recurred consistently in the software creation process from the construction stage. Instead, there exists an "urge to write code", to begin the construction process before fully determining the nature of the object to be built. While this technique works up to a point, particularly with smaller programs, it has a tendency to collapse with more complex systems. It can be seen, by analogy, that a building contractor can safely purchase roofing materials, wiring, plumbing fixtures, insulation, and electrical appliances for a house before the design is complete, but is likely to make some incorrect and irrevocable decisions in trying to assemble those components prior to the completion of the design.

Just as a builder must wait for the architect to complete the detailed plans for a building, so must the programmer wait for the "software architect" to complete the system design. This is a key principle in the achievement of a disciplined approach to software design and development.

..."

from "On the Meaning of Discipline in Software Design and Development" by Anthony I. Wasserman (Wasserman 1977).

Everything must fit together as a whole. A standard approach to developing a large software system is described by the standard development (red) line in figure 18.1 (Truex, Baskerville, and Klein 1999). The system is developed. It then undergoes a much lower cost maintenance period. Eventually the system is replaced with a new system.

But the universal patient record system, to be useful, is even more complex than this! Rather than the system being eventually replaced, you want a system that is continually replaceable, with parts of the system being replaced by improved components. Rather than the standard development line in figure 18.1, what would be preferable would be to have the system lifecycle that looks more like the distributed development (blue) line in figure 18.1 instead, with future maintenance phases consisting of component replacement.

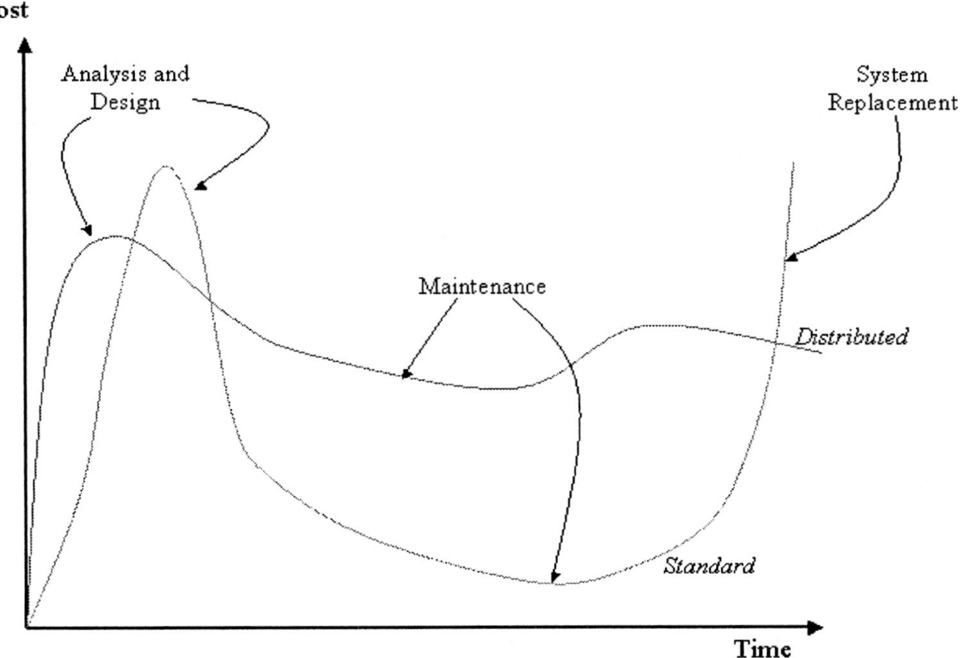

Figure 18.1 Standard vs. distributed development: software life cycles and costs over time (Turnlund 2004).

Also, because of the large size and complexity of the universal patient record, the universal patient record must be developed by people working on creation of the it in different geographic locations. This *distributed development* of the universal patient record adds complexity to the project management process, as most successful technology projects stem from close team interaction (Turnlund 2004).

And as difficult as it is to build a system, it is even more difficult to predict how the system will interact with its users. Its these interactions of the system with the users who use it that no one can possibly completely predict or figure out!

But these interactions with users are critical. Even the smallest little computer program which is used by many, many, users can have great effects on an organization. And even the largest system, which is not used at all by users, can be worthless.

In this respect, the automated patient medical record system and universal patient record have two possibilities:

1. They are something that gets in the way and no one wants to use them.
2. They help all mankind!

Which of these is true is completely determined by the users. Thus the users must be involved throughout the entire analysis, database design, program design, construction and maintenance of the system. The users do not only include physicians, but all these listed in section 4.2, including patients.

Now, one could compare the world with and without an automated patient medical record system and universal patient record system, and conclude that it would be much better to have these two systems than not. But these systems could be viewed in a completely different way:

Say, that even one thing goes wrong with the automated patient medical record system and universal patient record system, and as a direct result, a patient dies. You have lost the most precious thing in the world, for at least someone.

Therefore, it must be that these systems are done right. The only way this could be done is getting representatives of everyone who is remotely knowledgeable about the systems, including patients, physicians, nurses, lawyers, and software designers and other technical people who develop the system. After development of these systems and installation, then comes the hard part--preserving and protecting the system, especially from those in power who could destroy it (e.g., presidents, prime ministers, legislators, etc.)

If the Internet goes down, then all that happens is a person doesn't receive the information he or she was expecting. If the automated patient medical record system or universal patient record system go down a life could be lost—this is perhaps forgivable if it is just fate or due to an "act of God", but when it is the result of a sloppy programmer error, a design error, a power play of a politician or sabotage, then we as the people involved in the creation and implementation of the system are saying, "perhaps we didn't consider this project to be as important as we should have".

These systems potentially could save many lives. These systems could potentially be a huge waste of money if not done right. These systems are definitely not for anyone's competitive advantage—It could be that the automated patient medical record system and universal patient record system allow us to provide world wide medical care with the few physicians the world has, together with a world of trained caregivers, and a much larger world of untrained caregivers—to support all the patients of the world!

How can such complex systems be done with minimization of errors? One answer is that it must be done with the collaboration of many different categories of qualified people. Another answer is from the master of understanding the complex, Albert Einstein, "Everything should be made as simple as possible, but not simpler". And a third answer was presented in a previous chapter of this book—For both the automated patient medical record system and universal patient record system, "Build the infrastructure first!"

18.4 MEDICAL SOFTWARE DEVELOPMENT, DUE DILIGENCE, AND ETHICS

Civil engineers who design buildings, bridges and other structures are required by a state to have a civil engineering license to practice, and no such structure can be built without the review of a civil engineer. As a result, a civil engineer—whether self-employed or working for an employer--has the power, and in fact the duty, to refuse to sign off on a structure if there is potential of harm to the public from the building of that structure.

Patient care systems, such as the automated patient medical record system, also have the very real potential of causing harm—harm to patients—if they are not designed and programmed correctly.

...The IEEE Computer Society and the ACM have jointly developed *a code of ethics for software engineers* In this code of ethics, "the primacy of well-being and quality of life of the public is emphasized" (Gotterbarn, Miller, and Rogerson 1999). However, there are practical problems in applying such a code of ethics to software engineers:

Firstly, software engineering, unlike civil engineering, is not recognized as an engineering discipline by any state. And secondly, software engineering is not licensed by any state.

Perhaps, software engineering dealing with patient care systems should also become an established engineering discipline requiring a state license, with the state requiring that all patient care software systems be overseen by a software engineer. The software engineer would then have the power to refuse to sign off on any software project that could cause harm to patients.

18.5 THE TWO SIDES OF TECHNOLOGY

Technology could be a boon to healthcare, but also a hindrance.

On the one hand, technology and computer systems could provide more complete information on a patient, together with organization of this information, and filtering and search capabilities for this information. Technology through computer systems could provide a means for caregivers to communicate with other caregivers. And it could provide quick access to information anywhere, including to medical expertise where otherwise limited expertise would be available.

On the other hand, technology may require a caregiver to learn two ways of doing things, one when the technology is working and one when it is not. It requires an infrastructure to fix things when they go bad and an infrastructure to train users of systems. At its worst, technology may cause information on a patient to be totally unavailable, where it otherwise would be.

Technology could result in a large expense of money that could be used in better ways: on medical supplies, on additional caregivers. There are ongoing costs for electrical power or batteries and the infrastructure to support the system and train users.

Electrical power to support this technology, even in the supposed richest, most sophisticated, places in the world may be unreliable. In California, in one year, blackouts periodically brought down computer systems. In underdeveloped countries, this infrastructure for technology is even more unreliable.

And burning of the fossil fuel that produces much of this electricity may have devastating effects upon the health of humans on this planet. The UN has published a report (IPCC 2001) that predicts increased temperatures, more droughts, higher sea levels, and an increase in tropical cyclones in this century as a result of technology. And computer systems incorporate many dangerous—often carcinogenic—chemicals that can pollute the environment once scrapped, potentially causing new medical problems (Mitchell 2004).

But technology on a broader scale has produced a myriad of inventions that have enhanced human health, as varied as refrigerators and stoves, transportation and transportation networks, x-rays and cat-scans, sanitation plants, and computer networks and computer systems.

Although the use of computer technology in the poorer parts of developing countries may seem to some to be inappropriate, this may not be true. In developing nations, computer systems could potentially be hand-me-downs from developed nations (like old cars now are). And computer systems could be community appliances, shared by many people in a community (like television sets and telephones are in some places in China). In India, an inexpensive computer, referred to as the *Simputer™*, short for simple inexpensive mobile computer, is being developed that supports text-to-speech technology and sharing by people in who speak multiple languages and who may be illiterate (The Simputer Trust 2000).

But even in the remote areas of developed nations there are challenges. Reference (Goodman, Gottstein, and Goodman 2001) describes the barriers to making the Internet available to small villages in the Alaska and the Yukon and to encouraging people to use it.

A caregiver will want to use an automated patient medical record system if (1) it provided some overwhelming benefit to the caregiver, (2) the caregiver was sufficiently trained in its use, (3) there was sufficient bandwidth to make the system fast, and (4) if the system was available when needed. For caregivers in poor areas, an additional requirement would be that the system is paid for by someone other than the caregiver (Goodman, Gottstein, and Goodman 2001). Together, these are significant obstacles to implementing the universal patient record in developing countries.

18.6 PATIENT CARE WITHOUT THE PRETENSE OF PERFECTION

When it comes to healthcare, often anything is better than nothing.

Western medicine, or least that practiced in the United States, puts many restrictions on medicine. Only a physician can practice medicine. In order to practice medicine in a country or a state of the United States, the physician must be licensed in that country or state. The physician must be highly educated, and consequently is usually paid extremely well. To protect the patient, malpractice laws allow patients to sue physicians or other healthcare workers, further increasing the cost of medicine.

Implicitly, Western medicine assumes that medicine and practitioners must be "perfect" to practice medicine and puts on these restrictions to insure that medicine is done correctly all the time. But what is reality?

Use of the treatments and practices for diseases that produce the best outcomes for the least cost as determined by the best scientific evidence is called *evidence-based medicine*. There is a great controversy over what percentage of treatments are actually evidence-based. In Time magazine in 1998 (Thompson 1998), Dr. Robert Califf of Duke Med stated that "Only 15% of the decisions a doctor makes every day are based on evidence."

But there certainly are treatments that are of definite benefit, without which the patient might be damaged irreparably or later have a very poor quality of life. These "treatments" done by physicians and other "healthcare workers" would include the following:

- Prevention and early detection of diseases (e.g., through education, vaccinations, complaint-based physical assessments in the early stages of diseases, condoms, some types of preventive care for at-risk populations)
- Cure and control of potentially life-threatening and long-duration infections and other types of treatable diseases
- Setting broken bones, installing prostheses, fixing other structural problems
- Treating debilitating depression
- Prenatal care and the delivery of babies
- Prescribing and fashioning eye glasses to correct poor vision
- Insuring access to adequate water and food, including keeping teeth healthy so people can eat and food refrigerated so it does not spoil
- Insuring that drinking water and air is not polluted
- Insuring access to adequate shelter
- Insuring access to birth control and protection from sexually transmitted diseases
- Correcting cosmetic defects that cause the person to be treated as abnormal, such as cleft lip or facial injuries.

All of the above are health issues, but at least in Western medicine, not all of the above fall in the realm of medicine. David Werner's concept of village health care workers in the books *Where There is No Doctor* (Werner, Thuman, and Maxwell 1992) and *Where There is No Dentist* (Dickson, Blake, and Thompson 1983) does include all these elements of healthcare.

But, even with the above more all inclusive view of health care, there are problems in many countries, including very advanced ones: (1) In the United States, many people do not have access to the total of healthcare, in particular, to some forms of early detection of diseases. (2) In the other parts of the world, many people have virtually none of what is listed above.

Insuring that healthcare is "perfect" may be a delusion. Restricting healthcare to insure that it is "perfect" may result in more harm than it does good. If these restrictions cause healthcare to be too costly, are we not limiting healthcare for those who cannot afford it? If only physicians can practice medical care and only patients geographically located in the right place can have healthcare, aren't we severely limiting healthcare for most of the people in the world? The delusion of perfection may be harmful for people both in rich and poor nations.

There are too few physicians, nurses, and other healthcare workers in the world. Even in nations where this is not generally true, physicians and nurses tend to concentrate in cities, and rural areas are often underserved.

There is not enough knowledge about the most efficacious treatments. There is an inability to recognize patients that are at risk for diseases due to lifestyle, environmental factors, and family history.

By itself, a universal patient record may not solve these problems, but with a universal patient record there could be

- Enhanced communication between healthcare workers and physicians, no matter where they are located in the world,
- Enhanced knowledge of the patient's medical history and current medical conditions,
- Greater information on what constitutes the best treatments for a particular patient due to larger database of information on treatments and diseases,

- Greater ability to recognize patients who are a risk due of particular medical conditions due to their lifestyles, environment or family history, and thus greater ability to inform a patient of ways he could preserve his health,
- Greater recognition of the totality of what constitutes good health (e.g., good medical care, clean water, eye care and healthy teeth), and
- Greater ability to improve people's lives . . . many more people's lives.

One significant effect on quality of medical care may be socioeconomic status. Some studies have shown that health—as measured by morbidity rate for many different diseases (e.g., osteoarthritis, chronic disease, hypertension, cervical cancer) and by mortality rate—is highly correlated with *socioeconomic status* (Adler et al. 1999), where socioeconomic status is "a composite measure that typically incorporates economic status, measured by income; social status, measured by education; and work status, measured by occupation". This correlation of socioeconomic status with health is even the case at the upper levels of socioeconomic status. Thus, increasing socioeconomic status seems to be one way to significantly improve a community's health. One negative effect on social economic status is gender stereotyping that inhibits women's equal participation in many, if not most, societies (Cook 1999).

18.7 HUMAN AND MEDICAL ECOLOGY

Often, when we think of ecology, we think of animals and plants and their relationships in a wilderness area. Perhaps, we include man in the equation, often as destroyers or predators. Or perhaps we view ecology as man requiring other animals and plants in order to survive. But there are many other levels of human ecology, including those of pertinence to medicine.

As noted in the last section, if a person is cured of a waterborne disease and the polluted water that caused the disease is not cleaned up, then the disease is likely to reoccur. One form of human ecology is then, the person's physical environment.

But another form of ecology is the person's relationship with others, especially with his or her caregivers. If a paraplegic wife is cared for by her husband, physical ailments that incapacitate her husband can cause her to have additional physical ailments. If a child with a chronic disease loses her mother, then the child is likely to have more emotional problems, and perhaps also more physical ones. A person without any caregiver may die or become more sick because he or she has no one to turn to for help; even a treatable condition could cause greater ill health or even the person's death.

There is also an internal ecology within a human being. *Metastasis* is the spreading of disease from one part of the body to another, such as the spreading of cancer from one organ to another. But also, when one organ weakens, then another organ may weaken. It may be difficult to know the true disease, and after a while it may become irrelevant, as curing the diagnosed disease cannot cure the precursor.

Humans are members of a *physical ecology*, a *relationship ecology*, and an *internal ecology*. If any part fails, then others may also. We need some way of recording and recognizing these parts and interrelationships, so medical and human care can treat the most significant problems, and not just the secondary ones.

Internal ecology is an application of what is learned from a new field called systems biology. *Systems biology* is the study of how all of a human body's RNA, DNA, genes, proteins, cells and tissues function together to produce a living human being (Cohen 2004). (See section 17.5 for information on the interconnections of these areas.)

18.8 MEDICINE AND CULTURE

Medicine can also not be divorced from culture.

Clearly, most of the world views female mutilation that occurs in some African cultures abhorrent, while in the United States, male circumcision is considered medically beneficial. Some religious conservatives in the United States and Catholics in the Vatican want to fight HIV but not to do it in association with birth control. Acupuncture is generally not accepted as a form of anesthesia outside of China.

But cultural ideas also change over time, but often with lingering effects. For example, in the past in the United States, medicine and the rest of life had a pact: "Medicine could cure what was wrong with the body, but not what was wrong with the mind!" The mind was not the province of medicine—It was the province of religion, law, psychology, philosophy, and other ways of influencing human behavior and relationships. Each man had the "free will" to overcome his mental problems. Over time this has changed, first with psychotherapy and now medications treating mental problems—the latter making it clear that the mind cannot be disassociated from the brain.

Despite these changes, there is still a stigma in the United States with medicine treating the mind. There is the idea that if an individual cannot control his mind—such as controlling his anxiety or depression—that he has a character flaw. There is the fear that the individual will lose self-control because of the medication. There is the fear by the individual's relatives that the individual's personality could change, particularly that the relative would no longer be important in the individual's life.

For drugs that do not affect the mind, there are good, bad and mediocre drugs. For drugs that affect the mind, even if they have all the desired effects, they could have unintended consequences on relationships with others.

For caregivers, at least in the United States, it is important to remember that medicine involving the brain is different than medicine that involves other parts of the body. For drugs that affect the brain, the caregiver must be aware of the effects of these drugs on the patient's relationships with other individuals, or merely of the fear that these relationships could be affected.

If medicine is to become truly global with the help of a universal patient record, caregivers must understand that there are these differences in customs and philosophies between cultures.

Key Terms

a code of ethics for software engineers
distributed development
evidence-based medicine
infrastructure
internal ecology
physical ecology
relationship ecology
Simputer™
socioeconomic status
systems biology

Study Questions

1. What system is most comparable to the universal patient record? Research: When the computer and Internet were first created, what were the expectations for them?
2. What critiques of current medical care does the author present? What concerns the author have about a universal patient record?
3. How is building a software system like the automated patient medical record or universal patient record like building a house? What is "distributed development"?—Why does it apply to the universal patient record?
4. How are civil engineers who design buildings and software engineers who design software that supports medical care alike? Which occupation is more regulated? Which occupation is given more authority by the state?
5. What are health benefits and health risks of technology? What are some challenges in implementing technology solutions in developing countries?
6. Name ways in which Western governments restrict medical care? How might these restrictions affect the implementation of a universal patient record?
7. Discussion item: How does socioeconomic status contribute to good health?
8. The author contends that there are three levels of ecology connected with medical care. Give examples of each. "Internal ecology" is an application of what new field of study?
9. What are some cultural differences in the way healthcare is provided?
10. Discussion item: Why do some U.S. insurance companies refuse to provide health insurance for individuals who take antidepressant medication?(Pollitz, Sorian, and Thomas 2001)

APPENDIX

Healthcare Standards

APPENDIX OUTLINE

A.1 AN OVERVIEW

This chapter presents major *healthcare standards* that could be used with an automated patient medical record and universal patient record. Standards—or multiple sets of standards—exist for the following (Blair 1995):

- patient identifier (recommendations only at this time)
- provider identifier
- care site identifier
- health plan identifier
- employer identifier
- product and supply identifier
- computer to computer communication message formats
- clinical data representation
- patient chart content and structure
- medical terminology within the chart
- privacy, confidentiality and security
- performance measures within managed care
- clinical guidelines.

When any definitive standard is established or changed, this can cost large healthcare organizations millions of dollars in that they have to retrofit many existing computer software systems. Preparation for such changes in standards could involve many years of preparation. Some of these standards are imposed by government agencies and thus cannot be avoided.

There are a number of organizations, *standard development organizations (SDOs),* working on healthcare standards. These SDOs include ANSI (American National Standards Institute) that has developed healthcare standards for electronic commerce through EDI for Medicare via the X12 standard, part of the required HIPAA transaction set (CMS 2003) , the ASTM (the American Society for Testing and Materials) that produces a number of standards, including a standard for the CPR (ASTM 2003), the National Committee of Quality Assurance (NCQA) that produces an HMO "report card" (NCQA 2004), and the American Medical Association (AMA) that produces CPT-4 codes for reporting medical services and procedures. (*Electronic commerce* is the paperless exchange of business information using Electronic Data Interchange (EDI), electronic mail, electronic bulletin boards, electronic funds transfer and other similar technologies.)

Also there are organizations and groups that coordinate and promote standards established by other organizations. One organization working to coordinate standards from other organizations is the ANSI Health Informatics Standards Planning Panel (HISPP). Also, the Hewlett-Packard Company (now Agilent Technologies) formed the Andover Working Group for Interoperability (Elliott 1997) to build upon existing healthcare standards; the principal standards supported by the Andover Working Group are HL7, DICOM, ASTM for clinical lab data interchange (now ANSI/NCCLS LIS5-A), EDIFACT for international healthcare data interchange, HTML for information on the Internet, IEEE (Institute for Electrical and Electronic Engineers) P1073 for medical device communication with computer systems, including IEEE MIB for wave form communication, IEEE P1157, an object-oriented standard for exchange of data between hospital computer systems (JWP 1996) and ANSI ASC X12 for electronic data interchange standards for insurance. A follow-on group to the Andover Working Group is the Point-of-Care Connectivity Industry Consortium (Connectivity Industry Consortium 2001), that was organized to agree upon standards for communication between ordering, testing, recording of results and return of results for point-of-care applications; the standard established was POCT1-A (standing for "Point of Care Testing"). Another organization that focuses on automation of the patient medical record and supports groups who further this effort is the Computer-based Patient Record Institute (CPRI) (Steen, Detmer, and Dick 1997). The CEN/TC251 Technical Committee of Health Informatics is a European committee to improve the interoperability of computerized health care information systems in Europe (Värri 2003). Health Level Seven (HL7) is an ANSI accredited SDO in the clinical and administrative data domain, with standards including HL7, the HL7 RIM (Reference Information Model), and the Clinical Document Architecture (CDA) among others (Health Level Seven 2004).

There are also government organizations that promote or develop standards. These include the Health Care Financing Association (HCFA) that controls Medicare and Medicaid and supports standards for reimbursement. Also, there is the National Library of Medicine that supports the Unified Medical Language System (UMLS), a system linking together various medical vocabularies (U.S. National Library of Medicine 2003).

At the time of this writing, the most important changes in standards are a result of the Health Insurance Portability and Accountability Act of 1996 (HIPAA) (CMS 2004) under the control of HCFA. HIPAA mandates standards for healthcare organizations dealing with Medicare. Although some of these HIPAA mandates are primarily meant for transmission of Medicare payments through EDI (Electronic Data Interchange), administrative standards often cross over into the clinical area. But some mandates apply to all aspects of medical care: specifically, rules regarding "protected health information".

HIPAA (Amatayakul 2000) mandates standards for *claims transactions* including *coordination of benefits* information, a provider identifier, a healthcare organization identifier, a *provider taxonomy* (defining specialty areas for providers), and establishes requirements for security (including standards for an electronic signature) and for privacy. HIPAA also proposed a national patient identifier, but this was put on hold. HIPAA transactions standards would include use of *codes sets*, ICD-9-CM for diagnoses and inpatient care; CPT-4 for outpatient and physician care; and HCPCS for equipment, supplies, and injectable drugs. HIPAA security and privacy mandates apply to all clinical information. A *claim* is demand for payment in accordance with an insurance policy. *coordination of benefits* is the transmission of claims or payment information from any entity to a health plan for the purpose of determining the relative payment responsibilities of the health plan. A *transaction* is an electronic communication between two groups for medical or business reasons. An *electronic signature* is a code or symbol that is the electronic equivalent of a written signature and that can legally substitute for the written signature.

From reading this chapter, the reader should gain an appreciation and understanding of the importance of standards in healthcare. This chapter may not be up-to-date nor accurate at any point in time, so more definitive information should come from other more authoritative sources.

A.2 PATIENT IDENTIFIER

At one time, the U.S. government, though HIPAA, mandated that there be a standard unique health identifier for each individual (Appavu 1997) for the purposes of electronic commerce. This mandate has been put on hold indefinitely.

Different SDOs are developing requirements for such an identifier. ASTM's (American Society for Testing and Materials) E31.12 Subcommittee developed a *E1714 Guide for the Properties of a Universal Health Care Identifier* (ASTM 1995). (T. Scott Powers of Care Data Systems, Inc. and Dr. Paul C. Carpenter, MD, of Mayo Clinic have suggested that the Universal Health Care Identifier consist of a series of three universal/immutable values plus a checksum: 1) A 7 digit date code for the date of birth, 2) A 6 digit geographic code that relates to the place of birth, or entry into the healthcare system, 3) A 5 digit sequence code to identify people born on the same date, and the same geographic area, plus 4) a 4 digit checksum.)

A grant was awarded to Sequoia Software by the U.S. Commerce Department's National Institute of Standards and Technology (NIST) to create a Master Patient Index (Citizens' Council on Healthcare 1997). In the industry, a Master Patient Index is a cross-reference to all the patient identifiers that the various healthcare organizations and clinical information systems use for each patient. The author feels that eventual standardization on one universal patient identifier would be much less problematic with every source document having a local patient identifier storing the translation of the local identifier to the universal patient identifier. On the other hand, it would be extremely difficult to guarantee that each patient had a single unique universal identifier. A *master patient index* is a cross reference of all the identifiers that various information systems use to identify a person. Since a master patient index is often for an entire organization or enterprise, a master patient index is often called an *enterprise master patient index (EMPI).*

A.3 PROVIDER, SITE OF CARE, HEALTH PLAN, AND EMPLOYER IDENTIFIER

The U.S. government through HIPAA and the Department of Health and Human Services (HHS) has mandated that there be standard unique identifiers for health care providers, health plans, and employees (CMS 2004). These are respectively, the National Health Care Provider Identifier (NPI), the National Health Plan Identifier, and the National Standard Employer Identifier.

Along these lines, an industry-sponsored, non-profit, SDO, the Health Industry Business Communications Council (HIBCC), has developed site-of-care identifiers and provider identifiers for Electronic Data Interchange (EDI) transmission, mainly for purposes of financial reimbursement. A Health Industry Number (HIN) is assigned by HIBCC to every health care provider facility in the United States. It includes more than 290,000 identifiers including hospitals, nursing homes, HMOs, pharmacies and can not only identify specific health care facilities, but also specific locations or departments within them. An HIN Practitioner Database now comprises approximately 500,000 individual physicians and other prescribers. (HIBCC 2004).

In addition to provider identifiers, provider job descriptors for EDI have been developed through ANSI that will be used by HCFA. ANSI chartered the Accredited Standards Committee (ASC) X12 to develop standards for EDI. These standards include provider job descriptors referred to as Provider Taxonomy Codes (AMA 2003).

All healthcare professionals entitled to dispense, administer, or prescribe controlled drugs must have a *DEA registration number*, which they receive upon registration with the Drug Enforcement Administration (DEA) (DEA 2003).

A.4 PRODUCT AND SUPPLIER IDENTIFIERS

The HIBCC has developed a uniform bar code labeling standard for products shipped to hospitals, the Health Industry Bar Code (HIBC). The barcodes use Universal Product Number (UPN) codes. HIBCC is in charge of a repository for two UPN codes, HIBC-LIC codes and UCC/EAN codes, that are used for product bar codes to identify medical and surgical products and manufacturers. See references (HIBCC 2004) and (Roberts 2004).

The National Drug Code system identifies pharmaceuticals in great detail. The U.S. Federal Drug Administration (FDA) requires their use for reporting.

The Healthcare Common Procedure Coding System (HCPCS) are codes and descriptive terminology used for reporting the provision of supplies, materials, injections and certain services and procedures to Medicare for medical billing. (CMS 2004)

A.5 COMPUTER TO COMPUTER MESSAGE FORMATS

A number of computer communications standards are well established for computer to computer communication:

- **Between general purpose healthcare systems:** Standards for transactions for transmitting data about patient registrations, admissions, discharges, transfers, orders and results, master files, appointments scheduling, problem lists, etc.: HL7. A standard used by many vendors for communications between automated healthcare systems and recommended in this book for communication between the automated patient medical record system and other health organization clinical systems (Health Level Seven 1997-2003). The standard is message based and uses triggers—*Messages* are defined for various *trigger events*. The current version is *HL7 version 3 Reference Information Model (RIM)* describes this version in an object-oriented form, with explicit definitions of healthcare concepts and showing their relationships (HL7 2004).
- **Payers and providers:** Standards for transactions between payers and providers: ANSI X12 148, 270, 271, 276-278, 820, 834, 835, 837; EDI and EDIFACT, that are standards for electronic commerce over various types of networks. X12N codifies provider type and provider specialization for medically related providers; EDIFACT and X12N will coordinate their standards (CMS 2003). The National Council for Prescription Drug Programs (NCPDP) develops standards for information processing for the pharmacy services sector of the health care industry; NCPDP provides a standardized format for electronic communication of claims between pharmacy providers, insurance carriers, third-party administrators, and other responsible parties (NCPDP 2004).
- **Patient data:** Standards for transactions used to request and send patient data (tests, procedures, surgeries, allergies, etc.) between a requesting party and the party maintaining a database: ANSI X12 274 and 275 (request and response), which is compatible with HL7 (CMS 2003).
- **Clinical laboratory test results:** Standards for transferring clinical observations between independent systems: ANSI/NCCLS LIS5-A, HL7, and LOINC (Logical Observation Identifier, Names and Codes), a data base providing a set of universal names and ID codes for identifying clinical laboratory test results. The National Committee for Clinical Laboratory Standards has responsibility for defining standards for laboratory information systems, laboratory automation systems, and laboratory procedures and protocols. Some clinical laboratory standards have been transferred over to ANSI from ASTM. See references (ASTM 2003) and (LOINC 2003). An *observation* is a clinical statement about a subject, where the subject is usually a patient.
- **Clinical instrument to clinical instrument:** Standards for transferring information between clinical instruments: ANSI/NCCLS LIS2-A. These laboratory standards have been transferred over to ANSI from ASTM. For a list of some of the clinical instruments for which there are standards, see section 17.4.6. See reference (ASTM 2003).
- **Medical device with a hospital information system:** IEEE P1073, a family of standards for medical device communications with computerized hospital information systems (McCabe 2002).
- **Interfaces between point-of-care ordering systems and point-of-care testing devices or test reporting systems:** ANSI POCT1-A developed by the Point-of-Care Connectivity Industry Consortium. Also, the National Committee for Clinical Laboratory Standards has responsibility for defining standards for laboratory information systems, laboratory automation systems, and laboratory procedures and protocols, including for point-of-care (ANSI 2004).
- **Medical knowledge:** Standards for defining and sharing medical knowledge bases, including clinical guidelines: *Arden Syntax*, a method of encoding medical knowledge

and organizing it to make medical decisions such as diagnoses, interpretations, and generating medical alerts, was developed by the ASTM Subcommittee E31.14 and described in document E1460. The *Guidelines Elements Model (GEM)* enables structuring of a text document that contains a clinical guideline as an XML document that enables sharing of guidelines over the Internet; GEM is described in *E2210-02, Standard Specification for Guideline Elements Model (GEM)-Document Model for Clinical Practice Guidelines.* (ASTM 2003)

- **Medical chart information:** *IEEE Medix*—IEEE P1157 Medical Data Interchange (Medix) Committee composed of ASTM, HL7, NCPDP, DICOM, IEEE, X12N groups—an object-oriented standard for exchange of data between hospital computer systems, compatible with HL7 and DICOM which is a comprehensive specification for a health data exchange standard that its developers have stated has an objective of eventually supporting the transfer of the entire patient record (JWP 1996). *The Clinical Document Architecture (CDA)* is a document markup standard that specifies the structure and semantics of a clinical document that can include text, images, sounds, and other multimedia content and can be sent inside an HL7 message (Dolin et al. 2001).
- **Diagnostic images:** Standards for transfer of diagnostic image information: DICOM (Digital Imaging and Communications), a standard supported by all Picture Archiving and Communications Systems (PACS) vendors (DICOM 2004). A *diagnostic image* is one of a number of technologies (e.g., MRIs, x-rays, cat-scans) producing images of the internal body.

An international electronic business standard for communication of documents between businesses is also being developed: *ebXML* is a project to use XML to standardize the secure exchange of business data (ebXML 2003). EbXML was developed by the United Nations along with the Organization for the Advancement of Structured Information Standards (OASIS), an organization that promotes organizations trying to develop XML for electronic business use. EbXML could potentially be used for exchange of medical documents. EbXML was developed to replace the more costly EDI (electronic data interchange)—EDI had the complications of using private networks and required very detailed bilateral agreements between companies, most often using proprietary data formats.

A W3C standard is *Simple Object Access Protocol (SOAP)* to enable programs on different computers, even with different operating systems, to communicate using the Web with XML being the mechanism for information exchange (Gudgin et al. 2003). EbXML incorporates SOAP.

A.6 CLINICAL DATA REPRESENTATIONS

A clinical data representation, or *code set*, is a complete set of clinical representations and associated codes, with each representation defined by a code. Code sets exist for diagnoses, procedures, clinical test observations and drugs, among others. A *diagnosis* is an identification of the cause of a patient's illness or discomfort A *disease* is a pathological condition of the body that presents a group of clinical signs, symptoms and laboratory findings peculiar to it. A *procedure* is a series of steps by which a desired result is accomplished.

- **Diseases:** Codes based upon diseases used mainly for reimbursement purposes: ICD-9-CM (International Classification of Diseases) codes maintained by the World Health

Organization and DRGs (Diagnostic Related Groups) maintained by HCFA (the Health Care Financing Administration) (Rupp's Insurance & Risk Management Glossary 2002). A replacement coding scheme, ICD-10-CM expands on ICD-9, containing a larger number of categories for classification and includes further detail (NCHS 2003).

- **Procedures:** Codes used for classification of procedures for reimbursement and utilization review: CPT-4 (Current Procedural Terminology) codes maintained by the AMA (AMA 2004). ICD-9-CM is used for inpatient procedures. ICD10-CM-PCS is being developed as a replacement for procedure coding for ICD-9-CM (AHIMA 2004).
- **Multi-purpose:** Codes for various clinical purposes including pathological test results: SNOMED (Systematized Nomenclature of Human and Veterinary Medicine) maintained by the College of American Pathologists. SNOMED was created for indexing the entire medical record including signs, symptoms, diagnoses and procedures, and is thus a possible future standard for the computer-based patient record. (SNOMED International 2001-2003)
- **Laboratory observations:** Universal clinical test code database, containing codes for 6300 types of laboratory observations, including those for chemistry, toxicology, serology and microbiology: LOINC (Laboratory Observation Identifier Names and Codes) (LOINC 2003).
- **Mental disorders:** Codes for mental disorders: DSM-IV (Diagnostic and Statistical Manual of Mental Disorders). DSM-IV is being incorporated into ICD-10-CM, but ICD-10-CM is not expected to be adopted in the United States until the year 2006 at the earliest (Lehmann 2004).
- **Drug codes:** UPC format (Universal Product Code for identification at point of sale), National Drug Code (NDC) maintained by the FDA (Federal Drug Administration) (Roberts 2004).

A.7 PATIENT CHART CONTENT AND STRUCTURE

The ASTM Committee E31 on Healthcare Informatics has a number of documents on the content and structure of Electronic Health Records, including the following (ASTM 2003):

- *1284-97 Standard Guide for Construction of a Clinical Nomenclature for Support of electronic Health Records*
- *E1384-02a Standard Guide for Content and Structure of the Electronic Health Record (EHR)*
- *E1633-02a Standard Specification for Coded Values Used in the Electronic Health Record*
- *E1744-98 Standard Guide for View of Emergency Medical Care in the Computerized-Based Patient Record*
- *E1762-95 Standard Guide for Electronic Authentication of Health Care Information*
- *E1769-95 Standard Guide for Properties of Electronic Health Records and Record Systems*
- *E2017-99 Standard Guide for Amendments to Health Information*

- *E2171-02 Standard Practice for Rating-Scale Measures Relevant to the Electronic Health Record*
- *E2182-02 Standard Specification for Clinical XML DTDs in Healthcare*
- *E2183-02 Standard Guide for XML DTD Design, Architecture and Implemention*
- *E2184-02 Standard Specification for Healthcare Document Formats.*

The ASTM Committee E31 also has standards for other clinical systems that may communicate information to the CPR, including, but not limited to, the following (ASTM 2003):

- *E1239-00 Standard Guide for Description of Reservation/Registration-Admission, Discharge, Transfer (R-ADT) Systems for Electronic Health Record (EHR) Systems*
- *E1467-94(2000) Standard Specification for Transferring Digital Neurophysiological Data Between Independent Computer Systems*
- *E1713-95 Standard Specification for Transferring Digital Waveform Data Between Independent Computer Systems*
- *E1715-01 Standard Practice for An Object-Oriented Model for Registration, Admitting, Discharge, and Transfer (RADT) Functions in Computer-Based Patient Record Systems.*

The Health Level Seven (HL7) group has developed the Clinical Document Architecture, an XML-based model for the exchange of clinical (source) documents. It uses HL7 version 3 RIM semantics. See section 6.6.4.

The Health Level Seven (HL7) group is also in the process of creating of a model of Electronic Health Record (EHR) behavior by identifying an expected set of functions of such a system. The model is termed the HL7 Electronic Health Record-System Functional Model (HL7 EHR-S).The intent is to facilitate the communication between medical providers and vendors providing EHR systems, in that it would, according to Don Mon, Phd., "provide a common language for the provider community to help guide their planning, acquisition, and transition to electronic systems". (Himlin 2004)

A.8 MEDICAL VOCABULARIES AND TERMINOLOGY WITHIN THE CHART

Medical vocabularies are medical terms, including diseases, diagnoses, procedures, and codes for them. *Controlled medical (health) vocabularies* are the codes (e.g., ICD-9, CPT-4 or SNOMED). *Medical terminology* in this book are free text medical terms.

The ASTM Committee E31 on Healthcare Informatics has two standards documents on controlled health vocabularies (ASTM 2003):

- *E1284-97 Standard Guide for Construction of a Clinical Nomenclature for Support of electronic Health Records*
- *E2087-00 Standard Specification for Quality Indicators for Controlled Health Vocabularies.*

Current charts may use a variety of different free text medical terminology, making it hard for one caregiver to understand another caregiver's chart. The following are attempts to establish a common free text medical terminology.

The Convergent Medical Terminology (CMT) Project is a joint venture of the College of American Pathologists, the Kaiser Permanente Medical Care Program, the Mayo Clinic, and the

National Library of Medicine. A medical terminology was developed by combining terminology taken from a variety of computerized and non-computerized systems, including terminology from

- SNOMED
- ICD-9-CM
- CPT-4
- HCPCS
- LOINC.

This incorporation permits creation of a reference terminology useful for clinical medicine and through a semi-automated process which would relieve clinicians from the burden of coding their patient encounters. (Dolin 2002)

In addition, the National Health Service [United Kingdom], READ Codes—a UK clinical coding system—have been combined with SNOMED RT to form SNOMED CT (Clinical Terminology). Other specialized vocabularies will be integrated or mapped to SNOMED CT as necessary. (SNOMED International 2000)

For whatever medical terminology set is chosen—either free text or controlled medical vocabularies—section 7.7.6 identifies an approach to organizing this terminology to facilitate automated patient chart information retrieval.

The author believes that, besides medical terminology for health practitioners, that there should be a medical terminology for patients. See section 17.4.8.

A.9 PRIVACY, CONFIDENTIALITY AND SECURITY

The Health Insurance Portability and Accountability Act (HIPAA) of 1996 for Medicare and Medicaid programs includes requirements for security and privacy of claims and clinical information for individuals and mandates standards for electronic signatures (Amatayakul 2000). On December 20, 2000, U.S. Department of Health and Human Services Secretary Donna E. Shalala, announced privacy policies for a patient's personal medical records (Shalala 2000): "The new standards: limit the non-consensual use and release of private health information; give patients new rights to access their medical records and to know who else has accessed them; restrict most disclosure of health information to the minimum needed for the intended purpose; establish new criminal and civil sanctions for improper use or disclosure; and establish new requirements for access to records by researchers and others." The new rules allow "disclosure of the full medical record to providers for purposes of treatment", but protect against "unauthorized use of medical records for employment purposes".

But HIPAA security and privacy rules are even broader than this, especially for large healthcare organizations: HIPAA requires that various technical, physical and administrative security measures be combined to protect the privacy, integrity and availability of patients' medical records. Current information on HIPAA regulations can be found in reference (CMS 2004). Also see section 13.9.1 of this book.

Section 13.9.2 describes protected health information (PHI) as defined by HIPAA. *Protected health information (PHI)* is any information in any media that relates to "an individual's past, present, or future physical or mental health status, condition, treatment, service, products purchased, or provision of care", and in any way identifies the individual. HIPAA mandates that health organizations track the disclosure of PHI and maintain records that will, on demand, supply reports and disclosure statements on a patient's PHI to any patient who requests such a report. An individual has the right to receive an accounting of disclosures of PHI made by the health organization in the six years prior to the date on which the accounting was requested (164.528a(1)). Examples of what protected health information is and what it is not are given in reference (OFT 2003).

There are many other organizations providing input to the establishment of privacy, confidentiality, security and integrity standards for medical information in computer information systems. One of the most influential group is the *JCAHO (Joint Committee on Accreditation of Healthcare Organizations),* the primary healthcare accreditation organization, whose standards cannot be ignored; otherwise, a healthcare organization might lose its accreditation. JCAHO and *NCQA (National Committee for Quality Assurance),* an organization overseeing managed care organizations, jointly presented a privacy certification policy for member organizations based upon HIPAA mandates (Shilling and Hill 2004). JCAHO and NCQA require the following privacy protections:

- privacy protections for oral, written and electronic health information
- processes and practices respecting the use, disclosure, and secure storage of personal health information
- employee training in protecting personal health information
- consumer access to their own health information, and
- contracting between covered entities and their business associates.

An international initiative for establishment of criteria for security in corporate networks is "Common Criteria". The governments of Canada, Europe and the United States joined together in 1993 to produce an evaluation system for IT security products, with the ultimate goal of the evaluation criteria being accepted by the ISO as an international standard. ISO standard 15408 was the result. (Nortel Networks 2002)

A subcommittee of the ASTM, E31.17, has been meeting on Access, Privacy, and Confidentiality of Medical Records. Resulting publications are the following (ASTM 2003):

- *E1869-97 Standard Guide for Confidentiality, Privacy, Access, and Data Security Principles for Health Information Including Computer-Based Patient Records*
- *E1902-02 Standard Guide for Management of the Confidentiality and Security of Dictation, Transcription, and Transcribed Health Records*
- *E1985-98 Standard Guide for User Authentication and Authorization*
- *E1986-98 Standard Guide for Information Access Privileges to Health Information*
- *E1987-98 Standard Guide for Individual Rights Regarding Health Information*
- *E1988-98 Standard Guide for Training of Persons who have Access to Health Information*
- *E2084-00 Standard Specification for Authentication of Healthcare Information Using Digital Signatures*
- *E2085-00a Standard Guide on Security Framework for Healthcare Information*
- *E2086-00 Standard Guide for Internet and Intranet Healthcare Security*

A.10 PERFORMANCE MEASURES FOR MANAGED CARE PLANS

The *Health Plan Employer Data and Information Set (HEDIS)* is a standardized set of 60 performance measures for managed care plans, producing a managed care "report card", comparing one managed care organization versus others. HEDIS is controlled by the National Committee for Quality Assurance (NCQA). which is a non-profit organization dedicated to reporting the quality of managed care plans, including HMOs (NCQA 2004).

A.11 CLINICAL GUIDELINES AND EVIDENCE-BASED MEDICINE

The *National Guideline Clearinghouse* is a comprehensive database of clinical practice guidelines for treatment of a number of medical conditions in association with private and public healthcare organizations based upon the best available scientific evidence (NGC 1998-2004). Although the structure of these guidelines is not an official standard, it establishes a de facto standard for such guidelines.

Two ways of communicating clinical guidelines are the Arden Syntax and the Guideline Elements Model (GEM) using XML. Both standards were supported by the ASTM. GEM is described in the ASTM standards manual, *E2210-02, Standard Specification for Guideline Elements Model (GEM)-Document Model for Clinical Practice Guidelines* (ASTM 2003). To insure the quality and facilitate the implementation of clinical guidelines, the Conference on Guideline Standardization was convened in April 2002 to define a standard for guideline reporting (Shiffman et al. 2003). A *clinical guideline* or *clinical practice guideline* is a set of parameters related to a specific disease or medical condition that help clinicians make clinical decisions.

A.12 SUMMARY

This section presents a list of existing and emerging standards that might be useful in a future universal patient record and the automated patient medical record. Standards are constantly changing. Mandates for standards and widespread agreement on particular standards is expected in the future.

Key Terms

claim
clinical data representation
Clinical Document Architecture (CDA)
clinical guideline
clinical practice guideline
code set
controlled medical (health) vocabulary
coordination of benefits
DEA registration number
diagnosis
diagnostic image
disease
ebXML
electronic commerce
electronic signature
enterprise master patient index (EMPI)
Health Plan Employer Data and Information Set (HEDIS)
HL7 version 3 Reference Information Model (RIM)
Joint Committee on Accreditation of Healthcare Organizations (JCAHO)
master patient index
medical vocabulary
message
National Committee for Quality Assurance (NCQA)
National Guideline Clearinghouse
observation
procedure.
protected health information (PHI)
Simple Object Access Protocol (SOAP)
standard
standard development organization (SDO)
transaction
trigger event

Study Questions

1. What effect may changing a standard have on an organization. Discussion item: Why are healthcare standards important?
2. What are organizations called that create standards?
3. What standards can our HMO ignore without any penalty? What are they penalties for the other standards?
4. What healthcare identifiers did HIPAA originally mandate for electronic commerce with Medicare? Which id is no longer mandated? Discussion item: Why?
5. What is the industry standard definition for the Master Patient Index? What definition does this book use? What are the possible problems with each?
6. What is a message and a trigger event? What is an observation? What is a transaction? What standard network protocol uses these terms?
7. What are the commonly used codes sets in medical care? What is the difference between a code set and a controlled medical (health) vocabulary?
8. What is the difference between a medical vocabulary and a controlled medical (health) vocabulary?
9. What is HIPAA? What is protected health information (PHI)? What rights do patients have with respect to PHI?
10. What is JCAHO and what is NCQA? What is another name for the HMO report card?—Who is it for?
11. Discussion item: Contrast the approach taken by the HL7 EHR-S model to define an automated patient medical record and the one taken by this book.

Glossary

The following are medical and computer terms used in this book with their definitions. Terms specific to this book begin with the phrase, "In this book, . . ."

abnormal: A description for diagnostic findings, including clinical laboratory test results, meaning deviating from the normal. See "diagnostic findings".

acceptance testing: The process of comparing the end product of development with the current needs of its users; acceptance testing often involves operating the system in production for a pre-specified period.

access: To store or retrieve data from a storage device such as a disk or magnetic tape. To provide the capability to initiate an automated service on a system.

access point: A location in a medical center where there is an antenna that allows point-of-care computers to communicate via wireless with a server.

access to care: The ability of the patient to obtain the type of care needed at the time necessary.

ACR/NEMA: American College of Radiology and the National Electrical Manufacturers Association. This relationship was formed in 1982 to develop the DICOM standard for medical imaging. See "DICOM".

actionable information: Data that can be used by its receiver to immediately analyze and resolve a problem.

active window: A window is a rectangular box on the screen. The active window is the one currently being used, which appears on top of other windows.

activities of daily living: Activities usually performed in the course of a normal day of a person to meet basic needs, such as eating, toileting, dressing, bathing, teeth brushing and grooming. While a patient is in the hospital, nurses are responsible for insuring they occur.

activity: See "care activity".

actor: A UML concept represented by a stick figure that either represents a user of a system or an external system that needs information. See "United Modeling Language (UML)".

acuity: Intensity of nursing care required to meet the needs of a patient; higher acuity usually requires longer and more frequent nurse visits and more supplies and equipment.

acupuncture: A technique that relies on piercing parts of the body with needles to treat disease or relieve pain.

acute care: Short term care, as opposed to long-term, "chronic", care.

acute illness: Illness characterized by symptoms that are of relatively short duration, are usually severe, and affect the functioning of the patient in all dimensions; not "chronic".

adaptability: In this book, the quality and ease of an organization to adapt to new business needs.

addendum: An appendage to an existing document that contains supplemental information. The parent document remains in place and its content is altered by the addendum. For example, a clarification or correction to an interpretation of an anatomic pathology specimen might produce an addendum.

administration of medication: The process whereby a prescribed medication is given to a patient by one of several routes—oral, inhalation, topical or parenteral.

admission: The formal acceptance by a hospital of a patient who is to be provided room, board, and continuous nursing services in an area of the hospital where patients generally stay at least overnight.

admitting diagnosis: A statement of the provisional condition given as the basis for admission to the hospital for study.

admitting physician: The physician who admits the patient to the hospital. See "attending physician".

ADT (admission, discharge and transfer system): A clinical system for recording admissions to a hospital, discharges from a hospital and transfers within a hospital and maintains the hospital census.

advance directive: Written instructions a patient has prepared for medical personnel to inform them of the patient's wishes for treatments and care when the patient is incapacitated, especially regarding life-sustaining treatment if the patient's condition becomes irreversible. An advance directive is a legal document prepared when the individual is competent and able to make decisions.

adverse drug event (ADE): An unwanted or harmful side effect experienced following the administration of a drug or combination of drugs and suspected to be caused by the drugs.

advice nurse: A nurse who takes patient phone calls and advises the patient on medical conditions according to protocol; the advice nurse informs the patient when self care is appropriate and when a patient needs to come in and when the patient does not.

Agency for Health Care Policy and Research (AHCPR): An agency of the U.S. Department of Health and Human Services whose mission is to enhance the quality, appropriateness, and effectiveness of health care services and access to these services. AHCPR developed a clinical practice guidelines based upon "evidence-based medicine" that has been superseded by the *National Guideline Clearinghouse* database. See "*National Guideline Clearinghouse*".

agent: In this book, a way of categorizing and separating out a set of code and tables, interfaces between systems, databases, and user interfaces (possibly all spread across a number of different software systems), and administrative and operational procedures of employees implementing a business policy, so that the business policy could be implemented and changed by the people responsible for the business policy instead of relying totally on technical staff to do so.

aggregation: For databases, a relationship where one entity (engine) is "a part of" another entity (e.g., car).

AHCPR clinical practice guidelines: A set of clinical practice guides for various diseases available on-line on the Internet. Each set of guidelines has several versions: Clinical Practice Guidelines, Quick Reference Guides for Clinicians, and Consumer Guides. Examples of conditions for which there are guidelines are "acute pain management", "urinary incontinence", and "pressure ulcers in adults". This has been superseded by the *National Guideline Clearinghouse* database. See "*National Guideline Clearinghouse*".

AIDS: The disease acquired immunodeficiency syndrome. When HIV virus infection becomes advanced, it is referred to as AIDS. See "HIV".

alarm: A notification message for an abnormal result, panic result, or other result of a caregiver order that the caregiver wants to be notified about.

alert: A notification message describing a patient put in by one caregiver to later inform other caregivers. More urgent messages are alerts and less urgent messages are reminders

algorithm: A generic procedure consisting of a finite sequence of well-defined steps (instructions) for producing one or more outputs from a set of inputs. For example, a set of instructions on how to generically draw a graph with its axes on the screen.

allergy: A state of hypersensitivity induced by exposure to a particular antigen (allergen) resulting in harmful immunologic reactions on subsequent exposure.

alliance organizations: Healthcare organizations that HMOs contract with to share hospital space or medical office facilities.

alternate delivery systems: Health services provided as a less expensive substitute for care as an inpatient in a hospital. Examples within general health services include skilled and intermediary nursing facilities, hospice programs, and home health care.

alternative medicine: Acupuncture, naturopathy, care given by chiropractors or osteopaths, and other approaches to medical diagnosis and therapy that have not been developed by use of generally accepted scientific methods. Also called "complementary medicine".

ambiguous allergy: An allergy that is not clear cut (e.g., the allergy is not confirmed, the benefit of the substance causing the allergy outweighs its allergic side effects, the substance causing the allergic reaction only causes the reaction some of the time).

American Medical Association (AMA): A partnership of physicians and their professional associations dedicated to promoting the art and science of medicine and the betterment of public health.

ANSI (American National Standards Institute): A group that publishes many computing standards. The U.S. representative is the ISO (International Standards Organization). For example, ANSI has standards for the computer languages of COBOL and C.

ANSI ASC X12N: A federally mandated EDI format to be used by providers and payers who electronically transmit claims and related transactions to the federal government. ASC stands for Accredited Standards Committee.

ANSI Health Informatics Standards Planning Panel (HISPP): The primary organization working to coordinate healthcare standards being developed by other standard development organizations.

analog: A flow of information where things change smoothly and have an infinite number of values, as opposed to "digital".

analysis: The determination of the total effects of any addition, change or deletion to a project to the other aspects of the project (e.g., requiring a user to remember a status code could divert the caregiver's attention away from patient care).

analytic disease prediction: In this book, disease prediction based upon a patient having a known risk factor for a disease (e.g., smoking increasing the risk of lung cancer, a severe knee injury increasing the risk of osteoarthritis and knee replacement, the presence of the BRCA1 or BRCA2 genes increasing the risk of breast cancer) or alternatively, a patient having a protective factor against that disease. Analytic disease prediction is based upon analytic epidemiology studies. See "disease prediction", "risk factor", "protective factor", and "analytic epidemiology".

analytic epidemiology: A branch of epidemiology identifying the causations of diseases, also referred to as etiology. See "etiology".

anatomic pathology: An ancillary department that determines if tissues are in fact abnormal or diseased. Anatomic pathology deals with wet specimens, tissues, anything out of the body (a piece of bone, skin tissue, muscle, blood vessel, bullet). Anatomic pathology includes surgical pathology, cytology (study of cells), histology (microscopic structure of tissues) and autopsy (multiple body parts). Cytology deals with smears: vaginal, sputum, semen—fluids with cellular material.

ancillary services: Support services other than room, board, medical or nursing services to patients, including the following: clinical laboratory, x-ray, physical therapy, injection clinic, pharmacy, optical sales and hearing center.

Andover Working Group for Interoperability: A group of companies formed to build upon healthcare standards set up by the Hewlett-Packard Company. The principal standards supported are HL7, DICOM, ASTM for clinical lab data interchange, EDIFACT for healthcare data interchange, HTML for information on the Internet, and IEEE P1073 for medical device communication with computer systems.

angiography: X-ray with contrast material injected into blood showing arteries and veins.

application: A set of files (or databases), software, equipment, and procedures to support a set of related functions suited to the needs of an organization. Such functions may be related to a business, entertainment, science or engineering organizational need.

application database: Any database that is not meant to be used by all automated systems in an organization, containing data specific to a single automated system or to a set of related automated systems. See "corporate database".

application service provider (ASP): "A company that offers individuals or enterprises access over the Internet to application and related services that would otherwise have to be located in their own personal or enterprise computers . . . on a rental, pay-as-you-use basis." (searchWebServices.com 2003)

application server: A computer that runs an application. See "application".

application software: Software to support the needs of an organization. See "application" and "system software".

appointment: A scheduled outpatient meeting between a patient and a caregiver. Also, sometimes patients are also scheduled with a room, equipment, a class, etc. Making appointments minimizes wait time for patients and optimizes utilization of resources.

appointment clerk: A person who takes member phone calls and who may schedule an appointment.

arbitration: A dispute resolution process involving a hearing outside of court. The arbitrators, who are supposed to be neutral, hear a complaint and resolve the dispute. The resolution is final and binding to all parties.

architecture: See "system architecture".

archive: Archiving is the process of long-term storage and organization of data and documents. An archive is storage of patient data or other information on storage slower than standard on-line storage that can be retrieved but may require the requestor to wait a long period of time to retrieve it.

Arden Syntax: Standards for defining and sharing medical knowledge bases.

ASCII: American Standard Code for Information Exchange: ASCII is a 7 bit code with an 8th bit used for parity (ISO-7 code) used for defining displayable and non-displayable characters.

aspects: Modular units of code that describe a recurring property within a software system that can be defined once and used wherever needed in the software system, possibly in different objects, applications, or computer systems.

aspect-oriented programming: A programming paradigm providing modular units of code called aspects that can be used across objects, applications or computer systems.

assessment: A clinician's interpretation of the subjective and objective findings, including any tests, x-rays or procedures that are performed and thus an appraisal or evaluation of a patient's condition, based upon clinical and laboratory data, medical history, and the patient's account of symptoms.

association: For databases, a relationship existing between instances of entities (e.g., a company has a number of offices, a person works for a company).

association class: Data to describe a formal association (e.g., to describe a contract between an employee and employer).

ASTM (the American Society for Testing and Materials): A not-for-profit organization that provides a forum for members of various groups to meet on common ground and write standards for materials, products, systems and services.

ASTM E1384: ASTM standards for the content and structure of the Computer-Based Patient Record.

ASTM s E31.12 Subcommittee: An ASTM group meeting on standards for healthcare.

asynchronous communication: Irregularly timed communication where each character is sent independently. Synchronization of the clock of the receiver generally is achieved by adding start and/or stop bits to each character transmitted. See "synchronous".

attending physician: A physician directly responsible for the care of an inpatient. See "admitting physician"

audit: An official examination and methodical review of the medical record in all aspects of medical care, based upon established standards, usually done by trained medical staff unaffiliated with the healthcare organization.

audit trail: Computerized recording of transactions, the resources, or medical records, that were accessed and the identity of the user.

authentication: (1) computer science: In a computer system or network, the process of verifying that a person, organization, process or device seeking access to a computer system or network is who or what it claims to be; authorization of a person signing on to a system is often done at the time the person enters a user name and password. (2) medicine: Proof of authorship of a medical record entry, such as by a "digital signature".

authorization: (1) computer science: In a computer system or network, the determination by a security service of what access rights, if any, a person, organization, process or device seeking access has to a given device, application, process or information resource; (2) medicine: To use or disclose health information.

automated call distribution (ACD): A specialized telephone switching system that distributes incoming and outgoing calls to agents. See "call center".

automated medical record: Another term for the automated patient medical record.

automated patient medical record: Health care record stored in electronic format; patient medical records available over a network.

back up: The process of copying important software, data or documents onto some other media (magnetic tape, floppy disks, etc.) to guard against its loss should anything happen to the original.

backup: The media on which information is backed up. See "back up".

Balanced Scorecard: A management technique for measuring the future financial health of an organization or the financial benefits of a project. It does this by not only using financial figures to predict the future, but also by looking at positive aspects of an organization that would predict the financial health of the organization in the future.

bandwidth: The amount of information that can be handled by a device or system, usually measured in baud rate or bps. Also the range of frequencies that can be passed through a communication channel.

bar code: An array of rectangular marks and spaces in a predetermined pattern, usually used for automatic product identification or for input of encounter or other information on a scanned document.

batch processing: A mode of data processing where programs are put into queues to be processed off-line and where there is no user interaction.

baud: When transmitting data, the number of times the medium's "state" changes per second. A 2400 baud modem changes the signal it sends on the phone line 2400 times per second. Since each change in state can correspond to multiple bits, the actual bit rate of data may exceed the baud rate.

benefits: The services payable under a specific payer plan.

benign: Not malignant; not recurrent; favorable for recovery.

best practice guideline: A guideline for treating a medical condition that is based upon the best current scientific research, that produces the best outcome.

binary number: A number expressed in base 2. Internally, it is shown as a series of 1's and/or 0's and internally in the computer as on or off switches.

biomarkers: Cellular, biochemical, molecular, or genetic characteristics or alterations by which a normal, abnormal, or simply biologic process can be recognized, or monitored. (NIH 2004)

biometrics: The utilization of an anatomical or behavioral characteristic in order to verify the identity of an individual; an "authentication" technique for identification of a user of a computer.

bit: Short for "binary digit". A 0 or 1, on or off. Computers use bits in combination to represent data, numbers, characters.

bitmap: A pattern consisting of rows and columns of dots, or bits in memory, that correspond to pixels on a screen.

black box: With regard to computer software systems, everything seen by the users of the system. "Black box" is often used to describe testing, where "black box" testing is done without a knowledge of the internal workings of the system. See "white box" and "internal workings".

bps (bits per second): The speed at which bits are transmitted over a communications medium. This speed may exceed the baud rate.

blood pressure: The pressure exerted by the circulating volume of blood on the walls of the arteries, veins, and chambers of the heart. Systolic pressure is the highest level of blood pressure, which is the pressure exerted in the aorta and large arteries during systolic contraction of the left ventricle. Diastolic pressure is the minimum level of blood pressure, which occurs between contractions of the heart. A typical value for a young adult is 120 mm Hg during systole and 70 mm Hg during diastole.

board-certified: A physician or other healthcare professional who has passed a test given by their national specialty organization.

body surface area: The total area of skin on the entire or a particular part of the body, which is sometimes used in determining dosages of medications. Formulas exist based upon sex, height, weight, build. Body surface area is important in determining pediatric dosages, in determining the extent of burns and in determining radiation doses.

book: The act of making an appointment and recording it in a schedule.

bookmark: A recording of where a system user left off , allowing the user to return to that exact location.

border: A box around an object on a screen to mark its boundary.

bottleneck: A system component that limits the performance of an automated system. Such components include disk subsystems, memory, CPU's/processors, networks, buses, operating systems, databases, and transaction or application software.

brand-name: See "trade-name".

broadband: Transmission facilities with a bandwidth greater than those for voice grade facilities.

broadness: In this book, a description for a software system that is built to handle the automated as well as the previous non-automated environment to enable both previous business processes and new business processes to be handled at the same time.

browser: A tool that provides an Internet Web user interface to access HTML pages.

business analysis: A process which identifies the changes to be accomplished by a project or phase in terms of a mission, objectives and business requirements for the project or phase.

business mosaic: In this book, a set of interrelated projects and business capabilities that together perform important functions in an organization.

business policy: A set of rules and procedures for one aspect of running an organization; a policy to be applied throughout an organization via changes to workflows, systems and data kept for organizational business reasons.

business process reengineering (BPR): Means the same thing as reengineering. See "reengineering".

business requirement: A required characteristic of an organization at the end of a project.

button: In a graphical user interface (GUI), an object on the screen that the user can select, either by a mouse click or by an equivalent keyboard operation, sending a command to an application to trigger a specified action such as the start of a particular process.

byte: Eight bits forming a meaningful unit. It may represent an ASCII character or some other coded meaning to the computer. A computer's memory size is measured in megabytes where 1 megabyte is equal to 1,048,576 bytes.

C: A programming language developed in 1972 by Dennis Richie and Brian Kernighan of AT&T.

C++: An object-oriented extension of the C language developed by Bjarne Stroustrup of AT&T - Bell Labs.

calibration: The set of operations that establish, under specified conditions, the relationship between values indicated by a measuring instrument or measuring system, or values represented by a material measure or a reference material, and the corresponding values of a quantity realized by a reference standard.

call center: A bank of telephones in a managed care healthcare organization with appointment clerks and advice nurses who together (1) make appointments for the member, (2) give the member advice on medical care based upon protocols, including when self care is appropriate and when the patient should come in, and (3) connect the member with medical resources, including physicians and patient education.

capacity: The ability of an automated system, including computer, hardware, software and network systems, to handle the anticipated number of users and customers.

capitation: The payment of premiums or dues directly to the provider organization in the form of fixed periodic payment for comprehensive care, set in advance.

capture (data): The recording of data on a form or its entry into a computer.

care activity: Specific tasks to be performed (that one "does") in the care of a patient to arrive at a specific outcome in a clinical pathway.

caregiver: In this book, a healthcare organization employee in any way, directly or indirectly, providing care for a patient; also, any person who provides direct care to an individual (such as a child or a chronically ill person).

caregiver tracking: A tracker used to identify when a caregiver entered a room or left it. See "indoor positioning system".

care management: Aggregates encounters and other events into episodes for a particular occurrence of a medical condition, possibly across care settings, rather than just focusing on a single encounter or event of an illness or injury.

care notes: In this book, a caregiver's notes to him- or herself with encounters for a patient within the scope of care of a caregiver or care team. Such notes are less formal than other care documentation.

care path: An element of a clinical pathway representing a time period between two care activities.

care plan: A written framework that provides the direction of care for a patient.

care, primary: See "primary care".

care, secondary medical: Medical care of a patient by a physician acting as a consultant. The physician providing primary care usually refers the patient for this care.

care team: A group of caregivers who jointly care for patients. Care teams may be defined for one or all of the following reasons: (1) to identify nurse practitioners or physicians assistants who are supervised by a particular physician, (2) to identify other caregivers working with or supervised by the physician, (3) to identify to whom to send diagnostic test results if the ordering caregiver is unavailable, (4) to identify to whom to send clinical messages or e-mail if the recipient is not available, or (5) to identify physicians who will back up a physician if the latter physician is unavailable.

Cascading Style Sheets: Tags within HTML that create templates to control different aspects the HTML page's layout, including text font-faces, text line-heights, text styles (like bolding and italics), colors, and margins.

case: One instance of case management for a particular patient. A case is often assigned to a case manager.

case management: An organized system for delivering health care to an individual that includes assessment and development of a plan of care, coordination of services, referrals and follow-ups.

case manager: A person specifically assigned to oversee the case management of an individual for a particular case.

case notes: A set of notes developed by a case manager for a particular case.

CD-ROM: A term referring to storage of information on a CD (compact disc) using ROM (read-only-memory) format.

CD-RW: A term referring to storage of information on a CD (compact disc) using RW (read-write) format.

cell: The smallest unit of an organism that is capable of functioning independently, including a nucleus with genetic material, cytoplasm, various organelles, that is surrounded by a cell membrane.

CEN: European Committee for Standardization.

CEN/TC251: European Committee for Standardization, Technical Committee for Medical Informatics.

certified nurse-midwife: A healthcare practitioner who is educated, and who has acquired a national certification and a license within a state, in the two disciplines of nursing and midwifery.

certified registered nurse anesthetist: A registered nurse with training and certification in anesthesiology, who may substitute for an anesthesiologist in many surgical procedures.

change: In this book, in the context of a project, a modification in the way an agreement, workflow or automated system is implemented when the implementation matches the documentation of the implementation. See "error".

change control board: A group responsible for reviewing changes to controlled documents during a project.

change control process: A defined process to insure that important documents on which a project depends are not changed without careful consideration. Often a change control board is set up to agree upon or reject changes to these "controlled documents". See "controlled document".

character: Any symbol, letter, digit, or punctuation mark that can be typed on a keyboard.

character-based terminal: A type of data terminal that displays only alphanumeric or text characters (not common any more).

chart: See "medical record".

charting by exception: A charting methodology in which data is entered only when there is an exception from what is normal, from what is expected or from what was previously recorded. Such an approach may reduce time spent documenting.

chart room: A location storing patient medical records.

check box: A box where a pointing device can be put and with a button press a check mark can be entered or removed. A check sets an option. Where there are other check boxes, these check boxes remain as is. Compare this to a "radio button", where selecting one radio button turns another off.

checkpoint/restart: A technique associated with transactions where the state of the database is recorded at the start of a transaction, and if the transaction should abnormally terminate, then the database would be restored to that state.

chief complaint: The primary reason a patient is coming in for medical care.

chiropractor: A medical professional who treats disease based on the theory that disease is caused by interference with nerve function, and uses manipulation of the joints and the spine to restore normal function.

chronic condition: A condition that lasts a long time, or recurs frequently, and can be treated but not eradicated; opposite of "acute illness".

chronic disease: Illness that persists over a long period of time and affects the physical, emotional, intellectual, social and spiritual functioning of the patient.

chronic care management case: A case to track a patient who is being treated for a chronic condition over many encounters where there is likely to be long term continuing care.

CICS (IBM Corporation s Customer Information Control System): A widely used teleprocessing monitor (transaction processing system) for online application systems found on IBM mainframes.

claim: A demand for payment in accordance with an insurance policy.

client: A client process in a client-server architecture. A client is a program that issues processing requests to a server program in the same or a different computer. See "server".

client-server architecture: A network configuration in which decentralized client processes request services from centralized server processes.

clinical: Pertaining to a clinic or to the bedside; pertaining to or founded on actual observation and treatment of patients, as distinguished from theoretical or basic sciences.

clinical checking: Checking for patient drug allergies and for drug/drug, drug/food, drug/laboratory and other interactions.

clinical data repository (CDR): A database that combines clinical data related to a patient from various healthcare organization clinical systems. Example information is patient demographics, radiology data, laboratory data, medications, physician orders and H&P's. (In an automated patient medical record system, this is a portion of the information in the automated patient medical record.)

clinical data representation: A medical code set. See code set.

Clinical Document Architecture (CDA): A document markup standard that specifies the structure and semantics of a clinical document that can include text, images, sounds, and other multimedia content and can be sent inside an HL7 message (Dolin et al. 2001).

clinical epidemiology: The use of epidemiology in direct patient care.

clinical guideline: Same as "clinical practice guideline".

clinical images: Scanned medical documents producing images that can be stored on the automated patient medical record system along with completely automated documents. Clinical images can be displayed on the same monitors as the automated documents. See "medical images".

clinical information: Data contained in the patient record. Information may also include summary information such as found in CPR repositories: significant health problems, lab results, current medications, etc.

clinical laboratory: Health care professionals who perform a variety of laboratory tests that contribute to the diagnosis and treatment of disease. Areas covered by the clinical laboratory include hematology, clinical chemistry, immunology, immunohematology, and microbiology.

clinical laboratory information system: A clinical system that manages clinical laboratory data to support laboratory management, laboratory data collection and processing.

clinical pathway: A structured way to identify care activities and caregiver work flow needed to provide care for a category of person for preventive care or for a patient with a particular condition or disease. Paths through a clinical pathway can be adjusted for the particular needs of an individual patient. Also, clinical pathways for separate diseases can be combined into one clinical pathway.

clinical practice guideline: A set of parameters related to a specific disease or medical condition that help clinicians make clinical decisions.

clinical record: See "medical record".

clinical social worker (CSW): A person who possesses a master's or doctor's degree in social work, has performed at least two years of supervised clinical social work, and either: is licensed or certified as a clinical social worker by the State in which the services are performed, or in the case of an individual in a State that does not provide for licensure or certification, has completed at least 2 years or 3,000 hours of post master's degree supervised clinical social work practice under the supervision of a master's level social worker in an appropriate setting such as a hospital, SNF, or clinic.

clinical summary: A summary of clinical information about a patient, which may include demographics information, significant health problems, past encounters, primary care physicians and other significant caregivers, and medications.

clinical system: Information system that manages clinical data to support patient care and clinical decision making.

clinical trial: A scientifically rigorous investigation of new methods, materials such as medications, or procedures in the treatment of a particular disease or condition.

clinician: Someone who sees, evaluates, and treats patients, especially a physician, nurse practitioner, or physician assistant.

cluster: In computer science, a group of computers working together to share resources or workload; in epidemiology, an unusual aggregation of health events that are grouped together in time and space and that are reported to a public health unit.

clustering: The use of clusters.

code: The programming content of any application.

code set: The complete set of representations and codes, with each representation defined by a code.

coding scheme: A method of replacing each member of a vocabulary of names (such as a patient problem or diagnosis) by a number or "mnemonic".

co-insurance: A provision in an insurance policy, generally for health coverage in a PPO, that limits coverage to a certain percentage, typically 70-80%. The remainder is to be paid by the insured person is called co-insurance.

collaborative communication: In this book, communication while two or more caregivers have access to the automated patient medical record.

column: All the values from multiple rows in a database table corresponding to a particular data element in the table. See "data element".

commercial off-the-shelf (or COTS) software: Vendor software systems that are made to be sold to and used by multiple organizations.

Common Gateway Interface (CGI) processing: A protocol that enables a web server to pass a web user's request to an application program and to receive data to forward back to the user. For example, a program using CGI can read and write data files and produce different results each time (whereas a Web server by itself can only read data files).

communicable disease: Any disease that can be transmitted from one person or animal to another by direct or indirect contact.

communications protocol: Communications standards that identify how two computers coordinate the exchange of data.

community-based charts: When multiple facilities of a healthcare organization share the same set of paper patient medical records.

co-morbidity: An accompanying illness or disease that coexists with an already established medical diagnosis.

compiler: A program that translates programs written in a higher level computer language such as COBOL, C or C++, into code that a computer can execute. Compiled programs run faster than interpreted programs, such as those written in Java. See "interpreter".

complaint: A reason a patient is coming in for medical care.

complementary medicine: See "alternative medicine".

compliance, patient: "The extent to which the patient's behavior, in terms of taking medications, following diets, or executing life style changes, coincides with the clinical prescription"(Haynes, Taylor, and Sackett 1979) (Sackett et al. 1991).

compliance management: In this book, (1) advising a patient on community and health organization resources such as classes for making life style changes or (2) periodically contacting a patient to monitor, advise, and encourage the patient in complying with treatments and changes

component adaptability: In this book, the use of various strategies to procure, develop or structure a system or component of a system so that the system or component can more easily be replaced in the future by another equivalent system or component.

compression: An algorithm to transform and compact text or image data to minimize storage requirements or transmission time.

computed radiography: X-ray images captured in a computer, instead of on film.

computer: A device capable of accepting data, manipulating it in a prescribed way, and displaying or storing the results where it is instructed.

computerized provider order entry (CPOE): Automated ordering and return of results, which may be part of an automated patient medical record system.

computer language: The vocabulary and syntax of a set of symbols that may be used to tell a computer what it is to do.

computer-based patient record (CPR): An electronic patient record.

Computer-based Patient Record Institute (CPRI): An organization whose primary purpose is to promote automation of the patient chart.

computer telephony integration (CTI): The integration of computer applications with telephony applications by interfacing a computer system to a telephone system.

conceptual view: Models of systems, workflows, etc. which are vehicles for communication and for critique.

concurrency: (1) medicine: Multiple caregiver access to a patient's medical record, which may be for the same encounter, with possibly more than one update occurring at the same time. (2)

computer science: In database processing, the situation wherein multiple processes access the same database record at the same time for various database functions, which may include reading, updating, deleting, etc. In either case, concurrency rules must insure no loss or corruption of the data.

concurrent review: The investigation of patient care while it is in progress, with the intention of modifying that care if appropriate and determining if continued treatment is medically necessary.

conditional order: A type of medication where the medication is given based upon a condition occurring (e.g., the patient experiences pain).

conditional treatment case: In this book, a case developed by a primary care physician, urgent care physician, nurse practitioner, or advice nurse that may be later used to generate a treatment case, or may later be dispensed with.

confidentiality: The act of limiting disclosure of private matters; maintaining the trust that an individual has placed in one who has been entrusted with private matters; not disclosing information about a patient that is considered to be privileged and cannot be disclosed to a third party without the patient's consent.

consent: The agreement of an individual for a given action relative to the individual. This may be consent for treatment, special procedures, release of information, and advance directives. "Expressed consent" is written; "implied consent" is an action other than an expressed consent on the part of a patient that demonstrates consent; while "informed consent" is freely given consent that follows a careful explanation by a caregiver.

constraint: In this book, something that limits what could be done in a project. The most important constraints are time and money.

consultation: Process in which the help of a specialist is sought to provide advice or care for a patient. A request for a consultation is often accompanied by a referral; see "referral" and "referral letter".

content facilitator: In this book, a person who gathers information from domain experts to design and produce products of the project. See "domain expert".

content management system: A system for storing different types of unstructured content (such as Web content, office documents, scanned images and faxes, e-mail and rich media) and semi-structured content (such as printed reports) as well as structured content (XML and associated documents). See "document management system".

contingency plan: Plan of action to minimize or negate the adverse effects of a risk should it occur.

continuity of care: The coordination of care received by a patient over time, with care often given by multiple caregiver.

contraindication: Any condition, especially any condition of disease, which renders some particular line of treatment improper or undesirable.

control: An item that may appear within a window on a computer screen to allow the user to control the window. These include list boxes, input fields, buttons, check boxes, radio buttons, and others.

control chart: A control chart is a graph of data used in statistical process control that incorporates statistical content—a mean (average) and upper and lower statistical thresholds (control limits)—to guide interpretation and decision-making of the data. A "trend document" is a form of control chart. See "trend document".

controlled document: An important document created during a project that can not be changed without approval of a change control board within a change control process. Examples of such documents are documents to record project objectives and goals, business requirements, workflow requirements, system requirements, program specifications, user documentation. See "change control process".

controlled medical vocabularies: Codes for medical terms, diseases, diagnoses, and procedures. See "medical vocabularies".

controlled substance: A drug whose distribution and use is controlled by federal and/or state government regulation. Controlled substances, which may include narcotics, stimulants and sedatives, are divided into five classes called schedule I through schedule V. See "schedule I through V drugs".

Controlled Substances Act: The Controlled Substances Act (CSA), Title II of the Comprehensive Drug Abuse Prevention and Control Act of 1970, is the legal foundation of the U.S. Government's regulation of controlled substances.

conversion plan A document identifying how to convert data in existing and replaced production systems to produce the data for the new and changed production system databases. See "data conversion".

cooperative business objects (CBOs): Real world "business objects" used in a GUI interface of a computer system that are relatively independent from each other.

cooperative editing systems: "Multi-user systems where the actions of one user are instantaneously propagated to all the other participating users" (Ionescu and Marsic 2000)

coordination of benefits: The transmission of claims or payment information from any entity to a health plan for the purpose of determining the relative payment responsibilities of the health plan.

coordination of care: Methods to assist caregivers in coordinating their care of a patient.

copayment: Fixed monetary payments a patient makes per visit or prescription filled.

copy: (1) To copy information displayed on a computer screen and keep it so you can paste it somewhere else on the screen. (2) To make an exact copy of a file so you can place the duplicate in another location.

corporate database: A database sharing data across many systems in an organization to avoid redundant entrance of information and to insure that data in the organization is in a consistent format. See "application database".

co-sign: (1) Verbal medical orders from a physician may be entered and signed by a caregiver other than the physician (e.g., a registered nurse, physician assistant, pharmacist, respiratory therapist) but must be later co-signed by the physician (e.g., within 24 hours). (2) Medical or nursing students documentation (e.g., a progress note) may be co-signed by an instructor, indicating the instructors agreement with the information and acceptance of responsibility for the documentation.

cost-benefit analysis: Identification and evaluation of all costs and benefits associated with a particular project.

CPR repository: In this book, a national database containing a summary of a patient's clinical information in a format using national or international data standards. Possible information might include patient identification information, a patient problem list, patient practitioners, patient encounters, services (including medications, diagnostic tests, immunizations, procedures and therapies), assessments/exams, and care plans.

CPT (Physicians Current Procedural Terminology): A system describing medical and surgical procedures in a hierarchical format with six major sections, developed by the American Medical Association. The current version is CPT-4.

CPU (central processing unit): The part of a computer that controls all the other parts. The CPU fetches instructions from memory and decodes them. This may cause it to transfer data to or from memory or to activate peripherals to perform input or output. Sometimes just called the "processor".

credentialing system: A system that uses national databases to record or verify a healthcare practitioner's professional credentials. For example, a credentialing system may (1) verify that a healthcare practitioner has a license to practice, (2) record or verify hospital privileges, (3) verify DEA certification, (4) record board certification, (5) identify sanctions against licensure, and (6) identify Medicare/Medicaid sanctions.

crisis: See "panic".

critical pathway: See clinical pathway.

cryptographic techniques: Methods of concealing data by representing each character or group of characters by others.

CT (computed tomography) scan: A diagnostic test that combines the use of x-rays through the body from multiple angles, the resultant absorption values are analyzed by a computer to produce cross-sectional slices.

cursor: A flashing line, square, rectangle or other symbol on the computer screen that moves when you move the mouse or other pointing device and can also be moved around via characters or character combinations entered through the keyboard.

cut: To remove information displayed on a computer screen but keep it around so you can paste it back somewhere else on the computer screen.

data: Symbols that represent observations; often called raw data to emphasize that they are unprocessed. Data are processed and interpreted to yield "information".

database: The collection of permanently stored data used by one or more applications.

database administration: The tasks necessary to insure data integrity, non-redundancy of data, immediate up-to-dateness of data, integrity of the meaning of data as recorded in data dictionaries, security, and database software installation and upgrades.

database management system (DBMS): A scheme using "software" and sometimes "hardware" to store and retrieve large quantities of interrelated data by one or many different application programs. See "database", "application database", and "corporate database".

data communication: The sending, transmission and reception of information between different electronic systems.

data conversion: Converting data used in the current automated system to be used in the new automated system. See "conversion plan"

data dictionary: A database about data objects in a database, defining the use of each table in the database and the meaning of each row and data element (column) in each table in a database. See "meta-data".

data element: The smallest, meaningful piece of information in a business transaction or database. A data element may condense lengthy descriptive information into a short code. Equivalent to a data field in a paper document; a series of data elements are used to build a row in a relational database. See "field" and "column".

Data Flow Diagrams (DFDs): A structured analysis tool used to track the flow of data through an entire (business, software or other) system, identify transformations on data, and identify data repositories.

data independence: Changing data or data relationships within the database without having to make major changes to software that use the database.

data mining: Discovering useful relationships in data warehouses. See "data warehouse".

data model: A model of the logical data content of a system, expressed in terms of entities, relationships and attributes, such as may appear in an entity-relationship diagram.

data redundancy: Duplicated data in more than one place in the database.

data warehouse: A system for storing, retrieving and managing large amounts of data that planners and researchers can use without slowing down the day-to-day operations of the production database.

DEA license: License allowing a physician to prescribe controlled substances. See "Drug Enforcement Administration (DEA)".

deadlock: A situation wherein two or more processes are unable to proceed because each is waiting for one of the others to do something.

decoupling: Changing systems so they use industry standard connections so that any one system can be replaced by a different one using the same standards without having any effect on any of the other ones. See "component adaptability".

decryption: The transformation of cipher text back into plain text. See "encryption".

dedicated line: A permanent connection with a network.

deductible: The amount an individual must pay for health services each year before the individual's HMO or insurance company starts to pay.

Defense Advanced Research Projects Agency (DARPA): The U.S. federal government agency that was the originator of the Internet.

de-identification: Removing patient identifiers so that patient information can be distributed without breaking federal privacy rules.

demand management: An approach in HMOs to lowering medical costs by instructing the member in self-care, by "triaging" the patient to the most cost-effective caregiver for the member's complaint, and by coordinating the caregivers giving care to the patient. Demand management is important in an HMO because patient care is primarily paid for by a fixed capitation fee, rather than being paid for by a fee for each service given.

descriptive disease prediction: In this book, a method to predict disease by reviewing the medical records of a large number of persons over a long period of time and identifying those factors either singly or in combination that predispose a person to a particular disease. No determination is made as to whether these factors could be used as risk factors for the disease or not. Descriptive disease prediction could be done through a computer program doing pattern matching or using a data warehouse to do on-line analytic processing (OLAP). See “disease prediction”, “on-line analytic processing” and “descriptive epidemiology”.

descriptive epidemiology: A branch of epidemiology identifying patterns or trends in diseases and injuries.

desktop computer: A microcomputer using the traditional full-size case, monitor and keyboard that are designed to be used in a stationary “desk-centered” environment. See “portable computer”.

development system: An automated system used by the programmers, analysts and testers to develop, modify or test the system rather than one used by the organizational users of the system.

(medical) diagnosis (Dx): Identification of the cause of a patient’s illness or discomfort; identification of a specific disease or pathological process.

DSM-IV (Diagnostic and Statistical Manual of Mental Disorders): Diagnostic classification systems that allow consistent diagnoses of emotional illnesses published by the American Psychiatric Association.

diagnostic findings: The results of a diagnostic test. For clinical laboratory tests, diagnostic findings (results) are identified as “normal”, “out-of-range”, “abnormal”, “negative”, “positive”, and “panic” or “crisis”. In general, for results of diagnostic procedures outside of the clinical laboratory, results are “normal”, “abnormal”, “negative” or “positive”. Some results, such as x-rays, require interpretation by an expert to get the results and this description.

diagnostic image: One of a number of technologies producing images of the internal body including (1) x-rays, (2) fluoroscopy, (3) nuclear medicine, (4) angiography, (5) ultrasound (ultrasonography), (6) interventional radiology, (7) computed tomography, (8) magnetic resonance imaging (MRI) and (9) computed radiography.

diagnostic related group (DRG): A way of classifying patients for United States government reimbursement and sometimes to establish an initial care plan. Classification is based upon the following: primary and secondary diagnoses, primary and secondary procedures, and length of stay.

diagnostic tests: Clinical laboratory tests and other diagnostic procedures.

dialog box: A window that a GUI program displays to prompt a reply from a user. The dialogue box could consist of multiple controls, which may include list boxes, input fields, buttons, check boxes, radio buttons, etc. See “modal dialog box” and “modeless dialog box”.

differential diagnosis: Identification of a disease by comparison of the symptoms of two or more similar diseases.

DICOM (Digital Imaging and Communications in Medicine): A standard that has been developed by ACR/NEMA to meet the needs of manufacturers and users of medical imaging equipment for interconnection of devices on standard networks. The current version is DICOM-3.

digital: Information represented as discrete numeric values, such as 0 or 1, as opposed to analog. See "analog".

digital paper: Paper this is preprinted with thousands of tiny, nearly invisible dots which a special pen with a digital camera can read to record what was written and send to a computer.

digital signature: Cryptographic data that undeniably identifies a message with its sender.

dimmed: A menu option that a user can see but not choose. Dimmed items are usually shown in gray letters instead of black.

direct cause disease prediction: In this book, a theoretical approach to disease prediction where the total of a person's genetics and significant environmental factors are recorded enabling prediction of future diseases based upon analytic epidemiology studies. See "disease prediction" and "analytic epidemiology".

direct cut over: A way of phasing out an old automated system by turning off the old system the day the new system goes into operation.

direct manipulation: Transferring information from one window to another

directory: A listing of all the file names and subdirectories that are available on a computer system or on computers in a network.

discharge: Termination of a period of inpatient hospitalization through the formal release of the inpatient by the hospital; to release from care at a medical care facility by a physician or other medical care worker, such as from the hospital or emergency department.

discharge planning: Set of decisions and activities involved in providing continuity and coordination of care once the patient is discharged from a healthcare facility.

disclosure accounting: Disclosing to an individual an accounting of disclosures of protected health information (PHI) made by the health organization in the six years prior to the date on which the accounting was requested.

discrete event simulation: The modeling of a system (e.g., a work flow) as it evolves over time by a representation in which the state variables change instantaneously at separate points in time. These points in time are the ones at which an "event" occurs. The time between events is modeled statistically and the expected total time of the running of the system (the execution of a work flow) can be determined by running the model, randomly selecting time values within constraints, over and over again.

disease: A pathological condition of the body that presents a group of clinical signs, symptoms and laboratory findings peculiar to it.

disease map: In this book, a compedium of disease and aging progressions consisting of visualizations of different parts of the body that may vary according to aging, diseases, treatments, and chance. It also associates biomarkers and treatment decision points with these progressions and identifies possible and recommended treatments for the various types of diseases and at any point the probabilities of possible future progressions.

disease management: Identifying populations (patients) with particular acute and chronic diseases, such as diabetes, cancer, coronary artery disease or asthma, and introducing interventions throughout the life cycle of the disease that will both improve the quality of life and lower the costs associated with the disease process.

disease path: In this book, the visualization of the progression of a disease for an individual together with associated biomarkers, treatments, and treatment decision points.

disease prediction: In this book, any approach to predicting that a patient will get a disease, or to predicting when a patient will get a disease, when a disease will worsen, or when a treatment decision for a disease will need to be made, most often expressed in terms of the probability of that event happening compared to the probability of that event happening for the general population or for an applicable population group. This book identifies these forms of disease prediction: analytic disease prediction, direct cause disease prediction, descriptive disease prediction, and disease progression analysis.

disease progression analysis: In this book, determining the probable progression of a disease or progression to developing a disease for a particular patient by measuring a medical value or state for that patient over time that is predictive of the disease and comparing this progression of values or states with other patients who have developed the disease. Measurements could be recorded on a trend document. See "disease prediction" and "trend document".

disk: The most common high volume auxiliary storage medium for a computer system. Usually refers to a magnetic disk, but also refers to an optical disk.

disk mirroring: A method of fault tolerance for information stored on disks that involves writing the same information on two different disks with two different controllers. If one drive is lost or unavailable, the other is still available. See "fault tolerant".

distributed database: A database that is stored at multiple locations within a network either by partitioning the data or replicating the database.

distributed development: Doing a large project where project personnel are located in different parts of a country or of the world.

distributed facility group: In this book, the set of medical facilities of a healthcare organization handled by a particular computer system that is part of the automated patient medical record system, where the automated patient medical record system consists of a number of distributed computer systems, usually with each system each handling a different geographic location.

distributed system: Implementation of a single application system on multiple computer systems at different locations with the systems usually connected by a network.

DNA (Deoxyribonucleic Acid): A molecule in a chromosome which includes components called bases, with strings of bases serving as templates (genes) for creating polypeptides that fold into proteins. Normally, DNA is double stranded with the strands having complementary bases.

docking station: An addition to a portable computer, such as a laptop or pen computer, to add capabilities such as an AC power supply, full size monitor, CD-ROM drive, sound card, hard drive, a recharging unit, etc., to make the computer act more like a desk-top computer when it is being used in a designated fixed location.

document: A written, and sometimes pictorial, form of communication that permanently records information relevant to the health care of a patient.

document list: In this book, a list of medical documents associated with an encounter, where the medical document can be displayed by selecting it.

document type definition (DTD): A DTD defines the elements, attributes, entities and rules for creating one or more documents in a markup language (SGML, HTML, or XML). (For XML, XML DTDs are being replaced by XML Schema documents.)

documentation: Medical or computer documents. For computer systems, manuals, online help, README files and other instructions that come with a software package. See "document".

document list: A list of documents in a medical record for an identified patient.

document management system: A system that supports enterprise-wide on-line documentation (of any type) on an Intranet. A documentation management system enables enterprise wide creation, controlled access, review and update, routing and management of documents. See "content management system".

domain: The set of values allowed for a data element in a given column or for the set of data elements in a group of columns of a relational database.

domain expert: An expert in the project subject area (e.g., for an automated patient medical record, an expert in patient care and medicine).

domain name: An addressing construct on the Internet network used for identifying and locating computers on the Internet (e.g., "www.whitehouse.gov"), which can be translated by a name server into a numeric IP address. Domain names must be registered through an agency associated with ICANN (Internet Corporation for Assigned Names and Numbers),a private (non-government) non-profit corporation.

dosage: The determination and regulation of the size, frequency, and number of doses of medication or radiation for a patient.

dose: A quantity to be administered at one time, such as a specified amount of medication (e.g., 5 g. for 5 grams).

download: Transferring data or software from a central location to a remote location (e.g., your server or workstation) via a communications link.

drag: The action of using a mouse or other pointing device to select and move an object on the screen.

drag and drop: The action of using a mouse or other pointing device to select and move an object, placing it somewhere else on the screen.

drill down: For tree structured connected document such as hypertext, to go down from a higher level document to a lower level one by selection at the higher level.

drive: Any device that reads and writes information, such as a hard drive, floppy drive, CD-ROM drive, CD-RW drive, or tape drive.

drug allergy: Hypersensitivity to a pharmacological agent, with reactions that could range from those that are very mild (e.g., a rash) to those that very severe.

drug compendium: A listing of drugs and information about them used by healthcare practitioners who prescribe them. It is used to validate drug orders. It includes both HMO formulary and non-formulary drugs, enables clinical checking (drug interaction checking) and enables drug costing.

Drug Enforcement Administration (DEA): U.S. Government agency that is part of the U.S. Department of Justice that enforces drug laws and regulations including regulations concerning the legal manufacture and distribution of controlled substances. See "DEA license".

drug formulary: In this book, a listing of all the drugs a healthcare organization recommends, the most effective and least cost ones. Some managed care organizations charge more for non-formulary drugs, whereas in some managed care organizations non-formulary drugs are not covered at all.

drug interaction: Interactions of a drug with other drugs, with foods, with laboratory tests, or other interactions.

drug jumping: Going from physician to physician and/or facility to facility to get a prescribed medication, especially a narcotic or other controlled substance, and especially for a patient who is addicted to that drug.

DTD (Document Type Definition): See "XML DTD".

dumb terminal: A terminal consisting of a keyboard and display screen that cannot run applications itself but can receive and send character data to a mainframe

durable medical equipment (DME): Equipment leased or sold to patients for use in their homes (e.g., wheelchairs, walkers, canes).

durable medical equipment (DME) formulary: A database that lists and describes all durable medical equipment (DME) offered to patients within a healthcare organization. See "durable medical equipment".

durable power of attorney for healthcare: See "healthcare proxy".

DxPlain: An experimental system of clinical decision support provided by time shared telephone links, which was developed at Harvard University Massachusetts General Hospital in the late 1960s.

EBCDIC: Extended binary-coded decimal interchange code: A character-coding scheme found mostly in large-scale IBM computers.

E code: An injury code, sometimes used for an injury registry, with the injury registry being a database for recording injuries from which epidemiological studies can be done.

EDIFACT: EDI for Administration, Commerce, and Transportation (EDIFACT). An international UN-sponsored EDI standard primarily used in Europe and Asia. An alignment is envisioned between ANSI ASC X12N and EDIFACT EDI standards in the future to create a single EDI standard. The standard is used for the electronic interchange of structured data related to trade in goods and services.

effective: Producing the intended result.

efficacy: The ability to produce the desired effect.

electrocardiography (ECG or EKG): ECG is the graphic tracing of the variations in electrical potential of the heart.

electroencephalography (EEG) : A graphic tracing of the variations in electrical potential of the brain.

electronic commerce (E-commerce): The paperless exchange of business information using Electronic Data Interchange (EDI), electronic mail, electronic bulletin boards, electronic funds transfer and other similar technologies. ANSI ASC X12N standards are used in the U.S.

Electronic Data Interchange (EDI): The computer to computer exchange of business data in a standardized format between Trading Partners.

electronic health record (EHR): Another term for the automated patient medical record. Health care record stored in electronic format.

electronic medical record (EMR): Another term for the automated patient medical record. Health care record stored in electronic format.

electronic patient record: Another term for the automated patient medical record. Health care record stored in electronic format.

electronic signature: A code or symbol that is the electronic equivalent of a written signature and that can legally substitute for the written signature.

elective: Subject to the choice or decision of the patient or physician; applied to procedures that are advantageous to the patient but not urgent.

elective admission: An admission to the hospital that could be medically delayed without endangering the patient, such as for an elective surgery.

eligibility/coverage: Refers to the period of time a healthcare organization subscriber or dependent is entitled to benefits.

e-mail (electronic mail): The use of a computer network by individual users to send, store, and receive messages or documents to and from other individuals.

emergency: The sudden onset of a condition or an accidental injury requiring immediate medical or surgical care. See "prudent layperson standard".

emergency department (ED): A hospital area staffed and equipped for the reception and treatment of persons requiring immediate medical care.

emergency medical condition: A medical condition that with the absence of immediate medical treatment could be expected to (1) place the patient's health (or for a pregnant woman, the unborn child's health) in jeopardy, (2) seriously impair bodily functions, or (3) create serious dysfunction of any bodily organ or part.

EMTALA (Emergency Medical Treatment and Active Labor Act): A Federal law which gives all patients showing up at the emergency department, independent of their financial status, the right to receive a medical screening exam to determine whether an emergency medical condition exists, and, if so, to receive care to stabilize the condition and/or to be transferred to a more appropriate facility. See "emergency medical condition".

emulation: A program that runs a program that mimics something else (e.g., a program that mimics a dumb terminal).

encapsulation: Hiding data and methods within an object class from outside programmers to make the class easier to use.

encounter: A face-to-face interaction between a patient and a healthcare provider. In some cases this may also include an interaction via a phone call or television if this takes the place of the face-to-face interaction. Encounters could include all of the following: an inpatient stay, outpatient visit, emergency department visit, advice nurse call, a phone call between a patient and a physician, a home health visit, a skilled nursing facility (SNF) visit.

encounter status: An event that may logically precede, occur during or be a result of an encounter or potential encounter, or a result of a situation causing the encounter not to occur. For example, encounter statuses for an outpatient visit could be patient wait-listed, appointed, appointment canceled, appointment no show, patient registered, in the examination room, visit completed, diagnoses and procedures identified.

encounter synopsis: In this book, a summary of a patient encounter.

encryption: The transformation of confidential plain text into a cipher text in order to protect it from being read by a third party. See "decryption".

endemic: Present or usually prevalent in a population or geographical area at all times; said of a disease. This is opposed to "epidemic" and "sporadic".

end-stage renal disease (ESRD): A disease of the kidneys that ends up requiring either dialysis or renal replacement.

enhancement: Implementation of a change in an automated system. See "change".

enterprise management system: A package of software systems that together manage a distributed computer network, composed of possibly disparate computers, as if the distributed network was a mainframe system.

enterprise master patient index (EPMI): A master patient index for an enterprise. See "master patient index".

enterprise scheduling system: A multi-dimensional healthcare organization scheduling system that schedules patients with caregivers and resources (e.g., patients with caregivers, patients and caregivers with rooms—such as operating rooms, patients and caregivers with classes, patients and caregivers with equipment) and may provide information for charging for associated services, for automatic ordering of associated supplies, and for recording caregiver time for the caregiver payroll system.

entity: Something about which information is stored. An entity might be a tangible item, such as a patient, physician or room. An entity can also be intangible, such as what this book calls an agent.

entity-relationship (E-R) diagrams: A database analysis diagram that documents business entities about which database information will be stored that shows the relationships that exist between the entities.

entrance by exception : See "charting by exception".

epidemic: Occurring suddenly in numbers clearly in excess of normal expectancy; said especially of infectious diseases but applied also to any disease, injury, or other health-related event occurring in such outbreaks. This is opposed to "endemic" and "sporadic".

epidemiology: Study of the occurrence, distribution, and causes of disease and the application of this study to the control of health problems.

episode: "One or more healthcare services received by an individual during a period of relatively continuous care by healthcare practitioners in relation to a particular clinical problem or situation" (ASTM 2002).

episodic: Care handled by a single outpatient encounter, possibly including calling back the patient. Also see "acute care".

error: In this book, in the context of a project, an inconsistency between how a project agreement, a workflow or an automated system is implemented and how it is documented—the error may either be an error in the implementation or in the documentation. See "change".

error of commission: Mistake resulting from overdiagnosis or diagnosing a nonexistent health problem.

error of omission: Mistake resulting from failure of the caregiver to diagnose a health problem or disease.

essential business practice: Some aspect of the current environment and systems that must be preserved in a changed environment because it is essential for the proper functioning of the organization.

Ethernet: A local area network architecture (also known as the IEEE 803.2 standard) developed by the Xerox, Digital and Intel that operates at 10 Mbps and uses the CSMA/CD protocol for media access control. Ethernet is being extended to gigabit bandwidth.

etiology: A study of the causes of disease. Also see "analytic epidemiology".

event: Events are milestones one "sees" in a clinical pathway (e.g., patient has mammogram). Also, a term used in discrete event simulation to describe an instantaneous occurrence that may change the state of the system (e.g., patient enters waiting room, patient registers, patient comes into the exam room).

evidence-based medicine: Best treatments and practices for diseases that produce the best outcomes—sometimes for the least cost—as determined by the best scientific evidence.

exclusive searching: In this book, searching for exact matches and synonyms (e.g., a search for "myocardial infarction" would also find occurrences of "heart attack"). See "inclusive searching".

expected outcome: Expected condition of a patient at the end of therapy or the end of a disease process, including the degree of wellness and the need for continuing care, medications, support, counseling and education.

expert system: A program that structures knowledge from business experts (such as experts in the medical field on a particular medical condition) to advise other people on how to make decisions based upon that knowledge. For example, an expert system may be created to determine a diagnosis in a specialized medical field based upon patient parameters.

extranet: An intranet that is open to selective access by outside parties.

face sheet: A document that is created at the time of a hospital admission that is used to collect information for the admission that includes the name, address, birthdate, contact and other patient demographics information, and may include admitting diagnosis, admitting physician, attending physician, unit, room and bed location and assigned diagnostic related group.

facilitation: Establishing a group dynamic, helping make a group function effectively and efficiently.

facilitator: A process facilitator. See "process facilitator".

facsimile (fax): The transmission of images, usually over the telephone network. Images are scanned and transmitted on a bit basis over the telephone system and reconstructed at the receiving end.

fail-over recovery: When the primary server goes down, a backup server automatically takes over.

family history (FH): Facts about the health of the patient's parents, siblings, and other blood relatives that might be significant to the patient's condition. Part of the subjective part of a SOAP note.

family physician: A primary care physician for all members of a family.

FAQ (frequently asked questions): A list of the most commonly asked questions with answers that appear in a newsgroup on the Internet or are asked regarding a subject presented at a Web site (e.g., regarding HL7 at the Duke Web site discussing HL7). At the Web site, these FAQs are usually available via a hypertext selection.

fault tolerant: Systems that have redundancy built into their components so that component failures do not cause the system to fail. Rather, the system switches processing from a failed component to its backup.

feasibility study: A study based upon projected changes in the organization due to a project, evaluating whether the project can be done within the required budget and time with the required results.

feature analysis: Analyzing images or waveforms for features for purposes of automated diagnostic interpretation such as analyzing a mammogram for breast cancer.

FDA (Federal Drug Administration): FDA is a federal government public health agency, charged with protecting American consumers by enforcing the Federal Food, Drug, and Cosmetic Act and several related public health laws.

fee for service: Paid for on the basis of individual services provided (as opposed to a prepayment scheme such as capitation).

field: A discreet piece of information in a database, such as a first name, last name, street address, city address, state, or zip code. Fields are grouped together to make records or make rows in a table. See "data element".

file: A collection of information, stored in terms of records, especially a collection stored on an auxiliary storage medium, with a name for identification of the file. See "record".

file name: An assigned name given to a file to enable the user to retrieve the file by name.

file server: A server that stores the files for multiple users at other computers in a network.

file sharing: Allowing multiple end users or application programs to access the same files or databases. In some computer systems, this may include allowing users to access the same file or database at the same time.

filler: Used in HL7 to mean an application responding to an order or producing results. The ASTM term is a "producer".

filtering: A systematic approach to extracting information that a particular person finds important from a larger stream of information.

firewall filtering: Software and/or dedicated computer system that sits between an organization's internal network and the Internet and monitors all traffic from outside to inside, blocking any traffic that is unauthorized.

fix: A correction of an error in an automated system. See "error".

flexibility: In this book, a description for a software system that is built to be scalable to handle more advanced automated capabilities.

flow sheet: A inpatient nursing document to document the interventions used to meet the patient's needs, which may include the type of intervention, the time of care and the identity of the nurse administering care. Flow sheets generally are designed to limit the need for long written patient care notes by allowing information to be recorded either in graphics or table form with display of values for variables (e.g., temperature or respiration) as they change over time.

fluoroscopy: X-rays aided by use of a contrast material such as barium providing an outline of the structure of soft tissues including the esophagus, stomach and intestines.

font: A set of characters with a particular design and size.

foreign key: A data element in a table or data base that forms a primary key in some other table or data base.

formulary: A listing of items of a particular type that an healthcare organization recommends. Most often this is a drug formulary. Some managed care organizations charge more for non-formulary items, whereas some managed care organizations do not cover non-formulary items at all. See "drug formulary" and "DME formulary".

free text: Unstructured, uncoded representation of information in text format; for example, sentences describing the results of a patient's physical examination.

frequency: The number of occurrences of a periodic or recurrent process per unit time, e.g., administering a medication to a patient (e.g., p.r.n. is a frequency meaning "as necessary" and q.h. is a frequency meaning every hour).

FTP (file transfer protocol): A popular way to transfer files between computers on the Internet or via a TCP/IP network.

full-time equivalent (FTE): Effort equivalent to that of one full-time worker. For example, two half-time workers constitute an FTE.

function: The smallest discrete, complete set of code of an automated system that can be initiated by the user and run to completion to produce a single purpose set of results (e.g., a stand-alone function to look up patient demographical information about a patient, a function to issue an order for medication, or a function to make an appointment for a patient); a set of commands that produce a single output, named so the function can be called from many different program locations by name, with parameters to pass data to the function or from the function.

functional specification: A document describing a function within an automated system for use by the programmers and testers of the automated system. A "functional specification" describes the external design and describes the internal design of a function generically, while an "internal design specification" for a function describes the internal design more specifically in terms of the code, databases and interfaces for the function. See "internal design specification".

furnishing number: Together with his/her name and furnishing number, a nurse practitioner can furnish medications to essentially healthy patients under standardized procedures.

gate: A point where a project is to be re-evaluated for costs, feasibility and adherence to the goals of the organization.

gatekeeper: A physician, usually a primary care physician, responsible for overseeing and coordinating all aspects of a patient's care, through whom referrals to specialists must be preauthorized.

gene: A region of DNA (template of component bases) that specifies an RNA and consequently a protein.

gene expression: The genome's current functioning within the individual; turning on of a gene—although the genome serves as a template to create proteins, there are many regulatory controls turning on and off genes, thus controlling the creation of these proteins.

generalization: For databases, a relationship where one entity is a sub-type (e.g., dog) of another entity (e.g., animal)—also referred to as inheritance or an "is-a" relationship. See "inheritance".

generic drugs: Non-brand name drugs, with a name not protected by trade mark with the name usually descriptive of its chemical structure. When a generic drug is ordered its name is usually in lower case, whereas brand-name drugs are capitalized.

genome: The whole of the genetic information for an individual contained as DNA. See "DNA".

gesture: For a pen computer, entrance of information that is interpreted as a command to do something, rather than as character input, for example, to insert text at a certain location within text.

giga-: One billion or the closest multiple of 2 value to one billion. For example, a gigabit and a gigabyte respectively are 1,073,741,824 (2^{30}) bits and bytes.

glidepoint: The same as "touch pad".

global warming: An increase in average temperature on Earth, especially any increase caused by human activities.

goal: A target to be met and measured at a specific point in time that can be used to determine if and to what extent an objective or business requirement is being met. See "objective" and "business requirement".

graph: A picture created from a set of numbers. Popular graph types include line, bar, area and pie graphs.

GUI (graphical user interface): A user interface that makes use of every addressable pixel on the screen and thus makes it possible to create detailed visual symbols for user navigation, characters, pictures, and lines.

Graphical User Interface Design and Evaluation (GUIDE): A method for designing, evaluating and refining the design of GUI-based software systems.

grayscale: A graduated variation in the luminous output of a screen at a pixel location, with the variation expressed in terms of a bit value.

grid computing: Concurrently applying the resources of many computers in a network to a single problem that requires a great number of computer processing cycles or access to a large amount of data.

group communication: Concurrent view of documents by multiple users at the same time and possible updating at the same time.

groupware: Software that lets several people work with the same file at once. It also helps coordinate and manage activities, such as scheduling a meeting.

Guardian Angel system: A computer system for a high risk patient for use outside the healthcare organization, at home or away from home, that can be used to monitor the patient's health either via patient input or instrumentation input. The system can give advice, health education and therapy plans to the patient, inform the patient of appointments or inform the patient to schedule appointments. The system can alarm physicians or other caregivers of critical situations.

handheld computer: A pen computer that can be held in one hand

handwriting recognition: The technique by which a computer system can recognize characters and other symbols written by hand.

hard disk: A magnetic disk that provides relatively quick access to large amounts of data no matter where it is stored on the disk.

hardware: The mechanical and electronic components of a computer system.

HCPCS Medicare Level 2: HCFA Common Procedure Coding System, National Level II: codes and descriptive terminology used for reporting the provision of supplies, materials, injections and certain services and procedures to Medicare for medical billing.

header: The segment of data that indicates the start of an entity that is to be transmitted.

Health Care Financing Administration (HCFA): A U.S. Government agency responsible for the administration of Medicare and Medicaid.

healthcare proxy: A method of giving another person legal power to make medical decisions when you are no longer able to, also called a "durable power of attorney for healthcare".

healthcare services representative: In this book, an HMO employee to whom an HMO member could be assigned. A healthcare services representative would serve as an ombudsman who the member could call to resolve problems, to learn more about how the HMO functions and to learn more about the benefits provided to the member.

health care team records: During a patient's hospital stay, notes from other departments, such as physical and respiratory therapy.

Health Industry Business Communications Council (HIBCC): An industry-sponsored, nonprofit standards development organization (SDO), accredited member of the American National Standards Institute (ANSI), to facilitate electronic commerce by developing appropriate standards for information exchange among health care trading partners.

Health Industry Number (HIN): A number for Electronic Data Interchange (EDI) assigned by HIBCC to every health care provider facility in the United States. It includes identifiers for hospitals, nursing homes, HMOs, pharmacies and also specific locations or departments within them.

Health Maintenance Organization (HMO): A corporate entity (profit or non-profit) that provides comprehensive health care for members for a fixed periodic payment specified in advance. See "capitation".

Health Plan Employer Data and Information Set (HEDIS): A set of health care quality measures developed by the National Committee for Quality Assurance (NCQA) consisting of statistics on health care delivered by managed care plans, including preventive care and rates for certain surgical procedures.

help desk: A set of designated phone numbers to where users can call to seek advice on an automated system or to report errors in the system.

highlight: (1) In a GUI system, to select text or graphic data that is to be altered. For example, a highlighted item can be selected to be deleted or moved. (2) In a character-based system, showing text on the screen with higher intensity to make it stand out.

high-risk patient: A potential high utilizer of HMO services because of medical condition or age.

history and physical (H&P): Documentation of health history and physical examination. The purpose of the health history is to collect "subjective" data, what the person says about himself or herself. The physical examination collects "objective" data, a record of the clinician's examination of the patient and of diagnostic measurements.

history of present illness (HPI): The following information pertaining to the patient's illness: (1) the symptoms that are troubling the patient; (2) when the symptoms were first noted; (3) the patient's opinion as to the cause of the illness; (4) possible influences by any external factors; (4) any remedies that the patient may have tried; and (5) any medical treatment the patient may have been given. Part of the subjective part of a SOAP note.

HHS (The Department of Health and Human Services): A federal government agency that administers over 300 programs, including medical research, financial assistance, substance abuse treatment, Medicare and Medicaid, and Head Start.

HIPAA (The Health Insurance Portability and Accountability Act of 1996 for Medicare and Medicaid programs): A federal bill that includes standards for security and electronic signatures, provider identifiers and taxonomy, electronic transfers, and employer identifiers.

HISPP: See ANSI HISPP.

HIV: Human immunodeficiency virus, the cause of AIDS. See "AIDS".

HL7 (Health Level 7): Messaging standards for information exchange between disparate clinical, administrative and financial computer systems for the healthcare industry, developed by ANSI. "7" refers to the seventh level of the OSI / ISO interconnection reference model.

HL7 Electronic Health Record-System Functional Model (HL7 EHR-S): A Health Level Seven (HL7) group model of Electronic Health Record (EHR) behavior identifying an expected set of functions of such a system.

HL7 Reference Information Model (RIM): HL7's object-oriented information model of the healthcare domain.

HMO member: A person who pays a fixed periodic payment to an HMO in exchange for comprehensive health care.

HMO report card: See the "Health Plan Employer Data and Information Set (HEDIS)".

home health care: Skilled nursing and related care supplied to a patient at home.

home page: On the Internet World Wide Web, a screen related to a company, government organization or person that is identified and initiated by an Internet user entering a domain name or IP address in a browser or by user selection of a hyperlink on an Internet page that causes entrance of the domain name or IP address.

hospice care: Care specifically given to terminally ill patients—generally those with six months or less to live.

hospital: An establishment with an organized medical staff with permanent facilities that include inpatient beds and continuous medical/nursing services and that provides diagnosis and treatment for patients.

hospitalist: A physician who is a specialist in in-patient medicine, who takes responsibility for a patient's care from the personal care provider during the patient's entire hospital stay.

HSQ 2.0 (Health Status Questionnaire 2.0): A trade-name product of National Computer Systems, Inc., a survey to be filled out by a patient related to a particular medical condition that identifies the patient perception of his/her quality of life, and which can be used by healthcare providers to identify which treatments and physicians provide the best outcomes from the patients' point of view. It captures aspects of both physical and emotional health. It contains all items found in SF-36.

HTML (Hyper Text Markup Language): An SGML-based language used as a standard language for creation of Internet World Wide Web pages that can be used to incorporate hypertext links, text, graphics, sound and video.

HTTP (Hypertext Transfer Protocol): The protocol for transporting Web pages across the Internet.

hypertension: A condition where the patient has a higher than normal blood pressure.

hypertext: A method of linking different parts of a database where the database could consist of text, graphics, data files, video and sound, usually in a top-down tree like structure, that enables a user to display and navigate through the links depending upon his or her interests, jumping from one related topic to another, by enabling text to be selected to present a connected document. This structure is used extensively in the Internet.

hypothetico-deductive approach: A classical data collection and interpretation strategy followed by many physicians, nurse practitioners and other clinicians within the examination room or hospital room, applicable both for the outpatient and inpatient setting.

icon: A small pictorial representation of an object (for example, a patient, the patient chart, an appointment form) appearing as part of a screen using a graphical user interface.

IEEE (Institute for Electrical and Electronic Engineers): An association for professionals in electrical engineering and computing, which also establishes standards for electrical devices.

IEEE Medix: IEEE P1157 Medical Data Interchange (Medix) Committee. A object-oriented standard for exchange of data between hospital computer systems, compatible with HL7 and DICOM. MEDIX is a comprehensive specification for a health data exchange standard, which its developers have stated has an objective of eventually supporting the transfer of the entire patient record.

IEEE P1073: An IEEE family of standards for medical device communication with hospital information systems.

ICU (intensive care unit): An area of the hospital where there are critically ill patients who are closely monitored.

ICD (International Classification of Diseases): A hierarchical system published by the World Health Organization using three-digit codes describing procedures, health status, categories of diseases, disablements and reasons for contact with healthcare professionals. Because ICD-9 was not felt to be adequate, a set of clinical modifiers of two additional digits were added, known as ICD-9-M. A still newer set of codes is being developed, ICD-10-CM.

IETF (Internet Engineering Task Force): The standards body for the Internet community.

-ilities: What aspects can be used to implement, including reliability, availability, responsiveness, performance, security, and manageability.

immunization: The process of inducing or providing immunity artificially by administering a vaccine, toxoid or antibody containing preparation.

implementation: The action that must follow any preliminary thinking in order for a project to actually happen.

in-basket: A collection of a clinician's orders and results, e-mails, and clinical messages.

incident report: Document that describes any patient accident while the patient is on the premises of a healthcare institution.

inclusive searching: In this book, searching for exact matches and synonyms (like for exclusive searching) but in addition, searching for related items (e.g., a search for "urogenital" would find occurrences of "bladder" and "uterus"). See "exclusive searching".

indication: A sign or circumstance that points to or shows the cause, pathology, treatment, or issue of an attack of disease.

index: An object consisting of identified data elements in a relational database table that is used to control the order in which the table is accessed or stored.

indoor positioning system (IPS): A system that reads the signals from tags, for example worn by caregivers, to identify the position of the tag within a building. See "caregiver tracking".

information: "Data" processed in some way, usually by selection and formatting, so that it has meaning and may facilitate decision making.

information hiding: Hiding data from other programmers in order to protect the data from corruption and to simply the overall system structure.

information retrieval: A field of computer science that deals with the automated storage and retrieval of textual documents.

informed consent: Process of obtaining permission from a patient to perform a specific test or procedure after describing all the risks, side effects and benefits.

infrastructure: The underlying foundation or basic framework of a system which must be done before the functional part of the system can be done.

inheritance: (1) A relationship between object classes where an object class that inherits from another may share the data and methods of that other class. (2) For both databases and object classes an "is-a" relationship between two objects or entities (e.g., an "inpatient" is a "patient" and an "outpatient" is a "patient" and may both inherit from "patient").

injection: Act of introducing a liquid into the body by means of a syringe.

inpatient: Patient admitted for treatment within a hospital over the course of more than one day.

Inpatient Census: A patient list of all patients in rooms within a particular hospital unit at the current time, including patient identity and bed and room within the unit.

inpatient clinical summary: A summary of information during a patient's inpatient stay similar to the Kardex that is generated at the start of the inpatient stay based upon patient medical record information and disappears after discharge. See "Kardex".

Inpatient Clinician List: A patient list for an inpatient clinician (physician or nurse) listing all inpatients assigned to the clinician and role of the clinician (attending physician, admitting physician, primary care physician, nurse, etc.)

instance: Naming and using an object class to generate code.

integrated: In the context of an organization, all the employee workflows, automated systems, and other parts of the organization function well together, ideally meeting the totality of the objectives of the organization; in the context of a project, the project produces products that work together with pre-existing systems and employee workflows, and other projects, to support the organization.

Integrated Circuit Card (ICC): A credit care size plastic card containing a microprocessor. Also called a "smart card".

interactive voice recognition (IVR): A software application that accepts a combination of voice telephone input and touch-tone keypad selection and provides appropriate responses.

interface: The connection between any two components of a computer system and the protocols of information passed between the components. (Interfaces include connections between a user and an application, two computers, a computer and a hardware device such as a disk drive.)

interface engine: A hardware/software system used by the healthcare industry to support network communication and perform other functions. A typical interface engine provides a message queue, translates transmitted information, and stores the translated information on databases. Because interface engines are generally used in healthcare, they often support HL7.

interface plan: A recording of interfaces within an organization, identifying the interfaces required for each new automated system.

interface standard: Standard that specifies requirements concerned with the compatibility of products or systems at their points of interconnection.

interface testing: Validation of interfaces between the automated system and other automated systems. See "validation".

integration testing: Validation of functions and programs working together into subsystems and in the entire automated system. See "validation".

intermediate care: In this book, off-chart and strictly confidential counciling by a psychologist or clinical social worker (CSW) to either (1) provide the patient with a means to cope with a life situation, (2) refer the patient to appropriate medical care if this is necessary, or (3) suggest patient education classes to take.

internal design specification: A program specification to describe the code, databases and interfaces that implement a function or implement a capability within an automated system. See "functional specification".

internal workings: Used in this book for computer software systems to mean everything not seen by the users of the system. See "black box" and "white box".

Internet: Worldwide network of interconnected computers. Uses the TCP/IP communications protocol.

Internet Engineering Task Force (IETF): "A large open international community of network designers, operators, vendors, and researchers concerned with the evolution of the Internet architecture and the smooth operation of the Internet". (IETF 2004)

Internet service provider (ISP): A company that sells an account providing Internet access.

interpretation: Analysis of diagnostic images or test results for indications of abnormalities and possible disease.

interpreter: A program that reads computer source language code statements one by one, evaluating a statement, immediately executing the statement and advancing to the next statement. This is opposed to a compiler where the total of source language code statements making up a program are translated to a program in a form directly executable by the computer; a program in a form executable directly by the computer is said to be a program in "machine language". Machine language programs always run (execute) faster than interpreted programs. JAVA is a language where programs are interpreted within a browser.

interval: The lapse of time between two recurrences.

interventional radiology: Use of x-rays to help guide biopsy needles to evaluate tumors or place catheters for widening narrowed arteries and draining infections.

intervention: The act or fact of interfering so as to modify.

interview: Type of communication with a patient initiated for a specific purpose and focused on a specific content area.

intranet: A private computer network based upon the data communication standards of the public Internet.

intravenous (I.V.) therapy: Form of injection in which fluid is introduced directly into the vein.

I/O: Input/Output device. An external device connected to a computer to allow input or output of information, such as a disk, keyboard, mouse, screen or printer.

IP (internet protocol): Defines how each packet of a message travels across a TCP/IP network. IP assigns an address to each packet. See "TCP/IP".

IP addresses: A unique, numeric identifier used to specify hosts and networks on the Internet and TCP/IP networks. See "domain name".

ISO (International Standards Organization): An international group of experts that sets standards for technology. For example, ISO 9660 is a CD-ROM standard.

ISO/OSI interconnection reference model: International Standards Organization / Open System Interconnection Reference Model: A model for networks developed by the ISO to act as a framework for developing standards that will achieve the concept of an open network architecture. The model is a layered model with seven layers.

invasive: Referring to procedures that involve puncture, incision, or insertion of a foreign object, such as a needle or catheter, into the body.

Java: Interpreted, object-oriented programming language developed by Sun Microsystems. Derived from C++.

Java applets: Interactive pieces of code written in Java that may be downloaded from the Web at the same time as HTML pages.

Joint Committee of Accreditation of Healthcare Organizations (JCAHO): A private, nongovernmental agency that establishes guidelines for the operation of hospitals and other health care facilities.

JPEG (Joint Photographic Experts Group): Image compression technique. The amount of information lost depends on the level of compression.

Kardex: Trade-name for card-filing system that allows quick reference to the particular need of an inpatient for certain aspects of nursing care.

kilo- : One thousand or the closest multiple of 2 value to one thousand. For example, a kilobyte is 1024 (2^{10}) bytes and is represented by K such as 10K for ten kilobytes.

Labeler Identification Codes (LICs): Part of a uniform bar code labeling standard for products shipped to hospitals developed by the HIBCC. LICs identify manufacturers.

LAN (Local Area Network): A network of computers that uses direct cable connections or short wireless connections rather than telecommunications; thus, the computers are in a localized area (such as a building).

layer: A set of data in a network message with a header and trailer for a particular purpose and intervening data. A layer may be inside another layer. Headers and trailers are added to create a layer before the message is sent, and removed as it is received. For example, one layer may be used for routing the message through a complex telecommunications network; once the associated header and trailer is not needed it is removed.

laptop computer: A class of portable briefcase-sized computers with capabilities similar to desktop computers. See "portable computer".

legacy systems: Existing organizational systems.

length of stay (LOS): The number of days between admission and discharge of a hospital stay or other inpatient stay.

licensed practical nurse (LPN): A nurse who is licensed by a state board of nursing after completing an education program and passing the licensure exam who practices under the supervision of a registered nurse.

life care path: A clinical pathway identifying preventative care for a member over a long period of time, which may be used for long term preventative care, or alternatively, for a chronic disabling disease that must be tracked over a very long period of time.

limited parallel operation: A way of phasing out an old automated system by running the new system with real data to test and verify functionality, but the new system does not completely parallel the old system.

Linux: A Unix-type operating system that is intended to be free or low-cost. Linux is short for "Linus' Unix". See "Unix".

load balancing: Distributing processing and communications activity evenly among computers in a cluster so no computer is overloaded.

local system: In this book, a computer system that is a portion of a distributed automated patient medical record system for a healthcare organization that records patient clinical information for a set of healthcare organization facilities and performs all the functions of the automated patient medical record system for caregivers at these facilities.

locking: The process of prohibiting dual access to a file, database, record or field that has been accessed with the potential of change of the data. This is to prevent conflict or corruption of the data.

logical database design: A part of the design of a database where sets of data ("tables", "records" or "entities") making up the database are identified, the formats of data elements making up each entity are identified, and the relationships between the entities are identified.

log in or **log on:** To gain access to a computer system, usually by entering a user identifier and password.

log off: To sign off a computer system performing all clean-up processing necessary to not lose data and to restore the system to a consistent state.

LOINC (Logical Observation Identifier, Names and Codes): A set of names and ID codes for identifying laboratory and clinical observations.

longitudinal patient record: A life time patient record.

long term care: Non-acute hospital care, for chronic conditions (e.g. nursing homes, psychiatric institutions, geriatrics, etc.)

low-utilizer: A health organization member who seldom comes in for care.

machine language: The language characteristic of a particular computer.

magnetic resonance imaging (MRI): A technique using magnetic fields that produces anatomic images in multiple planes and may provide information on tissue characterization. A type of diagnostic imaging.

magnetic tape: A reel of pliable plastic, coated with magnetizable material on which may be recorded signals that represent data.

mainframe: A large, powerful, central computer, typically operated and maintained by professional computing personnel.

maintainability: A measure of how easy or hard it is to change the system without introducing new errors in the system or inconsistencies in the requirements.

maintenance: The process of changing an automated system after it has been delivered and is in use; also, changes to functionality in an automated system after the function has been implemented. Also called "software maintenance".

malignant: Tending to become progressively worse and to result in death.

malpractice: Injurious or unprofessional actions that harm another.

mammography: Diagnostic imaging examination of the breast for screening and diagnosis of breast disease.

managed care: An arrangement where a third-party payer (such as an insurance company, federal government, or corporation) mediates between physicians and patients, negotiating fees for service and overseeing the types of care given.

master file: Common reference files, such as clinical lab test codes, caregiver identifiers, etc., that must be synchronized across clinical systems.

Master Patient Index (MPI): In this book, a MPI is a set of patient identifiers, such as name, gender, date of birth, mother's maiden name, etc., which together can be used to uniquely and unambiguously identify a patient. In the healthcare industry, an MPI is a cross reference of all the identifiers that various information systems use to identify a person.

Medicaid: A U.S. government program that provides medical assistance for certain low-income individuals and families.

Medicare: A federal health insurance program designed to provide healthcare for the elderly and the disabled.

medical: Pertaining to medicine or to the treatment of diseases; pertaining to medicine as opposed to surgery.

medical assistant: A multi-skilled healthcare professional who performs a variety of clinical, clerical and administrative duties within a healthcare setting.

medical image: The same as "diagnostic image". Medical images usually require very high-resolution monitors to be displayed for diagnostic purposes. See "diagnostic image".

medical informatics: The use of computers in medical care.

medically necessary: Services or supplies that meet the following tests:

- they are appropriate and necessary for the symptoms, diagnosis, or treatment of the medical condition
- they are provided for the diagnosis or direct care and treatment of the medical condition
- they meet the standards of good medical practice within the medical community in the service area
- they are not primarily for the convenience of the plan member or a plan provider
- they are the most appropriate level or supply of service that can safely be provided.

medical record: A written transcription of information obtained from a patient, guardian or medical professional concerning a patient's health history, diagnostic tests, diagnoses, treatment and prognosis.

medical references: Used in this book to mean compendiums of information on medicine available on the Internet or an Intranet or otherwise available through an automated patient medical record system. Medical references include poisons information, AHCPR clinical practice guidelines, drug compendiums and formularies, the PDR and others.

medical screening exam: An examination that goes beyond the initial triage, utilizing ancillary services as necessary (lab tests, x-rays EKGs), to determine whether or not an emergency medical condition exists. See "emergency medical condition".

medical transcriptionist: Medical language specialist who transcribes dictation by physicians and other healthcare professionals in order to document patient care.

medical vocabularies: Medical terms, including diseases, diagnoses, procedures, and codes for them.

Medicare: A federal health insurance program for people over age 65, the disabled, and people with end-stage renal disease who require dialysis or transplantation.

medication administration record (MAR): In a hospital, a record of medication orders for a patient and documentation of their execution.

medication scheduler: In this book, a person who assists in creating patient medication schedules. See "patient medication schedule".

MEDLARS (MEDical Literature Analysis and Retrieval System): A computerized system of databases and databanks offered by the National Library of Medicine for medical literature retrieval, which includes specialized databases in health administration, toxicology, cancer, medical ethics and population studies.

Medline: An on-line bibliographic database of medical information.

MedWatch: A safety information and adverse event reporting program run by the United States government FDA. In turn, such suspected associations may be reported back to healthcare organizations.

mega-: One million or the closest multiple of 2 value to one million. For example, a megabyte is equal to 1,048,576 (2^{20}) bytes and is represented by Mb such as 10Mb for ten megabytes.

member: A individual who has a contract with an HMO to provide medical services for the individual for a capitation fee and possibly other payments such as co-pays or deductibles.

memory: The part of a system that holds program instructions and information being processed. See "RAM" and "ROM".

menu: A list of options from which a user chooses.

mentoring: In this book, caregivers randomly or selectively reviewing automated medical records, asking questions about the medical record, and discussing alternative medical practices in order to improve healthcare.

menu bar: A strip across the top of a window in a GUI system, listing all the menus available in that program.

message: The atomic unit of data transferred between systems, containing address information and content.

message queuing: Programs on separate computers with queues on each computer to store and then forward a message from one computer to another. Even though a computer or the network is down, the message will not be lost and will still eventually arrive. See "store-and-forward".

messaging: See "caregiver messaging system".

meta-data: Data that describes data objects in the database. Data about data. See "data dictionary".

metastasis: The change in location of a disease.

method: A routine within an object class.

microbiology: The science that deals with microorganisms, including algae, bacteria, fungi, protozoa and viruses.

microcomputer: A small computer generally with one user.

Micromedix: A product of the Micromedix company in Denver, Colorado that offers current, comprehensive reference libraries for toxicology, pharmacology, emergency and acute care, occupational medicine, chemical safety, and industrial regulatory compliance.

Microsoft Windows: A window system and user interface software released by Microsoft in 1985 to run on top of an older, character-based operating system, MS-DOS.

middleware: Software that mediates between an application program and a network, managing the interaction between disparate applications across heterogeneous computer systems.

milestone: A major event (often at the start of a stage) which is used to monitor the progress at a summary level of a project.

minicomputer: A computer with a size and computing capacity between that of the mainframe and the microcomputer.

minimal disclosure necessary: For protected health information only the minimum amount of information needed to satisfy an outside request is to be disclosed. See "protected health information".

(disk) mirroring: Writing data twice, once to each of two disk drives. If one drive fails, the other contains an exact duplicate of the data and the disk system can switch to using the mirrored drive with no lapse in user accessibility.

mission: A summary of the change to the organization expected to be produced by a project or a phase of a project.

mitigate a risk: To take whatever actions are possible in advance to reduce the effect of an identified risk in a project.

mnemonic: A code that serves as a representation and memorable abbreviation for some word or phrase.

mobile code: The transmission of code across a network from one computer system to another for execution on the second computer system.

modal dialog box: A dialog box that takes control of an application and requires the user to close the dialog box before continuing the application.

model: A simplified description of a complex process.

modeless dialog box: A dialog box that does not take control of the application, allowing the user to work within other dialog boxes while the dialog box is open.

module: Logical blocks of reusable code.

molecular biology: The study of genomes and cells.

molecular medicine: The use of molecular biology for medical purposes.

monitor: A television-type device that displays text and graphics generated by a computer;.

monitoring: (1) The process of continually checking, observing, recording or testing the operation of some procedure or one or several physiological parameters. (2) To observe a project or the results of a project in order to change the direction of the project when necessary.

monitoring systems: A system that monitors a patient, collecting large amounts of information, such as ECGs and Guardian Angel systems. Monitoring systems could potentially produce large volumes of information; therefore, much filtering of such information has to be done to determine the significant information to store.

morbidity: A diseased condition or state, the incidence of a disease or of all diseases in a population.

morbidity rate: The sickness rate, the number of people who are sick or have a disease compared with the number who are well.

mortality: Death rate in a given population.

mortality rate: The proportion of deaths in a population or to a specific number of the population.

mouse: A hand-manipulated computer input device used for pointing and drawing with computer programs. When the device is moved across a flat surface, a ball on the bottom causes the cursor to be moved on the screen.

multidisciplinary: Care across multiple medical departments.

multimedia: A blend of text, graphics, sound, animation and video.

multiplexing: Combining several signals for transmission on some shared medium (e.g. a telephone wire). The signals are combined at the transmitter by a multiplexor (a "mux") and split up at the receiver by a demultiplexor.

multiplicity: In a GUI system, allowing the user to work on two instances of an object at the same time (e.g., two different patient lists, two different clinical summaries).

multiprocessing: Executing tasks or programs on separate processors, thus allowing them to execute concurrently. Conversely, if tasks and/or programs share a processor, then processing switches between the various tasks and programs.

multiprogramming: A technique used in an operating system for executing several independent programs at the "same time", either on the same processor or multiple processors.

multitasking or **multithreading:** A technique used in an operating system for executing several tasks, either part of the same program or not, at the "same time", either on the same processor or multiple processors.

name server: In the Internet or TCP/IP networks, a computer that has both the software and the data required to resolve domain names to Internet Protocol (IP) addresses.

NANDA (North American Nursing Diagnosis Association) nursing diagnoses: A set of nursing diagnoses developed by a group, NANDA, that meets every two years. NANDA developed the following definition for nursing diagnosis: "Nursing diagnosis is a clinical judgment about individual, family, or community responses to actual and potential health problems/life processes. Nursing diagnoses provide the basis for selection of nursing interventions to achieve outcomes for which the nurse is accountable" (NANDA, 1990).

narcotic: An agent that produces insensibility or stupor, applied especially to the opioids, i.e. to any natural or synthetic drug that has morphine-like actions.

natal: Associated with one's birth.

National Drug Code (NDC): A drug code maintained by the FDA (Federal Drug Administration).

National Guideline Clearinghouse: A comprehensive database of clinical practice guidelines for treatment of medical conditions based upon the best scientific evidence developed in association with public and private healthcare organizations.

national healthcare system: A national government sponsored healthcare system.

National Library of Medicine (NLM): Located in Bethesda, Maryland, the world's largest repository of biomedical health sciences information.

National Patient Identifier (NPI identifier): A standard unique identifier mandated by the U. S. government for health plans and health care providers by the year 2000.

National Patient Identifier Assigning Authority: In this book, a national location to send information to uniquely identify a patient. The location will return either an existing national patient identifier for the patient or a new national patient identifier.

National Science Foundation: A U.S. federal government foundation that extended the Internet from a government network to a public network.

NCPDP (The National Council for Prescription Drug Programs): An organization that develops standards for information processing for the pharmacy services sector of the health care industry.

NCQA (National Committee for Quality Assurance): A non-profit oversight organization for the managed care industry.

NCQA database: A national database for evaluating HMOs, which includes information for generation of the HEDIS report, an HMO "report card".

need to know: A philosophy for granting security to a person. If the person does not "need to know" the information is his position, then he is not given the authority to view or access the information.

negative: Not affirming the presence of the organism or condition in question.

neonatal: Pertaining to the first four weeks after birth.

network: A system of interconnected computers and terminals.

network access point (NAP): Several major Internet connections that tie together Internet service providers. See "Internet service provider".

network layer: See "layer".

NIC (Nursing Intervention Classifications): A comprehensive classification of nursing interventions developed by a research team at the University of Iowa.

NIH: National Institutes of Health, a part of the U.S. Department of Health and Human Services.

NOC (Nursing Outcomes Classifications): A standardized terminology and criteria for measurable or desirable nursing-sensitive patient outcomes that result from nursing interventions. Links can be made between NOC outcomes and NANDA nursing diagnoses.

non-functional specification: A specification that describes not what the software will do, but how the software will do it (e.g., "all responses must be in 2 seconds").

normal: A description for diagnostic findings, including clinical laboratory test results. See "diagnostic findings". Performing proper functions; natural; regular.

normalization: A procedure for placing data elements in tables in databases according to a set of dependency rules so as to create stable data structures that minimize data redundancy and maximize data independence.

nosocomial: Pertaining to or originating in the hospital, said of an infection not present or incubating prior to admittance to the hospital, but generally occurring 72 hours after admittance; the term is usually used to refer to patient disease, but hospital personnel may also acquire a nosocomial infection.

n-tier: "n" refers to an integer that might be any value, while "tier" refers to a category of computer. Thus an "n-tier system" consists of "n" different categories of computers connected to each other. For example, a 3-tier system could include connected separate computers for the following: the workstation or presentation interface, the business logic, the database.

nuclear medicine: X-ray with tiny amounts of radioactive tracer material (radioisotopes) that are absorbed by an organ reveal how the organ works, rather than just its structure.

nurse: A profession concerned with the diagnosis and treatment of human responses to actual and potential health problems.

nurse practitioner (NP): A registered nurse who has completed an advanced training program in primary health care delivery, and may provide primary care for non-emergency patients, usually in an outpatient or community setting.

nursing assessment: The systematic collection of data related to the patient's nursing needs.

nursing diagnosis: Identification of a health problem made as a result of the nursing assessment.

nursing intervention: An action deliberately selected and performed to implement the nursing plan of care.

nursing plan of care: A written guideline for patient care that documents the patient's health needs determined by assessment and nursing diagnoses, priorities, goals and expected outcomes.

nursing unit: An area of the hospital serving a specific purpose (e.g., ICU, medical/surgical, respiratory, etc.) Also simply termed a "unit".

object: A term used in object oriented computing and analysis to mean a package of information and processes related to a definable entity.

object class: The name of an object, inheritance relationships of the object with other objects, together with the data and methods describing how the object is implemented.

object-oriented user interface (OOUI): A GUI interface using cooperative business objects.

object request broker (ORB): Software middleware that manages communication between objects.

objective: A future position of an organization expected from implementing changes in the organization. See "goal" and "strategy"; in medicine, a record of the clinician's examination of the patient and of diagnostic measurements—see section 4.4.1.3.

object-oriented design: A way of designing an application system by breaking the system program code into objects.

observation: A clinical statement about a subject, usually a patient. Examples are the following: clinical laboratory results, imaging studies, drug allergies.

observation visit: A visit where the patient is in for observation for possible admittance to the hospital, such as a pregnant woman having contractions.

obstacle: Any actual or potential hindrance to the successful completion of a project.

one off order: When there is a repeating medication order, a type of medication order where an extra dose is given this one time only.

on-line: Connected to and controlled by the computer.

on-line analytical processing (OLAP): A system software system to transform or limit data from data warehouses in order to discover patterns, trends and exceptions in business, medical or other operations. OLAP was a term coined by E.F.Codd in 1993.

on-line transaction processing (OLTP): A system software system to handle real-time transactions (e.g., making medical orders or appointments), requiring transaction management, extensive audit trails, routing, scheduling and administration. See "transaction".

open architecture: (1) Use of standardized technology and structures for hardware, operating systems, data bases, fault tolerances, and network and communications transport. (2) Program structure and hardware is compatible with the hardware and software of other vendors.

operating system: The master control program scheduling, running and providing services (such as file I/O, database processing, screen display or printer output) for application programs and other service programs. Popular operating systems are Linux, Windows XT, and Window 2000.

optical character recognition (OCR): A process wherein a printed page is scanned and the resulting image of the page, line, or part of a page is interpreted and translated into a sequence of characters.

optical disk: High-volume, slower speed and less costly storage than hard disk, using laser rather than electromagnetism to read and write data. Examples are CDs and DVDs.

order: A request for service from a clinician to an ancillary department for a particular patient, which may be sent from a clinical application where the order was created to another clinical application where the performing area is located.

order result responsibility group: In this book, a set of caregivers and/or print locations associated with a caregiver doing ordering at a particular ordering location identifying where, when and to whom alarm and order result information is to be sent beside to the ordering caregiver.

Organization for the Advancement of Structured Information Standards (OASIS): An organization that sponsors an initiative to develop industry-specific standards for XML and a registry and repository for specifications for these standards.

organizational objectives: Those things an organization needs to do to run the organization and have a quality organization. Also see "objective".

OSHA (U.S. Department of Labor Occupational Safety & Health Administration): A department of the U.S. government that enforces various healthcare regulations.

osteopathic physician: Doctor with training that places special emphasis on the relationship between the musculoskeletal system and the body's other systems.

outcome: Measurement of the impact of treatments, procedures or other care strategies on specific measures of a patient's health at the end of therapy. May include financial, clinical and patient satisfaction measures. Outcomes may be positive or negative.

out-of-range: A description for clinical laboratory test results. See "diagnostic findings".

out-of-area benefits (HMO): Benefits supplied by a plan to its subscribers or enrollees when they need services outside the geographic limits of the HMO. These benefits usually include emergency care benefits, plus low "fee for service" payments for non-emergency care.

outpatient: Patient who has not been admitted to a hospital but receives treatment in a clinic or facility associated with a hospital or in a medical office building.

overall clinical summary: A summary of clinical information for the patient including patient description information, a list of all encounters, significant health problems, and current medications.

overall design: Identifying how all products of a project could best fit together.

over-the-counter drug: Drug available to a consumer without a prescription.

packet switching: A method of passing information between any two points in a network in units (packets). The information to be passed is disassembled into packets on entry into the network, and packets then proceed individually by any available route to their destination. Before leaving the network, the packets are reassembled into their original form. TCP/IP and ATM use packet switching.

PACS (picture archiving and communication system): A software / hardware system for the management, acquisition, transmission, storage, retrieval and display of digitally acquired images which may include the following types of diagnostic images: CT scan, MRI, Ultrasound, Computed Radiography, Angiography, Mammography, Fluoroscopy and Nuclear Medicine.

panic: A description for diagnostic findings, including clinical laboratory test results. See "diagnostic findings".

Pap smear, Pap test, Papanicolaou test: A screening test for cervical cancer.

paradigm: A pattern or model of which all things of the same type are representations or copies.

parallel operation: A way of phasing out an old automated system by running both the old and new system concurrently and comparing results to verify both systems function alike.

parameter: (1) medicine: A variable whose measure is indicative of a quantity or function that cannot itself be precisely determined by direct methods; e.g., blood pressure and pulse rate are parameters of cardiovascular function, and the level of glucose in blood and urine is a parameter of carbohydrate metabolism. (2) computer science: Data passed between programs via a routine (aka a function, subroutine or procedure) or method.

parenteral: Not in or through the digestive system; typically refers to administering medications by injection.

password: A secret string of characters a user types to prove who he or she says she is, used for "authentication".

paste: To insert the last information that was cut.

past medical history (PMH): Any illnesses the patient has had in the past along with the treatments administered or operations performed. Part of the subjective part of a SOAP note.

pathogen: Any disease-producing microorganism.

pathology: Branch of medicine that treats the essential nature of the disease, especially the structural and functional changes in tissues and organs of the body caused by the disease.

patient: One who is sick with, or being treated for, an illness or injury.

patient-centered care: Used in this book to mean (1) care systems that center on patients, not caregivers, or (2) a situation where the patient is given full time care with the assistance of computers or monitoring systems, such as Guardian Angel systems. See "Guardian Angel systems".

patient case: In the book, a document that allows a case manager to track a patient over multiple encounters, whether or not the encounters are for a specific medical condition. It would consist of case notes and other case documents, as part of overall case management information.

patient clinical summary: Overall clinical summary or inpatient clinical summary. See "overall clinical summary" or "inpatient clinical summary".

patient demographics: Information that identifies, locates, or describes a patient.

patient education: Instruction to the patient and his/her family, for the purpose of improving or maintaining an individual's health status.

patient list: A list of patients of interest to a caregiver stored within the automated patient medical record system, usually automatically built from encounters and encounter statuses from other clinical systems.

patient (management) case: Documents to support the overall tracking by a case manager of high cost, high risk patients, such as elderly, frail Medicare or workers' compensation patients.

patient medical vocabulary: In this book, a medical vocabulary understandable to the patient.

patient medication schedule: In this book, a schedule for patients on when to take medications.

patient mentoring: In this book, a patient providing to another patient his or her experience in having a disease or in having a treatment for a disease.

patient profile: In this book, a quick summary of the attributes of the patient, preferrably created by the patient, which would be used locally within a healthcare organization only and would not be devulged to anyone outside the healthcare organization.

patient registry: In this book, a database and software system identifying all patients in the CPR repositories and identifying subscribing healthcare and other organizations, such as insurance companies, who are interested in each patient. Upon a patient encounter recorded in a CPR repository, a subscriber to the patient registry would be informed of the encounter. Also, a subscriber could request identification of all patient encounters for a patient and the CPR repositories containing the encounter information.

patient panel: A patient list for a caregiver of all patients for whom the caregiver is a primary care physician, case manager, or other defined relationship.

payback period: The amount of time it takes before a system will fully recover its investment (development) costs.

PDA: Stands for personal digital assistant. See "personal digital assistant".

peer review: The inspection by one or more physicians of the process and outcome of a patient's healthcare as recorded in the patient's medical record.

peer-to-peer: A network in which each party has equal capabilities and each can initiate a communication with the other.

pen computer: A small portable computer that mainly uses pen for input, with the user "writing" on the screen. See "portable computer".

peripheral: A physically independent device linked to a "CPU" and controlled by it. Examples are a terminal, printer, disc drive, or magnetic-tape drive.

performance: The total effectiveness of a computer system, including throughput, individual user response time, and availability.

performance and scalability plan document: In this book, a document that identifies required response time and other required performance characteristics, future projections of increases in number of customers handled by automated systems, bottlenecks identified so far, and contingency plans for resolving anticipated future performance problems.

personal physician: A primary care physician chosen by the patient or assigned to the patient who is responsible for overseeing and coordinating all aspects of the patient's care. See "primary care physician".

personal identification number: See PIN.

performance monitoring: Measuring the performance of an automated system while it is in operation.

performance testing: Testing the system for bottlenecks that could cause the system to take a long time to respond to users when many users are using the system. See "validation".

performing area: A location where an order can be sent to be put on a work list or to be transferred to a clinical system for execution of the order.

personal digital assistant (PDA): Also called "hand held computers", these are computers small enough to be carried around in a coat pocket or handbag.

Personal Health Record: A document similar to the CPR and to the Patient Clinical Summary that relies on patients to enter the medical information rather than the information primarily being generated from medical documents.

personal physician: A primary care physician chosen by a member to provide the bulk of his or her primary care.

pharmacist: Licensed professional who formulates and dispenses medications.

pharmacy: A place of business that specializes in preparing, identifying, and dispersing drugs.

pharmacy information system: Clinical system that deals with the pharmacy. Such systems can be linked to prescribing systems for electronic processing of a request for medication and can provide inventory control.

phase: In this book, a sub-project of a larger project.

phase in: A way of phasing out an old automated system by running the new system in a portion of the enterprise first, adjusting the way it works if necessary, and incrementally replicating it in other parts of the enterprise.

phone message: A message from a patient, e.g., from an advice nurse, to a physician or other caregiver, which may be saved in the patient medical record.

physical database design: A part of the design of a database where the logical database design is used to map the data in the database to physical files.

physical exam (PE): A recording of the results of a clinician's examination of the patient, which may, for example, include clinical laboratory and x-ray results. Usually findings for each of the major areas of the body are included under separate subheadings. Part of the objective part of a SOAP note.

physician: Health care professional who has the degree of Doctor of Medicine (MD) or Doctor of Osteopath (OD) and is licensed to provide medical, surgical and other treatment.

physician assistant (PA): A practitioner trained in aspects of the practice of medicine who works with or under the supervision of a physician to provide diagnostic and therapeutic care.

PDR (Physicians Desk Reference): A book updated every year by Medical Economics Data with cooperation of manufacturers that lists essential information on major pharmaceutical and diagnostic products.

pick list: A drop-down list of items, one of which can be selected, to fill in a text item.

pilot: Implementing a computer software system using a portion of the potential customers and users, such as at a single facility of an HMO.

PIN (personal identification number): A numeric value used to identify a particular user.

pixel: A point on a monitor screen that may be set on or to an identified color or shade of gray located in terms of a rectangular array of picture elements ("pixels") on a screen. The smallest addressable element on a display screen, located by horizontal and vertical position on the screen (x,y).

placer: The application (system or individual) originating a request for services (an order).

plan: Information regarding a clinician's treatment of an illness, including: (1) Prescribed medications along with exact dosages; (2) instructions given to the patient; (3) recommendations for hospitalization or surgery; and (4) any special tests that need to be performed.

platform: The hardware and software of a specific computer system.

plug-in: An "add-on" piece of software that enhances the capabilities of a browser application.

pointing device: A device a user can use to control the movement of the cursor on a display screen. Examples are mice, trackballs, touchpads and light pens.

point-of-care computing: Capturing and entering data at the locations where patients receive care, such as by bedside terminals or pen computers during the time of interviewing an outpatient.

point of service: Managed care plan that allows patients to see physicians not included in the plan for an increased fee.

point-to-point: A direct connection between two computers.

poison: Any substance that impairs health or destroys life when ingested, inhaled, or otherwise absorbed by the body in relatively small amounts.

pop-up menu: A list of options that appears on the screen when you click the right mouse button.

port: An input-output connection through which data flow can be directed.

portable computer: Designates a type of computer that is easily moved from place to place and that normally contains battery power to use on the go.

portability: The ability of a program to run on systems with different architectures.

porting: Moving software and data files to other computer systems.

positive: Indicating existence or presence of a condition, organism, etc.

postnatal: Occurring after birth, with reference to the newborn.

postoperative: Occurring after a surgical operation.

post partum: After childbirth, or after delivery.

post visit report: In this book, a report given to the patient at the end of the visit describing the results of the visit.

PPO (preferred provider organization): A method of health care financing where a network of physicians and others enter into an agreement with an insurer to provide health care services on a discounted fee schedule in exchange for the insurer sending patients their way.

pre-admission: The entrance of admission information at a time ahead of the admission, such as for an elective admission.

precision: A term used in information retrieval (searching) to mean retrieving only exactly what you need, limiting the number of items retrieved.

predictive modeling: A technique using mathematical and statistical algorithms based upon visit and patient medical record information to identify which HMO members would benefit the most from disease and other case management.

pre-existing condition: A medical condition that began before a plan member became covered under the plan.

prepayment: Payment in advance for health care, for example by fixed amounts monthly.

prescribe: To indicate the medicine to be administered.

prescription: Authorized order for medication, therapy, or a therapeutic device. It is signed by a physician or other practitioner licensed by law to prescribe such a drug, therapy or device.

preventive care: Interventions directed toward preventing illness and promoting health.

primary care: The first contact in a given episode of illness that leads to a decision regarding a course of action to resolve the health problem.

primary care physician: A generalist physician who is capable of overseeing and coordinating all aspects of a patient's care. A primary care physician is usually a family practitioner, general internist, pediatrician and sometimes an obstetrician or gynecologist. The primary care physician in an HMO initiates most referrals for specialty care. See "personal physician".

primary care provider: A primary care physician, or a generalist nurse practitioner or physician assistant who is supervised by a primary care physician. See "primary care physician".

primary key: A data element or group of data elements in a table or data base that can be used to uniquely identify a row of the table or record of the data base.

printer: A device for producing hard copy on paper of data from a computer.

priority: Each patient entering the emergency department must be appropriately assessed to identify a priority for the patient for treatment through a triage process. See "triage".

privacy: The right of individuals and organizations to establish when, how, and to what extent, information about themselves is transmitted to and used by others.

printer spooling: To send printouts to a storage file for a specific printer to be queued for later printing for that printer. This enables the program creating the printout to continue processing without waiting for the printer and for printouts to be saved even though the program has terminated or been interrupted.

p.r.n.: Abbreviation for "whenever necessary" used for prescriptions for a medication meaning to give the medication whenever it is necessary. A frequency.

probability density functions (pdf): A graph of the occurrence of a value (x) versus the probability of the value's occurrence (y). For example, the number of days it takes a simple fracture of a femur to heal versus the probability for each of those days. "pdfs" are generally shown as continuous functions interpreted from a set of sampled values.

problem: (1) Short for a "significant health problem". (2) Same as a "nursing diagnosis". A problem of a given individual can be described by formal diagnosis coding systems (e.g., DRG's, NANDA nursing diagnosis, ICD9, DSM, etc.) or by other professional descriptions of health care conditions affecting an individual.

problem list: (1) A list of significant health problems in a clinical summary. (2) A list of numbered patient problems used with the "problem-oriented medical record (POMR)" that provide a way to cross reference a problem with its manifestation in other places in the patient medical record.

problem-oriented medical record (POMR): A structured medical record fronted by a list of the patient's problems introduced by Dr. Lawrence Reed. All findings and treatments recorded are linked to the relevant problems. Within the POMR the SOAP note format was first introduced.

procedure: (1) medicine: A series of steps by which a desired result is accomplished. (2) computer science: A block of code which may be initiated (called) from many different programs with return to the next location in the calling program after completion; also called a "function" or "subroutine". A procedure may have parameters to pass data to the procedure or from the procedure.

process: A piece of code that can execute as a unit; the way a group agrees to function to be most productive.

process facilitator: A person who attends group meetings to help establish a group dynamic, making the group function effectively and efficiently.

producer: See "filler".

product: The final results of a project or phase remaining after the project or phase is complete.

production system: The automated system used by the day-to-day organizational users.

prognosis (Px): The clinician's opinion of what the outcome of the illness will be, the patient's chances of improvement or cures—often expressed as "good", "fair", "poor" or "guarded".

program: (1) Instructions coded in a computer language. (2) Loosely coupled but tightly aligned sets of projects aimed to deliver the benefits of part of a business plan or strategy.

program design language (PDL): A structured English description of the code for a module or routine which can be used to code it in a programming language.

programmer: A person who writes computer programs.

progress note: A document recording notes of the patient's progress. An initial medical examination is recorded in a History and Physical, subsequent encounters result in recording notes of the patient's progress.

progressive: Advancing; going forward; going from bad to worse; increasing in scope or severity.

project: A project, in a business environment, is: (1) a finite piece of work (i.e., it has a beginning and an end), (2) undertaken within defined cost and time constraints, and (3) directed at achieving a stated business benefit.

project constraints: Resource restrictions on the project determined by organizational management such as the project budget or the allowed number of workers of various types to accomplish the project.

project life cycle: The duration of a project, especially the sequence of defined stages in the project.

project management: "A systems approach to development and implementation of a defined set of inter-related products with the development and implementation described by a project plan breaking the development and implementation into tasks stated in terms of time, costs, resources, and performance parameters". (Gouse 1988)

project mission: A summary of the change to the organization expected to be produced by the project.

project objectives: The intended final positions of an organization after a project is completed. Also see "objective".

project plan: A description of events to come". (Wysocki and McGary 2003)

project strategy: A change in direction of an organization that is part of a project that is presumed to result in an objective or objectives of the organization being fulfilled. See "strategy".

proposal: A short document for the initial investigation of a proposed project, which usually identifies the impact of the project on the organization, broad estimates of benefits and costs, and expected time to complete.

protective factor: In this book, something that is done that protects against a specific disease—the opposite of risk factor. See "risk factor".

protected health information (PHI): Any information in any media that relates to "an individual's past, present, or future physical or mental health status, condition, treatment, service, products purchased, or provision of care", and in any way identifies the individual (e.g., combines medical information, gender, and geographic location to identify an individual)

protocol: (1) medicine: Written and approved plan specifying the procedures to be followed during an assessment or in providing treatment. (2) computer science: A set of rules for how two computers speak to one another through a network.

prototyping: The process of developing and interacting with a partial version of a system in order to gain user feedback and to evaluate feasibility.

prudent layperson standard: Emergency care is covered in a health care plan if the decision to go to the ED was one that an average person with average medical knowledge would make at the time.

psychiatry: The branch of medicine that deals with diagnosis and treatment of mental illness.

public health: Community efforts to improve the health of the community through health education, the detection and prevention of disease, and the control of communicable diseases.

pull-down menu: A list of options that is revealed when you select a menu name at the top of a window.

pulse: The regular, recurrent expansion and contraction of an artery produced by waves of pressure caused by the ejection of blood from the left ventricle of the heart as it contracts.

quality assurance (QA) group: A group responsible for validation and verification of an automated system after a change to the system.

quality manager: In this book, a person who evaluates the healthcare given by caregivers in a healthcare organization.

quality of service (QofS): The ability to differentiate between classes of network traffic and users and give the highest priority and error correction to the most critical messages.

queue: An ordered list in which items are inserted and later removed. Queues are usually FIFO, meaning an item put into the list first is removed first. In a LIFO list, an item that is put in last is removed first.

radio button: A circle where a pointing device can be put and with a button press the circle is filled in with black or returned to white. Setting to black sets an option. Where there are other radio buttons, other radio buttons are turned back to white. Compare this to a "check box".

radiology: The acquisition and analysis of medical images.

RAID: Short for "Redundant Array of Independent Disks". A method of using two or more standard, lower cost, disks for fault tolerance of information on the disks—Normally fault tolerance of information on disks requires expensive disk hardware. The most common types of fault tolerance supported by RAID technology are disk mirroring (referred to as RAID level 1) and striping (referred to as RAID level 5).

RAM (Random Access Memory): Memory area in a computer where information can be temporarily written and read for the execution of program.

random access: Reading or writing to a type of memory where every location of memory is equally available (e.g., RAM). This is opposed to sequential access. See "sequential access".

ROM (Read-Only Memory): Memory containing information written during the manufacturing process of a computer that physically cannot be overwritten.

Read Classification System (RCS) or **Read Code:** A coding system used in the United Kingdom that is a superset of several international classifications, including ICD-9, where this coding schedule is controlled by the NHS Centre for Coding and Classification. Read Codes cover such topics as occupations, signs and symptoms, investigations, diagnoses, treatments and therapies, drugs and appliances. Each clinical term in a clinical document is replaced by a Read Code when it is stored; when the clinical document is retrieved, the clinician is not presented with the code but with the clinical term.

reader: A person who can view a part of the automated medical record along with others. See "writer".

real-time: Occurring immediately.

recall: A term used in information retrieval (searching) to mean retrieving everything you need.

record: (1) computer science: A group of related fields or data elements about a person, place, thing or abstract concept. In a relational database, a row of a table. (2) medicine: Written form of communication that permanently documents information relevant to health care management.

reengineering: Rethinking and redesigning business processes to achieve quantum improvements in the performance of the business, which may be improvements in cost, quality, service or speed.

referential integrity: A database rule or constraint stating that every foreign key value in one table or database must either match a primary key in some other table or database, or it must be null.

referral: Sending or directing a patient for treatment with another caregiver or another medical department for consultation or service, usually where the "referred to" caregiver is a particular specialist physician or a caregiver in a specialty department and the "referring" caregiver is a primary care physician. A referral involves a delegation of responsibility, which should be followed up to ensure satisfactory care.

referral letter: A letter accompanying a referral, describing the reason and details of the referral.

reflex testing: An order generated automatically by some clinical laboratory systems if a test is out of range, usually to verify that the result is actual rather than due to equipment problems.

registered nurse (RN): In the U.S., a person who completed a prescribed course of study from an approved nursing education program and who has passed the National Council Licensure Examination for Registered Nurses (NCLEX-RN) exam.

regional system: In this book, a computer system that is a portion of a distributed automated patient medical record system that stores patient clinical summary information, handles communication outside the healthcare organization and interfaces with other healthcare organization clinical systems.

registration: Recording that a patient showed up for an outpatient visit and creation of a billing record for the visit.

registry: A voluntary or mandated government database for recording various disease and health problems, including cancer, AIDS, birth defects, diabetes, implants, organ transplants, measles, trauma and hazardous substances, from which epidemiological studies can be done.

regression testing: Testing after a program correction to insure that no previously-working function fails as a result of the correction. See "validation".

regressive testing: The same as "regression testing".

relational database: A database made up of tabular data structures that conforms to a set of formalized mathematically based rules described in terms of objects, operators that can be applied to these objects and a set of integrity rules.

relationship: How two entities are related. Common relationships are the following *is-a, is-part-of, causes, associated-with, equivalent-to, is-in.*

release: A fully functioning automated system or set of automated systems that is delivered to customers. See "release process".

release process: The process of keeping previous releases when delivering a new release to a customer so that the release can be backed out if necessary putting back the previous release. Releases are given version numbers. See "version" and "version control".

reliability: A measure of how well a software system provides the services expected of it by its users, including up time, accessibility and accuracy of stored information (e.g., patient medical record information), and speed in operation.

reminder: A notification message describing a patient put in by one caregiver to later inform other caregivers. More urgent messages are alerts and less urgent messages are reminders.

remote consultation: In this book, a consultation with a caregiver located in a different distributed facility group than that of the patient encounter. The significance is a technical one.

remote procedure call (RPC): A protocol that allows a program running on one computer to cause code to be executed on another computer without the programmer needing to explicitly code for this. An RPC is initiated by the caller (client) sending a request message to a remote system (the server) to execute a certain procedure using arguments supplied, and possibly returning results. It is a method for implementing the client/server model for distributed computing.

remote system: In this book, a computer system or combination of computer systems serving as part of the automated patient medical record system located in another healthcare organization or another region of a healthcare organization.

repeating orders: A type of medication order that is carried out at prescribed intervals.

request for information (RFI): A preliminary step to an RFP in which a company solicits a number of potential vendors for information about their products and services.

request for proposal (RFP): The publication by a prospective software purchaser of details of the required system in order to attract offers by vendors who can supply the software and services.

requirement: A required characteristic of the changed organization resulting from a project (a business requirement) or a required characteristic of a new or changed automated system resulting from a project (a system requirement).

requirements traceability: The ability to trace a requirement through the entire systems life cycle, e.g., to source code, data on databases, etc. See "traceability".

resolution: (1) The amount of information that a monitor can display, measured by number of pixels horizontally and vertically. (2) The quality of the images on a printed page, measured in dots per inch (dpi). (3) The amount of detail a scanner can detect, measured in dots per inch (dpi).

resource: A resource is any person, place or thing that must be reserved prior to its use.

respiration: Breaths per minute. Normal respiratory rates vary according to the age of the patient.

response: An action or movement due to the application of a stimulus (e.g., a response to a referral).

restore: To retrieve a backup and copy it back to a computer or computers to restore a previous state of the computer system.

results: See "diagnostic findings".

retroactive parallel operation: A way of phasing out an old automated system by using the old system for running the business and entering the same data in the new system whenever the day-to-day operations permit.

return on investment: Over the life of the project, the total costs as compared with the increased revenue that will accrue.

review of systems (ROS): A review of each body system with the patient (e.g., the respiratory system, the urogenital system) by asking the patient questions and by review of the patient chart. Part of the subjective part of a SOAP note.

RFI: Request for Information. A request from companies for information on a product.

RFP: Request for Proposal. A request for a proposal to implement a project.

RFQ: Request for Quote. A request for a quote (monetary cost) to implement a project.

risk factor: An environmental, psychological, physiological, or genetic element thought to predispose an individual to the development of a disease. The opposite of protective factor. See "protective factor".

risk management: Planning alternative measures if a prediction turns out to be wrong.

risk: A potential occurrence that may result in jeopardy to the success of a project.

RNA (ribonucleic acid): A molecule similar in structure to DNA that is single stranded. There are several types of RNA, but the most significant ones copy strings of bases of a DNA molecule in complementary form and are used to create polypeptides that fold into proteins.

room map: A type of patient list identifying rooms in a nursing unit, outpatient clinic or emergency department that identifies for each room, patients in the room and the caregivers in the room caring for patients.

route: The method by which the medication is given (e.g., sublingual, underneath the tongue).

router: A specialized computer that finds the best way to get an electronic message to its proper destination. It is an integral part of the Internet.

routine: General purpose code that may be used in many subsystems or in many programs, generally including the passing of data via input and output parameters associated with a routine name.

row: A particular entity occurrence or instance in a relational database table. A particular row contains a set of data elements each with a value, one data element for each column in the table. A row corresponds to a record in a non-relational database.

RSA encryption: A public key cryptography algorithm developed by mathematicians Rivest, Shamir and Adelman of MIT.

Russell-Soundex coding scheme: A method of encoding patient names phonetically, so entrance of a name would bring back all names that phonetically sound the same. Same as "**Soundex search**".

SAN (storage area network): A network to link storage devices (such as disk arrays, magnetic tape drives) to create a pool of storage, often using fiber channel technology.

SARS: The disease "severe acute respiratory syndrome", a respiratory disease characterized by fever, coughing and difficulty breathing.

scalable: Those characteristics of system structure that allow it to grow gracefully: the number of users or distributed computers or the data volume can be increased and the system still works and still works efficiently.

schedule: A type of date-oriented patient list for a particular caregiver listing patients with appointments that day and their times, may identify patients who have been registered, identifies unbooked time and identifies time where the caregiver does not normally see patients.

schedule I through V drugs: Controlled substances, which may include narcotics, stimulants and sedatives, are divided into five classes called schedule I through schedule V. Schedule I drugs are experimental and can be dispensed by a very limited number of institutions or are drugs that, on an emergency or temporary basis, have been determined to pose an imminent hazard to the public safety. Prescriptions for schedule II drugs must be written and may not be refilled. Prescriptions for schedule III and IV drugs may be written or oral but may only be refilled up to five times within 6 months. Schedule V drugs are less restricted but can be dispensed only to patients at least 18 years old; a patient must offer identification and have his or her name entered into a log maintained by the pharmacist.

screen pop: A technique, common with CTI, where the caller is identified before speaking to an agent allowing databases to be read to present caller information that 'pops up' on the agent's screen as the call arrives.

scope of care: Those care activities that a caregiver or care team together is allowed to perform.

script: A recording of the input actions of a user so they can mimic the user during performance and regression testing.

scroll: To move through a document using a scroll bar. See "scroll bar".

scroll bar: A bar at the edge of a window displaying a document the user can use to scroll (move) through the document.

search: A method of finding information in a document or database.

second opinion: To be seen by another physician to confirm a diagnosis, to help decide on a surgical procedure, or to get more information or another explanation of a medical condition.

security: Safeguards applied to an automated system to insure that it behaves as expected. The desired level of integrity, exclusiveness, availability and effectiveness to protect data from loss, corruption, destruction and unauthorized use; the means by which "privacy" and "confidentiality" are attained in computer systems.

selection: Identification of the relationship between types of data (e.g., patients and the patient's chart) so that selection of the first item could go to the second item.

selectivity: In pharmacology, the degree to which a dose of a drug produces the desired effect in relation to adverse effects.

sentinel event: JCAHO defines this as "an unexpected occurrence involving death or serious physical or psychological injury, or the risk thereof". (Moore 1998; Google 2004)

sequential access: Reading or writing to a type of memory where memory locations are ordered and a later memory location is not available until the earlier one is first available (e.g., a magnetic tape). This is opposed to random access.

server: A program that awaits and fulfills requests from client programs in the same or other computers. See "client".

server-based computing: A server-based approach to computing whereby an application's logic executes on the server and only the user interface is transmitted across a network to the client.

service level agreement (SLA): A contract between the end users of a system and the group running the system and/or the vendor providing the system that agrees upon a predefined level of service, in particular upon availability and performance levels.

service management system: System software that can measure system performance and record when it goes below a certain level (e.g., response time is too long); such systems could be used to evaluate compliance with service level agreements.

SF-12: Short Form Health Survey-12 Questions: A trade-name for a survey to be filled out by a patient related to a particular medical condition that identifies the patient perception of his/her quality of life that can be used by healthcare providers to identify which treatments and physicians provide the best outcomes from the patients' point of view. SF-12 is a survey of 12 questions.

SF-36: Short Form Health Survey-36 Questions: A trade-name for a survey with the same purpose as SF-12. It differs in that it is longer, having 36 questions to be answered by the patient.

SGML: Standard Generalized Markup Language: an international standard to enable the electronic exchange of documents between dissimilar systems. SGML is a language that can be used to create HTML or XML.

shared medical decision: Medical care where information regarding treatment outcomes are freely and accurately shared with the patient, so the patient can intelligently give his / her preferences on medical decisions.

side effect: A consequence other than the one(s) for which an agent or measure is used, as the adverse effects produced by a drug, especially on a tissue or organ system other than the one sought to be benefited by its administration.

sign: Objective finding perceived by an examiner, such as a fever, rash, abnormal reflex, or abnormal breath sound.

significant health problem: A current, permanent or long-lasting disease or medical condition. Significant health problems appear in "clinical summaries".

single log-on: See "single sign-in".

single (one-time) order: An order given only once.

single point (of) failure: An item that, if failed, would cause a failure of the system.

single sign-in: Users sign in to a system only once and are given access to multiple applications.

skilled nursing facility (SNF): An establishment with a nursing staff that bridges the gap between hospital and home for elderly patients who need skilled nursing care or rehabilitation services. It may be a separate facility or a distinct part of another facility such as a hospital.

slate computer: Same as a "tablet computer".

smart card: A credit care size plastic card containing a microprocessor. Also called an "Integrated Circuit Card".

SNMP (Simple Network Management Protocol): A TCP/IP-derived protocol governing network management and monitoring of network services. This is a common protocol, but some people have concerns about network security using this protocol.

SNOMED (Systematized Nomenclature of Human and Veterinary Medicine): Nomenclature covering the concepts of organism, disease, procedure, signs, symptoms and diagnosis, developed by the College of American Pathologists. It is intended for use in coding all content contained in electronic health records.

SOAP Notes: Notes on the care of the patient that is part of the patient medical record and is sequenced in the order of sections: subjective, objective, assessment, and plan. A "problem" section may be included before the "subjective" section. The SOAP note format was introduced by Dr. Lawrence Weed as part of a system of organizing the medical record called the problem-oriented medical record (POMR).

socioeconomic status: "A composite measure that typically incorporates economic status, measured by income; social status, measured by education; and work status, measured by occupation". See chapter 18.

social engineering: Tricking people to get around normal security procedures.

social history (SH): Information regarding the patient's eating, drinking, or smoking habits, the patient's occupation, and the patient's interests, if pertinent. Part of the subjective part of a SOAP note.

software: The components of a computer system other than hardware, including the program, documentation and the stored data to use the program.

software configuration management: The discipline of managing the evolution of large and complex software systems. See "version" and "version control".

software development life-cycle: The overall process of developing software systems through a multi-step process, including steps such as the following: concept, requirements, design, implementation, test, operation and maintenance.

software maintenance: The process of changing a system after it has been delivered and is in use; also, changes to functionality in an automated system after the function has been implemented. Also simply called, "maintenance".

solution: In this book, one of many different alternative ways of accomplishing all or part of a change.

solution alternative analysis: Comparing automated systems, hardware, software, or anything else based upon requirements.

Sonet (Synchronous Optical Network): A data communications standard resulting in a very high-speed network that operates over fiber optic cable.

sort: To arrange information in a specified order, such as alphabetical, numerical or chronological.

sound card: A hardware device in a computer that can be used to reproduce almost any sound from music to speech to sound effects. Can be used in conjunction with CD-ROM drives, microphones, speakers, MIDI devices for music reproduction, etc.

Soundex search: A method of encoding patient names phonetically, so entrance of a name would bring back all names that phonetically sound the same. Same as "**Russell-Soundex coding scheme**".

source document: An automated medical document making up part of and automated medical record, which may include a detailed patient care document created at the point of care or or a document created as a result of an ancillary service.

source document repository: A database to store source documents.

specialist: A physician who works in a department not providing primary care, also known as a "specialty care provider".

specialty: A classification of specialized fields of medical services, such as dermatology, urology, orthopedics, etc.

speech recognition system: Computer software that understands a user's voice so he / she does not have to type.

sponsor: A person who sees the usefulness of a project and who agrees to take ownership of the project.

spooling: See "printer spooling".

sporadic: Neither endemic nor epidemic; occurring occasionally in a random or isolated manner.

stage: The natural high level breakpoints in a project life cycle.

staging: Transferring patient clinical data from a remote to a local computer before it is needed, instead of at the time needed, so it will be there when it is needed, e.g., at the time of an encounter.

stakeholder: Any person or group who has an interest in a project. Typically some support the project, some are neutral, and some are antagonists.

standard: A set of guidelines and rules for a particular subject area set up by a committee whose members are authorities in the subject area in order to establish a commonality of computer software or hardware systems, healthcare procedures, etc., so that computer systems or people can communicate.

standard of care: The minimum level of performance accepted to ensure high quality of care to patients. Standards of care define the types of therapies typically administered to patients with defined problems or needs.

standard development organization (SDO): Organizations working on healthcare standards.

standards analyst: A person responsible for identifying or enforcing company and industry standards.

standing order: A type of medication order that is carried out until the physician cancels it.

STAT: Needed immediately.

STAT order: A type of medication order where the medication is given immediately and only once.

stateless: A method by which the server treats each request as a separate transaction. A World Wide Web server is a stateless server and thus it does not remember the caller of the previous request.

stay: Encounter(s) leading up to an inpatient admission (e.g., an ED visit where the patient is discharged to the hospital) together with the inpatient admission.

storage: A method of retaining data, text or graphics by preserving the information on hard drives, within the computer, floppy disks or other media.

store-and-forward: A communications approach wherein messages are transmitted to another node where they can be stored and forwarded at a later time to the recipient.

stored procedure: A set of procedural code stored in a database that is executed by the database software either on demand by an application program or when an associated database trigger is activated.

strategy: A change in direction of an organization that is presumed to result in an objective or objectives of the organization being fulfilled. See "objective".

striping: A method of fault tolerance for information stored on disks that involves using three or more disks and controllers and keeping the data on one disk and parity data on another disk. If data is lost, it can be reconstructed from data on the other disks.

structure chart: A hierarchical diagram that breaks a system into subsystems, subsystems into modules and modules into other modules and routines, which might also identify data flow.

structured coding constructs: Coding constructs that allow programmers to create code without GoTo statements, stopping programmers from creating very hard to understand programs (called "spaghetti code").

structured design: A way of designing an application system where the system program code if broken into subsystems, subsystems are broken into modules, and modules are broken into additional modules or routines.

Structured Query Language (SQL): A language that provides a user or program interface to relational database systems. It was developed by IBM in the 1970s and is an ISO and ANSI standard. It is often embedded in programs in other computer languages.

style guide: In this book, a guide to be used in the development of a particular user interface that defines screen display and input standards based upon business objects.

sublingual: Located beneath the tongue. May pertain to a medication and mean a "route".

subjective: Information given by the patient. See section 4.4.1.3.

subroutine: A series of instructions that together complete a specific task. A subroutine is named so that it can be called from many different program locations by name. A subroutine may have parameters to pass data to the subroutine or from the subroutine.

subspecialty: A specialty area within a particular medical discipline. For example, subspecialties within pediatrics might be the following: adolescent medicine, pediatric cardiology, pediatric critical care medicine, pediatric emergency medicine, pediatric endocrinology, pediatric gastroenterology, pediatric hematology-oncology, pediatric infectious diseases, neonatal-perinatal medicine, pediatric nephrology, pediatric pulmonology, and pediatric rheumatology.

subsystem: A major, largely independent, portion of code that defines an application that works in coordination with other applications to produce a coherent and complete major software system; a set of functions that are logically grouped together.

supervision: Designating or prescribing a course of action, or giving procedural guidance, initial direction, and periodic evaluation for individuals to whom tasks are delegated.

supervision, direct: Being physically present and immediately accessible to designate or prescribe a course of action or to give procedural guidance, direction and periodic evaluation.

surveillance system: A public health reporting system.

symptom: Any subjective evidence of disease or of a patient's condition, i.e. such evidence as perceived by the patient; a change in a patient's condition indicative of some bodily or mental state.

synchronous: Two or more processes dependent upon specific events occurring at the same time or in the same order.

synchronous transmission: Data communications in which characters or bits are sent at a fixed rate, with the transmitting and receiving devices synchronized; this eliminates the need for start and stop bits basic to asynchronous transmission and significantly increases data throughput rates.

synopsis: See "encounter synopsis".

system: Unit made up of separate parts or elements, where the parts rely on each other, are interrelated, have a common purpose, and together form a collective whole.

system architecture: The computers, the networks, the operating systems, the telecommunications, the database management systems and hardware, and other software and hardware necessary to support the applications.

system requirement: A required characteristic of a new or changed automated system due to a project.

system software: Any program that provides support to run the computer as opposed to an application program. See "application" and "application software".

system testing: The process at the end of development to validate that all the requirements have been satisfied by the automated system. See "validation".

system analysis: The process of assessing whether a particular task is suitable for computerization and developing the internal design of an automated system or developing any part of the collective internal design of the automated systems functioning together within an organization.

Systems Application Architecture (SAA) Common User Access (CUA): A definition and description of user interface standards developed by IBM for character-based systems, most using IBM's CICS. There are also equivalent GUI standards. These standards are seldom used any more.

systems biology: The study of how all of a human body's RNA, DNA, genes, proteins, cells and tissues function together to produce a living human being (Cohen 2004).

table: Information organized in rows and columns used for storing and retrieving data items in a relational database. Equivalent to a file.

tablet computer: A pen computer about the width and length of a standard, 8 ½" x 11", sheet of paper.

tailor: To have a system work differently for different users or categories of users.

tape: See "magnetic tape".

task: (1) For a project, an activity to be accomplished during a project. (2) For software, portions of code that can run concurrently, where these portions of code together make up a larger program; for example, a program can consist of a screen handling task and another task to do calculations when the screen handling program is not running.

TCP (transmission control protocol): Divides a message into packets and then reassembles the packets when they all arrive at the destination. TCP also checks that the packets of a message arrived error free. See "TCP/IP".

TCP/IP (transmission control protocol/Internet protocol): A set of standards for communicating among dissimilar computers, developed and supported by ARPA (Advanced Projects Research Agency) of the U.S. Department of Defense. This is the communications protocol for transferring data from one computer to another over the Internet.

team care: In this book, care by multiple caregivers over a period of time for a medical condition that results in a continuity of care for that condition.

telecommunications: The electronic transmission of information, including voice, data, video, image facsimile, telemetry, where there is a source that originates and encodes a message, a transmission medium, and a receiver that receives and decodes the message.

telemedicine: The use of interactive audio and visual links to enable remote healthcare practitioners to consult in "real time" with specialists in distant medical centers.

temperature: A measure of heat associated with the metabolism of the human body.

template: A document that provides the basic framework for another document.

tera- (e.g., terabytes): One trillion or the closest multiple of 2 value to one trillion. For example, a terabyte is equal to 1,099,511,627,776 (2^{40}) bytes.

terminal: A monitor with a screen and a keyboard or other input devices.

test bed: A smaller scale hardware and software system that mimics the automated system.

testing: Evaluation of a computer software system to determine if it meets the requirements for the system. Requirements to be tested are user requirements determined by talking to users and software requirements determined during the design of the system. Also called "validation". See "validation".

test plan: A description of test cases that will exercise a program or system to test its correctness.

therapy: The treatment of disease.

therapeutic substitution: The replacement of a prescribed medication with an entirely different medication of the same pharmacological or therapeutic class.

thin client: For server-based computing, a thin client is a low-cost, centrally-managed computer devoid of CD-ROM players, diskette drives, and expansion slots.

thread: For software, equivalent to a "task".

three-tier data architecture: A three-tiered system is partitioned into three separate processes: the user interface, business processing and database management. As opposed to a two-tiered system, the business processing is removed from the client and is placed on a separate application server. Each tier may have its own hardware and software architecture. Many companies use transaction processing (TP) monitors to distribute requests among multiple servers.

Token Ring: A networking architecture in the shape of a ring, where access to write to the network is controlled by a token that passes from station to station. The competing architecture is Ethernet, which is much more common.

tomography: The recording of internal body images at a predetermined plane by means of the tomograph; called also body section roentgenography.

tool bar or toolbar: In a GUI, a graphical strip appearing across the top of the screen, side of the screen or bottom of the screen containing icons on buttons that represent functions the user frequently invokes.

topical: Pertaining to a drug or treatment applied to the surface of a part of the body.

touch pad: A replacement for a mouse to move the cursor on the screen that works by sensing the user's finger movement and downward pressure. See "glide point".

toxicity: The quality of being poisonous, especially the degree of virulence of a toxic microbe or of a poison.

traceability: The ability to trace a requirement, project objective, or organizational business requirement through the entire systems life cycle, e.g., to source code, data on databases, etc. See "requirements traceability".

trackball: A replacement for a mouse that is an upside-down mouse that rotates in place within a socket.

trade-name: Proprietary names that are registered to protect the name for the sole use of the manufacturer holding the trademark (e.g., for drugs). Trade-name drugs are usually capitalized.

Trading Partners: Commercial entities that do business with each other using EDI.

trailer: The ending data segment of a set of data segments.

transaction: (1) A logical update that takes a database from one consistent state to another. (2) A module that performs a logical update of a database through an on-line transaction processing system. (3) An electronic communication between two groups for medical or business reasons.

translation: The process of turning instructions from messenger RNA, base by base, into chains of amino acids called polypeptides that then fold into proteins.

transcription: A process of transforming dictated or otherwise documented information into an electronic format.

transfer: Change in medical care unit, hospital, medical staff, or responsible physician of an inpatient after hospitalization.

treatment: To provide care to cure, improve or mitigate a medical condition.

treatment (management) case: In this book a case to track a treatment for a particular patient and usually non-chronic medical condition over a number of encounters where the condition is not likely to require long term continuing care.

trend document: In this book, a document that automatically records a value or values that a caregiver wants to track over time as the value(s) are input via other source documents. A trend document may include mean, minimum and maximum expected values and report out of bounds values to identified caregivers. See "control chart".

treatment decision point: A point in a disease before which therapy is either more effective or easier to apply than afterward.

treatment plan: An organized and documented approach to selecting care activities to treat a patient for an presumed or identified medical condition.

triage: Assessment of patients' medical problems to determine urgency and priority of care in the Emergency Department to determine which patient is to be seen next.

triage nurse: A nurse in the Emergency Department who triages patients.

Trustworthy Health Telematics (TrustHealth): An approach for caregiver security developed in Europe for the European Commission to provide personal smart cards (computer chips imbedded in credit cards) to caregivers to gain access to healthcare systems using RSA encryption algorithms.

two-phase commit protocol: An update approach in databases that results either in all database changes associated with a transaction being successfully made or all changes being successfully rolled back.

two-tier architecture: A user component and a database-server component. Most of the application—especially the user interface—runs on a desktop. The primary function of the server is to access databases. Two-tier systems usually have limited scalability—few applications can support more than 100 simultaneous users.

tunneling: A technology that enables one network to send its data via another network's connections. Tunneling works by encapsulating a network protocol with packets carried by the second network. For example, tunneling technology enables organizations to use the Internet to transmit data across a virtual private network (VPN).

ultrasound: Ultrasound is a technique by which sound waves are bounced into a person's body, and their reflections captured by a machine that transforms them into an image that can be read.

Unicode: A coding scheme for characters that provides a unique number for every character, no matter what the platform, no matter what the program, no matter what the language. Unicode is required within Java, XML, and all modern browsers.

unified messaging: Allowing messages to be text, fax, voice, graphics, picture, Internet page, or video, or any combination of these. See "messaging".

Uniform Resource Locator (URL): An address uniquely identifying a home page within the World Wide Web on the Internet.

uninterruptible power supply (UPS): A (battery powered) power supply that is guaranteed to provide working voltage to a computer regardless of interruptions in the incoming electrical power.

Unique Healthcare Identifier (UHID): An ASTM term for a unique patient identifier.

Unique Physician Identifier Number (UPIN): A number to identify providers for Medicare billing purposes. The UPIN identifier is being replaced by the National Patient Identifier (NPI identifier). See "National Patient Identifier".

Unique Product Number (UPN): Part of a uniform bar code labeling standard for products shipped to hospitals developed by the HIBCC. Two Universal Product Number (UPN) codes, HIBC-LIC codes and UCC/EAN codes, are used for product bar codes to identify med/surg products and manufacturers.

unit: See "nursing unit".

unit assistant: A healthcare professional who performs a variety of clinical, clerical and administrative duties within a unit, or section, of the hospital.

unit census: A patient list that identifies all admitted patients in a nursing unit.

unit testing: Validation of individual functions and programs. See "validation".

United Medical Language System (UMLS): A system linking together various medical vocabularies using semantic relationships, developed by the National Library of Medicine.

United Modeling Language (UML): An object modeling language for designing and describing application systems.

U.S. Standard Certificates of Birth and Death, and the Report of Fetal Death:

universal patient record: In this book, a possibly distributed patient medical record that electronically combines and summarizes all of a patient's medical information that is available to authorized caregivers and organizations via a network. It consists of the combination of all patient clinical information in CPR repositories and source document repositories, and all paper chart information in chart rooms, any of which, with the proper authority, can be located through the CPR repositories, and then ordered.

universal patient medical record: Same as "universal patient record".

universal precautions: The recommendations published by the Center for Disease Control, Atlanta, Georgia, for preventing transmission of infectious disease by blood or body fluids.

UNIX: Operating system developed by Bell Laboratories in the 1970s, now widely used in mini-computers and workstations. See "Linux".

UPC format (Universal Product Code for identification at point of sale): A bar code used for product identification. The code is sensed by laser / optical scanners.

upper management: Management of an organization who are responsible for the direction of the organization.

urgent care clinic: A facility that provides care for problems that need to be treated outside routine business hours but that are not serious enough to require Emergency Department care.

urgent condition: A condition that needs treatment within 24 hours.

usability: The extent to which a computer system is easy to learn and effective to use for the given business tasks and users.

usability testing: Validation during development, having users test an automated system during a simulation of production use of the system. See "validation".

use case: User workflow in terms of his or her task environment.

user: Someone who uses an automated system.

user interface: The part of a computer program that displays on the screen for the user to see and the user interactions it allows.

utility computing: Treating computing like an electric utility, telephone company, or other type of utility where computing service for a particular application is paid on a "pay-for-use" basis.

utilization review: The necessity, quality, effectiveness, or efficiency of medical services, procedures, and facilities.

vaccination: The introduction of vaccine into the body for the purpose of inducing immunity. Coined originally to apply to the injection of smallpox vaccine, the term has come to mean any immunizing procedure in which vaccine is injected.

validity: The extent to which data corresponds to the actual state of affairs or measures what it purports to measure.

validation: Testing an automated system at the end of development to determine if the system or component works as determined by the program specifications, vendor systems customization specifications or business policies specifications. See "testing".

VAN (value added network): Generally commercial networks that transmit, receive, and store EDI transactions on behalf of their customers.

variance: The differences between an expected outcome and an actual outcome of a care activity, either positive or negative.

variant: Variants of a program are two programs that function the same or nearly the same but differ slightly in some way; for example, two variants work exactly the same, but work under two different operating systems.

vBNS (very high-speed Backbone Network Service): One existing alternative version of the Internet, reserved for scientific applications, that can transfer data much faster than the current Internet.

vendors: Organizations that develop off-the-shelf hardware or software.

verification: "Human" examination of an automated system to compare it against system requirements or business requirements, including user interface requirements, to determine if the requirements are being fulfilled. See "validation".

version: A software system version is an instance of a system that differs in some way from other instances. Usually each version is identified by a decimal number "x.y" where "x" is an integer representing a "release" number that changes when there is a major new version, and "y" is an integer representing a more minor change within the identified release.

version control: Another term for the "release process".

VGA (Video Graphics Array): Color graphic format for monitors developed by IBM for PC compatible systems. The basic resolution is 640 x 480 pixels with 16 colors. Super VGA is an extension to the standard supporting resolutions of 1024 x 768 with 256 colors and 1280 x 1024 with 16 colors.

virtual machine interface: A program that executes computer-platform-independent code such as in Java on a specific computer platform.

virtual private network (VPN): A network that utilizes a public network such as the Internet as a secure channel for communicating private data. A VPN can be created using "tunneling".

virtual system: In this book, a local system that stores remote patient clinical information from CPR repositories and source document repositories so it can be staged.

visibility: The functionality in an application system provided to a particular user of an automated system or to a set of users with a particular staff position.

vision: In this book, a healthcare organization management's intelligent foresight into how the healthcare organization can best be improved to meet the future needs of its members, employees and outside organizations it does business with.

vital signs: A patient's temperature, pulse, respiration and blood pressure. Some medical people consider pain to be a fifth vital sign.

voice recognition system: See speech recognition system.

voice response unit (VRU): Same technology as "interactive voice recognition (IVR)".

VRML (Virtual Reality Modeling Language): Language used to represent and utilize three-dimensional objects on the World Wide Web.

wait list: A list of patients requiring outpatient appointments, which may include recommendations on when the appointment should take place and who the appointment should be with.

walkthrough: A group of people who meet to verify the correctness and acceptability of controlled documents or computer programs.

WAN (Wide Area Network): A public or private network that covers a wide geographic area.

WAPI (Wired Authentication and Privacy Infrastructure): A Chinese developed technology that describes how data transmitted over wireless networks should be encrypted to prevent unauthorized monitoring.

waveform: A continuous analog signal recorded as a line on paper, such as an ECG.

WDM (wave length division multiplexing): A technology which increases the capability of optical fiber by dividing a transmission channel into different wavelengths, each resulting in a separate channel.

WEP (wired equivalent privacy): An encryption standard for 802,11.

Web server: A computer that handles the display of information to users through the Internet.

well-formed requirement: "A statement of system functionality (a capability) that can be validated, that must be met or possessed by a system to solve a customer problem or to achieve a customer objective, and that is qualified by measurable conditions and bounded by constraints." (IEEE 1998). See section 2.7.

white box: With regard to computer software systems, everything seen by the users of the system and everything not seen by the users of the system, including behind the scenes hardware, the software, the databases, and the networks. "White box" is often used to describe testing, where "white box" testing is done with a complete knowledge of the system. See "black box" and "internal workings".

window: A rectangular part of a computer screen that contains a display different from the rest of the screen.

windowing: A display technique that uses multiple screen segments to display different items of information. The display can take two basic forms: tiling (breaking up the screen into discrete segments) and overlapping (producing a three-dimensional effect by having a screen segment overlap, and thus partially or fully obscure another segment).

Windows NT (Windows New Technology, NT) or **Windows XP** or **Windows 2000:** Microsoft's 32-bit operating system designed for workstations, servers and corporate networks. Other operating systems derived from Windows NT are Windows 2000 and Windows XP.

wireless communications: A term describing a computer network where there is no physical connection (either copper cable or fiber optics) between sender and receiver, but instead they are connected by radio.

word processor: Software that can be used to produce textual and other documents, including letters, reports, manuals and newsletters.

Work Breakdown Structure (WBS): A structured hierarchy of groupings of project elements—tasks, programs, phases, stages, etc.—which organizes and defines the total scope of a project.

worker s compensation: A state-mandated program requiring certain employers to pay benefits and furnish medical care to employees for on-the-job injuries.

workflow: The sequence of activities of a business, such as the business of providing medical care, often documented in a diagram in order to determine inefficient activities and inefficient usage of resources. See "business process reengineering".

workflow systems: Systems where a business is described by processes, discrete activities that make up the business practices of an organization or of a part of a business, and where these processes are analyzed.

work list: A list of orders for an ancillary department to complete.

workstation: A micro- or minicomputer system with a network attachment that is used for providing information, computation, and/or network services directly to an end user.

World Wide Web (WWW): A hypertext system that links together documents over the Internet. Sometimes just called the "Web".

World Wide Web Consortium (W3C): A standards body that controls both the structure of HTML and XML on the Internet.

writer: A person who can view and update that part of the automated medical record when it is being viewed.

WYSIWYG: Stands for "What You See is What You Get". A term to use graphical systems to display on the screen exactly what is printed.

XHTML (Extensible Hypertext Markup Language): The reformulation of HTML as an application of XML that could replace HTML in the future.

XLink: An extension to XML which enables you to create links within XML documents.

XML (Extensible Markup Language): Like HTML, an SGML-based language for defining document structures and elements for documentation management systems. XML supplements HTML (or XHTML) in the creation of web sites and serves as a way to define and transmit data. See "HTML" and "XHTML".

XML DTD (Document Type Definition): A document that describes the structure and data elements of an XML document; data descriptions are more limited than in an XML Schema. See "XML Schema".

XML Namespaces: An extension to XML which allow you to avoid namespace collisions when defining XML elements and attributes, especially when combining data from two different sources.

XML parser: Software that enables data values and data element names to be broken out from an XML document, for example, for storage on a database. A validating XML parser further validates the format of information on the XML document to be in the format identified by an XML DTD or Schema associated with the XML document.

XML Schema: A W3C-sponsered effort to define an alternative to DTDs for defining the structure and data elements of XML documents; within XML Schemas data elements can be described at a lower level than a DTD: byte, date, integer, user-defined, and others. See "XML DTD".

XPath: An extension to XML which allows you to use patterns to identify sections of an XML document.

XPointer: An extension to XML which extends XPath to allow you to address points in the document and ranges between points.

x-ray: Electromagnetic radiation for medical imaging.

XSL (Extensible Markup Language Stylesheet Language): Two facilities that facilitate the manipulation and display of information contained in XML documents: XSLT (XSL Transformations) a language for transforming XML documents into other XML documents or HTML documents, and XSL Formatting Objects, an XML vocabulary for formatting XML documents identifying templates for styles such as fonts, colors, and spacing for rendering including into HTML (similar to Cascading Style Sheets). See "Cascading Style Sheets".

XSLT: See "XSL".

X12N: See "ANSI ASC X12N".

Bibliography

Abdelhak, Mervat, Sara Grostick, Mary Alice Hanken, and Ellen Jacobs. 2001. *HEALTH INFORMATION: Management of a Strategic Resource,*. 2nd edition (January 15, 2001) ed: W. B. Saunders Company.

ACAAI. 2004. *Asthma Disease Management Resource Manual, October 7,1998* [Internet]. The American College of Allergy, Asthma & Immunology 1998 [cited January 2004]. Available from http://allergy.mcg.edu/physicians/manual/manual.html.

Adler, Nancy, Thomas Boyce, Margaret A. Chesney, Sheldon Cohen, Susan Folkman, Robert L. Kahn, and S. Leonard Syme. 1999. 13. Socioeconomic Status and Health: The Challenge of the Gradient. In *Health and Human Rights*, edited by J. M. Mann, S. Gruskin, M. A. Grodin and G. J. Annos: Routledge.

AHCPR. 2004. *Minutes: Vocabularies for Computer-Based Patient Records (NLM, 5-6 December 1994)*. Agency for Health Care Policy and Research 1994 [cited January 2004]. Available from http://www.nlm.nih.gov/lo/minvocab.html.

———. 2004. *AHCPR (Agency for Health Care Policy and Research) Clinical Practice Guidelines* 2004 [cited January 2004]. Available from www.ahcpr.gov/clinic/cpgonline.htm.

AHIMA. 2004. AHIMA Prepares Road Map to Guide Transition to ICD-10. *Journal of TxHIMA Article*.

Alberts, Bruce, Alexander Johnson, Julian Lewis, Martin Raff, Keith Roberts, and Peter Walter. 2002. *Molecular Biology of the Cell*. 4th edition (March 2002) ed: Garland.

Alison. 2004. *MYCIN: A Quick Case Study*. Heriot Watt University, Edinburgh & Scottish Borders, August 19, 1994 1994 [cited February 2004]. Available from http://www.cee.hw.ac.uk/~alison/ai3notes/section2_5_5.html.

AMA. 2004. *Healthcare Provider Taxonomy, Version 3.0.2* (July 2003). American Medical Association (AMA) 2003 [cited February 2004]. Available from http://www.adldata.com/Overview/taxonomy_302.pdf.

———. 2004. *CPT (Current Procedural Terminology)* [Internet]. American Medical Association, January 20, 2004 2004 [cited February 2004]. Available from http://www.ama-assn.org/ama/pub/category/3113.html.

Amatayakul, Margret. 2000. HIPAA - Fundamentals for the Newly Initiated (on the Internet). Paper read at 2000 HIPAA Conference, at McLean, VA.

Anderson, James G. 1997. Clearing the Way for Physicians' Use of Clinical Information Systems. *Communications of the ACM* 40 (8).

Anoto. 2000. *Anoto Web Site* [Internet]. Anoto 2004 [cited January 2000]. Available from http://www.anoto.com/.

ANSI. 2004. *eSTANDARDS STORE (Document#: POCT1-A)* [Internet]. American National Standards Institute 2004 [cited February 2004]. Available from http://webstore.ansi.org/ansidocstore/product.asp?sku=POCT1-A.

Appavu, Soloman I. 2004. *Analysis of Unique Patient Identifier Options:*

Final Report (November 24, 1997) [Internet]. The Department of Health and Human Services 1997 [cited February 2004]. Available from http://ncvhs.hhs.gov/app0.htm.

ASTM. 1995. E 1714 – 95, Standard Guide for Properties of a Universal Healthcare Identifier (UHID): ASTM.

———. 2004. *Namespaces in XML, World Wide Web Consortium 14-January-1999* 1999 [cited February 2004]. Available from http://www.w3.org/TR/REC-xml-names.

———. 2004. *ASTM XML Document Type Definitions (DTDs) for Health Care* [Internet], March 14, 2001 2001 [cited January 2004]. Available from http://xml.coverpages.org/astmHealthcare.html.

———. 2002. E 1633-02a Standard Specification for Coded Values Used in the Electronic Health Record.

———. 2002. E 2210 - 02: Standard Specification for Guideline Elements Model (GEM)--Document Model for Clinical Practice Guidelines: ASTM.

———. 2002. Standard Guide for Content and Structure of the Electronic Health Record (EHR): American National Standards Institute (ANSI).

———. 2003. *Volume 14.01, Healthcare Informatics; Computerized Systems and Chemical and Material Information*. June 2003 ed: ASTM International.

Baker, F. Terry. 1977. Structured Programming in a Production Programming Environment. In *Software Design Techniques*: IEEE Computer Society.

Baldwin, Fred D. 2004. *Well-Managed Care: Predictive modeling helps keep high-risk patients from becoming high-cost patients.* Healthcare Informatics-Online, August 2004 2004 [cited October 2 2004]. Available from http://www.healthcare-informatics.com/issues/2004/08_04/baldwin_care.htm.

Barlow, Linda. 2004. *The Spider's Apprentice: A Helpful Guide to Web Search Engines*. Monash Information Services, May 17, 2002 1996-2002 [cited January 2004]. Available from http://www.monash.com/spidap4.html.

Bates, David W., Lucian L. Leape, David J. Cullen, Nan Laird, Laura A. Petersen, Jonathan M. Teich, Elizabeth Burdick, Mairead Hickey, Sharon Kleefield, Brian Shea, Martha Vander Vliet, and Diane L. Seger. 1998. Effect of Computerized Physician Order Entry and a Team Intervention on Prevention of Serious Medication Error. *The Journal of the American Medical Association* 280 (15):1311-1316.

Becklin, Karonne J., and Edith M Sunnarborg. 1994. *Medical Office Procedures*: Glencoe.

Berman, Fran, Geoffrey Fox, and Tony Hey, eds. 2003. *Grid Computing: Making the Global Infrastructure a Reality*: John Wiley & Sons.

Birman, Alex, and John J. Ritsko, eds. 2004. *IBM System Journal: Utility Computing*. Vol. 43(1): International Business Machines Corporation.

Blair, Jeffrey S. 2004. *An Overview of Healthcare Information Standards*. Computer-based Patient Record institute 1995 [cited February 2004]. Available from http://www.hipaanet.com/cpri.htm.

Boehm, Barry. 1988. A Spiral Model of Software Development and Enhancement. *IEEE Computer* 21 (15):61-72.

Bolton, Fintan. 2001. *Pure Corba*. 1st edition (July 16, 2001) ed: SAMS.

Booker, Ellis. 2000. Enterprise Software Projects Rarely Satisfy. *InternetWeek*, March 28, 2000.

Bray, Tim, Jean Paoli, C. M. Sperberg-McQueen, and Eve Maler. 2004. *Extensible Markup Language (XML) 1.0 (Second Edition) W3C Recommendation* [Internet]. W3C, October 6, 2000 2000 [cited January 2004]. Available from http://www.w3.org/TR/REC-xml.

Buttrick, Robert. 1997. *The Project Workout: a toolkit for reaping the rewards from all your business projects*: Financial Times Prentice Hall.

Caglayan, Alper, and Colin G. Harrison. 1997. *Agent Sourcebook: A Complete Guide to Desktop, Internet, and Intranet Agents*. 1st edition (January 15, 1997) ed. John Wiley & Sons.

Campanale, Frank, and Brett Skakun. 1997. Behavioral Idiosyncrasies and How They May Affect Investment Decisions. *AAII (American Association of Individual Investors) Journal* XIX (9).

Champy, James, and Michael Hammer. 1993. *Reengineering the Corporation: A Manifesto for Business Revolution*. New York City: Harper Collins.

Chatterjee, Samir. 1997. Requirements for SUCCESS In Gibabit Networking. *Communications of the ACM* 40 (7).

Citizens' Council on Healthcare. 2004. *Instead of a National Patient ID Number. . .* (October 24, 1997) [Internet]. Citizens' Council on Healthcare 1997 [cited February 2004]. Available from http://www.cchconline.org/privacy/mpiart.php3.

Clark, David. 1998. Heavy Traffic Drives Networks to IP over Sonet. *Computer* 31 (12):17-20.

Cline, Gary. 1999. Testing the Performance of Enterprise Systems. Paper read at CMG 99 Conference (Computer Measurement Group), Better Computing Beyond 2000, December 5-10, at Reno, Nevada.

CMI. 2004. *Kaiser Permanente Wins Top National Disease Management Award*. Kaiser Permanent Care Management Institute (CMA) 2003 [cited January 2004]. Available from http://www.kpcmi.org/media/dmaa.html.

CMS. 2004. *Transaction Standards*. Centers for Medicare & Medicaid Services, January 31, 2003 2003 [cited February 2004]. Available from http://www.cms.hhs.gov/hipaa/hipaa2/regulations/hisbinv2.asp.

———. 2004. *Health Insurance Portability and Accountability Act of 1996 (HIPAA)* [Internet]. Centers for Medicare and Medicaid Services (CMS), October 16, 2002 2004 [cited January 2004]. Available from http://cms.hhs.gov/hipaa/.

———. 2004. *Healthcare Common Procedure Coding System (HCPCS)* [Internet]. Centers for Medicare & Medicaid Services 2004 [cited February 2004]. Available from http://www.cms.hhs.gov/medicare/hcpcs/default.asp.

———. 2004. *HIPAA Administrative Simplication - Identifiers* [Internet]. Centers for Medicare & Medicaid Services, January 23, 2004 2004 [cited February 2004]. Available from http://www.cms.hhs.gov/hipaa/hipaa2/regulations/identifiers/default.asp.

Cohen, Jon. 2004. Big-Picture Biotech. *Technology Review*, January 2004, 40-48.

Connectivity Industry Consortium. 2004. *Draft Technical Specifications* (January 2001). Connectivity Industry Consortium 2001 [cited February 2004]. Available from http://www.poccic.org/documents/index.html.

Conradi, Reidar, and Bernhard Westfechtel. 1998. Version Models for Software Configuration Management. *ACM Computing Surveys* 30 (2):232-282.

Cook, Rebecca. 1999. 17. Gender, Health and Human Rights. In *Health and Human Rights*, edited by J. M. Mann, S. Gruskin, M. A. Grodin and G. J. Annos: Routledge.

CSTB. 1997. *For the Record: Protecting Electronic Health Information*. Washington, D.C.: The National Academies Press.

Cule, Paul E., Kalle Lyytinen, and Roy C. Schmidt. 1998. A Framework for Identifying Software Project Risks. *Communications of the ACM* 41 (11):76-83.

Currey, Richard. 2003. Molecular Imaging: Changing the Face of Medicine. *Radiology Today*, February 3, 2003.

Dankel, Douglas D., and Giuliano Russo. 1988. Verification of Medical Diagnoses Using a Microcomputer. In *Microcomputer-Based Expert Systems*: IEEE Press.

Davis, Alison. 2004. *NIGMS Awards 'Glue Grant' to Study How Cells Move* [Internet]. NIGMS (National Institute of General Medical Sciences) part of NIH (National Institutes of Health), September 26, 2001 2001 [cited January 2004]. Available from http://www.nigms.nih.gov/news/releases/horwitz.html.

DEA. 2004. *Drug Registration* (August 27, 2003). U.S. Department of Justice, Drug Enforcement Administration 2003 [cited February 2004]. Available from http://www.deadiversion.usdoj.gov/drugreg/index.html.

Dickson, Murray, Michael Blake, and Joan Thompson. 1983. *Where There Is No Dentist*. (October 1983) ed: Hesperian Foundation.

DICOM. 2004. *Digital Imaging and Communications in Medicine (DICOM)* [Internet]. National Electrical Manufacturers Association (NEMA) 2004 [cited February 2004]. Available from http://medical.nema.org/.

Dismukes, Trey. 2004. *Wireless Security Blackpaper* [Internet]. Ars Technica: the pc enthusiast's resource 1998-2003 [cited January 2004]. Available from http://www.arstechnica.com/paedia/w/wireless/security-1.html.

Doenges, Marilynn E., Mary Frances Moorhouse, and Alice C. Geissler-Murr. 2002. *Nursing Care Plans: Guidelines for Individualizing Patient Care (Book with CD-ROM)*. 6th edition (March 2002) ed. Philadelphia: F A Davis Co.

Dolin, Bob. 2004. *Kaiser Permanente s Convergent Medical Terminology* (November 8, 2004). Kaiser Permanente 2002 [cited February 2004]. Available from http://www.snomed.org/Users_group/Presentations2002/SNOMED_at_KP/.

Dolin, Robert H., Liora Alschuler, Calvin Beebe, Paul V. Biron, Sandra Lee Boyer, Daniel Essin, Elliot Kimber, Tom Lincoln, and John E. Mattison. 2001. The HL7 Clinical Document Architecture. *Journal of the American Medical Informatics Association* 2001 (8):552-569.

Dowsey, Michelle M, Meredith L Kilgour, Nick M Santamaria, and Peter F M Choong. 1999. Clinical pathways in hip and knee arthroplasty: a prospective randomised controlled study. *Medical Journal of Australia* 170: 59-62.

ebXML. 2004. *ebXML: Enabling a Global Electronic Market*. Oasis 2003 [cited January 2004]. Available from http://www.ebxml.org/.

eEurope. 2004. *Open Smart Care Infrastructure for Europe v2: Smart Cards as Enabling Technology for Future-Proof Healthcare: a requirements survey* (OSCIE Volume 1 Part 4 (March 2003)). European Union, March 2003 2003 [cited January 2004]. Available from http://www.eeurope-smartcards.org/Download/01-4.pdf.

Elliott, Jeff. 1997. AWG Chooses Data Standard. *Health Informatics Online* (April 1997):100.

EMTALA Online. 2004. *Health Law Resource Center* [Internet]. Frew Consulting Group, Ltd. 1994-2003 [cited February 2004]. Available from http://www.medlaw.com/.

Express News Service. 2000. Now, doc-to-doc consultation on doctoranywhere.com. *Indian Express Newspapers Ltd.*, March 29, 2000.

Fayad, Mohamed, and Marshall P. Cline. 1996. Aspects of Software Adaptability. *Communications of the ACM* 39 (10):58-59.

Filman, Robert E., Stuart Barrett, Diana D. Lee, and Ted Linden. 2002. Inserting ilities by controlling communications. *Communications of the ACM* 45 (1):116-122.

Finkler, Steven A., and David M. Ward. 1999. *Essentials of Cost Accounting for Health Care Organizations (2nd Edition)*. 2nd edition (March 1999) ed: Aspen Publishers, Inc.

Forrest, Jane L., and Syrene A. Miller. 2002. Articles (Evidence-Based Decision Making). *The Journal of Contemporary Dental Practice* 3 (3):10.

Fowler, Martin. 2003. *UML Distilled: A Brief Guide to the Standard Object Modeling Language*. 3rd edition (September 19, 2003) ed: Addison-Wesley Pub Co.

Frakes, William B., and Ricardo Baeza-Yates. 1992. *Information Retrieval: Data Structures & Algorithms*: Prentice Hall PTR.

Franco, Pilar. 2004. *HEALTH: One Billion People Lack Medical Services* (June 9, 2000) [Internet]. Inter Press Service 2000 [cited February 2004]. Available from http://www.oneworld.org/ips2/june00/23_41_126.html.

Frieda, Andrew, Patrick W. O'Carroll, Ray M. Nicola, Mark W. Oberle, and Steven M.Teutsch. 1997. *CDC Prevention Guidelines: A Guide for Action*: Williams & Wilkins.

Fries, James F., and Stanford University colleagues. 2004. *Arthritis, Rheumatism and Aging Medical Information Systems (ARAMIS)--HAQ (Health Assessment Questionnaire) Page*, July 2003 2004 [cited January 2004]. Available from http://aramis.stanford.edu/HAQ.html.

Futrell, Robert T., Donald F. Shafer, and Linda I. Shafer. 2002. *Quality Software Project Management*. 1st edition (January 24, 2002) ed: Prentice Hall.

Gardner, Stephen R. 1998. Building the Data Warehouse. *Communications of the ACM* 41 (9):52-60.

Garfinkel, Simpson. 2002. *Web Security, Privacy and Commerce*. 2nd edition (January 15, 2002) ed: O'Reilly & Associates.

Garling, Andrew. 1996. *Stakeholder Presentation on a National Unique Patient Identifier, Work Group on Professional and Public Education (WPPE)*. Arlington, VA.: Computer-based Patient Record Institute Annual Meeting.

Gayek, P., R. Nesbitt, H. Pearthree, A. Shaikh, and B. Snitzer. 2004. A Web content serving utility. *IBM Systems Journal* 43 (1):3-4.

Gilb, Tom. 1988. *Principles of Software Engineering Management*: Addison-Wesley Publishing Company.

Gillooly, Caryn. 1998. Systems Mismanaged. *Information Week*, February 16, 1998, 46-48,52,56.

Gilman, Leonard, and Richard Schreiber. 1996. *Distributed Computing with IBM(r) MQSeries*. Book and CD-ROM edition (October 25, 1996) ed: John Wiley & Sons.

Goodman, Seymour E., James B. Gottstein, and Diane S. Goodman. 2001. Wiring the Wilderness in Alaska and the Yukon. *Communications of the ACM* 44 (6):21-25.

Google. 2004. *Google search engine* 2004 [cited February 2004]. Available from http://www.google.com.

Gotterbarn, Don, Keith Miller, and Simon Rogerson. 1999. Executive Committee IEEE-CS/ACM Joint Task Force on Software Engineering Ethics and Professional Practices. *Computer* 32 (10).

Gouse, Michael K. 1988. Overview of Project Management Applications. In *Project Management Handbook*, edited by D. I. Cleland and W. R. King: Van Nostrand Reinhold.

Gray, Jim, and Andreas Reuter. 1993. *Transaction Processing : Concepts and Techniques*. 1st edition (1993) ed: Morgan Kaufmann.

Grove, Andy. 1996. Taking on Prostate Cancer. *Fortune*, May 13, 1996, 54-72.

Gudgin, Martin, Marc Hadley, Noah Mendelsohn, Jean-Jacques Moreau, and Henrik Frystyk Nielsen. 2004. *SOAP Version 1.2 Part 1: Messaging Framework, W3C Recommendation 24 June 2003*. W3C 2003 [cited January 2004]. Available from http://www.w3.org/TR/SOAP/.

Hall, Elaine M. 1998. *Managing Risk: Methods for Software Systems Development*. 1st edition (February 5, 1998) ed: Addison-Wesley.

Harvard Medical School. 2000. Hepatitis C: The Silent Epidemic. *Harvard Men s Health Watch*, July 2000.

Haynes, R.B., D.W. Taylor, and D.L. Sackett. 1979. *Compliance in Health Care*. Baltimore: John Hopkins.

Health Level Seven. 2004. *HL7 web site* [Internet]. Health Level Seven, Inc. 1997-2003 [cited February 2004]. Available from http://www.hl7.org.

———. 2004. *About HL7* [Internet]. Health Level Seven 2004 [cited 2004]. Available from http://www.hl7.org/about/.

Hersh, William R. 1995. *Information Retrieval: A Health Care Perspective*. 1st edition (November 15, 1995) ed: Springer Verlag.

HIBCC. 2004. *Health Industry Number (HIN) System*. Health Industry Business Communications Council (HIBCC) 2004 [cited February 2004]. Available from http://www.hibcc.org/hin_sys.htm.

———. 2004. *Standards for Bar Coding*. Health Industry Business Communications Council (HIBCC) 2004 [cited February 2004]. Available from http://www.hibcc.org/barcodel.htm.

Himlin, Jonathan. 2004. *HL7 Announces March 18 Second Ballot Opening of Electronic Health Record - System Functional Model Draft Standard for Trial Use* (March 11, 2004). HL7.org 2004 [cited 2004]. Available from http://www.hl7.org/press/20040311.asp.

Hinden, Robert M. 1996. IP Next Generation Overview. *Communications of the ACM* 39 (6):61-71.

HIPAA. 2004. *Standards for Security and Electronic Signatures: Electronic Signature Standards*. HIPAAdvisory.com 2000-2003 [cited January 2004]. Available from http://www.hipaadvisory.com/regs/securityandelectronicsign/.

———. 2004. *Medical Privacy - National Standards to Protect the Privacy of Personal Health Information, United States Department of Health & Human Services* [Internet]. United States Department of Health & Human Services 2002 [cited January 2004]. Available from http://www.hhs.gov/ocr/hipaa/finalreg.html.

HL7. 2004. *HL7 Reference Information Model* [Internet]. Health Level Seven, Inc. 2004 [cited February 2004]. Available from http://www.hl7.org/library/data-model/RIM/modelpage_mem.htm.

HL7-Australia. 2004. *Clinical Document Architecture (CDA) Workshops* 2003 [cited January 2004]. Available from http://www.hl7-australasia.org/CDA.htm#CDA.

Holt, Ian James. 2003. *Genetics of Mitochondrial Diseases*. October 2003 ed: Oxford University Press.

Huang, Gregory T. 2004. Microsoft's Magic Pen. *MIT's Magazine of Innovation: Technology Review*, May 2004, 60-63.

Hughes, J. 2004. *Satisfaction with Medical Care: A Review of the Field (1991)* 1991 [cited January 2004]. Available from http://www.changesurfer.com/Hlth/PatSat.html.

Human Genome Project. 2004. *SNP Fact Sheet* [Internet]. Human Genome Project, January 12, 2004 2004 [cited January 2004]. Available from http://www.ornl.gov/sci/techresources/Human_Genome/faq/snps.shtml.

IEEE. 1998. IEEE Guide for Developing Systems Requirements Specification, IEEE Std 1233: Software Engineering Standards Committee of the IEEE Computer Society.

IETF. 2004. *The Internet Engineering Task Force Home Page*. IETF (Internet Engineering Task Force) 2004 [cited February 2004]. Available from http://www.ietf.org/.

Intel. 2004. *iSCSI: The Future of Network Storage* [Internet]. Intel Corporation 2002 [cited January 2004]. Available from http://www.intel.com/network/connectivity/resources/doc_library/white_papers/iSCSI_network_storage.pdf.

Ionescu, Mihail, and Ivan Marsic. 2000. An Arbitration Scheme for Concurrency Control in Distributed Groupware. Paper read at The Second International Workshop on Collaborative Editing Systems, An ACM CSCW'2000 Workshop, December 2000, at Philadelphia, PA.

Iowa Public Television. 2004. *Recombinant DNA: Example Using Insulin*. Explore More Project 2003 [cited January 2004]. Available from http://www3.iptv.org/exploremore/ge/what/insulin.cfm.

IPCC. 2001. Climate Change 2001: Impacts, Adaptation and Vulnerability. Geneva, Switzerland: IPCC (Intergovernmental Panel on Climate Change) Working Group II of the UN and WMO.

Iyer, Patricia W., and Nancy H. Camp. 1995. *Nursing Documentation: A Nursing Process Approach*: Mosby.

Janossy, James G., and Steve Samuels. 1995. *CICS/ESA Primer*. 1 edition (April 17, 1995) ed: John Wiley & Sons.

Jarke, Matthias. 1998. Requirements Tracing. *Communications of the ACM* 41 (12).

Johnson, Jeff. 2000. *GUI Bloopers: Don'ts and Do's for Software Developers and Web Designers*. 1st edition (March 17, 2000) ed: Morgan Kaufmann.

Johnson, Marian, and Nerudeab Naas. 1997. *Nursing Outcomes Classification (NOC)*: Mosby.

Johnson, Marion, Gloria Bulechek, Meridean Mass, and Sue Moorhead. 2000. *Nursing Diagnoses, Outcomes, and Interventions: NANDA, NOC and NIC Linkages*: Elsevier Science Health Science div.

Jones, Karen, and Peter Willett. 1997. *Readings in Information Retrieval*: Morgan Kaufmann.

Jones, Stephen R. 2004. *Microsoft Tablet PC Launch* (November 17, 2002). Reviews Online, Volico Web Consulting 2002 [cited January 2004]. Available from http://www.reviewsonline.com/tl01.htm.

JWP. 2004. *Trial-Use Standard for Health Care Data Interchange--Information Model Methods*. Joint Working Group for a Common Data Model (ASTM, DICOM, HL7, NCPDP, IEEE, X12N) 1996 [cited February 2004]. Available from http://www.meb.uni-bonn.de/standards/IEEE/JWG-MODEL/stdmain.pdf.

Kajii, Eugene H., and Jeffrey M. Leiden. 2001. Gene and Stem Cell Therapies. *JAMA (The Journal of the American Medical Association)* 285 (5):545-550.

Kaner, Sam, Lenny Lind, Catherine Toldi, and Sarah Fisk. 1996. *Facilitator's Guide to Participatory Decision-Making*: New Society Publishers.

Kaplan, Jack M. 1996. *Smart Cards: The Global Information Passport: Managing a Successful Smart Card Program*. January 1996 ed: International Thomson Publishing.

Kaplan, Robert S., and David P. Norton. 1996. *The Balanced Scorecard: Translating Strategy into Action*: Harvard Business School Press. Original edition, September 1996.

Kiessling, Ann A., and Scott. C. Anderson. 2003. Chapter 12- Neurogenerative Diseases. In *Human Embryonic Stem Cells: An Introduction to the Science and Therapeutic Potential*: Jones & Bartlett Pub.

King, William R. 1988. The Role of Projects in the Implementation of Business Strategy. In *Project Management Handbook*, edited by D. I. Cleland and W. R. Ring: Van Nostrand Reinhold.

Kit, Edward. 1995. *Software Testing in the Real World : Improving the Process*. 1st edition (November 7, 1995) ed: Addison-Wesley.

Kohli, Jagdish C. 1996. Unpublished Talk on "Emerging Medical Technologies—in the 1990s and beyond". Paper read at IEEE Oakland East Bay Communications Society, February 29, 1996, at Pacific Bell (SBC), San Ramon, CA.

Kohn, Linda T., Janet Corrigan, Molla S. Donaldson, and William C. Richardson. 2000. *To Err Is Human: Building a Safer Health System*: National Academy Press.

Kroeker, Kirk L. 2004. *Scientist Develop Breakthrough Internet Protocol* (March 15, 2004) [Internet]. TechNewsWord, March 18, 2004 2004 [cited March 15 2004]. Available from http://www.technewsworld.com/perl/story/33130.html.

Kuver, Polly Perryman. 2004. *The Off-The-Shelf Software Survival Guide Integrating Off-The-Shelf Software With Enterprise Systems*. (August 2004) ed: Auerbach Pub.

Law, Averill M, David W Kelton, W. David Kelton, and David M Kelton. 1999. *Simulation Modeling and Analysis (Industrial Engineering and Management Science Series)*. 3rd edition (December 30, 1999) ed: McGraw-Hill Science/Engineering/Math.

Lawrence, David. 2003. *From Chaos to Care: The Promise of Team-Based Medicine*. Reprint edition (September 30, 2003) ed: DaCapo Press.

Lee, John, and Ron Ben-Natan. 2002. *Integrating Service Level Agreements: Optimizing Your OSS for SLA Delivery*. 1st edition (July 15, 2002) ed: John Wiley & Sons.

Lehmann, Christine. 2004. Health Panel Urges Government To Adopt ICD-10 for Coding. *Psychiatric News (of the American Psychiatric Association)* 39 (1):5.

Leifer, Gloria. 1993. Less isn't more if you can't read it. *RN*, April 1993, 96.

Lemon, Sumner. 2004. *IEEE: Chinese security standard could fracture Wi-Fi* [Internet]. NetFlash! Network World Fusion's daily synopsis of key network IT news, 12/09/03 2003 [cited January 2004]. Available from www.nwfusion.com/news/2003/1209ieeechine.html.

Leyland, Valerie. 1993. *Electronic Data Interchange, A Management View*. Hertfordshire, UK: Prentice Hall.

Loeb, Stanley. 1992. *Better Documentation*: Springhouse Corporation.

———. 1995. *Mastering Documentation*: Springhouse Corporation.

LOINC. 2004. *Logical Observation Identifiers Names and Codes (LOINC)* [Internet]. The Regenstrief Institute 2003 [cited February 2004]. Available from http://www.loinc.org/.

Lozinsky, Sergio. 1998. *Enterprise-Wide Software Solutions: Integration Strategies and Practices*. 1st edition (January 15, 1998) ed: Addison-Wesley.

Lundy, Michael S. 1996. The Computer-Based Patient Record, Managed Care and the Fate of Clinical Outcomes Research. *Florida Family Physician*, January 1996.

Lyman, Jay. 2004. *Asia Looks for Lead on Next-Gen Internet* (December 31, 2004) [Internet]. TechnNewsWorld 2004 [cited March 28, 2004 2004]. Available from http://www.technewsworld.com/perl/story/32503.html.

Lynn, Joanne, Joan Harrold, and The Center to Improve Care of the Dying at George Washington University. 1999. *Handbook for Mortals: Guidance for People Facing Serious Illness*: Oxford University Press.

Margolis, S., and M. J. Klag. 1996. Hypertension. *The John Hopkins White Papers: The John Hopkins Medical Institutions, Baltimore, Maryland.*

Marks, Dr. James S. 2003. *The Burden of Chronic Disease and the Future of Public Health*: National Center for Chronic Disease Prevention and Health Promotion.

Marsan, Carolyn Duffy. 2003. IETF ponders internationalized e-mail. *NetworkWorldFusion*, November 24, 2003.

Martin, James, and Joe Leben. 1998. *Client/Server Databases: Enterprise Computing*. 1st edition (March 12, 1998) ed: Pearson Education POD.

Martin, Robert J., and Wilma M. Osborne. 1983. Guidance On Software Maintenance: National Bureau of Standards Publication.

McCabe, Karen. 2004. *IEEE Starts Work on Three Health Informatics Standards* (April 2, 2002) [Internet]. The Institute of Electrical and Electronics Engineers Standards Association (IEEE-SA) 2002 [cited February 2004]. Available from http://standards.ieee.org/announcements/hisstds.html.

McConnell, Steve. 1993. *Code Complete*: Microsoft Press.

Mearian, Lucas. 2004. Trumping Tape. *COMPUTERWORLD*, May 24, 2004.

MedWatch. 2004. *The FDA Safety Information and Adverse Event Reporting Program*. Department of Health and Human Services, January 2, 2004 2004 [cited January 2004]. Available from www.fda.gov/medwatch.

Meng, Maxwell V., and Rajvir Dahiya. 2002. Molecular Genetics. In *(American Cancer Society Atlas of Clinical Oncology) Prostate Cancer*, edited by P. R. Carroll and G. D. Grossfeld. Hamilton-London: BC Decker Inc.

Methvin, Eugene H. 1995. No Wonder Medicare and Medicaid Claims are Out of Control. *Reader's Digest*, September 1995, 91-97.

Michalowski, Jennifer. 2004. *NIH News Release: Protein Patterns May Identify Ovarian Cancer* [Internet]. NIH (National Institutes of Health) 2002 [cited January 2004]. Available from http://www.nih.gov/news/pr/feb2002/nci-07.htm.

Miller, Mark Steven, and M. T. Cronin. 2000. *Genetic Polymorphisms and Susceptibility to Disease*. 1st edition (August 15, 2000) ed: Taylor & Francis.

Miller, Sandra Kay. 2001. Aspect-Oriented Programming Takes Aim at Software Complexity. *Computer* 34 (4):18-21.

Mitchell, Robert L. 2004. Toxic Legacy. *Computerworld* 38 (5):19-21.

Moad, Jeff. 1996. Dose of Reality: The health-care industry is taking a shot at clinical information systems, but many are finding there are a few ailments to overcome. *PC Week*, February 12, 1996.

Moore, Connie, and Robert Markham. 2004. *Enterprise Content Management: A Comprehensive Approach for Managing Unstructured Content* (April 5, 2002). Giga Information Group, Inc. 2002 [cited January 2004]. Available from http://www.msiinet.com/html/pdfs/essecm3.pdf.

Moore, J. Duncan. 1997. The Inpatient's Best Friend. *Modern Healthcare*, March 25, 1996, 51-52.

———. 1998. JCAHO urges 'Do tell' in sentinel event fight. *Modern Healthcare*, March 2, 1998, 60-66.

Morrissey, John. 1997. Pressure for Privacy. *Modern Healthcare*, March 10, 1997, 6.

Morse, Stephen S., ed. 1996. *Emerging Viruses*. Reprint edition (June 1996) ed: Oxford Univ Pr on Demand.

Mullahy, Catherine M. 1998. *The Case Manager's Handbook, Second Edition*: Aspen Publishers, Inc.

Myriad. 2004. *Hereditary Cancer Testing*. Myriad 2004 [cited January 2004]. Available from http://www.myriad.com/med/index.htm.

Naur, P., and B. Randall. 1968. Software Engineering: A Report on a Conference Sponsored by the NATO Science Committee. Brussels, Belgium: NATO Scientific Affairs Division.

NCHS. 2004. *Classifications of Diseases and Functioning & Disability: About ICD-10-CM* (June 2003). National Center for Health Statistics 2003 [cited February 2004]. Available from http://www.cdc.gov/nchs/about/otheract/icd9/abticd10.htm.

———. 2004. *National Vital Statistics System* [Internet]. National Center for Health Statistics 2003 [cited January 2004]. Available from http://www.cdc.gov/nchs/vital_certs_rev.htm.

NCPDP. 2004. *ANSI Accredited: NCPDP Standard Claims Billing Version 2.0*. National Council for Prescription Drug Programs (NCPDP) 2004 [cited February 2004]. Available from http://www.hipaanet.com/hisb_ncpdp.htm.

NCQA. 2004. *NCQA: National Committee for Quality Assurance*

web site. NCQA: National Committee for Quality Assurance 2004 [cited January 2004]. Available from http://www.ncqa.org.

NDDIC. 2004. *Chronic Hepatitis C: Current Disease Management, NIH Publication No. 03-4230, February 2003* [Internet]. National Digestive Diseases Information Clearinghouse, part of the National Institutes of Health, Bethesda, MD, USA. 2003 [cited January 2004]. Available from http://digestive.niddk.nih.gov/ddiseases/pubs/chronichepc/index.htm.

NEMA. 1993. NEMA (National Electrical Manufacturers' Association) Standards Publication No. PS3.x, Digital Imaging and Communication in Medicine (DICOM). Washington, DC: National Electronic Manufacturers' Association.

Nemko, Marty.

NGC. 2004. *National Guideline Clearinghouse* [Internet]. Agency for Healthcare Research and Quality (AHRQ)

American Medical Association (AMA)

American Association of Health Plans-Health Insurance Association of America (AAHP-HIAA). February 9, 2004 1998-2004 [cited February 2004]. Available from http://www.guideline.gov/resources/guideline_index.aspx.

Niccol, Andrew. 1997. Gattaca, edited by A. Niccol: Columbia TriStar Pictures.

NICI Handwriting Recognition Group. 2004. *Pen & Mobile Computing* [Internet]. NICI Handwriting Recognition Group 1995 [cited February 2004]. Available from http://hwr.nici.kun.nl/unipen/.

NIDA. 2004. *Commonly Abused Drugs*. National Institute of Drug Abuse, National Institutes of Health, July 5, 2001 2001 [cited January 2004]. Available from http://www.nida.nih.gov/DrugsofAbuse.html.

Nielsen, Jakob. 1998. What is 'Usability'? *Design/Usability*, September 14, 1998.

NIH. 2004. *Medline Database* 2004 [cited January 2004]. Available from http://www.nlm.nih.gov.

———. 2004. *Web site*. National Institutes of Health 2004 [cited January 2004]. Available from www.nih.gov.

Nobel, Carmen. 2003. Microsoft Polishes Tablet PC. *eWEEK*.

Nortel Networks. 2004. *An Overview of the International Common Criteria for Information Technology Security Evaluation* [Internet, PDF]. Nortel Networks 2002 [cited February 2004]. Available from http://www.nortelnetworks.com/solutions/security/collateral/nn101441-0802.pdf.

NZ 0800 MEDBOOK. 2004. *YOUR PERSONAL HEALTH RECORD* [Internet]. Render-vue.com 2001 [cited February 16, 2004 2004]. Available from http://www.yourpersonalhealthrecord.com/.

O'Conner, Anahad. 2004. On the Trail of Diseases, Years Before They Strike. *New York Times*, May 11, 2004.

O'Conner, Eileen. 1999. Medical errors kill tens of thousands annually, panel says. *CNN.com*, November 20, 1999.

OFT. 2004. *New York Central HIPAA Coordination Project*. New York State Office for Technology (OFT) 2003 [cited February 2004]. Available from http://www.oft.state.ny.us/hipaa/Documents/AcctforDisclosure.htm.

Pastore, Michael. 2004. *Just What Is 'Content-Addressed Storage'?* [Internet]. IT Service Management Forum Conference & Expo 2003 [cited January 2004]. Available from http://www.internetnews.com/storage/article.php/2221281.

Patterson, D. A., G. Gibson, and R. H. Katz. 1987. A Case for Redundant Arrays of Inexpensive Disks (RAID), Report No. UCB/CSD 87/391: University of California, Berkeley, CA.

PCCM. 2004. *Clinical Pathways: What Is Everyone Looking For?* [Internet]. Pediatric Critical Care Medicine, July 22, 2003 2003 [cited January 2004]. Available from http://pedsccm.wustl.edu/CLINICAL/Pathways.html.

PDR-Staff, and Physicians. 2003. *2004 Physicians' Desk Reference with PDR Electronic Library on CD-Rom*. Edited by PDR-Staff. November 2003 ed, *Physicians' Desk Reference*: Thomson Healthcare.

Pedersen, Brian. 2004. *Infectious Diseases* [Internet]. LEO Pharma, January 31, 2004 2004 [cited January 2004]. Available from http://www.leo-pharma.com/w-site/leo/docs.nsf/0/b7a9847e34fcc86ec1256be500241b6e?OpenDocument.

Pfleeger, Shari Lawrence. 1988. Measuring Software Reliability. *IEEE Spectrum*:55-60.

Phillips, Ken. 1997. Unforgettable Biometrics. *P C Week.* 14 (45):96.

Pickar, Gloria D. 1993. *Dosage Calculations*: Delmar Publishers.

Pinto, Jeffrey K., and Dennis P. Sleven. 1988. Critical Success Factors in Effective Project Implementation. In *Project Management Handbook*: Van Nostrand Reinhold.

Pollitz, Karen, Richard Sorian, and Kathy Thomas. 2001. How Accessible is Individual Health Insurance for Consumers in Less-than-perfect Health?: Prepared for the Henry J. Kaiser Family Foundation by Georgetown University Institute for Health Care Research and Policy.

Pressman, R.S. 1992. *Software Engineering: A Practitioner's Approach, 2d ed.* New York,NY: McGraw-Hill.

Pyke, Jon. 2004. *The Workflow Management Coalition Web Site*. Workflow Management Coalition (WfMC) 2004 [cited January 2004]. Available from http//www.wfmc.org.

Raggett, Dave. 2004. *Getting started with HTML* [Internet]. W3C, February 13, 2002 2002 [cited January 2004]. Available from http://www.w3.org/MarkUp/Guide/.

Rajlich, Vaclav T., and Keith H. Bennett. 2000. A Staged Model for the Software Life Cycle. *Computer* 33 (7):66-71.

Reardon, Marguerite. 2004. *Next Net moves forward* (March 22, 2004) [Internet]. CNET News.com 2004 [cited March 27 2004]. Available from http://news.com.com/2100-1038-5177463.html?tag=sas.email.

Redmond-Pyle, David, Alan Moore, and David R. Pyle. 1995. *Graphical User Interface Design and Evaluation Guide*. 1st edition (June 26, 1995) ed: Prentice Hall PTR.

Richards, Edward P., and Katharine C. Rathbun. 1999. *Medical Care Law*. 1st edition (August 15, 1999) ed: Jones & Bartlett Pub.

Roberts, John J. 2004. *The National Drug Code (NDC) Encoded in the EAN.UCC System* [Word Document]. Federal Drug Administration 2004 [cited February 2004]. Available from http://www.uc-council.org/ean_ucc_system/membership/rso1kwdc.doc.

Rupp's Insurance & Risk Management Glossary. 2004. *diagnosis related group (DRG)* [Internet]. NILS Publishing 2002 [cited February 2004]. Available from http://insurance.cch.com/rupps/diagnosis-related-group.htm.

Sackett, David L, William M C Rosenberg, J A Muir Gray, R Brian Haynes, and W Scott Richardson. 1996. Evidence based medicine: what it is and what it isn't. *British Medical Journal* 312:71-72.

Sackett, David L., R. Brian Haynes, Peter Tugwell, and Gordon H. Guyatt. 1991. *Clinical Epidemiology: A Basic Science for Clinical Medicine*. 2nd edition (July 1991) ed: Lippincott Williams & Wilkins Publishers.

Schlier, F. 1996. The Impact of Demand Management on Health Care IT: Gartner Group.

Science Links. 2003. *Science Update: Color-Coded DNA*. AAAS (American Association for the Advancement of Science) 2002 [cited December 2003]. Available from http://www.sciencenetlinks.org/sci_update.cfm?DocID=108.

Scott, Lisa. 1996. Doctor's Orders: Providers Push for Remedies to Costly Drug Noncompliance. *Modern Healthcare*, April 15, 1996.

Scott, Ronald W. 2000. *Legal Aspects of Documenting Patient Care*. 2nd edition ed: Aspen Publishers, Inc.

searchWebServices.com. 2003. *whatis.com definition of "application service provider"* [Internet], September 19, 2003 2003 [cited September 2003]. Available from http://searchwebservices.techtarget.com/sDefinition/0,,sid26_gci213801,00.html.

Shalala, Donna E. 2004. *HHS Announces Final Regulation Establishing First-Ever National Standards to Protect Patients' Personal Medical Records* (Dec. 20, 2000) [Internet]. HHS News (U.S. Department of Health and Human Services) 2000 [cited February 2004]. Available from http://www.hhs.gov/news/press/2000pres/20001220.html.

Shiffman, Richard N., Paul Shekelle, J Marc Overhage, Jean Slutsky, Jeremy Grimshaw, and Aniruddha M. Deshpande. 2003. Standardized Reporting of Clinical Practice Guidelines: A Proposal from the Conference of Guideline Standardization. *Annals of Internal Medicine* 139 (6):493-498.

Shilling, Brian, and Charlene D. Hill. 2004. *JCAHO News Release: JCAHO, NCQA Establish Privacy Certification For Business Associates Program; Eight Organizations Commit to Surveys*. Joint Commission on Accreditation of Healthcare Organizations 2004 [cited February 2004]. Available from http://www.jcaho.org/news+room/news+release+archives/bap_6_16.htm.

Shortliffe, Edward H. 1990. Clinical Decision-Support Systems. In *Medical Informatics: Computer Applications in Health Care*, edited by E. H. Shortliffe and L. E. Perreault: Addison-Wesley Publishing Company.

Shortliffe, Edward H., and G. Octo Barnett. 2001. Medical Data: Their Acquisition, Storage, and Use. In *Medical Informatics: Computer Applications in Health Care and Biomedicine*, edited by E. H. Shortlife, L. M. Fagan, G. Wiederhold and L. E. Perreault: Springer-Verlag New York, Inc.

Signal Research Division. 2004. *The Role of Genes in Health and Disease* [Internet]. Signal Research Division, September 15, 1999 1999 [cited January 2004]. Available from http://www.signalpharm.com/scientific_background.html.

Sims, Oliver. 1994. *Delivering Cooperative Objects for Client-Server*. October 1994 ed, *IBM McGraw-Hill Series*: McGraw Hill Text.

SNOMED International. 2004. *SNOMED CT* [Internet]. College of American Pathologists (CAP), May 23, 2001 2000 [cited February 2004]. Available from http://www.snomed.org/snomedct_txt.html.

———. 2004. *SNOMED International*. College of American Pathologists (CAP), July 1, 2003 2001-2003 [cited February 2004]. Available from http://www.snomed.org/.

Solomon, Diane, and Ritu Nayar, eds. 2004. *Bethesda System for Reporting Cervical Cytology: Definitions, Criteria and Explanatory Notes*. New York City: Springer-Verlag. Original edition, March 2004.

Sommerville, Ian. 2000. *Software Engineering*. 6th edition (August 11, 2000) ed: Addison-Wesley Pub Co.

Sounder, William E. 1988. Selecting Projects That Maximize Profits. In *Project Management Handbook*, edited by D. I. Cleland and W. R. King: Nostrand Reinhold.

Spielberg, Alissa R. 1998. On Call and Online: Sociohistorical, Legal, and Ethical Implications of E-mail for the Patient-Physician Relationship. *The Journal of the American Medical Association* 280 (15).

Stahl, James E, Michael K Dempsey, Julian M Goldman, Warren S Sandberg, Marie T Egan, and David W Rattner. 2004. Evaluating a New Indoor Positioning System in a Clinical Setting: A Case Report.

Starfield, Barbara. 1998. Quality-of-Care Research: Intermal Elegance and External Relevance. *The Journal of the American Medical Association* 280 (11).

Steen, Elaine B., Don E. Detmer, and Richard S. Dick, eds. 1997. *The Computer-Based Patient Record: An Essential Technology for Health Care*. 1st edition (January 15, 1997) ed: National Academy Press.

Sternberg, Steve. 2004. Drug may block deadly gene: Find could be breakthrough for strokes, heart attacks. *USA Today*, February 9, 2004.

Strauss, James, and Ellen G. Strauss. 2001. *Viruses and Human Disease*. 1st edition (December 2001) ed: Academic Press.

Svenonius, Elaine. 2000. *The Intellectual Foundation of Information Organization (Digital Libraries and Electronic Publishing)*. 1st edition (April 18, 2000) ed: MIT Press.

swisstox.net. 2004. *More Gene Therapy Studies Are Suspended (orginally from Associated Press)* [Internet]. swisstox.net 2003 [cited January 2004]. Available from http://www.swisstox.net/en/news_e.php?st_lang_key=en&st_news_id=1112.

Swope, W. C. 2001. Deep computing for the life sciences. *IBM Systems Journal* 40 (2):248-264.

Szolovits, Peter, Jon Doyle, William J. Long, Isaac Kohane, and Stephen G. Pauker. 2004. *Guardian Angel: Patient-Centered Health Information Systems* [Internet] 1994 [cited January 2004]. Available from http://medg.lcs.mit.edu/ga/manifesto/GAtr.html.

TechTarget. 2004. *COLD* [Internet]. searchStorage.com Definitions 2000-2004 [cited January 2004]. Available from http://searchstorage.techtarget.com/sDefinition/0,,sid5_gci214402,00.html.

US Congress. 2004. Subcommittee on Health of the House Committee on Ways and Means. *Testimony of Francis J. Crosson, MD, Executive Director, The Permanente Federation, Kaiser Permanente*. March 18, 2004.

Thai, Thuan L., and Andy Oram. 1999. *Learning DCOM*. 1st edition (April 1999) ed: O'Reilly & Associates.

The Simputer Trust. 2004. *simputer: radical simplicity for universal access*. The Simputer Trust 2000 [cited February 2004]. Available from http://www.simputer.org/.

The Wellcome Trust. 1999. The cutting edge: SNPs and their medical application. *Wellcome News* (20 Q3 1999).

Thompson, Dick. 1998. More Science...And Much More Money. *Time*, Oct. 12, 1998.

Thorn, T. 1997. Programming Languages for Mobile Code. *ACM Computing Surveys* 29 (3).

Truex, Duane P., Richard Baskerville, and Heinz Klein. 1999. Growing Systems in Emergent Organizations. *Communications of the ACM* 42 (8):117-123.

TrustHealth. 2004. *Can you Trust Health Telematics?* European Commission 1997 [cited January 2004]. Available from http://www.ramit.be/trusthealth/.

Tsiaras, Alexander, and Barry Worth. 2002. *from Conception to Birth: a Life Unfolds*. 1st Edition ed: Doubleday.

Turnlund, Michael. 2004. Distributed Development: Lessons Learned. *Queue* 1 (9):26.

U.S. National Library of Medicine. 1994. Minutes of a Meeting Sponsored by

National Library of Medicine (NLM)
Agency for Health Care Policy and Research (AHCPR). Paper read at Vocabularies for Computer-Based Patient Records: Identifying Candidates for Large Scale Testing, at Lister Hill Auditorium,
National Library of Medicine, Bethesda, MD.

———. 2004. *United Medical Language System (UMLS)* [Internet]. U.S. National Library of Medicine, December 23, 2003 2003 [cited February 2004]. Available from http://www.nlm.nih.gov/research/umls/.

Unicode Consortium. 2004. *What is Unicode?* [Internet]. Unicode Consortium, January 20, 2004 1991-2004 [cited February 2004]. Available from http://www.unicode.org/standard/WhatIsUnicode.html.

UsabilityFirst. 2004. *Groupware: Links*. Usability First™, July 22, 2002 2002 [cited January 2004]. Available from http://www.usabilityfirst.com/groupware/cscw.txl.

Värri, Alpo. 2004. *CEN/TC251/WGIV - Technology for Interoperability in Health Care* (2003-06-11). Institute of Signal Processing, Tampere University of Technology 2003 [cited February 2004]. Available from http://www.cs.tut.fi/~varri/cenwgiv.html.

vBNS+. 2004. *Welcome to vBNS+ very high performance Backbone Network Service* [Internet]. MCI 2004 [cited January 2004]. Available from http://www.vbns.net/.

Voas, Jeffrey M. 1998. The Challenges of Using COTS Software in Component-Based Development". *Computer* 31 (6):44-45.

W3C. 2004. *World Wide Web Consortium Home Page* [Internet]. World Wide Web Consortium (W3C) 1994-2004 [cited February 2004]. Available from http://www.w3.org/.

———. 2004. *XSL Transformations (XSLT) Version 1.0, W3C Recommendation, 16 November 1999*. W3C 1999 [cited January 2004]. Available from http://www.w3.org/TR/xslt.

———. 2004. *XML Schema* [Internet]. W3C 2000-2003 [cited January 2004]. Available from http://www.w3.org/XML/Schema#dev.

Waegemann, C. Peter, and Claudia Tessier. 2002. Documentation Goes Wireless: A Look at Mobile Healthcare Computing Devices. *Journal of AHIMA (American Health Information Management Association)* 73 (8):36-39.

Walraven, Carl van, and MD C. David Naylor. 1998. Do We Know What Inappropriate Laboratory Utilization Is? *The Journal of the American Medical Association* 280 (6).

Wasserman, Anthony I. 1977. ON THE MEANING OF DISCIPLINE IN SOFTWARE DESIGN AND DEVELOPMENT. In *Tutorial on Software Design Techniques*, edited by P. Freeman and A. I. Wasserman: IEEE Computer Society.

Webopedia. 2004. *X.400* [Internet]. Webopedia, October 25, 2002 2002 [cited January 2004]. Available from http://www.webopedia.com/TERM/X/X_400.html.

Werner, David, Carol Thuman, and Jane Maxwell. 1992. *Where There Is No Doctor: A Village Health Care Handbook*. Revised edition (May 1992) ed: Hesperian Foundation.

Whitten, Neal. 1995. *Managing Software Development Projects: Formula for Success*. 2nd edition (April 24, 1995) ed: John Wiley & Sons.

Wilde, Erik, and David Lowe. 2002. *XPath, XLink, XPointer, and XML: A Practical Guide to Web Hyperlinking and Transclusion*. 1st edition (July 23, 2002) ed: Addison-Wesley Pub Co.

Wilson, Jennifer Fisher. 1997. Will demand management work? *American College of Physicians Observer*.

Wong, Jacqueline W. T., W. K. Kan, and Gilbert Young. 1996. ACTION: Automatic Classification for Full-Text Documents. *SIGIR Forum: The Special Interest Group on Information Retrieval, ACM Press*:26-41.

Wright, Sarah. 1997. Optical technique allows non-surgical biopsies: MIT.

Wysocki, Robert K., Robert Beck, and David B. Crane. 2000. How to Plan, Manage, and Deliver Projects on Time and Within Budget. In *Effective Project Management*: John Wiley & Sons, Inc..

Wysocki, Robert K., and Rudd McGary. 2003. *Effective Project Management: Traditional, Adaptive, Extreme*. 3rd edition (July 25, 2003) ed: John Wiley & Sons.

Yackel, Thomas R. 2002. Defining Performance and Quality Indicators for a Clinical Document Imaging Project. Master of Science, School of Medicine, Medical Informatics and Outcome Research, Oregon Health & Science University.

Yahoo. 2004. *Yahoo Web Site*. 2004 2004 [cited February 2004]. Available from http://www.yahoo.com.

Yeomans, Steven G. 1999. *The Clinical Application of Outcomes Assessment*. 1st edition (September 13, 1999) ed: McGraw-Hill Professional.

Index

B

C

D

E

F

I

N

P

S

T

U

Printed in the United States
40773LVS00003B/1

9 781581 125092